Intracranial and Spinal Dural Arteriovenous Fistulas

Xianli Lv
Editor

Intracranial and Spinal Dural Arteriovenous Fistulas

Springer

Editor
Xianli Lv
Department of Neurosurgery
Beijing Tsinghua Changgung Hospital
School of Clinical Medicine
Tsinghua University
Beijing, China

ISBN 978-981-19-5766-6 ISBN 978-981-19-5767-3 (eBook)
https://doi.org/10.1007/978-981-19-5767-3

This Springer imprint is published by the registered company Springer Nature Singapore Pte Ltd.
The registered company address is: 152 Beach Road, #21-01/04 Gateway East, Singapore 189721, Singapore

Preface

In 2006, professor Zhongxue Wu brought me into the field of endovascular neurosurgery. At that time, words like "neurointervention" was only found in some papers, and it had not been used to name a subspecialty. The term that I mostly saw and heard was Intervention Neuroradiology. It's also the name of a journal, which helps me a lot because it publishes papers that I like to read. Professor Pierre Lasjaunias was alive at the time, and his contributions to interventional neuroradiology made him my role model. Professor Marco Leonardi was a wonderful person who supported, encouraged, and trusted me in my darkest moments. Professor Karel terBrugge had been the editor-in-chief of Intervention Neuroradiology and I was very moved by his comments. Timo Krings strikes me as a very wise man. They are my role models and I am very grateful to them for their support. They have made outstanding contributions to the treatment of dural arteriovenous fistulas. Dural arteriovenous fistulas have intrigued me from the beginning because of their complexity. My doctoral dissertation was related to dural arteriovenous fistula. In recent years, the development of neurointervention has been very rapid and has matured into a discipline. The understanding and treatment of dural arteriovenous fistula have also undergone fundamental changes, from venous approach to arterial approach, to venous sinus recanalization and reconstruction. The advent of new catheters and embolic materials has provided more options for the treatment of dural arteriovenous fistulas. Because there has not been a monograph on dural arteriovenous fistula before, I edited this book. It is hoped that through this book, medical students and physicians in neurosurgery, neurology, and radiology will learn more about and understand this complex disease. Thanks to my teacher, professor Zhongxue Wu, who has been supporting me, trusting me, and shielding me from the wind and rain; otherwise, I would not be where I am today. Thanks to all the outstanding scholars who have contributed to the research of dural arteriovenous fistula. Thanks to Springer Nature and Stephanie Sibin for their hard work in making this book possible.

Beijing, China — Xianli Lv

Acknowledgements

This work was supported by Beijing Municipal Administration of Hospitals Incubating Program (PX2020039), Beijing, China and Tsinghua Precision Medicine Foundation (20219990008), Tsinghua University, Beijing, China.

About the Book

In memory of Academician Zhongcheng Wang

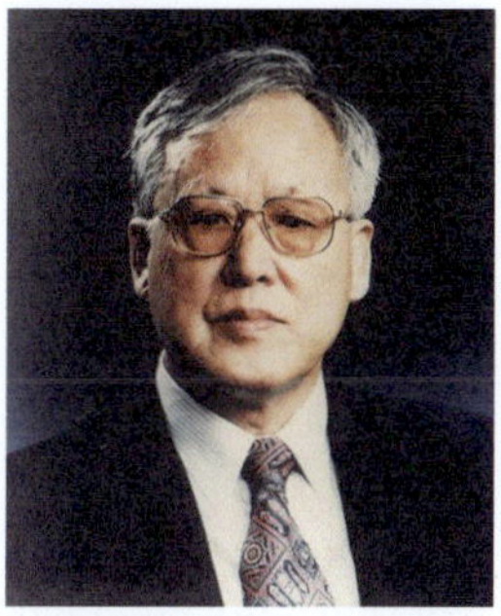

Prof. Zhongcheng Wang (20 December 1925–30 September 2012), Academician of Chinese Academy of Engineering

In memory of Prof. Pierre Lasjaunias and Prof. Marco Leonardi

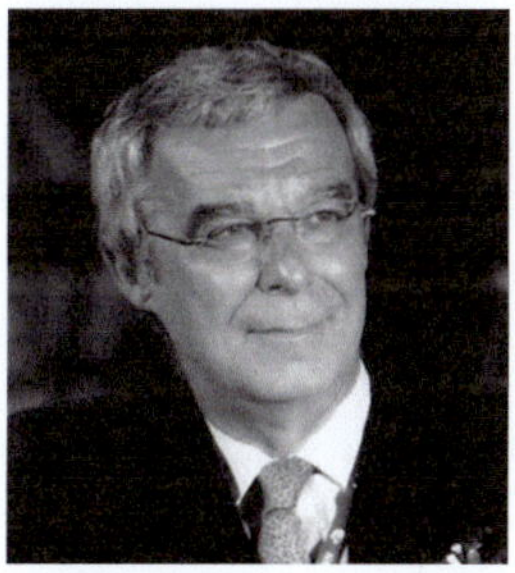

Prof. Pierre Lasjaunias (1948–2008), Head of Neurosciences at Bicêtre Hospital in Paris, France

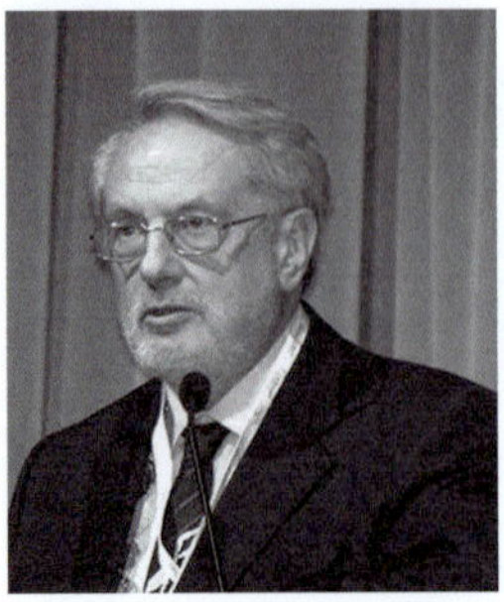

Prof. Marco Leonardi (1944–2017), Head of Neuroradiology, University of Bologna, Italy

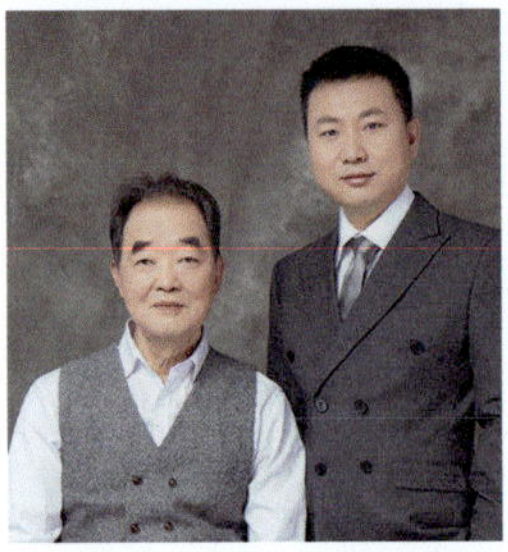

Thanks Prof. Zhongxue Wu (left), my great teacher, who is a human being of immense qualities, a man of incredible energy, and an extraordinary individual whom we will always love and admire.

Contents

About the Editor

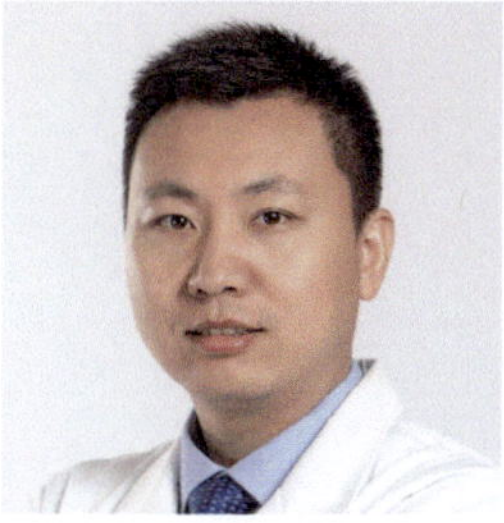

Xianli Lv, MD is an associate professor of neurointervention, Department of Neurosurgery, at Beijing Tsinghua Changgung Hospital, School of Clinical Medicine, Tsinghua University, in Beijing (China). His research focuses on neuroendovascular therapy of intracranial aneurysm, cerebral arteriovenous malformation, intracranial dural arteriovenous fistula, spinal vascular malformation, and pediatric cerebrospinal vascular malformation. He has authored 195 peer-reviewed scientific articles indexed in international databases and has published 5 books as editor. He is an editorial member of the journals: Interventional Neuroradiology, Stroke and Vascular Neurology, Journal of Neuroradiology, and The Neuroradiology Journal. He is also a deputy editor of Neuroscience Informatics and Frontiers in Neurology. Dr. Lv is the member of the World Stroke Organization (WSO) and the World Federation of Interventional Therapeutic Neuroradiology (WFITN) and consultant for BALT, Montmorency, France.

1 Classifications of Cranial and Spinal Dural Arteriovenous Fistulas and Their Endovascular Embolization

Huachen Zhang and Xianli Lv

Abstract

Dural arteriovenous fistula (DAVF) represents approximately 10–15% of all intracranial vascular malformations. DAVFs can be benign lesions, but the angioarchitecture of retrograde venous drainage or cortical venous reflux makes these lesions an aggressive high risk of neurological deficits and mortality caused by rupture or venous congestion. Endovascular embolization is the first line treatment for DAVF. Both transarterial and transvenous approaches have expanded the complex DAVFs that we can treat. The selection of endovascular approach depends on the angioarchitecture of the DAVF and experiences of neurosurgeons, the feeding arteries, lesion location, venous outflow direction. Surgery and stereotactic radiosurgery are used in few cases that endovascular approaches are impossible or unsuccessful.

Keywords

Cranial · Spinal · Dural arteriovenous fistula Pathology · Classification · Therapy

H. Zhang · X. Lv (✉)
Department of Neurosurgery, Beijing Tsinghua Changgung Hospital, School of Clinical Medicine, Tsinghua University, Beijing, China

1.1 Introduction

Dural arteriovenous fistulas (DAVFs) are the most common type of spinal vascular malformations (AVMs), but account for 10–15% of all intracranial arteriovenous malformations [1]. These abnormal connections between dural arteries and dural/pial veins can develop at everywhere of the dural mater. The most common places are transverse-sigmoid and cavernous sinuses, following tentorium, sagittal sinus, torcula, anterior cranial fossa, clivus, occipital foramen or dural sleeve of spinal nerve root [1, 2]. DAVFs cause a set of clinical signs and symptoms arising from venous congestion and pial venous rupture [1, 3, 4]. Patients with unruptured DAVFs may develop pulsatile tinnitus, bruit, headaches, visual changes, alterations in mental status, seizure, myelopathy, cranial nerve palsies and motor or sensory deficits depending on the location of the fistula [5–11]. The importance of venous drainage is well known when they distinguished between drainage directly into the dural sinuses and the pial veins in the clinical presentation of DAVFs (Table 1.1) [1, 3, 4]. The DAVF symptoms are produced by disruption of normal venous drainage causing changes in flow dynamics. Approximately 20–33% of DAVFs present with intracranial hemorrhage [6, 12].

CT scan is often useful for determining hemorrhage or oedema in DAVF diagnosis (Fig. 1.1). MRI can show parenchymal edema and flow void

X. Lv (ed.), *Intracranial and Spinal Dural Arteriovenous Fistulas*,
https://doi.org/10.1007/978-981-19-5767-3_1

Table 1.1 Previous classifications of DAVFs and Zipfel classification

Djindjian-Merland classification (1977) [8]	Borden classification (1995) [3]	Cognard classification (1995) [5]	Zipfel classification (2009) [28]	Symptoms
I, Drainage into a sinus	I, Venous drainage directly into dural venous sinus or meningeal vein	I, Venous drainage into dural venous sinus with antegrade flow	I, DAVFs drain directly into dural venous sinuses; spinal extra-dural AVM without perimedullary vein reflux	No symptom or tinnitus
		IIa, Venous drainage into dural venous sinus with retrograde flow	II, DAVFs drain into dural sinuses but also have retrograde drainage into ophthalmic and bridging veins; spinal extra-dural AVM with perimedullary vein reflux	Proptosis, chemosis, headaches, epilepsy, cognitive dysfunction, dementia, intracranial hemorrhage, myelopathy
II, Sinus drainage with reflux into cerebral veins	II, With cortical vein reflux	IIb, Venous drainage into dural venous sinus with cortical vein reflux		
III, Drainage solely into cortical veins	III, Cortical vein drainage	III, Venous drainage directly into cortical veins	III, DAVFs drain into pial veins and do not have dural sinus drainage; spinal DAVF drained with perimedullary vein only	Intracranial hemorrhage, myelopathy
IV, With supra or infra tentorial venous lake		IV, Type III with venous ectasias of the draining subarachnoid veins		
–	–	V, Spinal perimedullary vein drainage	II or III, Cranial or spinal DAVF	Intracranial hemorrhage, myelopathy

Cavernous fistula-modified Borden type I (petrosal sinus drainage) and II (ophthalmic vein drainage or cortical reflux)
Spinal DAVF-modified Borden type II (extradural dural fistula) and III (intradural dural fistula)

signals of venous hypertension, such as pial vein engorgement, dilated venous pouch or abnormal vascular enhancement [1] (Fig. 1.2). Susceptibility-weighted imaging can clarify arteriovenous shunting of DAVF by demonstrating hyperintense venous signal due to rapid wash-in of oxygenated blood [1] (Fig. 1.3). Cranial CT angiography (CTA) or MR angiography (MRA) can demonstrate engorged arterial or venous vessels, enhanced transosseous vessels or asymmetric sinuses.

Negative cranial CTA or MRA can not completely exclude the diagnosis of DAVF. Cerebral digital subtraction angiography (DSA) is the gold standard imaging to characterise the DAVF [1]. A full DSA, including bilateral internal carotid arteries (ICA), external carotid arteries (ECA) and vertebral arteries, is usually required to depict the DAVF. Superselective evaluation of smaller arteries is also helpful to clarify particular arterial feeders that can be choosen for embolization approach.

The Borden and Cognard classifications are the most well-known schemes to predict aggressiveness of intracranial DAVFs [3, 4]. The Borden classification system has unified spinal and intracranial DAVFs based on surgical practices [3]. The Borden classification

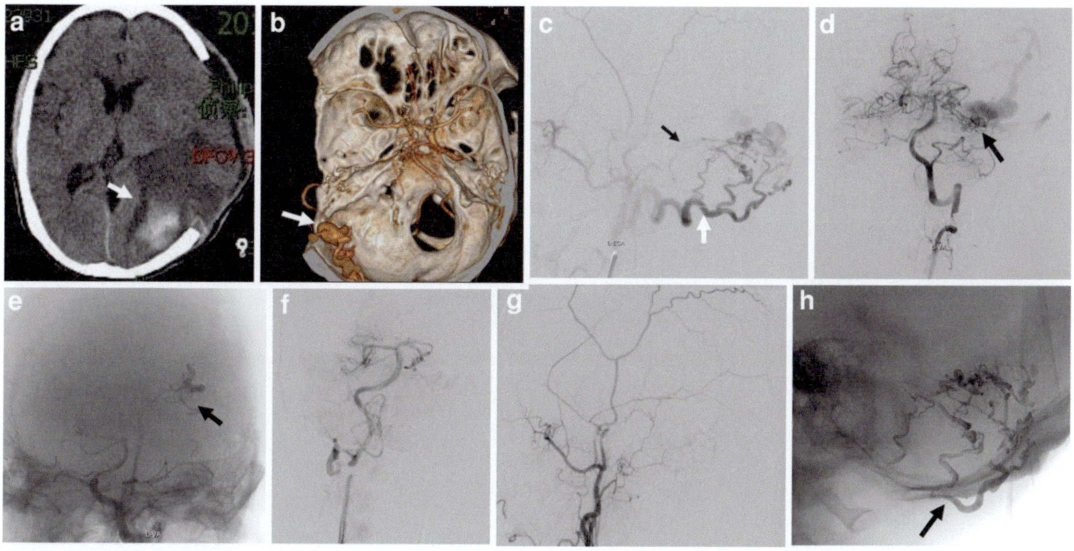

Fig. 1.1 A 63-year-old male patient presented with intracerebral hematoma. (**a**) CT scanning showing hematoma in left occipital lobe treated by surgery and decompression treatment (arrow). (**b**) CT angiography showing a giant venous ectasia of the left occipital lobe (arrow). (**c**) The left external carotid artery angiogram (lateral view) showing a Zipfel type 3 dural fistula supplied by the dural branches of the acending pharyngeal artery (black arrow) and the occipital artery (white arrow). (**d**) The left vertebral artery angiogram (frontal view) showing the dural fistula supplied by the temporal branches of the left posterior cerebral artery (arrow). The dural fistula was drained directly by cortical veins with a giant venous pouch. (**e**) Unsubtracted image (frontal projection) showed the posterior artery branches was embolized with Onyx firstly (arrow). (**f**) Control angiogram of the left vertebral artery (frontal view) showed the dural fistula was completely occluded. (**g**) Control angiogram of the left external carotid artery (lateral view) showed the dural fistula was completely occluded after left occipital artery embolization. (**h**) Unsubtracted image (lateral projection) showed the Onyx was injected to occlude the fistula via the occipital artery (arrow)

designates types I–III lesions as those with dural venous drainage without cortical venous reflux, dural venous drainage with cortical venous reflux, and cortical venous drainage without dural venous drainage, respectively. The Cognard classification designates types I, IIa, IIb, IIa + b, III, IV and V lesions as those antegrade dural venous drainage without cortical venous drainage (type I), retrograde dural venous drainage without cortical venous reflux (type IIa), antegrade dural venous drainage with cortical venous reflux (type IIb), retrograde dural venous drainage with cortical venous reflux (type IIa + b), cortical venous reflux without dural venous drainage (type III), cortical venous reflux with venous ectasias (type IV), and cervical perimedullary venous drainage (type V). Borden types II and III and Cognard types IIa, IIb, IIa + b, III, IV, and V DAVFs constitute aggressive lesions which must be treated [4].

The Borden and Cognard classifications have both focused chiefly on venous drainage direction of DAVFs excluding direct carotid cavernous

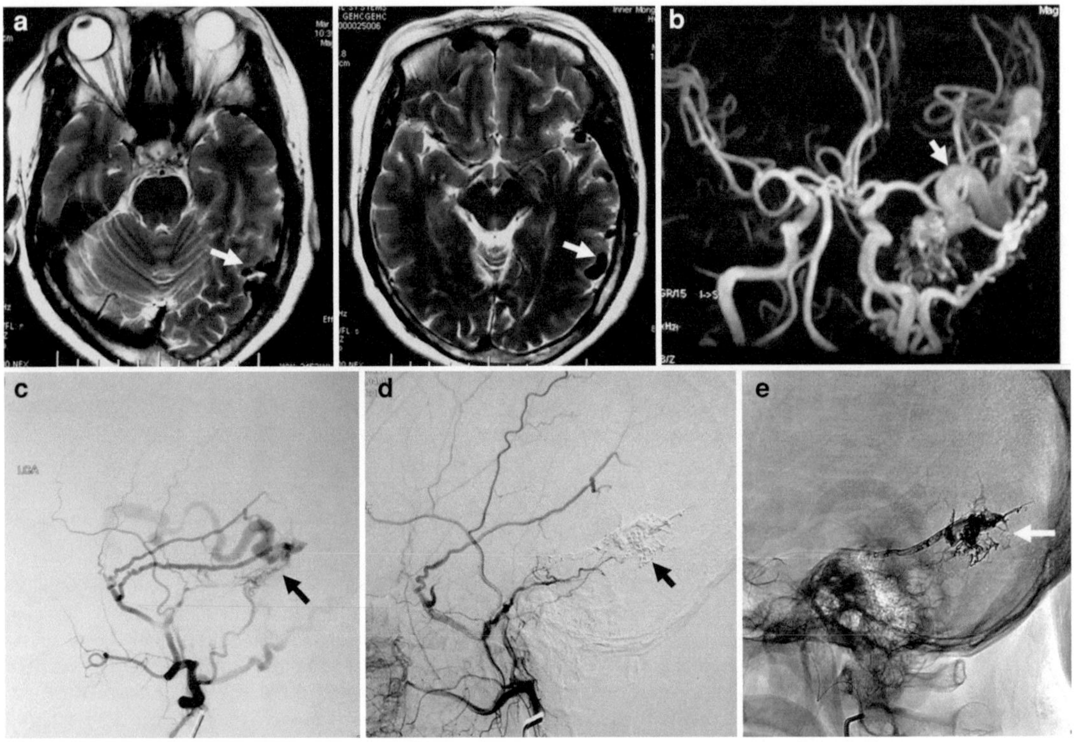

Fig. 1.2 A 50-year-old female patient presented with headaches. (**a**) Axial MR imaging, T2-weighted, showing flow void signals of cortical veins engorgement in the occipital lobe (arrow). (**b**) MR angiography (MRA) demonstrate engorged the left external carotid arteries and cortical veins of the left occipital lobe. (**c**) The left external carotid artery angiogram (later view) showing a Zipfel type 3 transverse sinus dural fistula (arrow) supplied by the middle meningeal artery branches and cortical vein drainage. (**d**) The left external carotid artery angiogram (lateral view) showed the dural fistula was completely occluded after Onyx embolization. (**e**) Unsubtracted image (lateral view) showing the Onyx cast after successful infusion through the middle meningeal artery (arrow)

fistulas [3, 4]. Though adequately predicting extent of venous flow and properly categorizing the lesions angioarchitecturally, these grades lack of correlation with patients' presentation, natural history, and hemorrhagic risk. While the Cognard system is more complicated to use, it can be changed. Therefore, Zipfel et al. proposed a classification of DAVFs based on natural history data, which is a modifier of the Borden grading system (Table 1.1) [13].

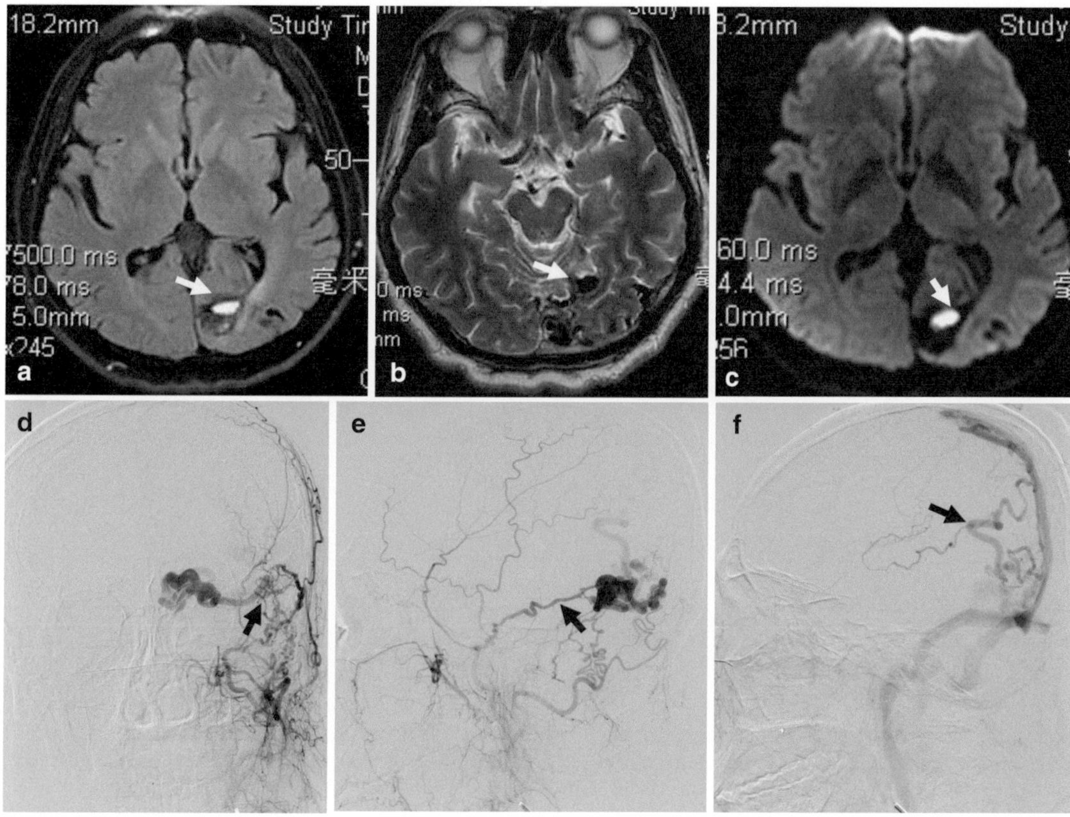

Fig. 1.3 A 59-year-old male patient suffered a second intracranial bleeding after 15 years of bleeding. (**a**) MR imaging, T1-weighted. (**b**) MR imaging, T2-weighted. (**c**) DWI MR imaging. Showing a subacute hemorrhage of the left occipital lobe and flow void signals of the engorged cortical veins. (**d**) the left external carotid artery angiogram (frontal view). (**e**) The left external carotid artery angiogram (later view). (**f**) The late phase of the left external carotid artery angiogram (later view). Showing a Zipfel type 3 dural fistula (arrow) supplied by the middle meningeal artery branches and cortical veins drainage

1.2 Zipfel Classification of DAVFs [13]

Type I DAVFs are those that drain into the dural sinus with antegrade venous flow, e.g. the flow of the veins draining from the parenchyma or spinal cord into the dural sinuses or epidural veins is anterograde, a carotid cavernous fistula (CCF) without cortical or superior ophthalmic vein (SOV) reflux.

Type II DAVFs drain into dural sinus with retrograde venous flow, a CCF with SOV reflux without cortical reflux. Intracranial type II DAVFs can drain into spinal perimedullary veins (Fig. 1.4).

Type III DAVFs are those that drain into the pial veins and the spinal coronal or perimedullary veins, a CCF with cortical drainage (Fig. 1.5). Type III spinal DAVFs can drain intracranially.

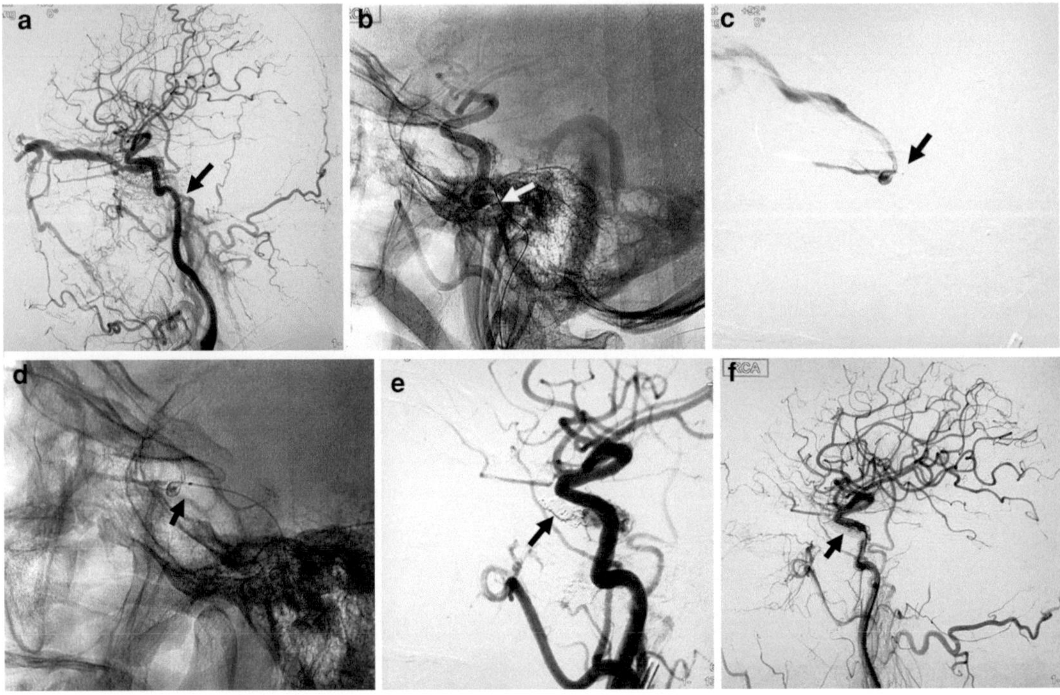

Fig. 1.4 A 46-year-old male patient presented with 6 months of right-sided proptosis. Transvenous embolisation of a right Zipfel type II cavernous sinus dAVF with Onyx and microcoils. (**a**) Lateral projection pre-embolisation angiogram, right carotid artery injection, showing multiple dural feeders arising from the external carotid artery and the internal carotid artery draining into superior ophthalmic vein and inferior petrosal sinus (arrow). (**b**) Unsubtracted lateral view showing successful catheterization of the inferior petrosal sinus (arrow). (**c**) Selective injection showing the Echelon-10 microcatheter positioned within the origin of the superior ophthalmic vein (arrow). (**d**) Unsubtracted lateral view showing successful deployment of microcoils within the origin of the superior ophthalmic vein (arrow). (**e**) Lateral view of the carotid artery injection showing successful deployment of microcoils within the origin of the superior ophthalmic vein (arrow). (**f**) Lateral view of the carotid artery injection showing successful occlusion of the dural fistula after Onyx injection (arrow)

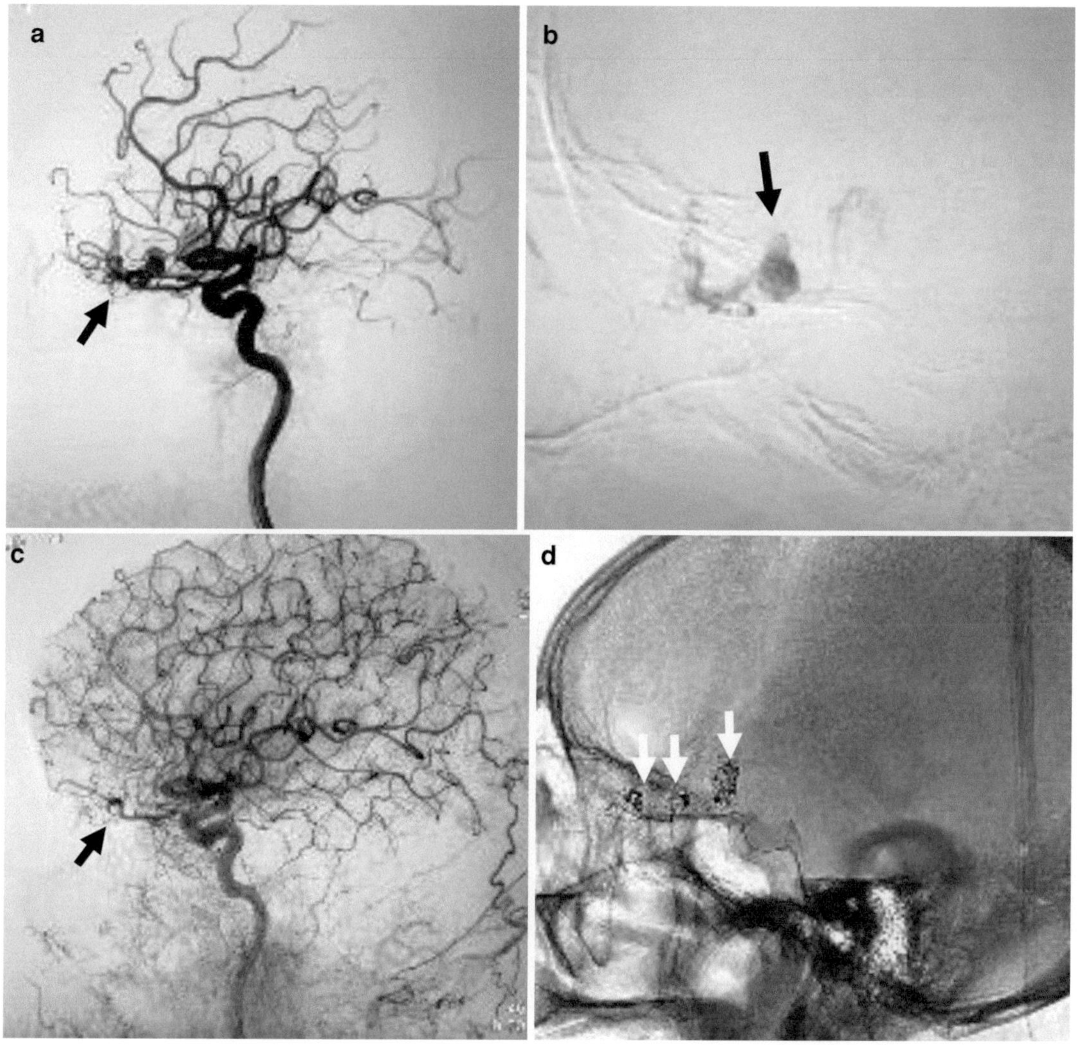

Fig. 1.5 A 55-year-old male patient presented with headaches. (**a**) The left internal carotid artery angiogram (later view) showing a Zipfel type 3 dural fistula arising from the anterior cranial fossa (arrow) supplied by the ethmoidal arteries arising from the ophthalmic artery and cortical vein ectasia. (**b**) Superselective angiography showing the microcatheter positioned through the left ophthalmic artery and the large venous pouch (arrow). (**c**) The left internal carotid artery angiogram (lateral view) showed the dural fistula was completely occluded after Onyx embolization. (**d**) Unsubtracted image (lateral view) showing the Onyx cast after successful infusion the venous pouch (arrows)

1.3 Endovascular Approaches

Endovascular approach is the first-line treatment for most DAVFs. The mainstay for endovascular treatment involves occlusion of the arteriovenous shunts and its initial venous components while preventing adverse effects [14]. Inappropriate embolisation could cause sudden changes of the flow dynamics in its venous drainage and potentially worsen the patient outcome (Fig. 1.6). Therefore, it is imperative to have comprehensive understanding of the arterial and venous components prior to initiating treatment [15].

The fistulous connection can be approached by either transarterial or transvenous approaches. Detachable balloons, polyvinyl alcohol, silk

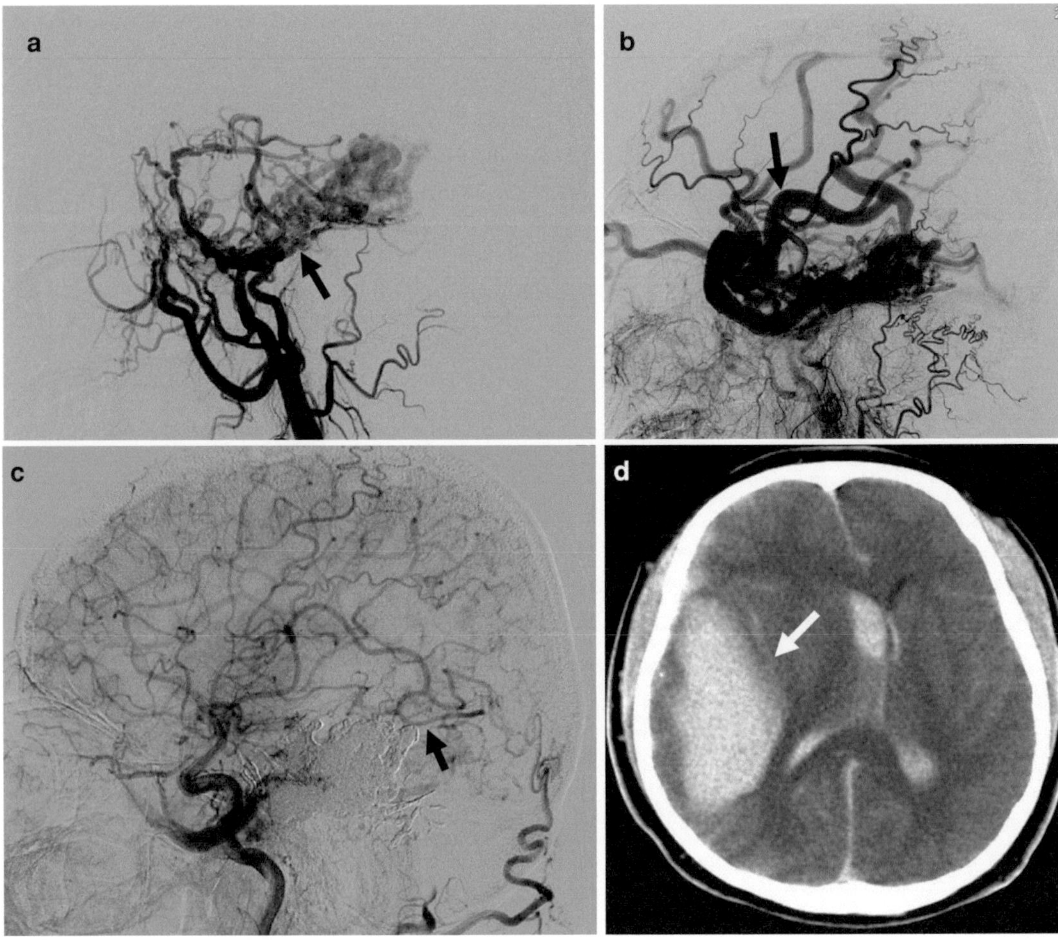

Fig. 1.6 A 47-year-old male patient presented with headaches. (**a**) The right external carotid artery angiogram (later view) showing a Zipfel type 3 dural fistula arising from the middle cranial fossa (arrow) supplied by the dural branches arising from the middle meningeal artery. (**b**) The late phase of the right external carotid artery angiogram (later view) showing the dural fistula drained by multiple dilated cortical veins. (**c**) The right carotid artery angiogram (lateral view) showed the residual fistula supplied by the middle cerebral artery after Onyx embolization (arrow). (**d**) The patient was in coma half an hour after embolization. CT scanning showed a large intracerebral hematoma (arrow)

sutures, microspheres and detachable microcoils were used for treatment of cerebral AVM and DAVFs in the past decades. However, they have been widely replaced by current embolic agents, including *n*-butyl-2-cyanoacrylate (nBCA, glue,Trufill, DePuy Synthes, Raynham, MA) and Onyx (Medtronic, Irvine, CA) [15]. Recent advancements have introduced newer embolic agents, such as Squid (Emboflu, Switzerland), precipitating hydrophobic injectable liquid (PHIL; MicroVention, Aliso Viejo, California) [15–17]. Flow diverters, such as the pipeline embolisation device (Medtronic Neurovascular, Irvine, California), have been reported to treat direct or indirect CCF, in which arterial feeder were ICA or its dural branch, a type of DAVF [18]. Endothelialisation of the flow-diverting stent allowed for occlusion of the CCF.

Endovascular approaches for DAVF embolization include transarterial, transvenous or a combination of both techniques. Endovascular DAVF embolization is often done under general anesthesia to decrease patient motion. Heparinised saline flushes are routinely used to prevent catheter-associated thrombosis and embolic events. Various imaging techniques, including superselective angiography through microcatheter, three-dimension angiography, roadmapping and negative roadmapping, are often used to obtain clear images throughout the procedure [19].

1.4 Transarterial Embolization

Transarterial approach is the preferred treatment for DAVFs, in which transvenous approach is limited. In transarterial embolization, microcatheters are tracked over microwires to distal locations in feeding arteries, with the goal of getting the microcatheter as close to the fistula point as possible. Different liquid embolic agents can be used: nBCA, Onyx, Squid or PHIL. Injection of an embolic agent through a compatible microcatheter. Advantages of transarterial embolisation include decreased complications specific to commonly used transvenous approaches (e.g., venous perforation from catheterisation and bleeding from premature venous occlusion), ability to save functional venous system, decreased chance of flow redirection into an alternate venous pathway and avoidance of post-treatment de novo DAVF formation from venous hypertension [20].

1.4.1 nBCA

Before the appearance of Onyx, nBCA was widely used as "glue" for the embolisation of DAVFs [20, 21]. NBCA can quickly solidify when it comes in contact with blood. Ethiodol (ethiodised oil) must be added to nBCA for radiopaque and identifiable on fluoroscopy [22]. The concentration of nBCA is an important consideration as it changes the extent of its penetration before polymerisation. A mixture with high nBCA-to-Ethiodol ratio (high concentration of glue) polymerises more rapidly to embolize more proximal targets. A mixture with low nBCA-to-Ethiodol ratio can achieve more distal penetration. NBCA of 25–33% concentrations are commonly used.

Prior to nBCA injection, the microcatheter must be advanced to the fistula point and helps successfully deliver the glue to the fistulous collateral networks [20]. Microcatheter angiography is obtained to help extimate the optimal glue concentration according to the flow velocity. Prior to injecting the nBCA and Ethiodol mixture, the microcatheter should be flushed with non-ionic solution of 5% dextrose, to prevent glue polymerisation within the microcatheter. The glue is then injected under negative road map as either a continuous column or a bolus [23]. Depending on the position of the microcatheter and the distance to the target vessel, 5% dextrose can be simultaneously injected through the guide or distal intracranial support catheter to promote more distal penetration of the glue [21]. After nBCA embolisation, it is important to rapidly remove the microcatheter to prevent the catheter from being entrapped to the vessel.

1.4.2 Onyx

Onyx is the preferred option for DAVF embolization. It is a liquid mixture of ethylene–vinyl alcohol copolymer (EVOH) suspended in dimethyl sulfoxide (DMSO). Catheters and syringes involved in the procedure must be DMSO compatible. Tantalum powder is added for radio-opacity. Before use, the Onyx mixture must be shaken for 20 min to evenly distribute the tantalum and obtain uniform radio-opacity [24]. When onyx is in contact with blood, it will precipitate into a non-adhesive substance with a characteristic "lava" flow pattern, resulting in blood vessel occlusion. After an in-depth understanding of the anatomy and hemodynamics of the fistula, the microcatheter must be flushed with DMSO before the injection of Onyx. The negative roadmap imaging is used to inject Onyx under direct visualization to identify any premature leaks. The injection speed can be customized to optimize vessel penetration. Once Onyx reflux is observed, the injection should be stopped for about 30–90 s to allow Onyx to solidify before next injection. When the Onyx reflux forms an ideal plug around the tip of the microcatheter, it can push Onyx into the fistula. Multiple control angiograms are usually necessary during the entire operation to carefully monitor the progress of the embolization. Since the injection of Onyx needs to be very precise, it is not uncommon for treatment with a single pedicle to last more than an hour or to divide the embolization into multiple stages. After embolization, the microcatheter can be removed from the Onyx cast by continuous gentle traction. The ability of prolonged Onyx injections allows curative embolization of DAVF with multiple feeders that form a complex vascular network with a single injection, especially when Onyx reaches the venous side [14, 25–27] (Fig. 1.7). Therefore, endovascular Onyx embolization has shown a higher DAVF cure rate than nBCA [28].

1.4.3 PHIL and Squid

PHIL is an iodinated copolymer dissolved in DMSO and will precipitate to form a non-adhesive substance when it contacts with blood. The agent can be used immediately (without shaking) because the radiopaque iodine is covalently bonded to the compound. Since it does not contain tantalum, very few artifacts can be seen in the postoperative follow-up CT scan. The agent can penetrate into blood vessels less than 10 μm. PHIL can be used in three concentrations, the lowest concentration is most commonly used for DAVF embolization. PHIL is currently not available for commercial use in China, but an active trial is underway to evaluate its effectiveness in the treatment of AVM. Leon et al. describes the use of PHIL in eight cases using Apollo (Medtronic) or Marathon (Medtronic) microcatheter to treat five skulls and three spinal

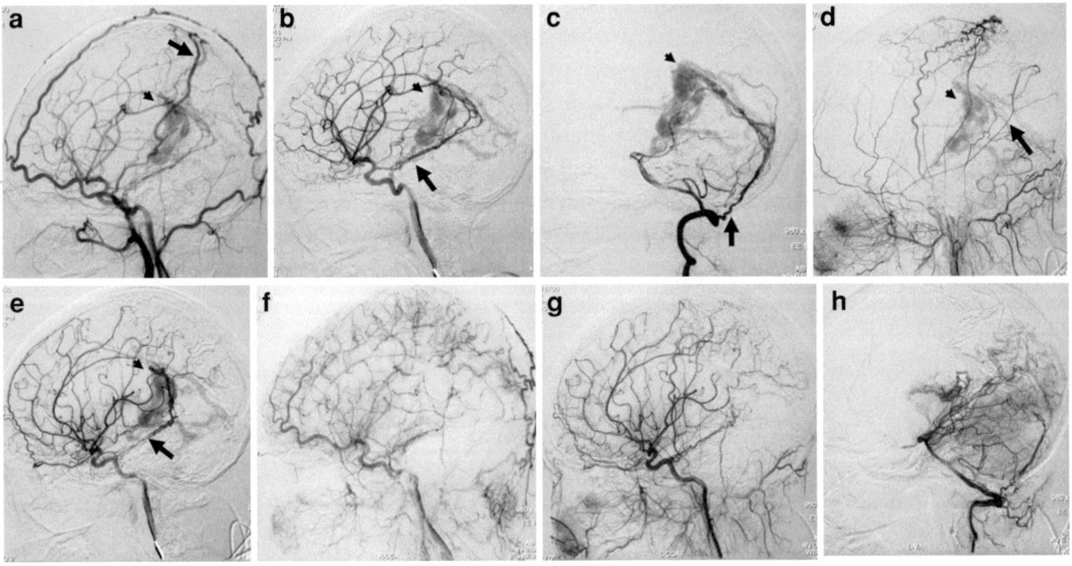

Fig. 1.7 A 29-year-old female patient presented with headaches. (**a**) The right external carotid artery angiogram (lateral view). (**b**) The right internal carotid artery angiogram (lateral view). (**c**) The right vertebral artery angiogram (lateral view). (**d**) The left external carotid artery angiogram (lateral view). (**e**) The left internal carotid artery angiogram (lateral view). Showing a Zipfel type 3 tentorial dural fistula multiple arterial feeders arising from bilateral middle meningeal arteries (arrow), bilateral meningohypophyseal arteries (arrow), and bilateral posterior meningeal arteries (arrow), draining into dilated pial veins (arrowhead). Post-embolization angiograms. (**f**) The right carotid artery angiogram (lateral view). (**g**) The left carotid artery angiogram (lateral view). (**h**) The left vertebral artery (lateral view). Showing the dural fistula was completely occluded after transarterial Onyx embolization

cords DAVF [29]. Laming et al. reported that Apollo, Marathon and Headway Duo (MicroVention, Tustin, California, USA) microcatheters are used in 30 PHIL embolization procedures [30].

Squid is another liquid embolic agent used to treat DAVF, but it is not currently on the market in China. Squid is an ethylene vinyl alcohol copolymer, available in two versions: Squid 12 and Squid 18 (Emboflu, Switzerland). Squid has 30% less tantalum content than Onyx and has micronized tantalum, which may help to better observe the structure behind the embolic material and provide a more uniform solution than Onyx [30, 31]. Akmanjit et al. reported a case series of nine cases of DAVF treated with Squid and Sonic detachable microcatheter [31]. Much like Onyx, the Squid is injected in a "plug and push" manner. In their case series, they used a higher density Squid 18 for initial plug formation and a lower viscosity Squid 12 for distal penetration. Gioppo et al. reported the use of Squid with the Headway Duo microcatheter (MicroVention, Tustin, California, USA) to treat a complex case of DAVF [17].

1.5 Transvenous Approach

In the transvenous method, the catheters are retrogradely inserted into the affected sinus or the affected pial vein to occlude them using a microcoils, liquid embolic agent, or a combination of them (Fig. 1.4). For the transvenous approach, appropriate patient selection is essential to achieve complete occlusion and avoid complications. The selected sinus or pial vein should fully participate in fistula drainage, not in normal cerebral venous drainage, and the venous access should be completely occluded for proper treatment [32]. When the DAVF is supplied by many small tortuous artery, the transvenous approach is preferred because of the lack of transarterial access. When the DAVF is only supplied by the branch directly from the ICA or the vertebral artery, when the DAVF is supplied by the dangerous extracranial to intracranial anastomosed artery, or when the DAVF is supplied by the nutrient arteries of the cranial nerve, the transvenous embolization should be considered [33, 34]. The transvenous route is the first-line treatment for indirect CCF, in which dangerous anastomosis, arteries supplying cranial nerves, and very small supply arteries supplying fistulas are very likely to be involved [34, 35].

Various approaches are used to achieve transvenous access. A transvenous access can be established through the femoral vein, the internal jugular vein, or directly puncture the draining venous pouch under the guidance of drilling, craniotomy, or ultrasound [36, 37]. In the case of a thrombotic sinus, the transvenous approach can be can be achieved by recanalization of the closed venous segment, such as traversing the ipsilateral occluded inferior petrosal sinus to access the trapped cavernous sinus or traversing the occluded sigmoid sinus to access an isolated transverse sinus [38, 39]. In this method, neurointerventionists need to carefully manipulate the catheter and guide wire to avoid the risk of thrombosis sinus or vein perforation [39]. Sometimes the contralateral approach can also be used, such as the contralateral jugular vein can be used to pass through torcula to the sigmoid sinus [40]. The trapped sinus can also be directly punctured by drilling or craniotomy [36]. The direct access to the trapped cavernous sinus in the indirect CCF can be achieved by a transforaminal approach via foramen ovale or transorbital puncture [41, 42]. The hybrid angio-operating room is the ideal choice for this type of combined endovascular surgical method.

Coil embolization is very effective for filling and occluding affected sinuses or venous pouch, especially an isolated transverse sinuses [24, 33]. Sometimes it is necessary to combine Onyx with coils to help seal the associated sinus or venous pouch [33, 43, 44]. Some authors prefer the "dual catheter technique," one is a proximal microcatheter used to deploy the coils, and the other is a distal microcatheter used to inject Onyx after coiling [33].

For ethmoidal or anterior cranial fossa DAVF, the blood supply arteries are usually small and very tortuous, making it difficult or impossible to perform a safe superselective transarterial catheterization [45]. In these cases, transvenous coil or Onyx embolization may be safe when there is an uncurved draining vein that allows the catheter to enter the venous pouch [45, 46]. Albuquerque and colleagues describe transvenous Onyx embolization for the treatment of high-risk transverse sigmoid sinus DAVF, in which a microcatheter is passed through the sinus into the venous pouch and positioned to the arterial ostium [45]. In these cases, Onyx penetrates into multiple arterial suppliers, and a small amount of reflux enters the venous pouch [45]. According to this report, this technique is safe when there is a venous pouch or an isolated sinus.

When a DAVF flows directly into the transverse sigmoid sinus and there is no venous pouch, the possibility of Onyx reflux to the normal sinus is high. A large amount of reflux to the normal sinuses can cause pulmonary embolism or inadvertent sinus thrombosis. In these cases, reconstructive transvenous balloon-assisted embolization was introduced as an option. For this technique, a microcatheter and a DMSO-compliant balloon are simultaneously guided to the affected transverse sigmoid sinus [47]. After the balloon is inflated, Onyx 18 is injected around the balloon and slowly penetrates into the blood suppliers resulting in complete occlusion of DAVFs [47]. In this technique, the preservation of normal cortical veins, such as Labbé vein and normal bridging vein, is essential to prevent complications such as venous infarction and cerebral or cerebellar hemorrhage [48]. It is also possible to temporarily block the main feeding artery during the Onyx embolization of the fistula venous pouch, especially in treatment of direct CCF [49]. When the venous drainage of the brain depends on the transverse sinus of the fistula, the use of a stent to reconstruct the transverse sinus, with or without transarterial Onyx embolization may be a good choice [50].

1.6 Stereotactic Radiosurgery

Stereotactic radiosurgery (SRS) is usually reserved as the last resort option for the treatment of DAVF. Endothelial cell damage and thrombosis are considered to be the main mechanism of DAVF occlusion caused by radiation [51]. Like SRS for the treatment of brain AVM, the occlusion of DAVF may take 1–3 years, and there is still a risk of bleeding during this incubation period [52–54]. When endovascular treatment and surgery fail, it can also be used as a supplementary treatment [52] (Fig. 1.8). When intravascular or surgical methods are too dangerous or fail, SRS can be used for high-risk DAVF [51]. According to reports, 50–93% of DAVFs are completely occluded and treated with SRS [52, 53, 55]. After SRS treatment, the complete occlusion rate and symptom improvement rate of indirect CCF are higher than them of the DAVF of the transverse and sigmoid sinuses [53]. According to reports, the average incubation period of DAVF closure after SRS is 23 months [54]. After SRS of DAVF, the annual rebleeding rate is reported to be as high as 2.6% [55], but this will depend on the initial fistula grade. For follow-up, MRI is recommended once a year, and angiography must be performed to accurately confirm complete DAVF occlusion [52, 53]. Complications include cranial nerve palsy, cerebral edema, latent hemorrhage and radiation effects [52, 53, 55].

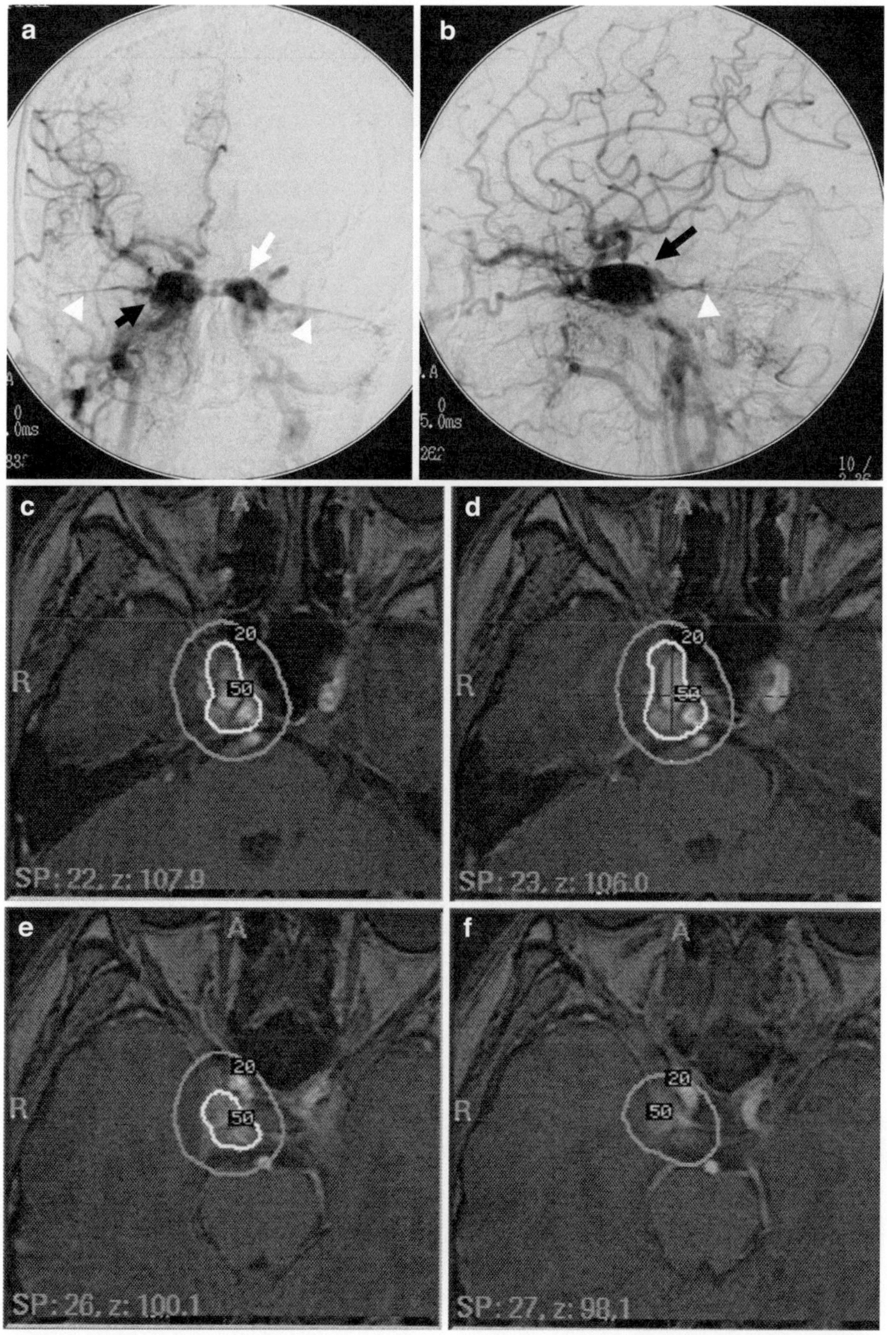

Fig. 1.8 A 53-year-old male patient presented with 2 months of bilateral proptosis. (**a**) Frontal projection angiogram, right carotid artery injection. (**b**) Lateral projection angiogram, right carotid artery injection. Showing multiple dural feeders arising from the external carotid artery and the internal carotid artery draining into superior ophthalmic vein (black arrow), contralateral cavernous sinus (white arrow) and superior petrosal sinus (white arrowheads). The right Zipfel type II cavernous sinus dAVF was treated with radiosurgery employing a dose of 19 Gy to the 50% isodose line, as seen on axial views of planning MRI T1-weighted sequence with contrast (**c**–**f**)

1.7 Surgery

Although endovascular techniques are generally considered the first-line treatment for DAVFs, surgery is still an effective and safe alternative [56]. For a DAVF in the transverse sigmoid sinus, surgery involves extensive exposure of the involved sinus by separating and coagulating the dural arteries and arterialized cortical veins [56]. If the affected sinus is not functional and is not involved in normal brain venous drainage, it can be completely removed. Care must be taken to avoid massive blood loss during surgery, especially in complex fistulas with highly developed and hypertrophic arterial networks. In surgical treatment of non-sinus DAVF, the cortical draining vein is disconnected from the fistula point by clip or coagulation [56, 57]. Frameless stereotactic navigation helps to locate the fistula connection during craniotomy [58]. Occlusion of the DAVF during surgery is usually confirmed by indocyanine green angiography with or without intraoperative DSA [59].

Surgery is usually considered when the endovascular method fails to completely cure the disease, such as such as DAVF in the anterior fossa [60, 61] (Fig. 1.9). According to reports, the long-term morbidity and mortality rate of DAVF surgery is as high as 13% [58]. The main complications of surgery include infection, hydrocephalus, cerebrospinal fluid leakage, stroke, cranial nerve palsy, and severe blood loss [58]. Preoperative embolization before surgery can help reduce blood loss during surgery.

1.8 Endovascular Management Based on Zipfel Classification of DAVFs [13]

Cranial and spinal DAVFs are classified into three types based on Zipfel et al.'s classification scales [13]. Zipfel et al. proposed a modified Borden classification based on natural history data correlating symptoms with outcome in 2009 [13]. The Zipfel classification designates types I, II, and III lesions as those with dural venous drainage without venous reflux, dural venous drainage with venous reflux, and cortical venous drainage, respectively. Zipfel type I lesions exhibit a benign clinical course. Patients harboring type II lesions usually present intracranial hypertension. Hemorrhagic ruptured occurred in more than 30% of patients harboring type III DAVFs. Type II and III spinal DAVFs exhibiting drainage into spinal perimedullary veins might present progressive myelopathy in all of cases. Some spinal DAVF patients characterized by spasticity of muscular hypertonia caused by the upper motor neuron syndrome.

Zipfel type I DAVFs can be treated by TAE and major sinus drainage needs to be preserved (Fig. 1.10). Because of the benign nature, DAVFs without venous reflux (type I) are often managed

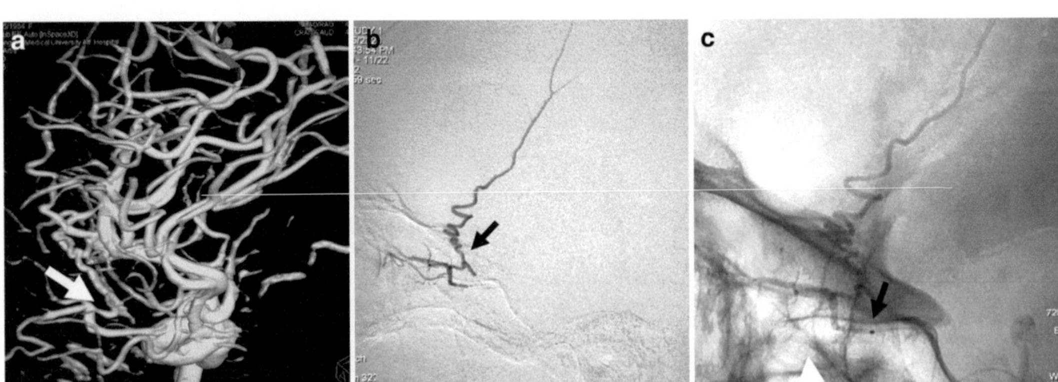

Fig. 1.9 A 54-year-old female patient presented with subarachnoid hemorrhage caused by a Zipfel type III dAVF supplied by the right ophthalmic artery. (**a**) 3-D reconstruction of the right internal carotid artery injection demonstrated a modified Borden type III dAVF supplied by the ophthalmic artery (arrow). (**b**) Lateral super selective injection of the right ophthalmic artery showing the arteriovenous shunt (arrow). (**c**) Unsubtracted image demonstrated the microcatheter tip (arrow) and the modified Borden type III dAVF in the right anterior cranial fossa

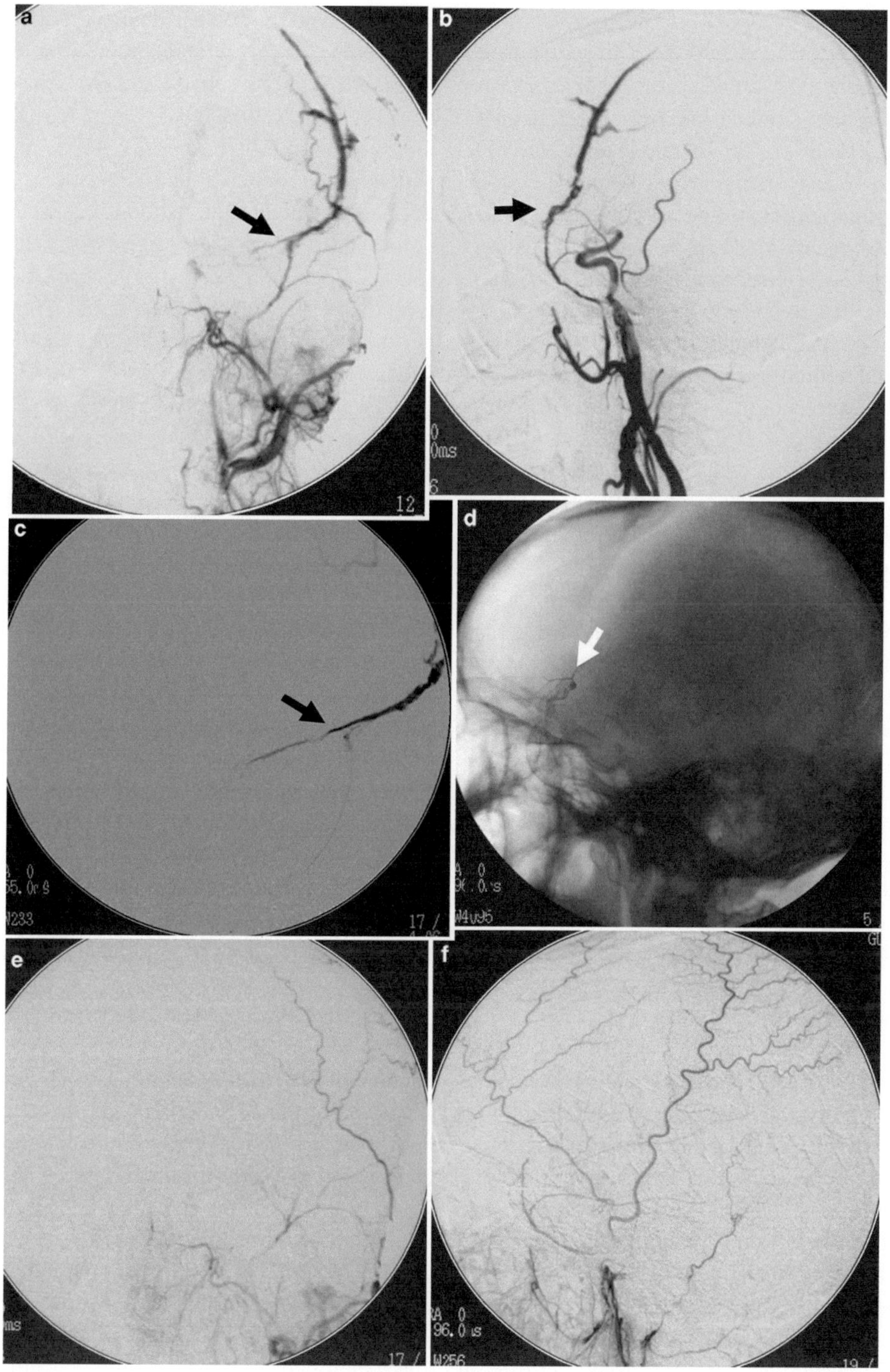

Fig. 1.10 A 38-year-old male patient presented with 3 years of pulsatile tinnitus. Transarterial Onyx embolisation of a left sphenoid parietal sinus dAVF. (**a**) Frontal projection pre-embolisation angiogram, selective the left external carotid artery injection. (**b**) Lateral projection pre-embolisation angiogram, selective the left external carotid artery injection. Showing arterial feeder arising from the middle meningeal artery (arrow), draining into sphenoid parietal sinus. (**c**) Superselective angiogram showing the microcatheter within the middle meningeal artery (arrow). (**d**) Unsubtracted lateral view showing Onyx cast after single infusion through the middle meningeal artery. Final digital subtraction angiography of the left external carotid injection, frontal view (**e**) and lateral view (**f**), showing no residual dAVF

conservatively. Compression therapy is sometimes used for these DAVFs. Compression of ipsilateral carotid artery or occipital artery is performed by contralateral hand for more than 20 min, three times a day. Contrast to type I DAVFs, which are usually benign, types II and III DAVFs presented a high proportion of worse clinical status before treatment. Their pathophysiology was consistent as venous congestion and hypertension. Type II and III DAVFs can be successfully treated with endovascular treatment. Since being associated with moderate risk for type II DAVFs, endovascular techniques should be used in selective patients (Fig. 1.11). When the venous drainage could be sacrificed safely, the DAVF can be cured by the venous obliteration. Type III DAVFs are usually cured by TAE embolization of the pial draining vein.

Classifications developed by Borden et al. and Cognard et al. have both inadequately distinguish between anterior and posterior drainage in the cavernous sinus region, which is the most common location [62–66]. Cavernous sinus DAVFs drained only inferior petrosal sinus and spinal extradural DAVFs only involving epidural venous plexus is defined as Zipfel type I DAVFs. Type I DAVFs are often asymptomatic or bruits. Cavernous sinus DAVFs that drain retrogradely into the intraorbital/ophthalmic veins with or without reflux to the Sylvian veins are classified as type II DAVFs because the intraorbital veins corresponds to dural sinuses [64] (Fig. 1.12). Spinal DAVFs that drain into the epidural venous plexus with reflux to the perimedullary veins are classified as type II DAVFs because the epidural plexus corresponds to dural sinuses and the intradural perimedullary veins are pial veins. Intraorbital arteriovenous fistula exhibit an exceedingly low incidence and prevalence, presenting chiefly with proptosis and chemosis and also is classified as Zipfel type II. There are two specific locations, such as the orbit and the spine. The intra-orbital veins are located between the orbital periosteum and ocular nerves sheath dura and the spinal epidural veins are located in the spinal canal between the spinal periosteum and meningeal dura [3]. Thus, the intraorbital venous plexus and spinal epidual veins correspond to the dural sinuses.

Zipfel type III DAVFs are drained directly into pial veins with or without giant venous pouch (Cognard type III and IV and Borden type III) because their natural history and treatment are the same as for other type III DAVFs. In type III patients, the venous pouch can cause subarachnoid hemorrhage, supratentorial ventricular dilatation and trigeminal neuralgia and facial nerve spasm. Cognard type V DAVFs can be Zipfel type II or III as those lesions drained into spinal perimedullary veins indirectly or directly [7, 9] (Fig. 1.13). The most common group of type III DAVFs are tentorial [12, 67] (Fig. 1.14). The most common spinal DAVFs are type III DAVFs supplied by dural branches of a radicular artery and drained into the perimedullary veins [68]. Spinal DAVFs drained into intradural spaces causing myelopathy.

When a DAVF drains into a major dural sinus that cannot be safely occluded, it is often difficult to cure the DAVF, especially if it has multiple fistulas [69]. The hemorrhagic complication risk of a major dural sinus sacrifice combined with the benign natural history of type I or II DAVFs makes this procedure an unwarranted option. When the sinus must be preserved and the arterial supply cannot be completely eliminated, our treatment goal should aim to restore the hemodynamic of brain or spine circulation, e.g. the arteriovenous shunts can be significantly reduced by endovascular embolization.

Type III DAVFs can be fed by vessels that also supply important structures [70]. DAVFs of the tentorium are fed by meningohypophyseal trunk branches of the ICA. DAVFs at the anterior cranial fossa are fed by the ethmoidal branches of the ophthalmic artery. Spinal DAVFs are fed by dural branches of the radicular arteries adjacent to the radiculomedullary arteries. When these arteries are embolized, there are potential risks of neurological deficits. Inadvertent embolization of the cavernous and petrosal branches of the middle meningeal artery, which triumphantly emerges into the middle cranial fossa through foramen spinosum, may precipitate infarctions of the trigeminal and facial nerves [71–73]. As to the cavernous sinus DAVFs, the cause of hemorrhagic or venous infarction complications are

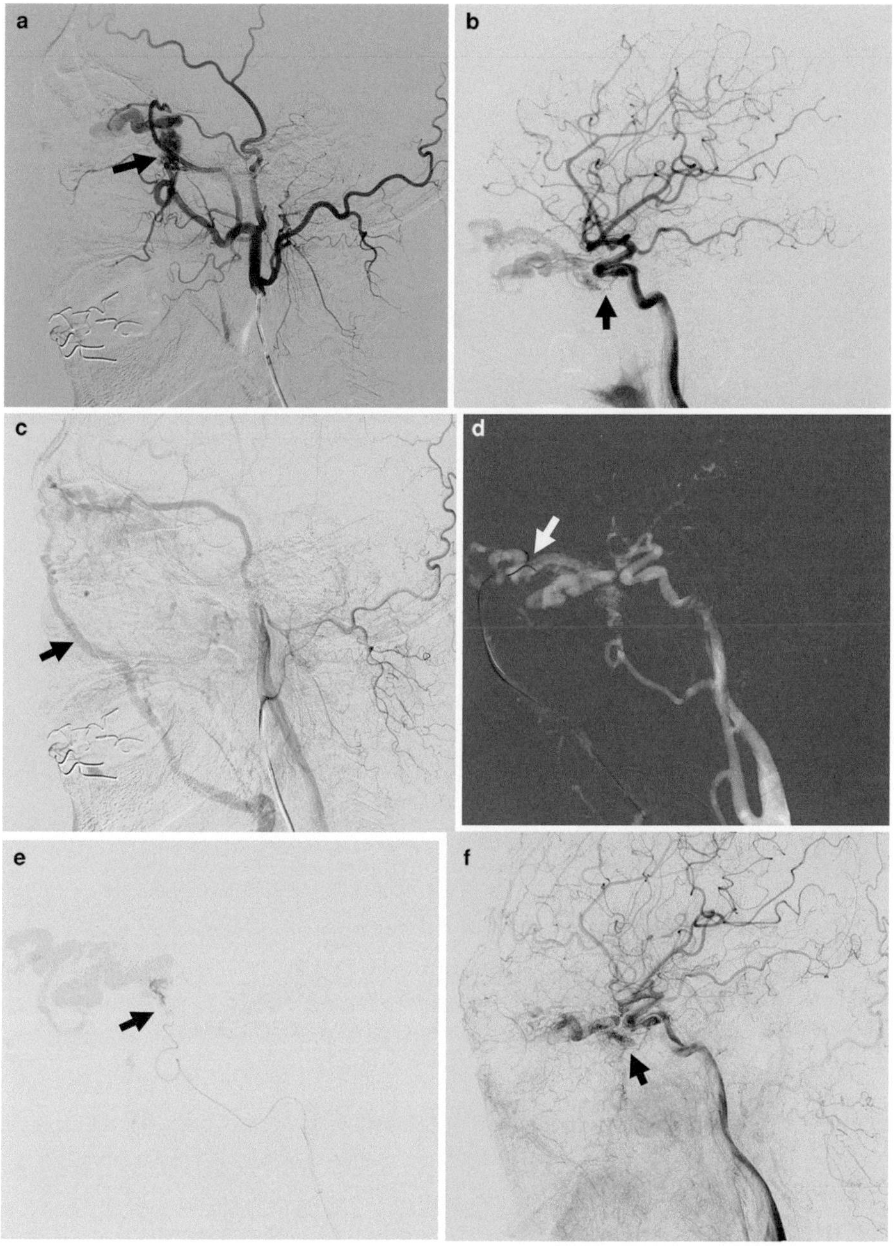

Fig. 1.11 A 45-year-old male patient presented with congestion of the right bulbar conjunctiva, exophthalmos, and right palpebral edema. (**a**) Arterial phase of a lateral view on selective right external carotid arteriography before treatment. Sphenopalatine and infraorbital arteries branched from the maxillary artery and the middle meningeal artery (arrow), exhibiting inflow to the shunt site via aggregated blood vessels. The entire shunt was visualized from the artery of the superior orbital fissure. Outflow to the ophthalmic veins was observed. (**b**) Arterial phase of a frontal view on right internal carotid arteriography before treatment. A portion of the shunt was visualized from small dural branches (arrow) from the cavernous segment of the internal carotid artery. (**c**) Venous phase of a lateral view on right carotid arteriography before treatment. The main drainers outflowed to the front are superficial temporal vein and facial vein (arrow) mediated by the angular vein. (**d**) Under roadmap, the transvenous treatment through the facial vein to the superior ophthalmic vein was attempted, but failed to access the fistula site because of the tortuous angular vein (arrow). (**e**) Selective angiography through a Marathon microcatheter guided to the area adjacent to the shunt at the periphery of the artery of the superior orbital fissure (arrow). The shunt and drainer were visualized. (**f**) Late phase of a lateral view on the right carotid arteriography after surgery showing a small residual arteriovenous shunt from the small dural branches (arrow) from the cavernous segment of the internal carotid artery

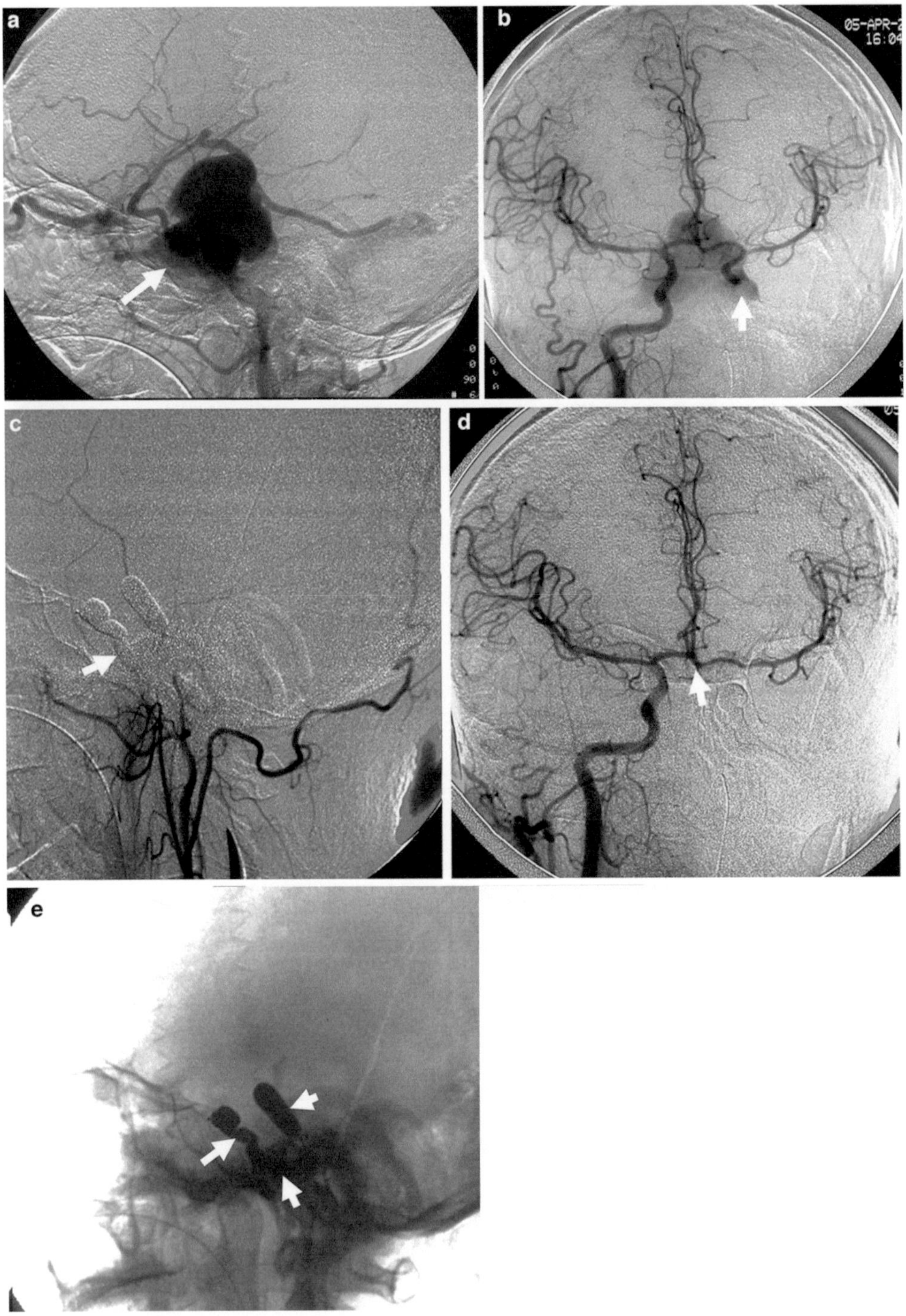

Fig. 1.12 A large carotid-cavernous fistula was treated with detachable balloons. (**a**) Left carotid artery angiogram (lateral view) showing a Zipfel type III carotid-cavernous fistula supplied by the internal carotid artery (arrow). (**b**) Right carotid artery angiogram (frontal view) showing the blood flow reflux from the contralateral carotid artery circulation (arrow). (**c**) The carotid artery angiogram (lateral view) showing the internal carotid artery and fistula was complete occluded (arrow). (**d**) Control angiogram (frontal view) showing there was no blood flow to the dural fistula. (**e**) Unsubtracted image (lateral view) showing the balloons

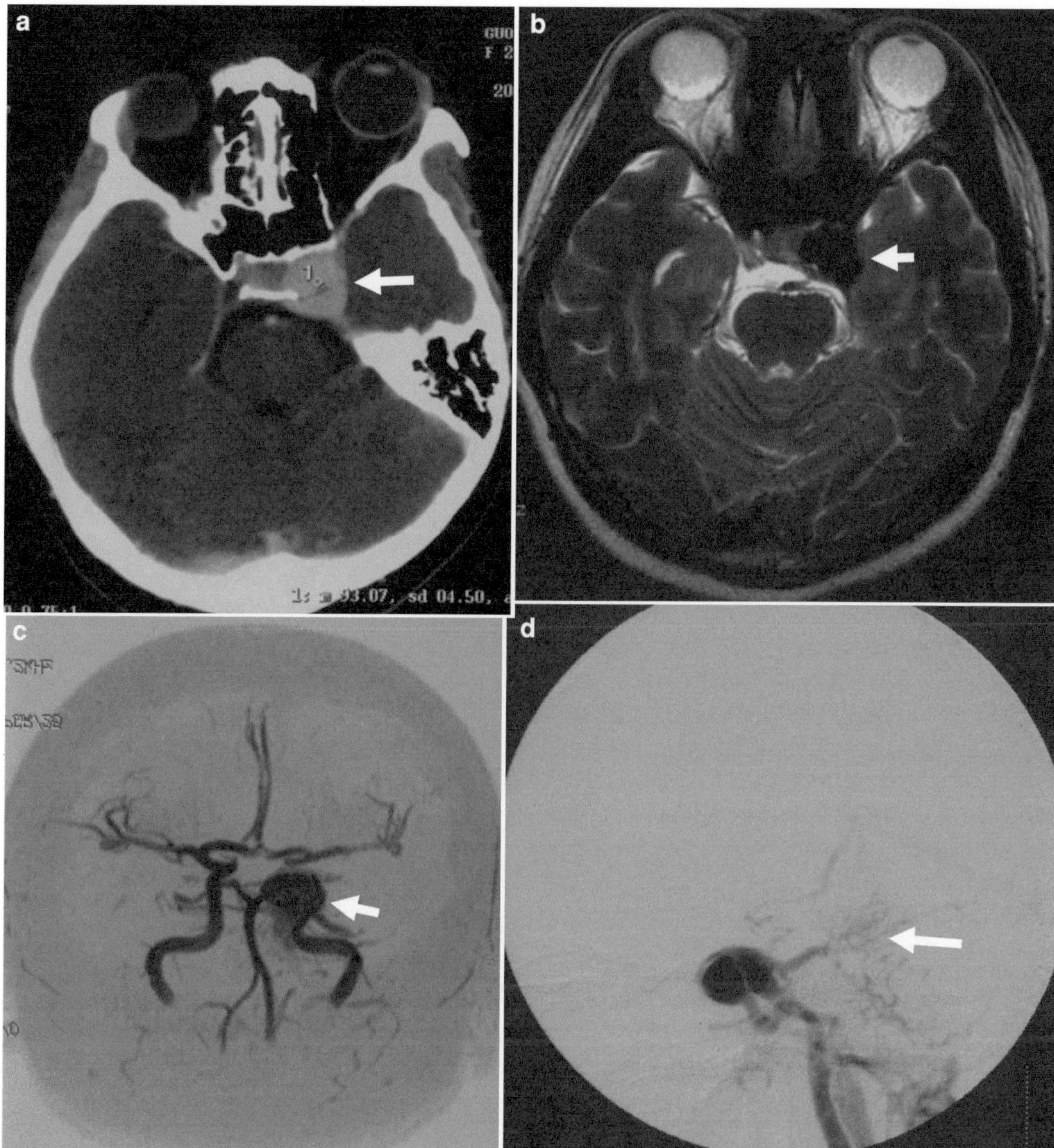

Fig. 1.13 A 24-year-old female patient presented with the left oculomotor nerve palsy and intracranial bruits. (**a**) Cranial CT scanning showing a hyperdensity lesion at the left parasellar location (arrow). (**b**) MR imaging showing a flow void signal at the left parasellar location (arrow). (**c**) MR angiography demonstrating engorged left cavernous sinus. (**d**) Left carotid artery angiogram (lateral view) showing a Zipfel type III carotid-cavernous fistula supplied by the internal carotid artery drained to brain stem and cerebellar veins

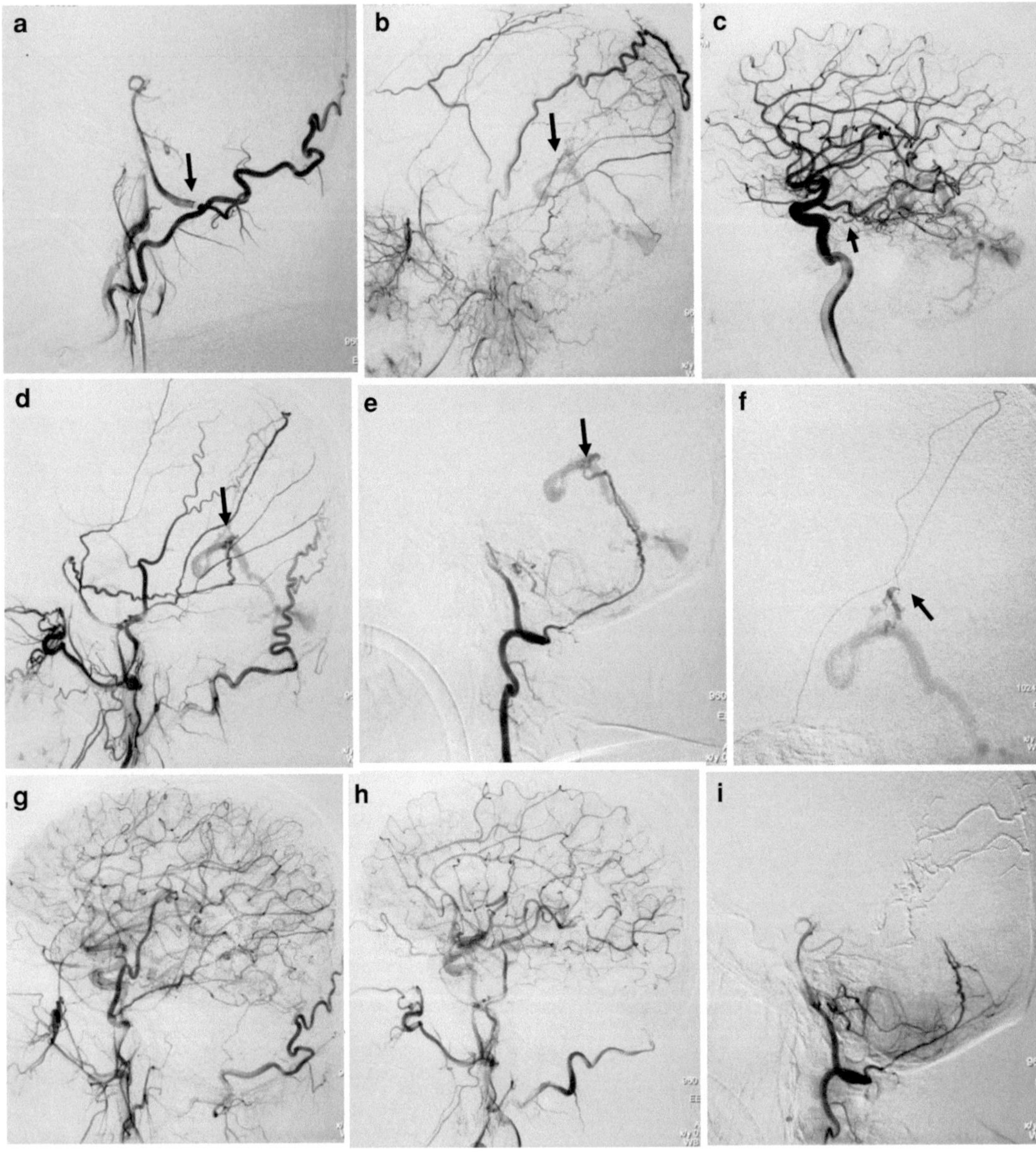

Fig. 1.14 A 53-year-old male patient presented with dizziness. (**a**) Lateral projection pre-embolisation angiogram, selective right external carotid artery injection, showing the occipital artery anastomosed to the vertebral artery with the transosseous vessel (arrow). (**b**) Late phase of the lateral projection pre-embolisation angiogram, selective right external carotid artery injection. (**c**) The lateral projection pre-embolisation angiogram, selective right internal carotid artery injection. (**d**) The lateral projection pre-embolisation angiogram, selective left external carotid artery injection. (**e**) The lateral projection pre-embolisation angiogram, selective left vertebral artery injection. Showing multiple arterial feeders arising from the bilateral middle meningeal artery (arrow), right meningohypophyseal artery (arrow) and left posterior meningeal artery (arrow), draining into a common channel (arrow). (**f**) Selective injection showing the Marathon microcatheter positioned within the arteriovenous shunt (arrow). Postembolisation lateral angiograms, (**g**) right carotid artery injection, (**h**) left carotid artery injection and (**i**) left vertebral artery showing no residual dAVF

attributed to the venous perforations or hemodynamic changes in direction of venous drainage [65, 74, 75]. Among patients harboring pial artery supply, giant venous pouch and high volume Onyx injection in one session constituted the chief causes of hemorrhagic complications [76]. When collateral arteriovenous shunts exist between dural and pial arterial suppliers, the injection force can cause Onyx reflux across these collateral vessels into the brain, which requires special attention during DAVF embolization.

1.9 Conclusions

Endovascular treatment is usually the first-line treatment of DAVF. Before intervention, it is necessary to have a complete understanding of the vascular structure of the fistula. This includes identifying blood supply arteries, fistula connection points, venous drainage pathways, and venous flow direction. According to the location and anatomical structure of the fistula, the intravascular approach is carried out from the artery, vein or combined access. Surgery and SRS remain as alternative treatment options, especially when endovascular methods are unsuccessful or considered dangerous. Follow-up angiography is needed to confirm the long-term occlusion of DAVF and the durability of treatment. The Borden and Cognard classifications do not explicitly cover cavernous DAVF, which is a very common type of DAVFs. In this study, based on the understanding of vascular structure and natural history of DAVFs, the Zipfel classification was proposed to guide the proper evaluation of DAVF and the treatment of these lesions.

References

1. Djindjian R, Merland JJ. Superselective arteriography of the external carotid artery. Berlin: Springer; 1978.
2. Lv X, Wu Z, Li Y. Innervation of cerebral dura mater. Neuroradiol J. 2014;27(3):293–8.
3. Borden JA, Wu JK, Shncart WA. A proposed classification for spinal and cranial dural arteriovenous fistulous malformations and implications for treatment. J Neurosurg. 1995;82:166–79.
4. Cognard C, Gobin YP, Pierot L, Bailly AL, Houdart E, Casasco A, Chiras J, Merland JJ. Cerebral dural arteriovenous fistulas: clinical and angiographic correlation with a revised classification of venous drainage. Radiology. 1995;194:671–80.
5. Alexander MD, Halbach VV, Hallam DK, Cooke DL, Ghodke BV, Dowd CF, Amans MR, Hetts SW, Higashida RT, Meyers PM. Long-term outcomes of endovascular treatment of indirect carotid cavernous fistulae: superior efficacy, safety, and durability of transvenous coiling over other techniques. Neurosurgery. 2019;85(1):E94–E100.
6. Bernstein R, Dowd CF,Gress DR. Rapidly reversible dementia. Lancet. 2003;361:392.
7. Jin H, Lv X, Li Y. Transarterial Onyx embolization of jugular foramen dural arteriovenous fistula with spinal venous drainage manifesting as myelopathy-a case report and review of the literature. Interv Neuroradiol. 2016;22(5):579–83.
8. Li T, Lv X, Wu Z. Endovascular treatment of hemifacial spasm associated with a petrosal DAVF using transarterial Onyx embolization: case report. Interv Neuroradiol. 2012;18:69–73.
9. Lv X, Yang X, Li Y, Jiang C, Wu Z. Dural arteriovenous fistula with spinal perimedullary venous drainage. Neurology India. 2011;59:899–902.
10. Lv X, Jiang C, Li Y, Yang X, Wu Z. Isolated oculomotor nerve palsy in interventional neuroradiology. Eur J Radiol. 2010;74:441–4.
11. Lv X, Zhang J, Li Y, Jiang C, Wu Z. Dural arteriovenous fistula involving the transverse sigmoid sinus presenting as chemosis: a case report. Neuroradiol J. 2008;21:428–32.
12. Cognard C, Januel AC, Silva NA Jr, Tall P. Endovascular treatment of intracranial dural arteriovenous fistulas with cortical venous drainage: new management using Onyx. AJNR Am J Neuroradiol. 2008;29:235–41.
13. Zipfel GJ, Shah MN, Refai D, Dacey RG Jr, Derdeyn CP. Cranial dural arteriovenous fistulas: modification of angiographic classification scales based on new natural history data. Neurosurg Focus. 2009;26(5):E14.
14. Macdonald JHM, Millar JS, Barker CS. Endovascular treatment of cranial dural arteriovenous fistulae: a single-centre, 14-year experience and the impact of Onyx on local practise. Neuroradiology. 2010;52:387–95.
15. Sirakov SS, Sirakov A, Minkin K, Hristov H, Ninov K, Penkov M, Karakostov V, Orlov K, Gorbatykh A, Kislitsin D, Raychev R. Initial experience with precipitating hydrophobic injectable liquid in cerebral arteriovenous malformations. Interv Neuroradiol. 2019;25(1):58–65.
16. Varadharajan S, Ramalingaiah AH, Saini J, Gupta AK, Devi BI, Acharya UV. Precipitating hydrophobic injectable liquid embolization of intracranial vascular shunts: initial experience and technical note. J Neurosurg. 2018;129(5):1217–22.

17. Gioppo A, Faragò G, Caldiera V, Caputi L, Cusin A, Ciceri E. Medial tentorial dural arteriovenous fistula embolization: single experience with embolic liquid polymer SQUID and review of the literature. World Neurosurg. 2017;107:1050.e1–7.
18. Castaño C, Remollo S, García-Sort R, et al. Treatment of Barrow type 'B' carotid cavernous fistulas with flow diverter stent (Pipeline). Neuroradiol J. 2017;30:607–14.
19. Mossa-Basha M, Chen J, Gandhi D. Imaging of cerebral arteriovenous malformations and dural arteriovenous fistulas. Neurosurg Clin N Am. 2012;23:27–42.
20. Nelson PK, Russell SM, Woo HH, et al. Use of a wedged microcatheter for curative transarterial embolization of complex intracranial dural arteriovenous fistulas: indications, endovascular technique, and outcome in 21 patients. J Neurosurg. 2003;98:498–506.
21. Moore C, Murphy K, Gailloud P. Improved distal distribution of n-butyl cyanoacrylate glue by simultaneous injection of dextrose 5% through the guiding catheter: technical note. Neuroradiology. 2006;48:327–32.
22. Guedin P, Gaillard S, Boulin A, et al. Therapeutic management of intracranial dural arteriovenous shunts with leptomeningeal venous drainage: report of 53 consecutive patients with emphasis on transarterial embolization with acrylic glue. J Neurosurg. 2010;112:603–10.
23. Baharvahdat H, Ooi YC, Kim WJ, Mowla A, Coon AL, Colby GP. Updates in the management of cranial dural arteriovenous fistula. Stroke Vasc Neurol. 2019;5(1):50–8.
24. Kirsch M, Liebig T, Kühne D, et al. Endovascular management of dural arteriovenous fistulas of the transverse and sigmoid sinus in 150 patients. Neuroradiology. 2009;51:477–83.
25. Nogueira RG, Dabus G, Rabinov JD, et al. Preliminary experience with onyx embolization for the treatment of intracranial dural arteriovenous fistulas. AJNR Am J Neuroradiol. 2008;29:91–7.
26. Jiang C, Lv X, Li Y, et al. Endovascular treatment of high-risk tentorial dural arteriovenous fistulas: clinical outcomes. Neuroradiology. 2009;51:103–11.
27. Cognard C, Januel AC, Silva NA, et al. Endovascular treatment of intracranial dural arteriovenous fistulas with cortical venous drainage: new management using Onyx. AJNR Am J Neuroradiol. 2008;29:235–41.
28. Rabinov JD, Yoo AJ, Ogilvy CS, et al. ONYX versus n-BCA for embolization of cranial dural arteriovenous fistulas. J Neurointerv Surg. 2013;5:306–10.
29. Leyon JJ, Chavda S, Thomas A, et al. Preliminary experience with the liquid embolic material agent PHIL (precipitating hydrophobic injectable liquid) in treating cranial and spinal dural arteriovenous fistulas: technical note. J Neurointerv Surg. 2016;8:596–602.
30. Lamin S, Chew HS, Chavda S, et al. Embolization of intracranial dural arteriovenous fistulas using PHIL liquid embolic agent in 26 patients: a multicenter study. AJNR Am J Neuroradiol. 2017;38:127–31.
31. Akmangit I, Daglioglu E, Kaya T, et al. Preliminary experience with squid: a new liquid embolizing agent for AVM, AV fistulas and tumors. Turk Neurosurg. 2014;24:565–70.
32. McConnell KA, Tjoumakaris SI, Allen J, et al. Neuroendovascular management of dural arteriovenous malformations. Neurosurg Clin N Am. 2009;20:431–9.
33. Natarajan SK, Ghodke B, Kim LJ, et al. Multimodality treatment of intracranial dural arteriovenous fistulas in the Onyx era: a single center experience. World Neurosurg. 2010;73:365–79.
34. Suzuki S, Lee DW, Jahan R, et al. Transvenous treatment of spontaneous dural carotid-cavernous fistulas using a combination of detachable coils and Onyx. AJNR Am J Neuroradiol. 2006;27:1346–9.
35. Alexander MD, Halbach VV, Hallam DK, et al. Long-term outcomes of endovascular treatment of indirect carotid cavernous fistulae: superior efficacy, safety, and durability of transvenous coiling over other techniques. Neurosurgery. 2019;85:E94–100.
36. Caplan JM, Kaminsky I, Gailloud P, et al. A single burr hole approach for direct transverse sinus cannulation for the treatment of a dural arteriovenous fistula. J Neurointerv Surg. 2015;7:e5.
37. Layton KF. Embolization of an intracranial dural arteriovenous fistula using ultrasound-guided puncture of a pericranial venous pouch. Proc (Bayl Univ Med Cent). 2009;22:332–4.
38. Wong GKC, Poon WS, Yu SCH, et al. Transvenous embolization for dural transverse sinus fistulas with occluded sigmoid sinus. Acta Neurochir. 2007;149:929–36.
39. Naito I, Iwai T, Shimaguchi H, et al. Percutaneous transvenous embolisation through the occluded sinus for transverse-sigmoid dural arteriovenous fistulas with sinus occlusion. Neuroradiology. 2001;43:672–6.
40. Komiyama M, Ishiguro T, Matsusaka Y, et al. Transfemoral, transvenous embolisation of dural arteriovenous fistula involving the isolated transverse-sigmoid sinus from the contralateral side. Acta Neurochir. 2002;144:1041–6.
41. Dashti SR, Fiorella D, Spetzler RF, et al. Transorbital endovascular embolization of dural carotid-cavernous fistula: access to cavernous sinus through direct puncture: case examples and technical report. Neurosurgery. 2011;68:75–83.
42. Gil A, López-Ibor L, Lopez-Flores G, et al. Treatment of a carotid cavernous fistula via direct transovale cavernous sinus puncture. J Neurosurg. 2013;119:247–51.
43. Shi Z-S, Loh Y, Gonzalez N, et al. Flow control techniques for Onyx embolization of intracranial dural arteriovenous fistulae. J Neurointerv Surg. 2013;5:311–6.
44. Bhatia KD, Wang L, Parkinson RJ, et al. Successful treatment of six cases of indirect carotid-cavernous fistula with ethylene vinyl alcohol copolymer (Onyx) transvenous embolization. J Neuroophthalmol. 2009;29:3–8.

45. Albuquerque FC, Ducruet AF, Crowley RW, et al. Transvenous to arterial Onyx embolization. J Neurointerv Surg. 2014;6:281–5.
46. Spiotta AM, Hawk H, Kellogg RT, et al. Transfemoral venous approach for Onyx embolization of anterior fossa dural arteriovenous fistulae. J Neurointerv Surg. 2014;6:195–9.
47. Kerolus MG, Chung J, Munich SA, et al. An Onyx tunnel: reconstructive transvenous balloon-assisted Onyx embolization for dural arteriovenous fistula of the transverse-sigmoid sinus. J Neurosurg. 2018;129:922–7.
48. Lv X, Jiang C, Liang S, Wang J. The variant with the absence of the superior petrosal venous and sinus: a potential pitfall of transvenous balloon-assisted embolisation of Borden type II transverse-sigmoid dural arteriovenous fistula. Interv Neuroradiol. 2019;25(4):474–7.
49. Ye M, Zhang P. Transvenous balloon-assisted Onyx embolization of dural arteriovenous fistulas of hypoglossal canal. Neuroradiology. 2018;60:971–8.
50. Levrier O, Métellus P, Fuentes S, et al. Use of a self-expanding stent with balloon angioplasty in the treatment of dural arteriovenous fistulas involving the transverse and/or sigmoid sinus: functional and neuroimaging-based outcome in 10 patients. J Neurosurg. 2006;104:254–63.
51. See AP, Raza S, Tamargo RJ, et al. Stereotactic radiosurgery of cranial arteriovenous malformations and dural arteriovenous fistulas. Neurosurg Clin N Am. 2012;23:133–46.
52. Cifarelli CP, Kaptain G, Yen C-P, et al. Gamma knife radiosurgery for dural arteriovenous fistulas. Neurosurgery. 2010;67:1230–5.
53. H.-C. Y, Kano H, Kondziolka D, et al. Stereotactic radiosurgery with or without embolization for intracranial dural arteriovenous fistulas. Neurosurgery. 2010;67:1276–85.
54. Koebbe CJ, Singhal D, Sheehan J, et al. Radiosurgery for dural arteriovenous fistulas. Surg Neurol. 2005;64:392–8.
55. Söderman M, Edner G, Ericson K, et al. Gamma knife surgery for dural arteriovenous shunts: 25 years of experience. J Neurosurg. 2006;104:867–75.
56. Collice M, D'Aliberti G, Arena O, et al. Surgical treatment of intracranial dural arteriovenous fistulae: role of venous drainage. Neurosurgery. 2000;47:56–66.
57. Thompson BG, Doppman JL, Oldfield EH. Treatment of cranial dural arteriovenous fistulae by interruption of leptomeningeal venous drainage. J Neurosurg. 1994;80:617–23.
58. Kakarla UK, Deshmukh VR, Zabramski JM, et al. Surgical treatment of high-risk intracranial dural arteriovenous fistulae: clinical outcomes and avoidance of complications. Neurosurgery. 2007;61:447–57.
59. Schuette AJ, Cawley CM, Barrow DL. Indocyanine green videoangiography in the management of dural arteriovenous fistulae. Neurosurgery. 2010;67:658–62.
60. Giannopoulos S, Texakalidis P, Mohammad Alkhataybeh RA, et al. Treatment of ethmoidal dural arteriovenous fistulas: a meta-analysis comparing endovascular versus surgical treatment. World Neurosurg. 2019;128:593–9.
61. Oh SH, Choi JH, Kim B-S, et al. Treatment outcomes according to various treatment modalities for intracranial dural arteriovenous fistulas in the Onyx era: a 10-year single-center experience. World Neurosurg. 2019;126:e825–34.
62. Casasco A, Guimaraens L, Negrotto M, Vivas E, Díaz LP, Aleu A. A new subtype of intracranial dural AVF according to the patterns of venous drainage. Interv Neuroradiol. 2021;27(1):121–8.
63. Kim DJ, Kim DI, Suh SH, Kim J, Lee SK, Kim EY, et al. Results of transvenous embolization of cavernous dural arteriovenous fistula: a single-center experience with emphasis on complications and management. AJNR Am J Neuroradiol. 2006;27:2078–82.
64. Lv X, Jiang C, Li Y, Lv M, Wu Z. Endovascular treatment of dural fistulas with the venous outflow of laterocavernous sinus. Eur J Radiol. 2010;75:e129–34.
65. Nakagawa I, Wada T, Nakagawa H, Hironaka Y, Kichikawa K, Nakase H. A rare brainstem hemorrhage during transvenous embolization of a cavernous dural arteriovenous fistula. J Clin Neurosci. 2012;19:589–92.
66. Wakhloo AK, Perlow A, Linfante I, Sandhu JS, Cameron J, Troffkin N, Schenck A, Schatz NJ, Tse DT, Lam BL. Transvenous n-butyl-cyanoacrylate infusion for complex dural carotid cavernous fistulas: technical considerations and clinical outcome. AJNR Am J Neuroradiol. 2005;26:1888–97.
67. Lv X, Jiang C, Li Y, Yang X, Wu Z. Transarterial embolization of tentorial dural arteriovenous fistulas with Onyx-18. Neuroradiol J. 2008;21:406–14.
68. Lv X, Wang G, Wang J. Craniospinal vascular diseases and endovascular neurosurgery. New York: Nova Science Publisher; 2021.
69. Lv X, Jiang C, Li Y, Liu L, Liu J, Wu Z. The limitations and risks of transarterial Onyx injections in the treatment of grade I and II DAVFs. Eur J Radiol. 2011;80:e385–8.
70. Lv X, Jiang C, Li Y, Wu Z. Results and complications of transarterial embolization of intracranial dural arteriovenous fistulas using Onyx-18. J Neurosurg. 2008;109:1083–90.
71. Gatto LAM, Saurin F, Koppe GL, Demartini Z Jr. Facial palsy after embolization of dural arteriovenous fistula: a case report and literature review. Surg Neurol Int. 2017;8:270.
72. Lv XL. Accessory meningeal artery: emphasis on its intracranial distribution. J Cerebrovasc Dis. 2019;2(1):1–3.
73. Lv X, Jiang C, Zhang J, Li Y, Wu Z. Complications related to percutaneous transarterial embolization of intracranial dural arteriovenous fistulas in 40 patients. Am J Neuroradiol. 2009;30:462–8.

74. de Carvalho JC, Machin FJ, Manzanera LS, Andaluz JB, Nogues SH, Soriano NP, et al. Intraventricular hemorrhage after dural fistula embolization. Braz J Anesthesiol. 2017;67:199–204.
75. Piippo A, Niemela M. Hemodynamic changes caused by the occlusion of dural arteriovenous fistula. World Neurosurg. 2013;80:e211–2.
76. Liu P, Chen X, You W, Li Y, Lv M, Lv X. Hemorrhagic risk factors of endovascular onyx embolization of intracranial dural arteriovenous fistulas. Interv Neuroradiol. 2020;26(5):643–50.

2 Pediatric Intracranial Dural Arteriovenous Fistulas: Review of the Literature and Case Report

Sergey Yakovlev, Nikolay Kobiakov, and Anna Shulgina

Abstract

Pediatric intracranial dural arteriovenous fistulas (dAVFs) are a group of rare pathological vascular malformations. dAVFs account for 5.7–10% of all intracranial vascular malformations in pediatric population. Pediatric dAVFs have a more aggressive clinical course compared with adult dAVFs. Pediatric dAVFs have been classified into three types: dural sinus malformation (DSM), infantile dAVF and adult-type dAVF. Most pediatric dAVFs tend to be considered congenital. The presentation of pediatric dAVFs depends on the hemodynamic symptoms including high-flow steal, venous drainage occlusion and mass effects. Pediatric dAVFs may be dormant for a long time prior to the occurrence of progressive symptoms. A multimodal imaging approach is essential in the evaluation of the venous system. When a vascular malformation is suspected, special imaging studies are necessary for verification of intracranial hemorrhage, identification of zones of venous infarction and ischemia. The goal of treatment of dAVFs is to prevent the occurrence of intracranial hemorrhage or neurological deficits. The aim is to occlude the fistulous communication and arterial feeders. The treatment strategies currently available are endovascular embolization, surgery, stereotactic radiosurgery, or a combination of these. Pediatric dAVFs can have an unsatisfactory prognosis, even with timely and appropriate treatment; however, with the ongoing development of embolization materials and techniques, improved treatments and prognoses are increasingly likely. The extent of brain damage acquired during the existence of functioning dAVF, as well as the need for surgical treatment of hydrocephalus, are among the factors that have to be considered to evaluate long-term results of treatment and prognosis.

Keywords

Intracranial dural arteriovenous fistulas · Pediatric dAVF · Dural sinus malformation · Infantile dAVF · Adult-type dAVF

2.1 Introduction

Intracranial dural arteriovenous fistulas (dAVFs) are a group of pathological vascular malformations that are defined by an abnormal connection between dural arteries and cerebral venous sinuses, dural or cortical veins. dAVFs account

S. Yakovlev · N. Kobiakov · A. Shulgina (✉)
N.N. Burdenko National Medical Research Center for Neurosurgery, Moscow, Russia
e-mail: ashulgina@nsi.ru

X. Lv (ed.), *Intracranial and Spinal Dural Arteriovenous Fistulas*,
https://doi.org/10.1007/978-981-19-5767-3_2

for 10–15% of all intracranial arteriovenous diseases and are rare in the pediatric population, with a reported incidence of 5.7–10% [1].

Dural arteriovenous fistulas are rare in pediatric population, and have higher morbidity and mortality when compared to adult dAVFs, with a reported mortality rate greater than 25% [2]. Common manifestations of dAVFs in neonates are signs of right-sided heart failure due to volume overload and signs of increased intracranial pressure. In older children, focal neurological deficits may also be observed [3]. Pediatric dAVFs are caused by congenital sinus wall development defects in the sigmoid and transverse sinuses and the confluence of sinuses. This differentiates this pathology form adult dAVFs, where most cases are caused by thrombosis of a dural venous sinus as a consequence of traumatic injury, a hypercoagulability disorder or iatrogenic sinus injury [4].

dAVFs are vascular malformations with an aberrant connection between an artery supplying the dura and either a dural venous sinus or a cortical vein. dAVF may have variable complexity: a single or multiple feeder arteries, as well as different patterns of venous drainage. Pediatric dAVFs may form during early fetal development, similarly to vein of Galen malformations, or be acquired later in development. Most dAVFs possess mature arterial and venous angioarchitecture, so these dAVFs likely form no earlier than during the third month of intrauterine development. In congenital dAVFs venous sinuses are massively enlarged, unlike in acquired dAVFs in adults, which corresponds to their fetal origin: due to arterio-venous high-flow shunting the venous sinuses retain abnormal enlargement instead of regressing. Similar to acquired adult-type dAVFs, venous thrombosis may promote dAVF formation during fetal development [5].

2.2 Pediatric dAVF Classification

The classification of pediatric dAVFs proposed by Lasjaunias et al. defines three subtypes: congenital dural sinus malformations (DSM), infantile dAVF and adult-type dAVF [1, 6, 7].

2.2.1 Dural Sinus Malformation

DSMs are rare congenital anomalies that manifest as focally enlarged bulging dural sinus deformities (Fig. 2.1) [3, 9]. The DSMs are lined with immature endothelium, which predisposes these lesions to spontaneous thrombosis. The pathogenesis of DSMs is linked to dysregulation of dural sinus development. Overgrowth of the sinus wall is followed by aberrant venous confluence formation in the epidural space, resulting in formation of giant venous lakes, subsequent thrombosis and venous drainage remodeling. These cause additional limitations on brain venous drainage, which cannot be resolved until the venous drainage of the brain is diverted. Possible alternate outlets are via sylvian veins into the cavernous sinus and ophthalmic vein; inferior petrosal sinus into the jugular bulb, or the pterygoid venous plexuses directly.

Two subtypes are recognized in DSMs. First, torcular DSMs, where the confluence sinuum is replaced by a massive venous lake [10]. These are characterized by slow-flow mural arteriovenous shunting. Hemorrhagic infarction may be observed, resulting from spontaneous thrombosis or hypoplasia of either jugular bulb [8]. Lesions involving the jugular bulb and latero-posterior sinuses are the second form of DSM. High-flow arteriovenous shunting is characteristic of these lesions.

The natural history of DSMs varies depending on where the deformed sinus is located anatomically: midline lesions affecting the torcula are associated with worse prognosis compared to lateral localizations. Torcular DSMs disrupt deep venous drainage, thus hemorrhagic infarction secondary to spontaneous thrombosis may be observed [1, 6]. The lateral type DSMs have more collateral drainage, which is frequently linked to a better prognosis.

DSMs may be diagnosed both prenatally and after birth and exhibit similar imaging features, implying a shared origin [1]. Around 20% of DSM cases can be diagnosed in utero [11]. DSM may be detected on ultrasound or MRI as a cystic lesion in the posterior fossa corresponding to an

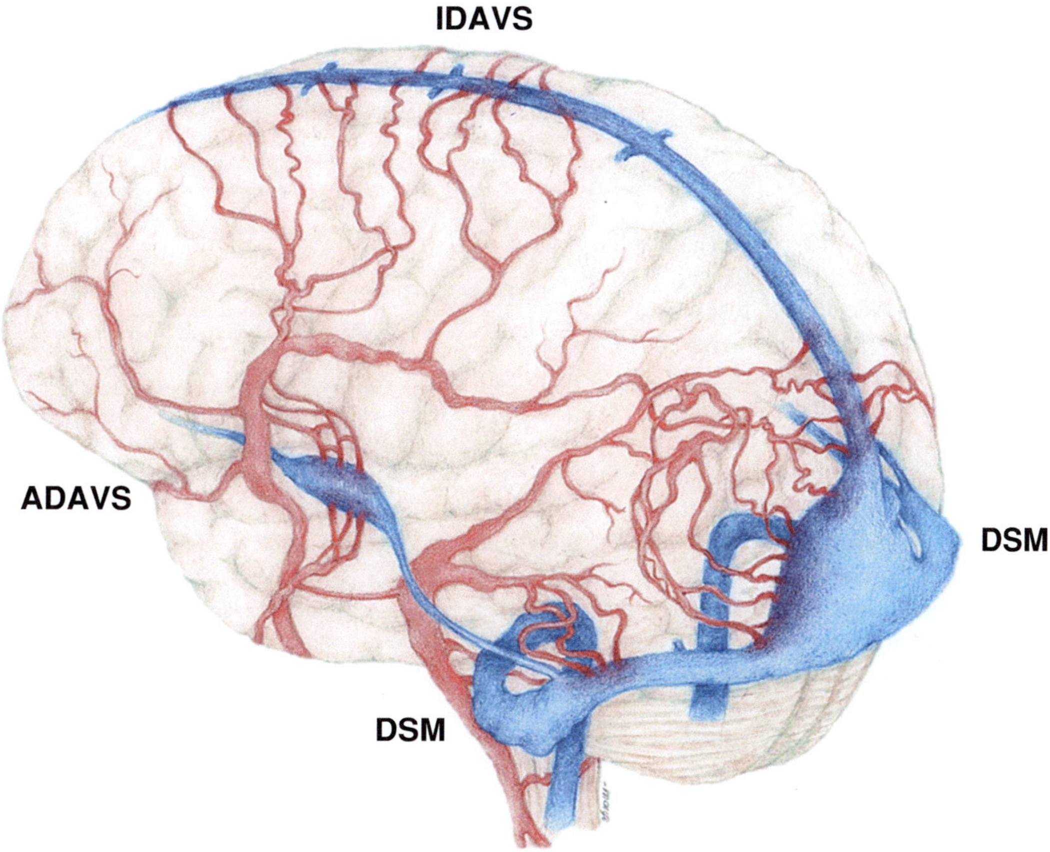

Fig. 2.1 Pediatric dAVS. IDAVS—infant dural arteriovenous shunt without venous lakes or sinus malformations; DSM—dural sinus malformation that involved confluence of sinuses (with giant dural lakes) and sigmoid sinus; ADAVS—adult dural arteriovenous shunt in the cavernous sinus. (Modified from [8])

enlarged bulging venous sinus as early as at 20 weeks pregnant [1, 6].

The disease commonly manifests during first months of life. Typical presentation includes well-tolerated congestive heart failure, increased head circumference, hydrocephalus, evidence of distended extracranial veins, intracranial hemorrhages and seizures. A cranial bruit, dilated scalp veins, or proptosis may be observed in older children [1, 9].

2.2.2 Infantile dAVFs

The most common variant of pediatric dAVFs are infantile dAVFs [9]. These are high-flow, low-pressure dural shunts, that drain into enlarged sinuses without lakes or sinus malformations. Infantile dAVFs may be multifocal; there are also reports of consecutive occurrence of multiple infantile dAVFs. As long as sinuses are patent and there is craniofugal flow with minimum hemodynamic impediment, progressive neurological deficits do not occur [9, 12]. These lesions are more commonly diagnosed in older children. Persistent high-flow low pressure blood flow in the large sinuses causes formation of pial AVFs at the brain surface close to the dural shunts, with the draining vein emptying into the abnormal sinus.

Infantile dAVFs typical manifestations include cranial nerve deficits, as well as increased head circumference and neurocognitive delay, which are caused by venous hypertension and relative venous ischemia. If the cavernous sinus is involved, proptosis, extraocular motor nerve palsies and enlarged facial vein may be observed.

2.2.3 Adult-Type dAVFs

The onset of all adult-type dAVFs is typically secondary to venous thrombosis [13]. Unlike DSMs and infantile dAVFs, that are caused by abnormal angiogenesis, adult-type dAVFs are thought to represent a localized angiogenic response to the thrombosis. Adult-type dAVFs are low-flow arteriovenous shunts that occur within the walls of normal-sized sinuses. Cavernous sinus and, rarely, the sigmoid sinus are typically involved. Adult-type dAVFs are strictly unifocal. Intracranial bruit is the characteristic symptom of adult-type dAVFs, thus the diagnosis in children may be elusive. In children, adult-type dAVFs are most commonly diagnosed by magnetic resonance imaging.

They are most frequently encountered in the cavernous sinus and, rarely, in the sigmoid sinus. Multifocality has not been described in these lesions. The diagnosis of adult-type dAVFs is difficult as children rarely complain of an intracranial bruit. Diagnosis is usually made by MRI/MRA. Because spontaneous regression is common, the prognosis is usually favourable [3].

2.2.4 Other Classifications

A topographic classification of dAVFs by location may be beneficial in designing a therapeutic approach, however it is more clinically relevant to describe these lesions by their venous drainage pattern. The first classification of dAVFs according to venous drainage pattern was proposed by Djindjian and Merland in 1978 (Table 2.1) [14]. A similar approach was described by Borden (Table 2.2) [15]. Cognard et al. later improved this classification by establishing a link between clinical presentation and angiographic results (Table 2.3) [16]. All three of these classifications focus on the dAVFs' venous outflow characteristics and how they relate to presentation.

Table 2.1 Djindjian classification of dAVFs by venous drainage (1978)

Type I	Drainage into a sinus
Type II	Sinus drainage with reflux into cerebral veins
Type III	Drainage solely into cortical veins
Type IV	With supra- or infratentorial venous lake

Table 2.2 Borden classification of dAVFs (1995)

1.	Venous drainage directly into the dural venous sinus or meningeal vein
2.	Venous drainage into dural venous sinus with cortical venous reflux
3.	Venous drainage directly into subarachnoid veins (cortical venous reflux only)

Table 2.3 Cognard classification of dAVFs (1995)

I	dAVF draining into a sinus, with a normal antegrade flow direction
II	dAVF draining into a sinus. Insufficient antegrade venous drainage and reflux.
IIa	Retrograde venous drainage into sinus(es) only
IIb	Retrograde venous drainage into cortical vein(s) only
IIa + b	Retrograde venous drainage into sinus(es) and cortical vein(s)
III	Draining directly into a cortical vein without venous ectasia
IV	Draining into a cortical vein with a venous ectasia >5 mm in diameter and three times larger than the diameter of the draining vein
V	Intracranial dAVFs draining into spinal perimedullary veins

Distinguishing between fistulae with and without retrograde leptomeningeal or cortical venous drainage is critical, as these two types of dural fistulae have different natural history, which necessitates different therapeutic regimens [4].

2.3 Pathogenesis

The pathogenetic mechanisms behind pediatric dAVFs are still unclear. There is ongoing debate about whether pediatric dAVFs are congenital or acquired lesions. The majority of pediatric dAVFs are congenital. Pediatric dAVFs, for example, have been linked to dural sinus malformations, and an unknown trigger has been proposed as the source of chronic posterior sinus enlargement and bulging, sinus wall hypertrophy, and the development of aberrant venous spaces, all of which can lead to dAVF [17–19].

The pathophysiology of dAVFs is explained by two major concepts. One postulates that dAVFs form from "latent" connections between external carotid circulation and dural venous circulation that are opened as a reaction to persistent venous hypertension. A second hypothesis proposes that angiogenic factors produced as a direct response to sinus thrombosis or resulting from tissue hypoxia drive the formation of new vascular channels. Although the exact cause of dAVFs is unknown, it is thought that a combination of arterialized turbulent flow, progressive venous hypertension and sinus lumen stenosis and venous reflux precipitates progressive veno-occlusive disease, which can lead to the melting brain syndrome. Chronic venous hypertension causes irreparable brain injury with encephalomalacia and white matter petrification in the melting brain syndrome. This condition, which is usually bilateral and symmetric, is caused by a localized decrease in cerebral blood flow resulting from retrograde venous hypertension [1, 20].

Syndromes resulting from inherited defects, such as hereditary hemorrhagic telangiectasia syndrome, craniofacial arteriovenous metameric syndrome, and cavernous malformations, have been linked to pediatric dAVFs [21–23]. These findings back with the theory that pediatric dAVFs are inherited. Additionally, genetic-phenotypic mutations may be present in pediatric dAVFs. Grillner et al. described a variety of intracranial high-flow AVFs with RAS p21 protein activator 1 (RASA1) mutations in 2016, including one case with a large DSM with dAVF between the meningeal arteries and the deformed superior sagittal sinus [24]. Srinivasa et al. described a case of a 9-year-old patient with dAVF who had a frameshift mutation in the phosphatase and tensin homologue tumor-suppressor gene (PTEN) in 2006 [25].

Adults with cerebral sinus thromboses may develop dAVFs. In rare cases, pediatric dAVFs can be caused by cerebral sinus thromboses, like adult dAVFs. Morales et al. reported the first confirmed case of adult-type dAVF in children in 2010 [26]. A 5-month-old girl presented with a ruptured aneurysm; extensive subarachnoid hemorrhage and a right sigmoid sinus thrombosis were observed, which lead to development of a new adult-type dAVF. Data by Walcott et al. (2013), suggests that adult-type dAVFs in children occur fairly often. Furthermore, numerous dAVFs may form at the same time [23].

dAVFs may be iatrogenic, occurring as a result of endovascular intervention. Bai et al. described the case of a 7-year-old male who had a totally embolized cerebral arteriovenous fistula; nonetheless, venous hypertension as a resulting hemodynamic alteration following the embolization lead to formation of multiple de novo dAVFs [27]. Paramasivam et al. reported four examples of de novo dAVF formation after embolization of pial arteriovenous fistulas in 2013 [28]. The significant slowing of blood flow in the draining vein or sinus postoperatively promoted thrombosis and localized venous hypertension, which triggered the dAVFs pathogenesis [8].

2.4 Natural History

Although the natural course of pediatric dAVFs is still partially unknown, it has been determined that in absence of early treatment dAVFs may cause substantial complications. Unlike in adult patients, in children with dAVFs typical early manifestations include increased head circumference, elevated intracranial pressure and cardiac failure, among other symptoms [29]. Later in the course of the disease, pediatric dAVF may rupture, presenting as subarachnoid or intracerebral hemorrhage. Other late manifestations of pediatric dAVFs include focal neurological deficits which develop as a response to impaired cerebrospinal fluid resorption, decreased venous drainage or arterial steal phenomenon [8].

Intracranial dAVFs in pediatric population have a more aggressive clinical course compared with adult dAVFs, with a reported mortality rate greater than 25%. However, pediatric dAVFs typically have a period of stable disease, where the most common manifestation is well-tolerated congestive heart failure [2, 30]. The disease exacerbation is caused by thrombosis of the draining vein or continued growth of the dAVF that disrupts the hemodynamic equilibrium [25]. Spontaneous thrombosis is rare in congenital pediatric dAVFs. dAVFs located in cavernous sinus are rare in pediatric patients [31]. Occlusion may occur after partial embolization of pediatric dAVFs [32].

2.5 Clinical Manifestations

There is slight male predominance in pediatric dAVFs, which is most apparent in infantile-type dAVFs [8]. All three types of dAVFs (DSM, infantile and adult-type dAVFs) may occur in neonates. DSMs are usually diagnosed prenatally or manifest shortly after birth. Infantile type dAVFs are discovered in infancy and early childhood. The incidence of adult-type dAVFs increases with age [7]. The manifestations of pediatric dAVFs is determined by hemodynamic alterations (cavernous capture and pial reflux), including high-flow steal; presence of sinus thrombosis leading to blockage of venous drainage; as well as degree of mass effect [33]. Infants and neonates rarely suffer hemorrhage as a first manifestation of a dAVF [32]. Before the onset of progressively increasing symptoms, pediatric dAVFs may be latent for a long time. There are two possible explanations to this phenomenon: persistence of high flow within the pial-induced shunts and gradual outlet restriction during skull base growth and development with stenosis or occlusion of jugular bulb.

2.5.1 Symptoms of High-Flow Arteriovenous Shunts

2.5.1.1 Pediatric DSM with dAVF

The typical clinical manifestations include heart failure, increased intracranial pressure, macrocrania, neurocognitive delay and seizures, which bear great similarity with intracranial high-flow pial arteriovenous fistulas [18]. The triad of macrocrania, cranial bruit and signs of severe cardiac failure is a classic manifestation of DSM with dAVF. A case of a DSM with dAVF in a neonate was reported by Ross et al. in 1986. The patient presented with macrocrania and congestive heart failure. The feeding arteries included numerous branches from external and internal carotid artery, giant dural lakes in the posterior sinuses were observed. The patient died shortly after birth [34]. A case of DSM with a high-flow dAVF in an 8-month-old boy was described by Prasanna et al. in 2011. The disease manifested with symptoms of respiratory distress, seizure, cardiac murmur and facial nevus with dilated veins. A cranial bruit located predominantly in the right frontal region was also noted [35].

2.5.1.2 Infantile dAVF

Infantile dAVF is the most common high-flow pediatric dAVF. Patients may present with symptoms of a high-flow shunt initially; however, in general, these symptoms develop gradually in infantile dAVF [8, 22, 30, 36]. Albright et al. reported a case of torcular infantile dAVF [37]. The disease manifested at 5 months after birth with macrocrania; the patient was unable to walk at 14 months, and at 23 months developed a loud heart murmur, a cranial bruit and thrill. No severe neurological deficits were observed. The symptoms may be mild or well-tolerated, even though the clinical onset is frequently observed during the first years of life. Infantile dAVF clinical manifestations may be especially convoluted in cases when veins distal to the AVF are involved. A report by Thiex et al. (2010), describes an 11-month-old child with a torcular dAVF. The patient had increased head circumference resulting from obstructed venous drainage, a captured cavernous sinus and posterior cortical venous drainage via the cavernous sinus into the superior ophthalmic, facial and scalp veins [38].

2.5.2 Symptoms from Retrograde Venous Drainage

In adults, the arterial supply of dAVFs is typically from the meningeal arteries, while the venous drainage may be direct (into the dural venous sinuses) or via the cortical and meningeal veins.

The pattern of venous drainage serves as a basis for widely used Cognard and Borden dAVF classifications. Borden type II and III and Cognard Type IIb, IIa + b, III and IV lesions involve direct or indirect reflux into the cortical veins that causes more aggressive presentations, including hemorrhage and neurological deficits [39]. Similar considerations apply to pediatric dAVFs. For example, even in DSM with low-flow torcular dAVF cerebral venous drainage may be compromised in case of spontaneous thrombosis in the dural lake or dysplastic sinus lumen, which may result in venous infarction and/or intraparenchymatous bleeding. In 2006, Srinivasa et al. reported a case with a DSM and dAVF [25].

For example, in DSM located on the midline, because spontaneous thromboses may occur in the dural lake and dysplastic sinus, even if the dAVF is slow-flowing, cerebral venous drainage may be compromised and may lead to subsequent venous infarction and intraparenchymatous hemorrhage. A case of DSM with a high-flow infantile dAVF was described by Srinivasa et al. in 2006 [25]. The patient had macrocrania and seizure shortly after birth, but the disease remained stable until 9 years of age, when thrombosis in the sigmoid sinus occurred, which rerouted the majority of cerebral venous drainage into the orbital veins; resulting in persistent headaches.

2.5.3 Symptoms of Cavernous Sinus Involvement

In pediatric patients, the adult-type dAVFs typically occur in older children and are almost exclusively located in the cavernous sinus or sigmoid sinus. The adult type dAVFs are frequently relatively small, occasionally partially thrombosed; and may be secondary to another local event [33]. The symptoms are similar to cavernous dAVFs in adults and include venous hypertension, proptosis and chemosis. In 1995, Yamamoto et al. reported the case of a 5-week-old boy with a congenital indirect caroticocavernous fistula [31]. This patient had an objective bruit, abducens nerve palsy, chemosis, gradually progressing proptosis, and dilated conjunctival veins. Similar cases were described by Konishi et al. in 1990 [40] and Cohen et al. in 2008 [41]. Rarely, the cavernous sinus may be involved in cases of dAVFs of different location, when the draining vein or sinus is occluded. This may lead to facial venous distension and pulsatile proptosis, among other symptoms.

2.5.4 Other Symptoms

The arteriovenous shunt may compromise the cerebral fluid circulation leading to hydrocephalus if a dAVF size is substantial. A case of a DSM with dAVF in a neonate was reported by Ross et al. in 1986 [34].

If a dAVF size is giant, the arteriovenous shunt may compress the cerebrospinal fluid circulation pathway, which results in hydrocephalus. In 1986, Ross et al. reported a neonatal case of DSM with dAVF [34]. This patient had giant dural lakes in the torcular region that impaired the venous drainage which caused venous hypertension and hydrocephalus. Hydrocephalus resolved following interventional embolization treatment.

2.6 Diagnostics

A multimodal imaging approach is essential in the evaluation of the venous system. Prenatal doppler ultrasound imaging and magnetic resonance imaging (MRI) combined with clinical examination are the methods of choice for suspecting vascular malformation. Doppler ultrasound and MRI provide an excellent overview of anatomy without ionizing radiation exposure.

When a vascular malformation is suspected, special imaging studies, e.g., computed tomography and magnetic resonance angiography, are necessary for verification of intracranial hemorrhage, identification of zones of venous infarction and ischemia.

Digital subtraction angiography (DSA) remains a gold standard technique with highest spatial resolution. Super-selective catheterization of bilateral external carotid, internal carotid, and vertebral arteries is done to complete the assessment. It is used for preoperative planning and to guide interventional procedures [42].

2.7 Treatment

The purpose of treating dAVFs is to avoid neurological implications or occurrence of intracranial hemorrhage. This is achieved by occlusion of feeder arteries and disruption of fistulous communication [43].

The general principles of pediatric and adult dAVFs are similar, with several important modifications [8]. During the occlusion of adult dAVF, the draining sinus may also be occluded; which should generally be avoided in children because of venous system immaturity. In pediatric dAVFs the goal is to disrupt the fistulous connection without compromising the draining sinus [44, 45].

The treatment strategies currently available are endovascular embolization, surgery, stereotactic radiosurgery, or a combination of these. To date, the treatment of pediatric dAVFs is primarily accomplished via endovascular embolization using both transarterial and transvenous approaches. Surgical resection of involved dural sinus wall or stereotactic radiosurgery is a second-line treatment [43].

2.7.1 Endovascular Treatment

dAVF treatment method of choice is endovascular intervention. Alternative approaches, including surgery and radiosurgery, are used in case endovascular treatment fails, or when endovascular intervention is technically difficult or impossible because of fistula angioarchitecture. Hetts et al. prefer the use of coils over liquid embolic agents for treatment of pediatric dAVFs. Systemic nontarget embolization with liquid embolic agents may worsen cardiopulmonary distress and be clinically devastating. More recent reports have described successful use of a combination of coils, liquid adhesive embolic agents and ethylene vinyl alcohol copolymer (Onyx) for treatment of complex pediatric dAVFs [38, 46].

The complicating factors for endovascular treatment of pediatric intracranial arteriovenous shunts include the presence of high-flow fistulas, tortuous cerebral feeding arteries, a limited femoral artery access site, contrast agent volume restrictions and risks of general anesthesia in a critically ill newborn. Open surgery and radiosurgery also have special considerations in neonates. Open surgery is complicated by small total circulating blood volume and chronic heart failure. Stereotactic radiosurgery is limited to frameless approaches in young patients with open cranial sutures and also is ineffective in large caliber dAVFs [9].

Endovascular treatment of intracranial arteriovenous shunts is performed under general anesthesia, through either transarterial or transvenous approach. There are reports of uncommon approach via umbilical catheterization. The transvenous approach is associated with higher morbidity and mortality risk and results in worse neurological outcomes [47, 48]. Most commonly used embolization materials for pediatric dAVFs include *n*-butyl-2-cyanoacrylate (glue), Onyx, Squid, precipitating hydrophobic injectable liquid and detachable microcoils. Flow-diverting stents are also used in treatment of pediatric dAVFs [49].

For high-grade dAVFs with direct cortical venous drainage (Cognard grades III–V) or situations where a transvenous approach is impractical, a transarterial approach is a favored method. Transarterial route has advantages such as a lower likelihood of flow switching to another venous conduit, the ability to preserve a functional venous system, and the prevention of post-treatment de novo dAVF formation caused by venous hypertension. It also avoids complications of transvenous approaches, such as abducens nerve palsy following the catheterization of the superior petrosal sinus. In order to reduce the rate of complications, the microcatheter must be advanced as close as possible to the fistula. Onyx was shown to be advantageous to glue because of higher success rates and lower operator dependency. Retrograde filling of liquid embolic agent with proximal vascular occlusion and infarction is a serious complication of transarterial approach that should be avoided [43, 49].

When transarterial approach is associated with high risks, a transvenous route is chosen. Possible indications include small tortuous feeder arteries, arterial supply of dAVF by branches straight from internal carotid or vertebral artery, or when feeder arteries also supply the cranial nerves. The transvenous approach is a method of choice for Type I and II dAVFs of hypoglossal canal as well as indirect carotid cavernous fistulas.

A transvenous approach is preferred when transarterial access is dangerous. This could be due to the following reasons: small tortuous arterial feeders, arterial supply of dAVF by branches directly from the internal carotid artery or vertebral artery, or when the feeder arteries are also nutrient arteries of cranial nerves. Therefore, the transvenous approach is the first line of treatment of an indirect carotid cavernous fistulas and type I and II dAVFs of the hypoglossal canal. The main risk of transvenous approach is vein rupture, resulting in hemorrhage and cerebral infarction. Transvenous embolization may also alter cerebral venous drainage, which can lead to intracranial hypertension [43, 49].

Surgery is often only used when endovascular treatments have failed to completely eradicate the lesion. Surgery is a first-line treatment option in few specific locations, such as anterior fossa dAVFs (ethmoidal dAVFs). Major complications of surgical intervention include infection, hydrocephalus, hemorrhage, cerebrospinal fluid leak, stroke, and cranial nerve palsies.

When endovascular therapy and surgery have failed to treat dural AVF, stereotactic radiosurgery is the final treatment option. dAVF occlusion by radiation occurs through endothelial cell damage and following thrombosis. The occlusion after of stereotactic radiosurgery is observed only after several months, which is the main limitation of this treatment modality. Complications include cranial nerve palsies, brain edema, radiation effect and hemorrhages in latent period before occlusion develops [49].

Iodinated contrast dosage limitations for pediatric cerebral angiography have not been well studied. The widely accepted dose limits currently used are 7 mL/kg, the maximum of 16.8 mL/kg is also reported. According to recent data, the risks of diagnostic digital subtraction angiography (DSA) in children is lower than 3%, however, the rate of intraprocedural complications of endovascular intervention in children is up to 24% [50–53].

Treatment with anticoagulants is used to prevent spontaneous thrombosis in pediatric dAVF patients. Anticoagulation therapy for DSM improves outcomes even when intracranial hemorrhage is present [8, 11]. Lv et al. propose low molecular weight heparin in dose of 0.2 mL/day subcutaneously for 3 days following endovascular embolization of DSM [9].

Outcomes of treatment for pediatric dAVFs are poor [9]. Barbosa et al. reported an overall mortality rate of 38% in 2003 [3]. The overall reported rate has dropped to 26% in 2010, however, it is unclear whether this was due to improved embolization techniques or a lack of follow-up in newer studies [9].

There are attempts to compare results of treatment of pediatric intracranial dAVF across different studies [1, 13, 23]. However, these studies try to compare outcomes of treatment of dAVFs of varying locations (including the torcula, transverse sinus, superior sagittal sinus and cavernous sinus) pooled into the same cohort based on single institution experience.

The cohorts in these studies differ in mean age at presentation, severity of clinical manifestations of the disease, treatment modalities used. Thus, the data from these studies does not reliably represent the results of treatment and prognosis in specific dAVFs by location, even in cases when total embolization is achieved. Lasjaunias et al. note that some dAVFs are lethal even 10 years after onset, indicating the importance of cautious long-term follow-up [54].

Case Report

Patient B, 1 year old.

Since birth, the child has an increase in the head circumference and a psychomotor delay. MRI showed extensive dAVF in the torcular and right lateral sinus.

DSA showed that the main afferents of the fistula were the hypertrophied posterior meningeal artery, arised from the right vertebral artery, as well as the three terminal branches of the hypertrophied left middle meningeal artery. The outflow was carried out into a giant spherically expanded confluence of sinuses, from which no obvious outflow was observed (Fig. 2.2).

The fistula was occluded with microcoils and adhesive glue (*n*BCA).

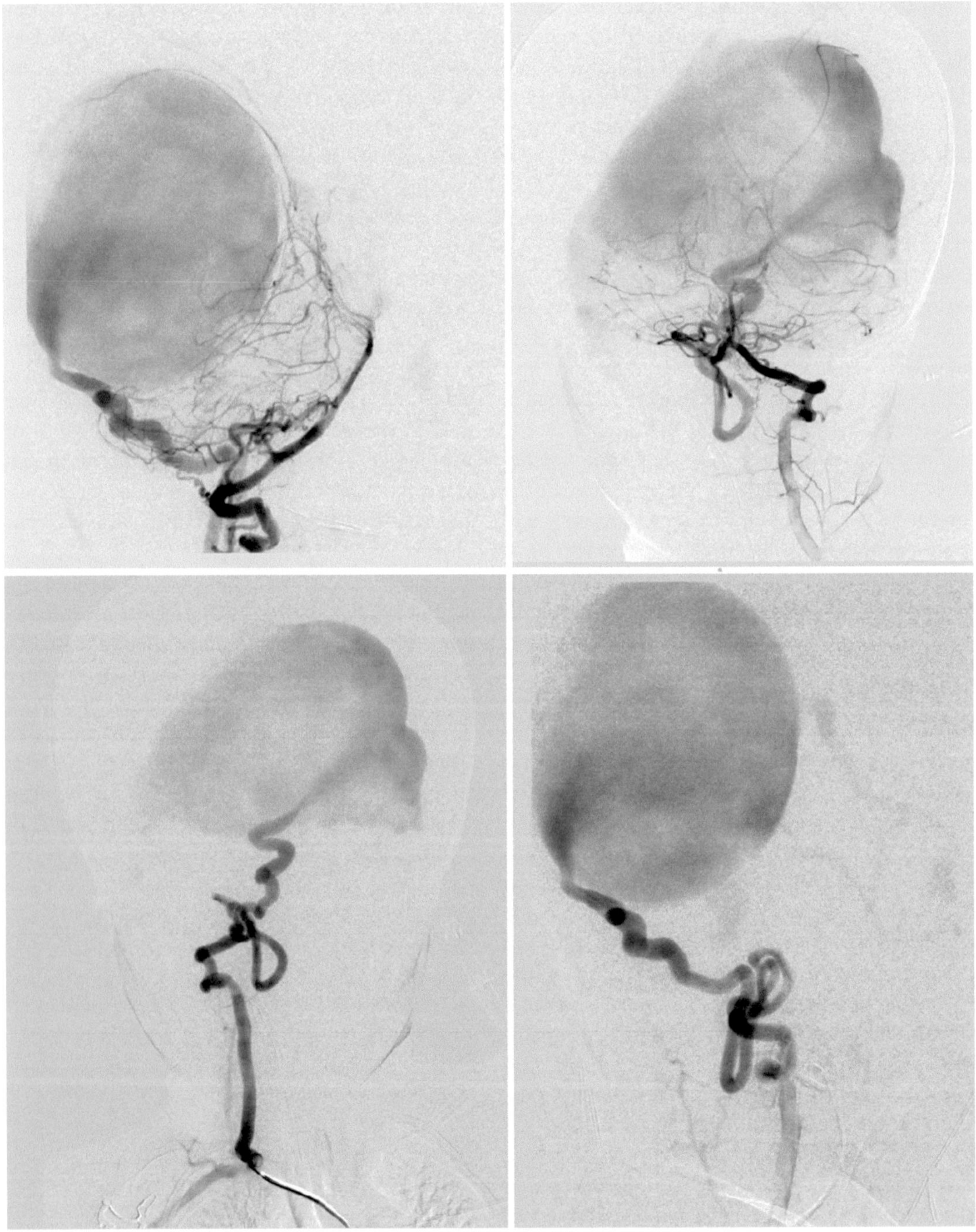

Fig. 2.2 DSA of the patient B—an extensive dAVF in the torcular and right lateral sinus

Control DSA showed residual contrasting of the fistula from the left middle meningeal artery (Fig. 2.3). An additional occlusion of the fistula with microcoils was performed.

Control DSA showed total disconnection of the fistula (Fig. 2.4).

The postoperative period was uneventful and the patient was discharged from the hospital three days after surgery. The patient was followed regularly every year—condition remained satisfactory. Control MRI showed the signs of thrombosed confluence of sinus.

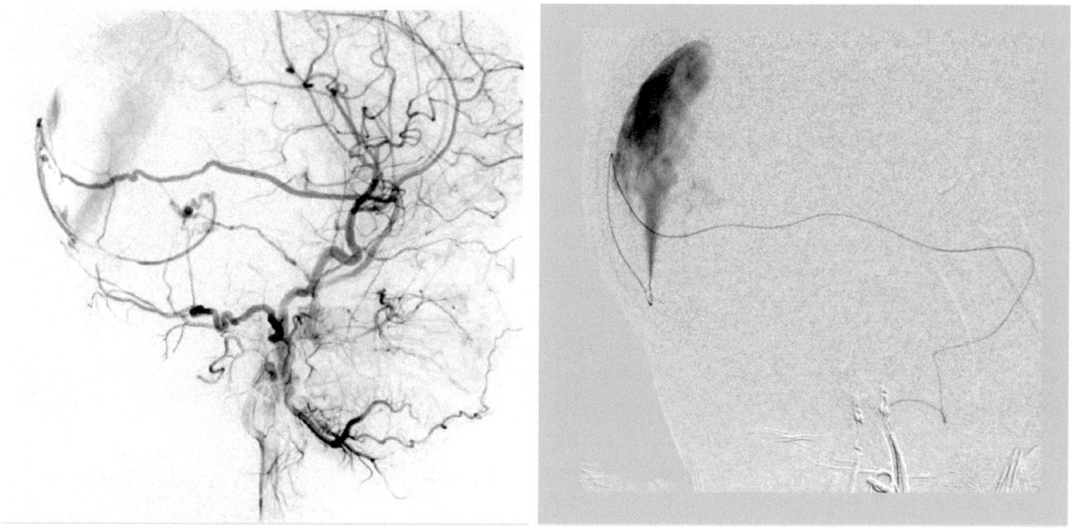

Fig. 2.3 Occlusion of the fistula—residual contrasting from the left middle meningeal artery

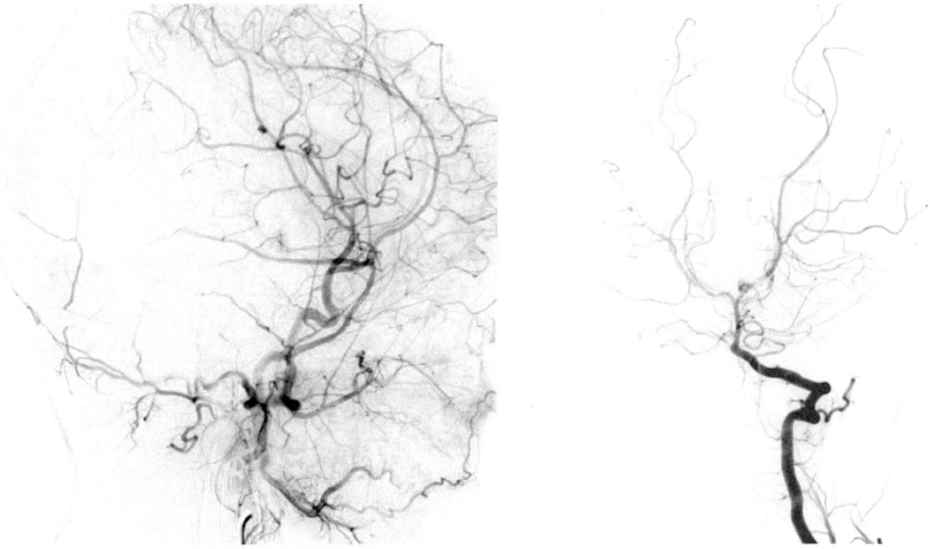

Fig. 2.4 Control DSA after total occlusion of the fistula

2.8 Conclusion

Dural arteriovenous fistulas are uncommon in pediatric population; most of them manifest during the neonatal period. The manifestation may be obscure and the diagnosis is revealed through imaging.

Common manifestations of dAVFs in neonates and infants ≤1 year of age are signs of right-sided heart failure due to volume overload and signs of increased intracranial pressure and hydrocephalus. In older children, focal neurological deficits may be observed. These lesions continue to have a significant morbidity rate because of intricate angioarchitecture. Compared to other forms of cerebral arteriovenous fistulas, children with dAVFs typically experience worse long-term outcomes. The treatment is necessary in symptomatic patients to stop the long-term effects of venous hypertension.

The first-line treatment for dAVF is typically endovascular. A thorough study of the fistula angioarchitecture is necessary before the procedure. This includes locating the feeding arteries, the point of fistulous connection, the venous drainage pathways, and the direction of venous flow. Depending on the location and structure of a fistula, endovascular treatment is performed through arterial, venous, or combined approach. Surgery and stereotactic radiosurgery, to a lesser extent, continue to be alternative treatment modalities, particularly when endovascular treatment is ineffective or deemed risky. Even with prompt and adequate treatment, pediatric dAVFs can still have a poor prognosis; however, as embolization techniques and materials continue to advance, better treatments and prognoses are becoming more and more likely. The extent of brain damage acquired during the existence of functioning dAVF, as well as the need for surgical treatment of hydrocephalus, are among the factors that have to be considered to evaluate long-term results of treatment and prognosis. Further careful follow-up and accumulation of experience of pediatric dAVF treatment are necessary to achieve satisfactory results and improve prognosis.

References

1. Hetts SW, et al. Pediatric intracranial dural arteriovenous fistulas: age-related differences in clinical features, angioarchitecture, and treatment outcomes. J Neurosurg Pediatr. 2016;18(5):602–10.
2. Appaduray SP, et al. Pediatric dural arteriovenous malformations: report of 3 cases. J Neurosurg Pediatr. 2014;14(1):16–22.
3. Barbosa M, et al. Dural sinus malformation (DSM) with giant lakes, in neonates and infants. Review of 30 consecutive cases. Interv Neuroradiol. 2003;9(4):407–24.
4. Lv X, et al. Transverse-sigmoid sinus dural arteriovenous fistulae. World Neurosurg. 2010;74(2–3):297–305.
5. Garcia-Monaco R, et al. Multifocal dural arteriovenous shunts in children. Childs Nerv Syst (Germany). 1991;7(8):425–31.
6. Yang E, et al. Imaging features and prognostic factors in fetal and postnatal torcular dural sinus malformations, part II: synthesis of the literature and patient management. J Neurointerv Surg. 2018;10(5):475–9.
7. Lasjaunias P, et al. Anatomoclinical aspects of dural arteriovenous shunts in children: review of 29 cases. Interv Neuroradiol. 1996;2(3):179–91.
8. Yu J, et al. Therapeutic progress in pediatric intracranial dural arteriovenous shunts: a review. Interv Neuroradiol. 2016;22(5):548–56.
9. Lv X, Jiang C, Wang J. Pediatric intracranial arteriovenous shunts: advances in diagnosis and treatment. Eur J Paediatr Neurol. 2020;25):29–39.
10. Liby P, Lomachinsky V, Petrak B. Jugular bulb dysmaturation in torcular dural sinus malformation: clinical images and review of literature. World Neurosurg. 2019;127:434–5.
11. Jagadeesan BD, et al. The role of percutaneous embolization techniques in the management of dural sinus malformations with atypical angioarchitecture in neonates: report of 2 cases. J Neurosurg Pediatr. 2015;16(1):74–9.
12. Guo L, Liu T, Lv X. Endovascular embolization of dural arteriovenous fistula in a child presented with slight conjunctival hyperemia. Childs Nerv Syst. 2019;35(12):2435–7.
13. Kincaid PK, et al. Dural arteriovenous fistula in children: endovascular treatment and outcomes in seven cases. AJNR Am J Neuroradiol. 2001;22(6):1217–25.
14. Djindjian R, Merland J-J. Super-selective arteriography of the external carotid artery. 1st ed. Berlin: Springer; 1978. p. 554.
15. Borden JA, Wu JK, Shucart WA. A proposed classification for spinal and cranial dural arteriovenous fistulous malformations and implications for treatment. J Neurosurg (USA). 1995;82(2):166–79.
16. Cognard C, et al. Cerebral dural arteriovenous fistulas: clinical and angiographic correlation with a revised classification of venous drainage. Radiology (USA). 1995;194(3):671–80.

17. Herman TE, Siegel MJ. Congenital dural arteriovenous fistula at torcula herophili. J Perinatol. 2007;27(11):730–1.
18. Crowley RW, et al. Combined surgical/endovascular treatment of a complex dural arteriovenous fistula in 21-month-old: technical note. J Neurosurg Pediatr. 2009;3(6):501–6.
19. de Haan TR, et al. A case of neonatal dural sinus malformation: clinical symptoms, imaging and neuropathological investigations. Eur J Paediatr Neurol. 2008;12(1):41–5.
20. Lasjaunias P. Vascular diseases in neonates, infants and children. 1st ed. Berlin: Springer; 1997. 707 p.
21. Ratliff J, Voorhies RM. Arteriovenous fistula with associated aneurysms coexisting with dural arteriovenous malformation of the anterior inferior falx. Case report and review of the literature. J Neurosurg (USA). 1999;91(2):303–7.
22. Bun YY, et al. Endovascular treatment of a neonate with dural arteriovenous fistula and other features suggestive of cerebrofacial arteriovenous metameric syndromes. Childs Nerv Syst (Germany). 2009;25(3):383–7.
23. Walcott BP, et al. Dural arteriovenous fistulae in pediatric patients: associated conditions and treatment outcomes. J Neurointerv Surg (England). 2013;5(1):6–9.
24. Grillner P, et al. A spectrum of intracranial vascular high-flow arteriovenous shunts in RASA1 mutations. Childs Nerv Syst (Germany). 2016;32(4):709–15.
25. Srinivasa RN, Burrows PE. Dural arteriovenous malformation in a child with Bannayan-Riley-Ruvalcaba syndrome. AJNR Am J Neuroradiol. 2006;27(9):1927–9.
26. Morales H, et al. Documented development of a dural arteriovenous fistula in an infant subsequent to sinus thrombosis: case report and review of the literature. Neuroradiology (Germany). 2010;52(3):225–9.
27. Bai Y, et al. De novo multiple dural arteriovenous fistulas and arteriovenous malformation after embolization of cerebral arteriovenous fistula: case report. Childs Nerv Syst (Germany). 2012;28(11):1981–3.
28. Paramasivam S, et al. De novo development of dural arteriovenous fistula after endovascular embolization of pial arteriovenous fistula. J Neurointerv Surg (England). 2013;5(4):321–6.
29. Toma AK, et al. Cerebral arteriovenous shunts in children. Neuroimaging Clin N Am (USA). 2013;23(4):757–70.
30. Geibprasert S, et al. Infantile dural arteriovenous shunt draining into a developmental venous anomaly. Interv Neuroradiol. 2007;13(1):67–74.
31. Yamamoto T, et al. Spontaneous resolution of symptoms in an infant with a congenital dural caroticocavernous fistula. Neuroradiology (Germany). 1995;37(3):247–9.
32. Johnson JN, et al. Developmental outcomes for neonatal dural arteriovenous fistulas. J Neurosurg Pediatr (USA). 2009;3(2):105–9.
33. Iizuka Y, et al. Neonatal dural arteriovenous fistula at the confluence presenting with paralysis of the orbicularis oris muscle. Neuroradiol J. 2013;26(1):47–51.
34. Ross DA, Walker J, Edwards MS. Unusual posterior fossa dural arteriovenous malformation in a neonate: case report. Neurosurgery (USA). 1986;19(6):1021–4.
35. Prasanna Karanam LS, Baddam SR, Joseph S. Role of endovascular embolisation in treatment of pediatric dural arteriovenous fistula: a case report with a review of the literature. Neurology (India). 2011;59(6):917–8.
36. Reig AS, et al. Eight-year follow-up after palliative embolization of a neonatal intracranial dural arteriovenous fistula with high-output heart failure: management strategies for symptomatic fistula growth and bilateral femoral occlusions in pediatric patients. J Neurosurg Pediatr (USA). 2010;6(6):553–8.
37. Albright AL, Latchaw RE, Price RA. Posterior dural arteriovenous malformations in infancy. Neurosurgery (USA). 1983;13(2):129–35.
38. Thiex R, et al. The use of Onyx for embolization of central nervous system arteriovenous lesions in pediatric patients. AJNR Am J Neuroradiol. 2010;31(1):112–20.
39. Piippo A, et al. Characteristics and long-term outcome of 251 patients with dural arteriovenous fistulas in a defined population. J Neurosurg (USA). 2013;118(5):923–34.
40. Konishi Y, et al. Congenital fistula of the dural carotid-cavernous sinus: case report and review of the literature. Neurosurgery (USA). 1990;27(1):120–6.
41. Cohen JE, et al. Endovascular treatment of congenital carotid-cavernous fistulas in infancy. Neurol Res (England). 2008;30(6):649–51.
42. Mankad K, et al. Correction to: Venous pathologies in paediatric neuroradiology: from foetal to adolescent life (Neuroradiology (2020), 62, 1(15–37), https://doi.org/10.1007/s00234-019-02294-x). Neuroradiology. 2020;62(7):903.
43. Yadav V, et al. Rare occurrence of dural arteriovenous fistula in a child: multi-modality imaging and literature review. Radiol Case Rep. 2021;16(4):879–83.
44. Tsai LK, Liu HM, Jeng JS. Diagnosis and management of intracranial dural arteriovenous fistulas. Expert Rev Neurother. 2016;16(3):307–18.
45. Berenstein A, et al. Endovascular management of arteriovenous malformations and other intracranial arteriovenous shunts in neonates, infants, and children. Childs Nerv Syst. 2010;26(10):1345–58.
46. Cognard C, et al. Dural arteriovenous fistulas as a cause of intracranial hypertension due to impairment of cranial venous outflow. J Neurol Neurosurg Psychiatry. 1998;65(3):308–16.
47. Lv X, et al. Transvenous retrograde AVM embolization: indications, techniques, complications and outcomes. Interv Neuroradiol. 2017;23(5):504–9.
48. Mendes GAC, et al. Transvenous embolization in pediatric plexiform arteriovenous malformations. Neurosurgery (USA). 2016;78(3):458–65.

49. Baharvahdat H, et al. Updates in the management of cranial dural arteriovenous fistula. Stroke Vasc Neurol. 2020;5(1):50–8.
50. Lin N, et al. Safety of neuroangiography and embolization in children: complication analysis of 697 consecutive procedures in 394 patients. J Neurosurg Pediatr (USA). 2015;16(4):432–8.
51. Hoffman CE, et al. Complications of cerebral angiography in children younger than 3 years of age. J Neurosurg Pediatr (USA). 2014;13(4):414–9.
52. Wolfe TJ, et al. Pediatric cerebral angiography: analysis of utilization and findings. Pediatr Neurol (USA). 2009;40(2):98–101.
53. Burger IM, et al. Safety of cerebral digital subtraction angiography in children: complication rate analysis in 241 consecutive diagnostic angiograms. Stroke (USA). 2006;37(10):2535–9.
54. Lasjaunias P, Ter Brugge KG, Berenstein A. Surgical neuroangiography: clinical and interventional aspects in children. Berlin: Springer; 2006. p. 1–979.

3 Pediatric Dural Arteriovenous Shunts

Huachen Zhang and Xianli Lv

Abstract

Pediatric dural arteriovenous shunts (DAVS) have clinical presentations, angiographic characteristics and natural histories that differ from those described in adults. Pediatric DAVS were categorized into three types: dural sinus malformations; infantile dural arteriovenous shunts; adult-type dural arteriovenous shunts. Therapeutic strategies and outcomes were variable depending on different subtypes. Proper diagnosis is mandatory for optimal therapeutic strategies within appropriate therapeutic windows. This chapter will discuss their clinical characteristics, classifications, angioarchitecture, and endovascular treatment.

Keywords

Vascular malformation · Pediatrics · Fistula · Congenital · Dural shunts

H. Zhang · X. Lv (✉)
Department of Neurosurgery, Beijing Tsinghua Changgung Hospital, School of Clinical Medicine, Tsinghua University, Beijing, China

Abbreviations

ADAVS	Adult-type dural arteriovenous shunt
AVS	Arteriovenous shunt
DAVS	Dural arteriovenous shunt
DSM	Dural sinus malformation
DVA	Developmental venous anomaly
EVT	Endovascular treatment
IDAVS	Infantile-type dural arteriovenous shunt
SS	Straight sinus
SSS	Superior sagittal sinus
VGAM	Vein of Galen aneurysmal malformation

3.1 Introduction

Pediatric dural arteriovenous shunts (DAVS) only account for 10% of the children referred with intracranial vascular malformations, of which developmental venous anomalies are the most frequent (Fig. 3.1) [1, 2]. They present specific clinical courses and angiographic characteristics which differ from those in adults. Therefore, the descriptions and classifications of pediatric DAVS should be stressed [3–5]. The unfavorable natural history and clinical outcomes after management reported in the literature attest the complexity of this type DAVFs [6, 7]. Unfavourable outcome occurred in more than 50% of untreated dural sinus malformation (DSM), in 83.3% of

X. Lv (ed.), *Intracranial and Spinal Dural Arteriovenous Fistulas*,
https://doi.org/10.1007/978-981-19-5767-3_3

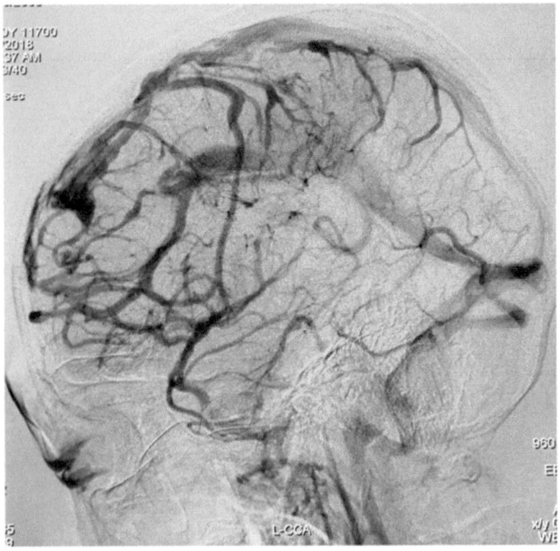

Fig. 3.1 An 11-year-old girl presented with headaches. Lateral left carotid angiogram, venous phase, shows the frontal developmental venous anomaly (DVA) with dilated and tortuous frontal and sylvian veins and inferior sagittal sinus

untreated infantile dural arteriovenous sinus (IDAVS). Hetts (2016) described 21 children of dural arteriovenous fistula (DAVF) treated with 38% with complete obliteration, 70% good outcomes, 19% complications, and 27% mortality rates [1]. Terada described 10 cases reported as DSM: 8 patients underwent EVT, while 1 with spontaneous shunt occlusion was managed conservatively [8]. A favorable outcome was obtained in 44% and unfavorable in 55% of cases.

3.2 Classification and Description of Arteriovenous Shunts

Lasjaunias first described the various types of pediatric DAVSs and their complex natural history [6]:

- DSM typically occurs antenatally, in neonates or infants, often affects the torcular herophili or lateral sinus, with giant dural lakes with or without AVS. Spontaneous thrombosis may further restrict cerebral venous drainage and subsequently lead to intraparenchymal hemorrhagic infarction.
- IDAVS is acquired high-flow low-pressure lesions with multiple DAVSs draining into enlarged sinuses mostly found in older infants and young children.
- ADAVS is acquired and architecturally similar to adult dural fistulas; they mostly affect the cavernous sinus area in older children.

3.3 Angiographic characteristics

Selective angiography properly defined the vascular anatomy of each DAVS subtype in agreement with Lasjaunias [6, 7]:

- *DSM* are characterized by a giant dural sinus lake, with or without multiple DAVS.
- *IDAVS* are angiographically characterized by multifocal high-flow shunts vascularized by six to seven arteries and draining into enlarged dural sinuses with or without sigmoid stenosis or occlusion. Cortical venous reflux was seen in all cases.
- *ADAVS* are para- or cavernous, the superior sagittal sinus (SSS), the transverse sinuse or the torcular lesions caused by thrombosis of the involved sinus or vein of Galen aneurysmal malformation (VGAM) treatment. The architecture of ADAVS is simpler vascularized by one to five dural arteries with or without pial venous reflux.

3.4 Treatment

Surgical morbidity and mortality are high in complex lesions [1, 9]. Surgery is contraindicated due to the extension and multiplicity of the AVS. Surgical ventricular shunting in the presence of hydrocephalus is not recommended [9]. The objective of endovascular treatment (EVT) in such cases should be the correction (even partial) of the venous sinus disorder. These multifocal and high flow fistulas prevented the use of radiotherapy.

All patients had diagnostic angiographies followed during the same session by EVT under general anesthesia. Except for the selected DSM, transvenous routes are not for the neonates. Transarterial routes is indicated for near all cases. Transumbilical approaches are only available for 7–10 days [10–13]. After that, they have to be removed to avoid infection. Direct puncture or exposure/puncture of carotid artery are also possible if the femoral routes cannot be used [11].

In neonatal cases, catheterization of the umbilical cord is performed just after delivery to neonatologists. They put a floppy cord catheter. In intervention, we prepare 4F catheter and sheath system. The sheath is curved by heat to follow the anatomy of the cord. As for the curve, exposure to steam will make a sheath as you expect. The Oval Foreman is always open in neonates. Thus, from femoral or umbilical vein to right atrium and then to left atrium is easy. Transcardiac, i.e., from left atrium to left ventricle and then aorta is not simple and not the work for neurointerventional doctor. Talented pediatric cardiologists can do this with a special device (Fig. 3.2).

The arterial and venous phases of both internal carotid and vertebral arteries are carefully studied. Treatment options included trans-arterial or transvenous DAVS embolization using Onyx (ev3, Medtronic), detachable coils or Glue [14–16]. Interventional procedures were usually staged with an interval between procedures of 1–3 months.

The possibility of an effective transvenous embolization is a chance for DAVS to slow down the progression of the disease, perhaps even extend patients' life. Furthermore, if during staged embolization of a DAVS, one should definitely control this abnormal flow as much as possible to avoid focal or general hydrovenous disorders that can lead to catastrophes [17].

Associated pial AV shunts and associated arterial aneurysms represent additional potential causes for hemorrhage [18]. Flow-related aneurysms are seldom encountered in children and they were noted on the middle meningeal artery, although the lesions were supplied by multiple feeders.

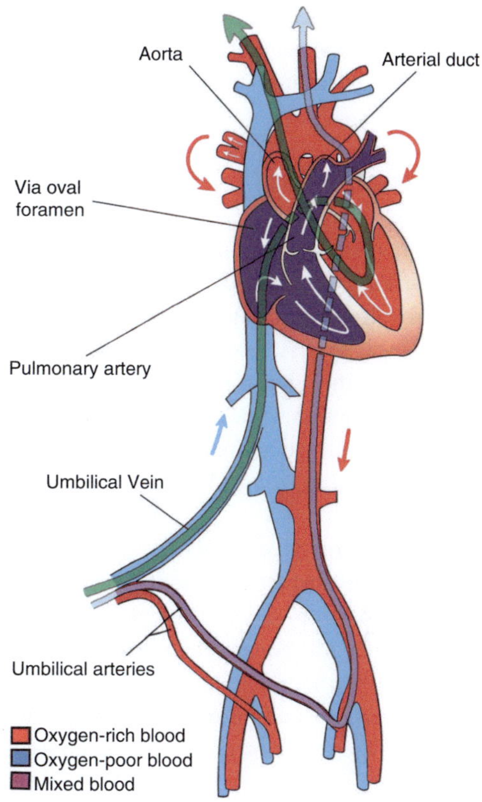

Fig. 3.2 Illustration of transumbilical approaches. A purple line with an arrowhead shows the transumbilical arterial approach. A green line with an arrowhead shows transumbilical venous, transcardiac arterial approach

Adjuvant therapies by steroids were given after each embolization with Onyx, and anticoagulation was delivered when the venous drainages were markedly modified compared with pre-EVT.

3.5 Predictors of Poor Neurological Outcome

Initial poor clinical status, spontaneous hemorrhage, and brain damage are significantly associated with poor clinical outcome [19–21]. IDAVS had poorer outcomes than ADAVS or DSM. Delay in diagnosis and treatment induced poor neurological evolution. Regardless of the subtype, better outcomes will be obtained if treatment was more rapidly performed after diagnosis. Midline lesion location (SSS and torcular) and pial venous reflux are not associated with poor outcome.

3.6 Dural Sinus Malformations

DSM are congenital lesions that may be discovered antenatally by ultrasound or MRI characterized by focally dilated and bulging dural sinus ectasias [7, 22, 23]. As described by Okudera, the formation of the dural sinuses start around 4 months of gestation while the transverse sinuses that grow laterally and medially to reach the primitive torcular at around 5–6 months of gestation [24].

The growth and development of dural sinuses are mainly related to that of the dura mater [25]. Because connection of the superficial middle cerebral veins with the cavernous sinus, and the connection of the superior petrosal sinus with the cavernous sinus, usually are not yet established before birth, the venous circulation related to the marked flow from the rapidly growing hemispheres is mainly directed towards the transverse sinus via the tentorial sinus [26]. These findings demonstrate the prenatal existence of a large venous-like-pockets phase of the fetal sinuses, which secondarily remodel during pre- and postnatal processes [27]. Intra-sinusal septations and pouches are formed that extend from the transverse sinuses towards the convexity or tentorial dura. By 6–7 months of gestation, the fetal sinus walls started to ossify and the periosteum was then clearly identified [27]. Surrounding the bone, loose collagen fibers transformed into extensive collagen fibers which formed the dural sinuses. The torcular corresponds to involution of the fetal tentorial venous plexus.

In DSM, the remodelling seems not to occur properly and the sinus remains expanded for reasons which are currently unclear [24]. It could be hypothesized that one of the intrasinusal venous pouches does not regress normally but continues to grow after connection of the transverse sinus and the torcular. The diverticulum of the sigmoid sinus in adults may actually be their remnants [28].

DSM is not always associated with AVS, but AVS influences the natural history of the DSM, which without AVS evolve more favorably than those with AVS [2, 29]. It has been emphasized that the affected sinus thrombosis plays a role in AVS formation [30]: because spontaneous thrombosis belongs to the potential evolution of the disease, this phenomenon occurring in utero could promote AVS formation.

Sigmoid sinus malformations usually associate with occlusions of the ipsilateral jugular bulb even frequently associated with contralateral sigmoid sinus stenoses or occlusions [24]. AVS located in the torcular area were usually of lower flow velocity than those located in superior sagittal sinus or sigmoid sinus [30]. These findings could point to different pathogenetic origins at various stages of development.

Other mechanisms, either genetic or epigenetic, could be involved in the pathogenesis of DSM. Associations between cervicofacial venous malformations, dural venous sinus abnormalities and cavernomas have been reported and described to correspond to a metameric syndrome [31–34]. One patient with a DSM affecting the SSS presented a capillary malformation-arteriovenous malformation syndrome type 1 related to RASA 1 mutation [35].

DSM without AVS (even diagnosed antenatally) has been reported to spontaneously occlusion with favorable clinical outcomes [7, 17, 18, 36]. DSM with AVS can be diagnosed antenatally (on fetal Doppler and confirmed on MRA) and has a poorer prognosis. Severe neurological morbidity or death have been reported in 41% of DSM with AVS cases, which is why the distinction between these two entities must be made [1, 8, 17, 18, 24].

The combination of AVS, venous reflux, and sinus stenosis result in cerebral venous congestion responsible for diffuse or focal brain damage, cortical/subependymal atrophy, hydrocephaly, and hemorrhages. White matter calcification is the marker of chronic venous ischemia. Because of their midline location and absence of alternative drainage routes, DSM involving the torcular is particularly prone to parenchymal injury in the territory of the deep venous system since reflux in the straight sinus is frequently associated. This feature can also be seen in lateralized lesions in cases of associated contralateral sigmoid stenosis or thrombosis, potentially increasing the risk of venous restriction [7, 37, 38]. Therefore, DSM with AVS is aggressive lesion requiring prompt treatment [17, 18].

In DSM presentations, severe neonatal heart failure is rare [7, 39]. The mean age at which diagnosis of the DSM is 8 months [8]. Macrocrania is frequently detected (58.8%). Neurological symptoms are seizures, developmental delay, behavioral disorders and more rarely intracranial hypertension. Hemorrhage as primary event is uncommon in accordance with previously published data [1].

MRI and MRA are recommended as long as intracranial vascular malformations are suspected. If the DSM is discovered antenatally by ultrasound, we recommend completing the assessment by MRI and MRA every week to evaluate both lesion and brain. The poor prognostic factors reported in the literature include venous pouch arterialization, ventriculomegaly (considered to be related to hydrovenous disorders), and parenchymal damage [23]. A better outcome seems to be correlated to spontaneous decrease of the size of the venous pouch on subsequent controls and intra-saccular thrombi, signs of a favorable regression of the DSM. For severe brain damage or melting brain syndrome therapeutic abortion can be envisaged. MRI and MRA should be performed rapidly after birth to determine the lesion and the aspect of the brain. We took into consideration several factors for our therapeutic strategy: lesion location, brain damage and relationships with normal veins.

Anatomical cure of the DSM is not the primary goal to reach [15]. Treatment is mainly meant to preserve brain maturation and obtain normal neurological development. A stepwise EVT based on angioarchitecture is usually performed, designed to preserve cerebral venous drainage, progressively occlude the various AVS and allow proper sinus remodelling. Our preferable embolic materials to manage DSM with AVS are coils, Onyx and glue [15].

The choice of the right moment to perform the treatments (optimal therapeutic window) is crucial to obtain favorable clinical outcome. Early embolization is mandatory if the MRI/MRA findings as described above are considered at risk for irreversible brain lesions and if the baby presents aggressive symptoms [7, 20]. Asymptomatic neonates with favorable angioarchitecture (slow flow AVS, absence of sinus stenosis or venous reflux) can be treated around 5–6 months after birth. They will have to be followed up precisely in the meantime by monthly clinical examination and by MRI/MRA performed every 3 months. Any early sign of developmental delay, progressive increase of the head circumference or hydrocephalus will prompt endovascular treatment at this stage. Trigemino-cardiac reflex, which mainly presented with decreasing heart beat rate during Onyx injection, can developed and should be noted [15, 40].

3.7 Infantile Dural Arteriovenous Shunts

IDAVS are acquired multifocal, low-pressure, high-flow dural shunts, complex in their angioarchitecture, draining into abnormal dural sinuses that are enlarged but not malformative and that remain patent for a long time. There may be no occurrence of progressive neurological deficits as long as dural sinuses are patent, which explains why the majority of these lesions are identified in older children rather than earlier in life [1, 2, 21, 41]. The persistence of high flow and low pressure in the large dural sinuses creates the presence of pial AVFs induced by venous sump at the surface of the brain in the vicinity of the dural shunts [2]. Unlike congenital vascular malformations, these dural shunts display mature arterial and venous configurations. IDAVS is considered to be due to diffuse unregulated angiogenic activities, for which the initial trigger is unknown [42]. Dural sinus thrombosis has been reported in a majority of the cases even if pathogenesis remains unclear [21, 41, 42].

The macrocrania and neurocognitive delay are often the initial symptoms because of the overall impact of the venous hypertension and the relative venous ischemia. The proptosis, extraocular motor nerve palsies, and facial vein enlargement are usually caused by the venous reroute of the cavernous sinus. Severe clinical symptoms of IDAVS include hemorrhage, seizures and intracranial hypertension, related to the significant hemodynamic impairment [6]. Lesion progression is indeed dictated by venous outlet restriction and AVS and this poor prognosis is in line with what was previously described by Lasjaunias [39].

A pulsatile bruit heard at auscultation of the head in a macrocephalic child suggests the existence of an intracranial vascular problem. CT or better MRI should be rapidly obtained to confirm the diagnosis. The presence of an objective but nonsubjective intracranial bruit suggests that it always belonged to the natural acoustic environment of the child, which is probably present at birth [1].

Early or delayed treatment will be proposed according to the symptoms of the lesion. Not finding the lesion early and not treating it in due time may lead to severe neurocognitive disorders. IDAVS can be partial and early recurrence of the shunts near the embolised regions is common. Variant dural sinuses are involved and transvenous sacrifice of these may be feasible in selective cases. The multifocal nature of the AVS makes surgery a limited option. The missed or overlooked optimum moment for treatment will result in failures to obtain a normal maturation process, which is considered as a therapeutic failure or complication [15]. Symptoms respond partially to transarterial embolisation, but recur rapidly. Therefore, the long-term prognosis is poor with neurological deterioration in early adulthood [43, 44].

3.8 Adult-Type Dural Arteriovenous Shunts

ADAVS is very rare condition in children with few reported cases [45, 46]. In the majority (83.6%) of ADAVS occurring secondarily in VGAM-treated patients, distant from the VGAM shunt itself, dural sinus thrombosis is observed [47]. ADAVS is considered as a focal post thrombotic sprouting angiogenic response, which is unlike IDAVS that result from diffuse unregulated angiogenic activity [42, 47, 48].

Treatment is mandatory for lesions with venous reflux and potential hemorrhagic risk, as well as ophthalmological symptoms in cavernous localization cases (Fig. 3.3). ADAVS discovered fortuitously after VGAM treatment are benign and have not exhibited unfavorable outcome in literature. They will be followed up and managed according to their clinical presentations.

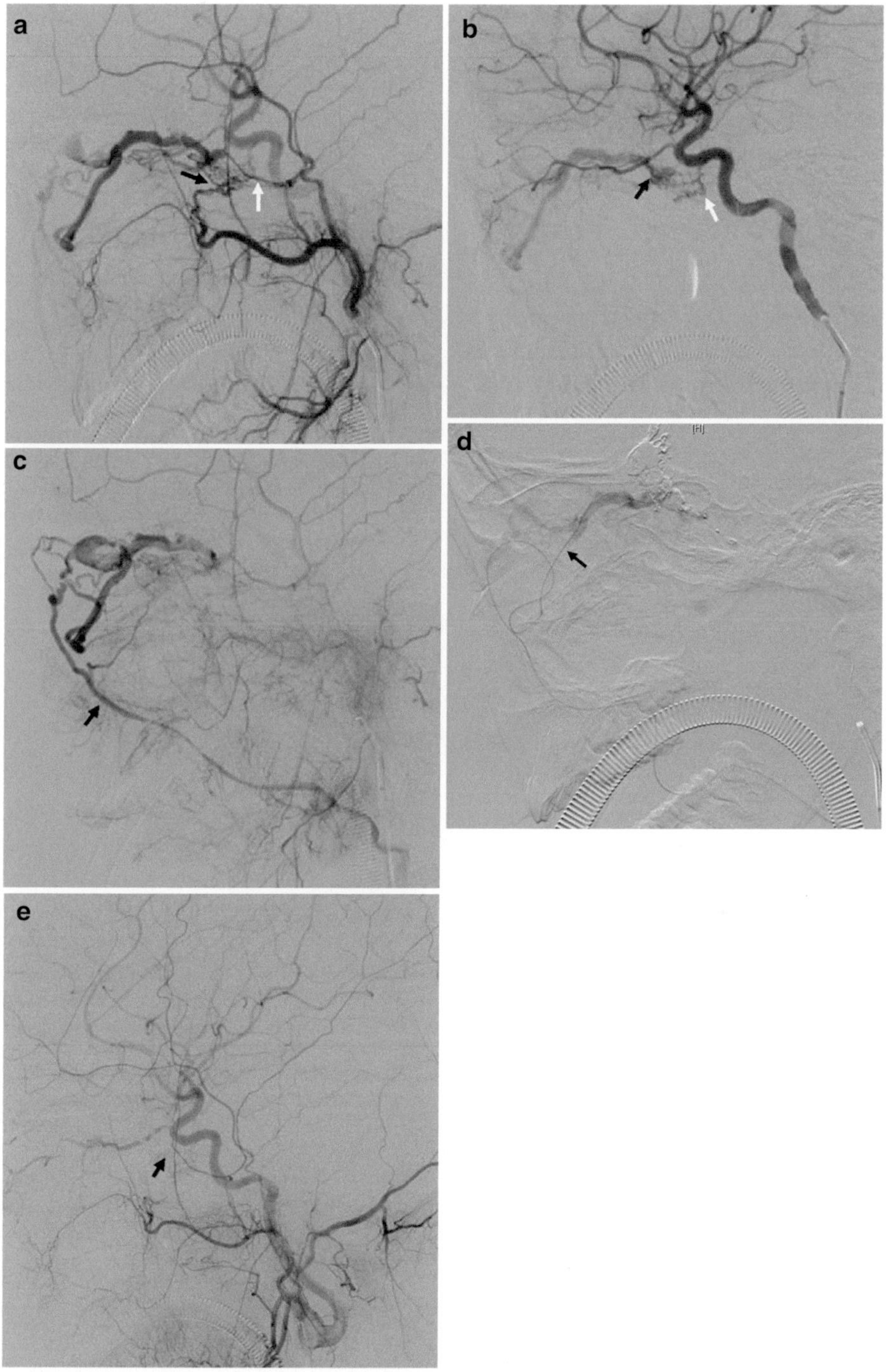

Fig. 3.3 A 9-year-old girl presented with proptosis and chemosis of the left eye. (**a**) Left external carotid artery angiogram, lateral view, shows an adult-type DAVS at the cavernous sinus region supplied by the anterior branch of the meningeal artery (white arrow) and the artery of foramen rotundum (black arrow). (**b**) Left internal carotid artery angiogram, lateral view, shows the adult-type DAVS at the cavernous sinus region supplied by the inferolateral trunk (white arrow) and drained by the ophthalmic vein (black arrow). (**c**) Venous phase of the left external carotid artery angiogram, lateral view, shows the venous drainage of facial vein (black arrow). (**d**) Superselective angiogram shows the microcatheter was retrogradely navigated through the facial vein, ophthalmic vein to the AVS (black arrow). (**e**) Control angiography of the left carotid artery confirmed the obliteration of the DAVS after Onyx embolization (black arrow). The patient improved clinically with complete resolution of the symptoms

3.9 Conclusion

Recognizing subtypes of pediatric DAVS is mandatory to optimize therapeutic strategies: DSM with AVS patients require early management and EVT can achieve a good outcome. IDAVS is the major challenges and associated with a high morbidity and mortality despite EVT. ADAVS has a less aggressive outcome and EVT is dictated by angioarchitectural factors similar to those in adults. A definitive understanding of the pathogenesis of these lesions is key to improve their management.

Acknowledgement Thanks Zhongyin Ye, at School of Medicine and School of Clinical Medicine, Tsinghua University, Beijing, for providing Fig. 3.2.

References

1. Hetts SW, Moftakhar P, Maluste N, et al. Pediatric intracranial dural arteriovenous fistulas: age-related differences in clinical features, angioarchitecture, and treatment outcomes. J Neurosurg Pediatr. 2016;18:602–10.
2. Garcia-Monaco R, Rodesch G, Terbrugge K, Burrows P, Lasjaunias P. Multifocal dural arteriovenous shunts in children. Childs Nerv Syst. 1991;7:425–31.
3. Cognard C, Gobin YP, Pierot L, et al. Cerebral dural arteriovenous fistulas: clinical and angiographic correlation with a revised classification of venous drainage. Radiology. 1995;194:671–80.
4. Borden JA, Wu JK, Shucart WA. A proposed classification for spinal and cranial dural arteriovenous fistulous malformations and implications for treatment. J Neurosurg. 1995;82:166–79.
5. Zhang H, Zhu K, Wang J, Lv X. The use of a new classification in endovascular treatment of dural arteriovenous fistulas. Neurosci Inform. 2022;2:100047. https://doi.org/10.1016/j.neuri.2022.100047.
6. Lasjaunias P, Magufis G, Goulao A, et al. Anatomoclinical aspects of dural arteriovenous shunts in children. Review of 29 cases. Interv Neuroradiol. 1996;2:179–91.
7. Barbosa M, Mahadevan J, Weon YC, et al. Dural sinus malformations (DSM) with Giant Lakes, in neonates and infants. Review of 30 consecutive cases. Interv Neuroradiol. 2003;9:407–24.
8. Terada A, Komiyama M, Ishiguro T, Niimi Y, Oishi H. Nationwide survey of pediatric intracranial arteriovenous shunts in Japan: Japanese Pediatric Arteriovenous Shunts Study (JPAS). J Neurosurg Pediatr. 2018;22:550–8.
9. Walcott BP, Smith ER, Scott RM, Orbach DB. Dural arteriovenous fistulae in pediatric patients: associated conditions and treatment outcomes. J Neurointerv Surg. 2013;5:6–9.
10. Komiyama M, Nishikawa M, Kitano S, Sakamoto H, Miyagi N, Kusuda S, Sugimoto H. Transumbilical embolization of a congenital dural arteriovenous fistula at the torcular herophili in a neonate. Case report. J Neurosurg. 1999;90(5):964–9.
11. Komiyama M, Terada A, Ishiguro T. Neurointerventions for the neonates with brain arteriovenous fistulas: with special reference to access routes. Neurol Med Chir (Tokyo). 2016;56(3):132–40.
12. Koutsouras GW, Rahmani R, Schmidt T, Silberstein H, Bhalla T. Coil and Onyx embolization of a torcular herophili dural arteriovenous fistula in a full-term neonate with advanced heart failure using a transumbilical approach. J Neurosurg Pediatr. 2018;23(1):80–5.
13. Oshiro T, Nakayama O, Ohba C, Ohashi Y, Kawakubo J, Nagamine T, Komiyama M. Transumbilical arterial embolization of a large dural arteriovenous fistula in a low-birth-weight neonate with congestive heart failure. Childs Nerv Syst. 2016;32(4):723–6.
14. Ye Z, Hao J, Zhang L, Lv X. Development of bilateral subdural hematoma after endovascular embolization of a dural sinus malformation. Childs Nerv Syst. 2022;38(1):211–5.
15. Lv X, Jiang C, Wang J. Pediatric intracranial arteriovenous shunts: Advances in diagnosis and treatment. Eur J Paediatr Neurol. 2020;25:29–39.
16. Guo L, Liu T, Lv X. Endovascular embolization of dural arteriovenous fistula in a child presented with slight conjunctival hyperemia. Childs Nerv Syst. 2019;35(12):2435–7.
17. Yang E, Storey A, Olson HE, et al. Imaging features and prognostic factors in fetal and postnatal torcular dural sinus malformations, part I: review of experience at Boston Children's Hospital. J Neurointerv Surg. 2018;10:467–70.
18. Yang E, Storey A, Olson HE, et al. Imaging features and prognostic factors in fetal and postnatal torcular dural sinus malformations, part II: synthesis of the literature and patient management. J Neurointerv Surg. 2018;10:471–5.
19. Liby P, Lomachinsky V, Petrak B, et al. Torcular dural sinus malformations: a single-center case series and a review of literature. Childs Nerv Syst. 2020;36:333–41.
20. Appaduray SP, King JA, Wray A, Lo P, Maixner W. Pediatric dural arteriovenous malformations. J Neurosurg Pediatr. 2014;14:16–22.
21. Souza MP, Willinsky RA, Terbrugge KG. Intracranial dural arteriovenous shunts in children. The toronto experience. Interv Neuroradiol. 2003;9:47–52.
22. Komiyama M, Ishiguro T, Kitano S, Sakamoto H, Nakamura H. Serial antenatal sonographic observation of cerebral dural sinus malformation. AJNR Am J Neuroradiol. 2004;25:1446–8.

23. Rossi A, De Biasio P, Scarso E, et al. Prenatal MR imaging of dural sinus malformation: a case report. Prenat Diagn. 2006;26:11–6.
24. Okudera T, Huang YP, Ohta T, et al. Development of posterior fossa dural sinuses, emissary veins, and jugular bulb: morphological and radiologic study. AJNR Am J Neuroradiol. 1994;15:1871–83.
25. Tischfield MA, Robson CD, Gilette NM, et al. Cerebral vein malformations result from loss of Twist1 expression and BMP signaling from skull progenitor cells and dura. Dev Cell. 2017;42:445–61.
26. Knosp E, Müller G, Perneczky A. Anatomical remarks on the fetal cavernous sinus and on the veins of the middle cranial fossa. In: Dolenc VV, editor. The cavernous sinus. Vienna: Springer; 1987. https://doi.org/10.1007/978-3-7091-6982-7_7.
27. Chow MSM, Wu SL, Hui V, Chow TCH, Yew DT. Revisit the cavernous sinus from fetus to adult-new and old data. Anat Rec (Hoboken). 2018;301(5):819–24.
28. Li B, Lv X, Wu Z, et al. Stent-assisted coil embolization of a transverse-sigmoid sinus diverticulum presenting with pulsatile tinnitus. Turk Neurosurg. 2016;26(4):632–4.
29. Hetts SW, Keenan K, Fullerton HJ, et al. Pediatric intracranial nongalenic pial arteriovenous fistulas: clinical features, angioarchitecture, and outcomes. AJNR Am J Neuroradiol. 2012;33:1710–9.
30. Herman JM, Spetzler RF, Bederson JB, Kurbat JM, Zabramski JM. Genesis of a dural arteriovenous malformation in a rat model. J Neurosurg. 1995;83:539–45.
31. Brinjikji W, Mark IT, Silvera VM, Guerin JB. Cervicofacial venous malformations are associated with intracranial developmental venous anomalies and dural venous sinus abnormalities. AJNR Am J Neuroradiol. 2020;41:1209–14.
32. Brinjikji W, Nicholson P, Hilditch CA, Krings T, Pereira V, Agid R. Cerebrofacial venous metameric syndrome-spectrum of imaging findings. Neuroradiology. 2020;62:417–25.
33. Brinjikji W, Flemming KD, Lanzino G. De novo formation of a large cavernoma associated with a congenital torcular dural arteriovenous fistula: case report. J Neurosurg Pediatr. 2017;19:567–70.
34. Manjila S, Bazil T, Thomas M, Mani S, Kay M, Udayasankar U. A review of extraaxial developmental venous anomalies of the brain involving dural venous flow or sinuses: persistent embryonic sinuses, sinus pericranii, venous varices or aneurysmal malformations, and enlarged emissary veins. Neurosurg Focus. 2018;45:E9.
35. Grillner P, Soderman M, Holmin S, Rodesch G. A spectrum of intracranial vascular high-flow arteriovenous shunts in RASA1 mutations. Childs Nerv Syst. 2016;32:709–15.
36. Robertson F. Torcular dural sinus malformation. J Neurointerv Surg. 2018;10:423.
37. Friedmann DR, Eubig J, McGill M, Babb JS, Pramanik BK, Lalwani AK. Development of the jugular bulb: a radiologic study. Otol Neurotol. 2011;32:1389–95.
38. Saliou G, Dirks P, Sacho RH, Chen L, terBrugge K, Krings T. Decreased superior sagittal sinus diameter and jugular bulb narrowing are associated with poor clinical outcome in vein of Galen arteriovenous malformation. AJNR Am J Neuroradiol. 2016;37:1354–8.
39. Lasjaunias P, ter Brugge K, Berenstein A. Surgical neuroangiography: clinical and interventional aspects in children. Berlin: Springer; 2006.
40. Lv X, Wang G, Wang J. Craniospinal vascular diseases and endovascular neurosurgery. New York: Nova Science; 2021.
41. Geibprasert S, Krings T, Pereira V, Lasjaunias P. Infantile dural arteriovenous shunt draining into a developmental venous anomaly. Interv Neuroradiol. 2007;13:67–74.
42. Roccatagliata L, Bracard S, Holmin S, Soderman M, Rodesch G. Pediatric intracranial arteriovenous shunts: a global overview. Childs Nerv Syst. 2013;29:907–19.
43. Yu J, Lv X, Li Y, Wu Z. Therapeutic progress in pediatric intracranial dural arteriovenous shunts: a review. Interv Neuroradiol. 2016;22:548–56.
44. Pan HC, Sheehan J, Huang CF, Yang DY. Two consecutive dural arteriovenous fistulae in a child: a case report of successful treatment with gamma knife radiosurgery. Childs Nerv Syst. 2007;23:1185–90.
45. Livi F, Ndoro S, Caird J, Crimmins D. Indirect cavernous carotid fistula in a 12-year-old girl. J Surg Case Rep. 2016;2016. https://doi.org/10.1093/jscr/rjw095.
46. Robert T, Sylvestre P, Blanc R, et al. Thrombosis of venous outflows of the cavernous sinus: possible aetiology of the cortical venous reflux in case of indirect carotid-cavernous fistulas. Acta Neurochir (Wien). 2017;159:835–43.
47. Paramasivam S, Niimi Y, Meila D, Berenstein A. Dural arteriovenous shunt development in patients with vein of galen malformation. Interv Neuroradiol. 2014;20:781–90.
48. Bhogal P, Yeo LL, Henkes H, Krings T, Soderman M. The role of angiogenesis in dural arteriovenous fistulae: the story so far. Interv Neuroradiol. 2018;24:450–4.

A Small Tentorial Dural Arteriovenous Fistula with a Venous Aneurysm in the Pons Mimicking a Cavernous Angioma

4

Huachen Zhang and Xianli Lv

Abstract

Background: Intracranial dural arteriovenous fistula (DAVF) is a rare lesion.

Case Description: A 54-year-old man presented with sleep disturbances, double vision and a left blepharoptosis. CT and magnetic resonance imaging showed a nodular mass, surrounded by edema located in the pons with a homogeneous contrast enhancement and confirmed the diagnosis of cavernous angioma. But DSA demonstrated a small, modified Borden III tentorial DAVF after a failure of surgical resection. Endovascular embolization was curative, and the symptoms and imaging improved dramatically.

Conclusions: To our knowledge, this is the first report of a DAVF that mimicked a cavernous angioma. The turbulence flow or partially thrombosed venous aneurysm can be confused with cavernous angioma, which can have similar radiographic features. It is mandatory to consider the possibility of a thrombosed venous aneurysm for a correct differential diagnosis.

Keywords

Dural arteriovenous fistula · Brain stem · Cavernous angioma

H. Zhang · X. Lv (✉)
Department of Neurosurgery, Beijing Tsinghua Changgung Hospital, School of Clinical Medicine, Tsinghua University, Beijing, China

4.1 Introduction

Intracranial dural arteriovenous fistulas (DAVFs) are rare. The rough detection rates of DAVF are reported to be 0.29 per 100,000 adults per year in populations [1]. The tentorium is the most frequent location of aggressive DAVFs [2]. DAVFs at the tentorium with retrograde leptomeningeal venous drainage can cause aggressive neurologic symptoms such as intracranial hemorrhage [2]. In some cases, DAVF is accompanied by enhanced lesions in the brainstem and might mimic a brainstem tumor in magnetic resonance imaging (MRI) scans [3]. We present a case of tentorial DAVF with a nodular mass in the pons mimicking a cavernous angioma.

4.2 Case Presentation

A 54-year-old man[presented with sleep disturbances for 12 months, double vision and a left blepharoptosis for 4 months. On cranial CT scanning showed a hyperdense mass in in the brain stem. The Magnetic Resonance Imaging (MRI) showed a nodular mass, located in the pons, with max diameter of 1.0 cm, that was hypointense in T1, heterogeneous hyperintense in T2 with perilesional edema posteriorly. After gadolinium, the mass showed a homogeneous impregnation (Fig. 4.1). Neurologic examination showed the left oculomotor nerve palsy. The

X. Lv (ed.), *Intracranial and Spinal Dural Arteriovenous Fistulas*,
https://doi.org/10.1007/978-981-19-5767-3_4

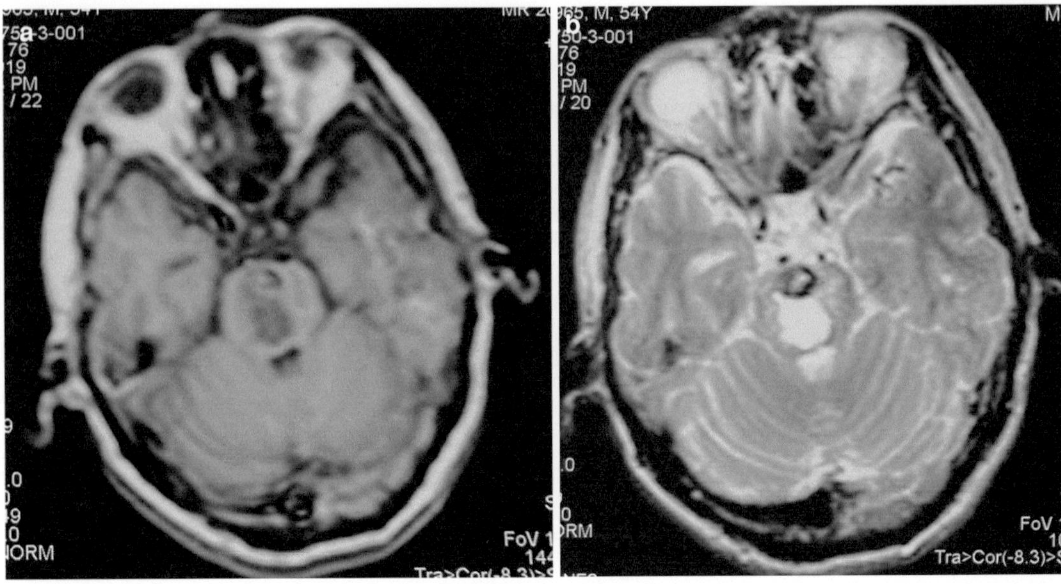

Fig. 4.1 (**a**) T1-weighted image showing a hypointensity lesion in the pons. (**b**) T2-weighted image exhibiting heterogeneous hyperintense in the pons. The lesion seemed like bleeding cavernous angioma

diagnosis of cavernous angioma bleeding was confirmed. The patient underwent surgery using a posterior fossa craniotomy and a venous pouch appeared like a blackberry was found after removement of the hematoma. An arteriovenous shunt was identified under indocyanine green (ICG) fluorescence and the operation was aborted (Fig. 4.2). The patient sustained an uneventful recovery and his neurological deficits gradually improved over the first week after surgery.

A postoperative DSA confirmed a small DAVF and transarterial Onyx embolization was performed to cure it (Fig. 4.3). The cerebral angiogram revealed the DAVF supplied by the dural branches of the right internal and external carotid arteries. The shunt point was located medial part of the tentorium. Drainages into the transverse vein of the pons and a venous aneurysm was observed. Transarterial Onyx embolization was performed via the right middle meningeal artery and the right meningohypophyseal trunk. Marathon microcatheters (Medtronic, California, USA) were used. Cerebral angiography after embolization showed that the DAVF had completely disappeared. After the treatment, the patient's symptoms improved dramatically. She was discharged with no neurologic deficit except for a slight oculomotor nerve disorder. The patient had a good recovery, without neurological deficit and discharged 3 days later.

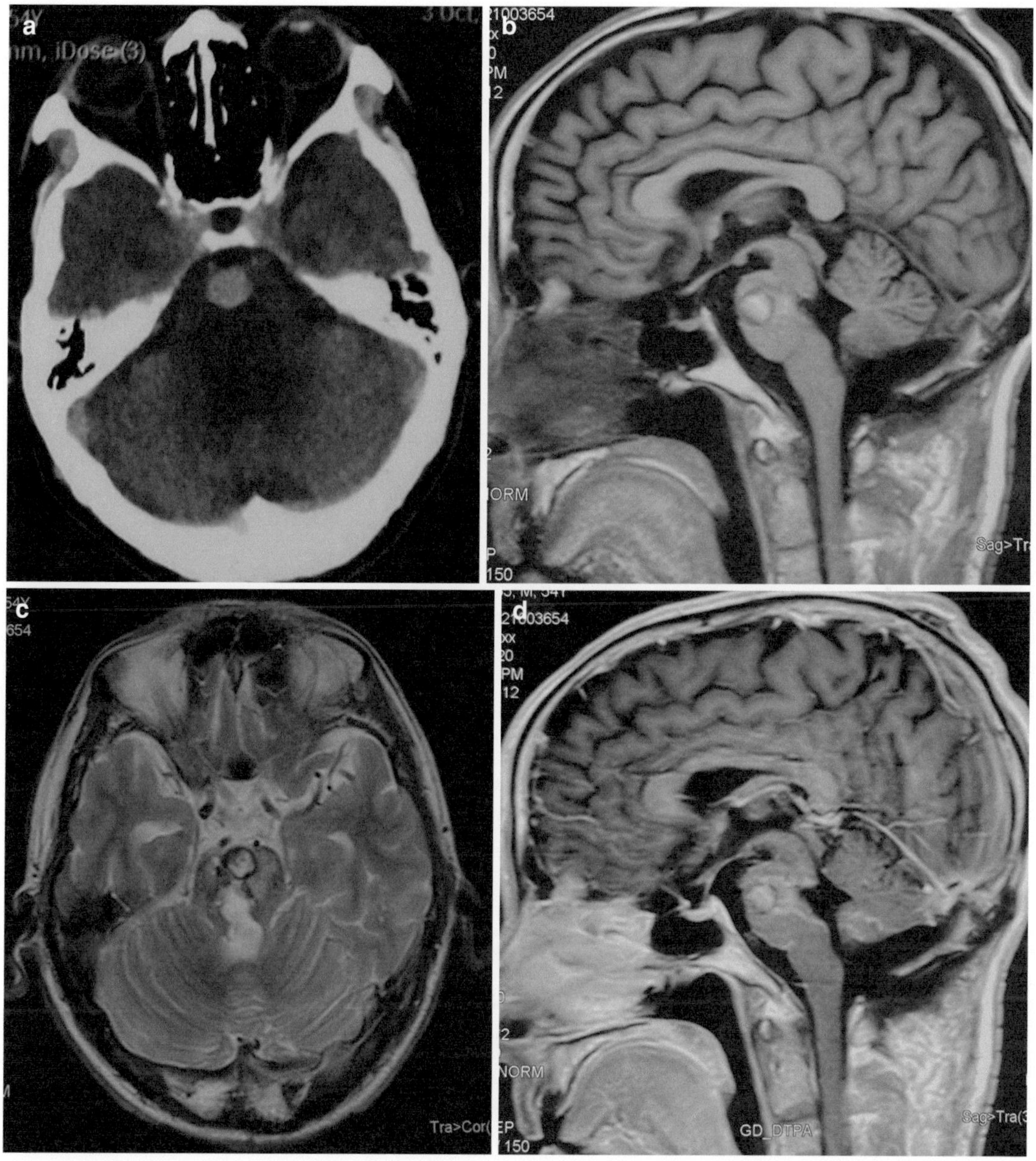

Fig. 4.2 Post-surgery CT and MRI examinations. (**a**) Axial CT image showing a hypointensity lesion in the pons. (**b**) Sagittal view of T1-weighted image showing a heterogeneous hyperintense lesion in the pons. (**c**) Axial T2-weighted image exhibiting heterogeneous hyperintense in the pons. (**d**) Sagittal view of T1-weighted image with gadolinium showing an enhanced lesion in the pons

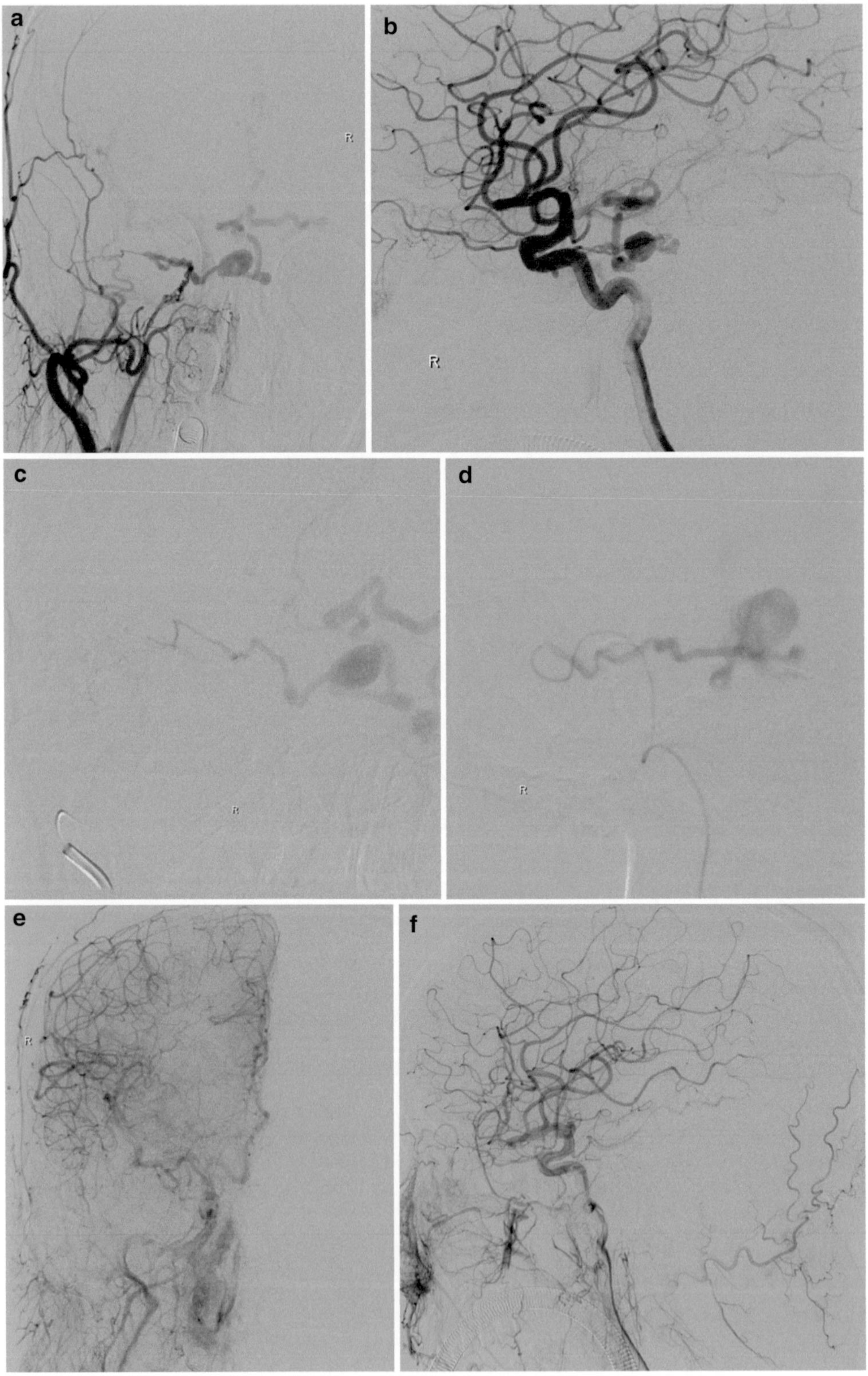
a
R
b
R
c
R
d
R
e
R
f

4.3 Discussion

To our knowledge this is the first report of a DAVF associated venous aneurysm that mimicked a cavernous angioma. This suggests that DAVF and cavernous angioma might have a similar radiological appearance in certain cases, despite they are separate pathological entities. The CT scan features in venous aneurysm include high-density attenuation in the venous lumen. The MRI features include appearance of various signal intensities of turbulent blood flow, enhancement and perilesional edema on T2-weighted images [4]. The diagnosis is more difficult only based on MRI examination and a misdiagnosis was made, in fact the neurosurgeon must be conscious of the limits of CT and MR imaging in identifying venous aneurysms associated with arteriovenous shunts.

DAVF with pial veins drainage causing brain edema and enhanced lesions on MRI that may be mistaken for tumors at the first consultation [5]. Different degrees of densities can be demonstrated for venous aneurysm as a consequence of different patterns of blood flow in them [6]. In the present case, obvious signs of a DAVF on MRI was not observed before surgery. The operator did evacuate the hematoma and careful exploration of the blackberry-like lesion; no clear nidus was initially identified and only a dubious area, which looked like a residual small clot tightly adhering to one of the cavity's wall, was seen.

Under ICG fluorescence, the blackberry-like structure, composed of multiple fluorescing spots, started becoming bright and gained a full fluorescence in the venous phase, it was rather in keeping with a small arteriovenous shunt and ruled out a possible diagnosis of cavernous angioma. The peculiar behavior of the lesion after dye infusion may be due to the fact that the small afferent vessels did not supply a high blood flow to the lesion. This made the venous aneurysm resembling a cavernous angioma. In the present case, the appearance after ICG infusion confirmed an AV shunt. The intraoperative video may be useful to neurosurgeons to realize, and hence recognize during surgery, how a small arteriovenous shunt in the context of a previous deep hemorrhage can present, despite unusual and peculiar appearance.

Endovascular embolization is the first-line curative therapy for DAVFs [7]. This dramatically improved the symptoms and imaging findings. The brainstem edema and enhanced lesion disappeared after the procedure and symptoms resolved completely after successful treatment.

4.4 Conclusion

This suggests that cavernous angioma and DAVF might have a similar MRI appearance in certain cases. The venous aneurysm can be confounded with intracranial lesions or cavernous angioma, which can have similar radiological features. When the lesion is located on the brain stem, it is important to have completely DAVF in mind as one of the differential diagnosis.

Fig. 4.3 (**a**) Right external carotid artery angiography (frontal view) demonstrates a dural arteriovenous fistula associated with a large venous aneurysm. The shunt point is located in the medial part of the tentorium. Drainages into the retrograde leptomeningeal venous drainage to the brainstem is observed. (**b**) Right internal carotid artery angiography (lateral view) demonstrates a dural arteriovenous fistula associated with a large venous aneurysm. The shunt point is located in the medial part of the tentorium. Drainages into the retrograde leptomeningeal venous drainage to the brainstem was observed. (**c**) Selective angiography from the right middle meningeal artery (frontal view) showing retrograde leptomeningeal venous drainage to the brainstem. (**d**) Selective angiography from the right meningohypophyseal artery (lateral view) showing retrograde leptomeningeal venous drainage to the brainstem. (**e**) The right common carotid artery angiography (frontal view) after treatment showing disappearance of the dural arteriovenous fistula. (**f**) The right common carotid artery angiography (lateral view) after treatment showing disappearance of the dural arteriovenous fistula

References

1. Elhammady MS, Ambekar S, Heros RC. Epidemiology, clinical presentation, diagnostic evaluation, and prognosis of cerebral dural arteriovenous fistulas. Handb Clin Neurol. 2017;143:99–105.
2. Pan DH, Wu HM, Kuo YH, Chung WY, Lee CC, Guo WY. Intracranial dural arteriovenous fistulas: natural history and rationale for treatment with stereotactic radiosurgery. Prog Neurol Surg. 2013;27:176–94.
3. Nambu K, Misaki K, Yoshikawa A, Kamide T, Nambu I, Sasagawa Y, Uchiyama N, Nakada M. Cavernous sinus dural arteriovenous fistula with an enhanced lesion in the brainstem mimicking a malignant tumor. World Neurosurg. 2020;140:13–7.
4. Zhang H, Liang S, Lv X. Intra-aneurysmal thrombosis and turbulent flow on MRI of large and giant internal carotid artery aneurysms. Neurosci Informatics. 2021;1(4): 100027. https://doi.org/10.1016/j.neuri.2021.100027.
5. Lv X, Li Y, Jiang C, Zhang J, Wu Z. Venous infarction associated with a sigmoid sinus dural arteriovenous fistula: case report. Neuroradiol J. 2008;21:579–83.
6. Pinker K, Stavrou I, Knosp E, Trattnig S. Are cerebral cavernomas truly nonenhancing lesions and thereby distinguishable from arteriovenous malformations? MRI findings and histopathological correlation. Magn Reson Imaging. 2006;24(5):631–7.
7. Liu P, Chen X, You W, Li Y, Lv M, Lv X. Hemorrhagic risk factors of endovascular onyx embolization of intracranial dural arteriovenous fistulas. Interv Neuroradiol. 2020;26(5):643–50.

5 Endovascular Treatment for Traumatic Internal Carotid Cavernous Fistula: Current Difficulties and Solutions

Kun Hou, Xianli Lv, Yunbao Guo, and Jinlu Yu

Abstract

Traumatic internal carotid-cavernous fistulas (TICCF) are uncommon, and endovascular treatment (EVT) is the first-line treatment for most TICCF cases. The EVT techniques for TICCF need a complete understanding. Therefore, we performed a review. At the same time, some illusive educational cases were provided. In this review, the following were discussed: the angioarchitecture of TICCF, the EVT principle, the transarterial EVT technique, the transvenous or combined transarterial EVT techniques, the EVT of bilateral and recurrent TICCFs, and the complications and prognosis of EVT. We considered that a deep understanding of the EVT strategy for TICCF was necessary and that a good prognosis could be obtained.

Keywords

Traumatic internal carotid cavernous fistula · Endovascular treatment · Review

K. Hou · Y. Guo · J. Yu (✉)
Department of Neurosurgery, First Hospital of Jilin University, Changchun, China
e-mail: jlyu@jlu.edu.cn

X. Lv
Department of Neurosurgery, Beijing Tsinghua Changgung Hospital, School of Clinical Medicine, Tsinghua University, Beijing, China

5.1 Introduction

During craniomaxillofacial trauma, shearing forces and/or bony spicules can lead to weakness of the muscular wall of the internal carotid artery (ICA) or cause an ICA laceration, producing an arteriovenous shunt from a high-flow ICA into a low-flow cavernous sinus (CS), and a traumatic internal carotid-cavernous fistula (TICCF) occurs [1]. TICCF belongs to Barrow type A and often occurs within a few weeks (often in 8 weeks) after the trauma [2].

TICCFs have been reported to occur in 0.2% of patients with craniocerebral trauma and in up to 4% of patients who have a skull base fracture [3]. Previously, in China, TICCF was common; now, due to legislation making the use of protective gear and restraint devices in vehicles compulsory, TICCF is not so common [4]. Untreated TICCFs will lead to visual loss, neurologic deficits, intracranial hemorrhage, etc. [5, 6]. Spontaneous regression of TICCFs is extremely rare [7, 8]. Therefore, active treatment is necessary.

Currently, endovascular treatment (EVT) is the first-line treatment for most TICCF cases. However, due to the anatomic complexity of the CS, the ICA tortuosity and the presence of high-flow communication make TICCF closure challenging. Currently, there is not a complete and thorough understanding of the EVT techniques for TICCF to improve the treatment success.

X. Lv (ed.), *Intracranial and Spinal Dural Arteriovenous Fistulas*,
https://doi.org/10.1007/978-981-19-5767-3_5

Therefore, this review is important, and some educational cases are also illustrated.

5.2 Angioarchitecture of TICCF

5.2.1 Feeding Artery

Most commonly, the ICA is the only feeding artery, and the cavernous ICA is particularly prone to rupture owing to its tethering by dural rings at its entry and exit points to and from the CS region [9]. According to Debrun et al.'s classification of the course of the ICA in the CS and adjacent skeletal structures, it can be divided into five segments: C1, anterior ascending segment; C2, anterior genu segment; C3, horizontal segment; C4, posterior genu segment; C5, posterior ascending segment [10]. Ruptures are most commonly located on the proximal and middle ICA in the CS, which appears to be more vulnerable to injury [11]. Tears can be classified as small, medium or large [11]. An incomplete tear can result in a delayed rupture [12].

In addition, when the ipsilateral ICA is occluded, retrograde feeding to the TICCF can be seen, including the anterior communicating artery (AcomA) from the contralateral ICA and the ipsilateral posterior communicating artery (PcomA) from the posterior circulation [13]. Rarely, the external carotid artery (ECA) can be recruited as the feeder due to long-term venous hypertension and thrombosis in the CS [14, 15]. The feeding arteries of TICCF are shown in Fig. 5.1.

5.2.2 CS State and Fistula

CS is a structure that is 2 cm long, 1 cm wide and 1.3 cm tall [16]. It is an extradural space that is in direct continuity through the clivus and the basiocciput with the epidural space of the spinal canal [17]. The bilateral CS communicates via the anterior and posterior circular sinuses. CS is maintained by multiple sinusoids, allowing the venous blood flow to be quite slow and be of low pressure (Fig. 5.2a, b). In TICCF, high-pressure arterial blood directly flowed into the CS, leading to the CS, and its tributaries were remodeled and dilated (Fig. 5.2c, d).

According to the shunt volume from the ICA into the CS, TICCFs can be classified into high-,

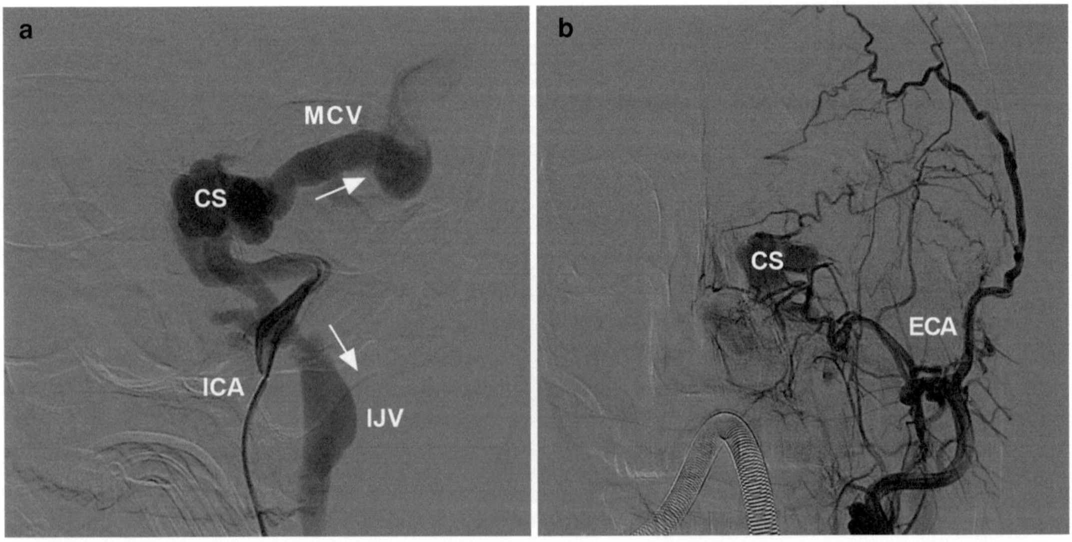

Fig. 5.1 Feeding arteries of TICCF. (**a**) An arterial early-phase DSA of the ICA showed the TICCF, and the MCV was dilated. (**b**) Arterial phase DSA of the ECA showed that the ECA supplied the TICCF. *Abbreviations*: *CS* cavernous sinus, *DSA* digital subtracted angiography, *ECA* external carotid artery, *ICA* internal carotid artery, *IJV* internal jugular vein, *MCV* middle cerebral vein, *TICCF* traumatic internal carotid cavernous fistula

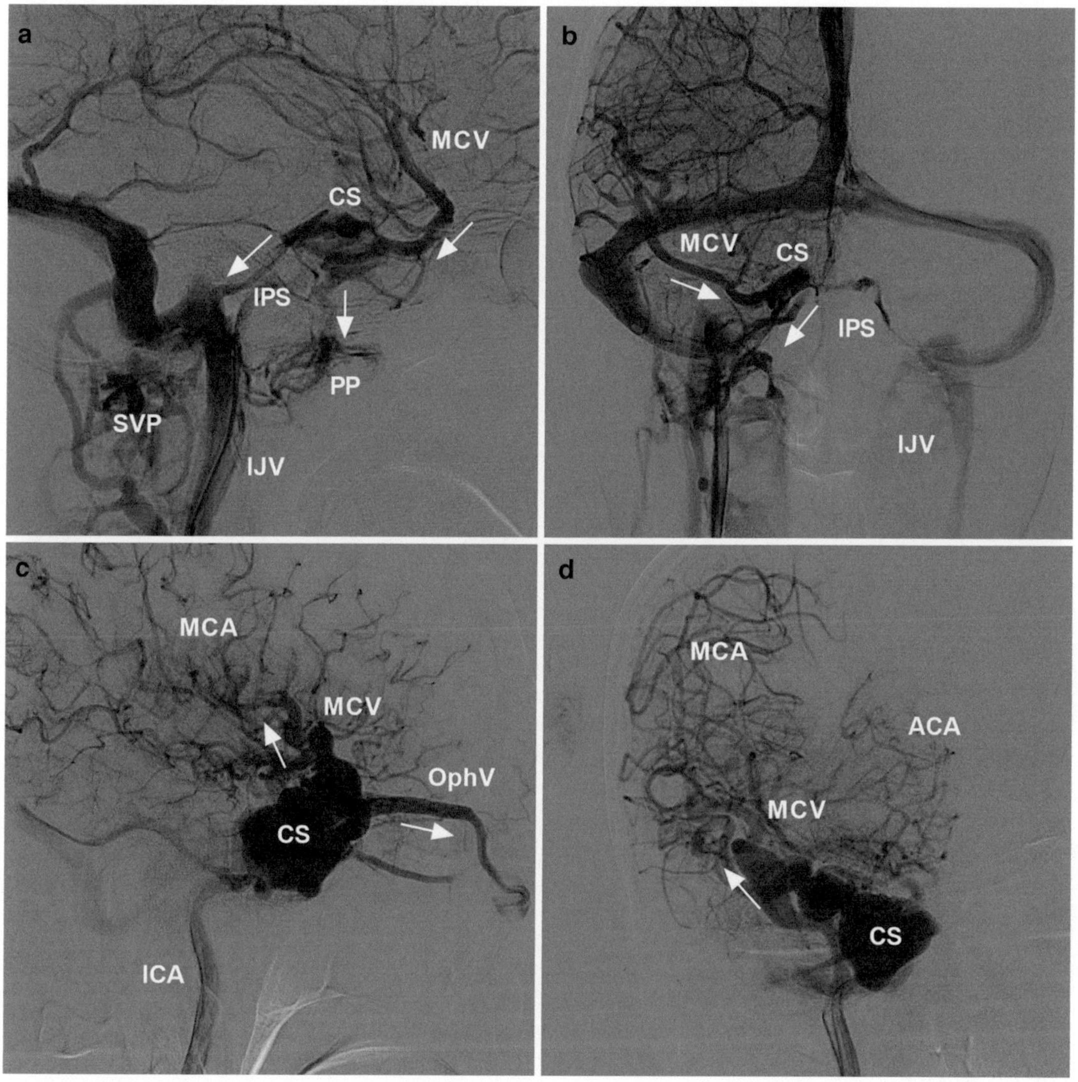

Fig. 5.2 Venous drainage of CS in a normal state and with TICCF. (**a**, **b**) A venous-phase DSA of the ICA showed that the normal CS accepted the blood flow from the MCV (arrow) and drained to the IPS (arrow) and PP (arrow). (**a**) Shows the lateral view, and (**b**) shows the anterior posterior view. (**c**, **d**) Arterial-phase DSA of the ICA showed, in TICCF the high-pressure arterial blood flow into the CS, the blood flow of MCA (arrow) and OphV (arrow) reversed, the MCA and ACA can be seen, (**c**) was lateral view, (**d**) was the anterior posterior view. *Abbreviations*: *ACA* anterior cerebral artery, *CS* cavernous sinus, *DSA* digital subtracted angiography, *ICA* internal carotid artery, *IJV* internal jugular vein, *IPS* inferior petrous sinus, *MCA* middle cerebral artery, *MCV* middle cerebral vein, *OphV* ophthalmic vein, *PP* pterygoid plexus, *SVP* suboccipital venous plexus, *TICCF* traumatic internal carotid cavernous fistula

intermediate- and low-flow types [18]. In high-flow TICCF, the entire shunt volume enters the CS without the filling of intracranial vessels. In intermediate-flow TICCFs, both the TICCF and the ipsilateral intracranial arteries are supplied with blood from the ICA. In low-flow TICCF, only mild arteriovenous shunting into the CS exists [19].

These dilated structures and the high-low shunts often make the TICCF angioarchitecture unclear. Therefore, it is necessary to slow the blood flow for better delineation of the fistula site. Injection of the ICA and manual compression of the ipsilateral common carotid artery are helpful. It is feasible to perform the maneuver using a balloon-guiding catheter to replace manual compression [20]. In addition, vertebral artery/contralateral ICA injections while occluding or compressing the ICA proximal to the site of the fistula can help visualize the exact site of the fistula by displaying retrograde AcomA and PcomA filling [21].

5.2.3 Draining Path

Normal CS receives blood flow anteriorly from the ophthalmic veins (OphVs) and superiorly from the sphenoparietal sinus, cortical veins and middle meningeal vein; it drains posteriorly into the inferior petrosal sinus (IPS) and superior petrosal sinus (SPS) and basilar plexus of veins, inferiorly into the pterygoid plexus via emissary veins (Fig. 5.2a, b). In TICCF, the hemodynamic pressure caused dilation and arterialization of the CS and draining veins, even presenting with a monstrous size. The blood flow in the OphVs and sphenoparietal sinus and cortical veins are reversed (Fig. 5.2c, d) [22, 23]. Due to the communication of the anterior and posterior circular sinuses, contralateral or bilateral drainages of the TICCF are common [23, 24].

5.2.4 Relationship Between Symptoms and Venous Drainage

The TICCF symptoms depended on the shunt degree and the route of venous drainage. The symptoms included CS high-pressure congestion and the flow-related water-hammer effect, retrograde venous drainage and arterial steal [25]. Due to the communication of both CSs, the symptoms may occur on the opposite side of the fistula or bilaterally [23, 24].

High-pressure congestion in CS can result in headache in 25–84% of patients with TICCFs and cranial nerve compression in 17–44% of patients [3]. Cranial nerve III was compressed against the CS roof, cranial nerve IV was compressed against the tentorial edge, and cranial nerve VI was compressed against the petroclinoid ligament [26, 27]. The first affected nerve is usually cranial nerve VI because it crosses through the CS, while cranial nerves III and IV are protected inside the dural duplication of the CS.

High-pressure congestion of the OphV system can result in proptosis in 72–98% of patients with TICCFs, chemosis in 55–100% of patients and pulsatile bruits in 71–80% patients. The other symptoms include progressive visual loss in 18% of the patients with TICCFs and eye pain [3]. Superficial and deep venous systems may be in a congestive state, resulting in focal neurological deficits, seizures and venous infarction; even intracranial hemorrhage can occur in 0.9–2.6% of TICCFs [3, 11, 28, 29]. The presence of a subarachnoid venous pouch has been described as an indicator of a high risk of bleeding [11].

Under high pressure, the CS can rupture into the fractured sphenoid sinus; the pterygoid plexus can also rupture, resulting in bleeding of the mouth, nose (epistaxis), or ears [30, 31]. The steal phenomenon can cause life-threatening or fatal complications when the collateral circulation from the circle of Willis is insufficient [32].

Rarely, CS can drain into the posterior fossa vein via the SPS draining to the lateral mesencephalic vein or cervical cord perimedullary vein via the basal vein of Rosenthal and into the deep vein, resulting in venous infarction of the brainstem, basal ganglia and spinal cord, and this will produce the corresponding deficits [33–38]. However, although many TICCFs experience venous drainage to the posterior fossa, the associated complications remain an uncommon finding.

5.3 EVT Principle and Choices

The EVT principle's goal is to occlude the shunt and preserve the ICA, and the CS has to be sacrificed and accept the packing [39]. Early EVT is necessary, which could reduce the morbidity of a deteriorating visual acuity [40]. In the presence of retrograde cortical venous and vital organ drainage, it is essential to obliterate this portion of the drainage first, avoiding disastrous consequences. A complete EVT is the ideal goal. It is helpful to convert the high-flow to a low-flow, low-pressure TICCF, which may lead to a spontaneous resolution due to the thrombosis [41]. However, retrograde cortical venous drainage or vital organ drainage is not permitted.

EVT includes transarterial or transvenous embolization (TAE/TVE) and reconstructive or deconstructive techniques. The endovascular devices included detachable balloon, coil, liquid embolic agents (Onyx (Medtronic, Irvine, California, USA) and NBCA glue), covered stent and flow diversion (FD), etc. [23, 24, 42–46]. Liquid embolic agents have rarely been solely used, and they are often combined with coils under the protection of the balloon [47, 48].

If ICA reconstruction is difficult or impossible, deconstructive sacrifice of the ICA has to be performed. In addition, when all EVTs had failed, a direct surgical approach with/without vascular reconstructive surgery has to be the last resort [49, 50].

5.4 Transarterial EVT Technique

In TAE, the microcatheter needed to be advanced carefully into the CS to deliver the embolic materials, and these include reconstructive and deconstructive techniques.

5.4.1 Reconstructive with Detachable Balloon or Coils

Currently, the standard treatment is still the use of a detachable balloon as a simple, effective and inexpensive method (Fig. 5.3). Approximately 85% of TICCFs can be successfully treated [51]. However, the rate of failure and recurrence can increase to 10% due to the failure of its delivery into CS, early detachment, rupture of the balloon caused by bone fragments, balloon displacement after it has been detached, etc. [25]. In large fistulae with high flow and CS enlargement, multiple balloons may be required, and their treatment may be complicated.

When a balloon was not available or if balloon catheterization had failed, coiling is also a good choice, especially for a small fistula, and the coils may be adjusted or even removed if the placement is not optimal. If the fistula was large, stent or balloon-assisted coiling is helpful (Fig. 5.4) [47, 52–55]. If coiling cannot occlude the TICCF, liquid embolic agents can also be added [56]. The coils should be placed first and can provide a framework for the liquid embolic agents. According to our experience, the microcatheter to cast Onyx should be placed deeper in the CS, and this can avoid the reflux of Onyx into the ICA, which could cause penetration into the CS compartment (Fig. 5.5). Certainly, a temporary balloon should be placed across the fistula to avoid the distal migration of liquid embolic material [52, 53].

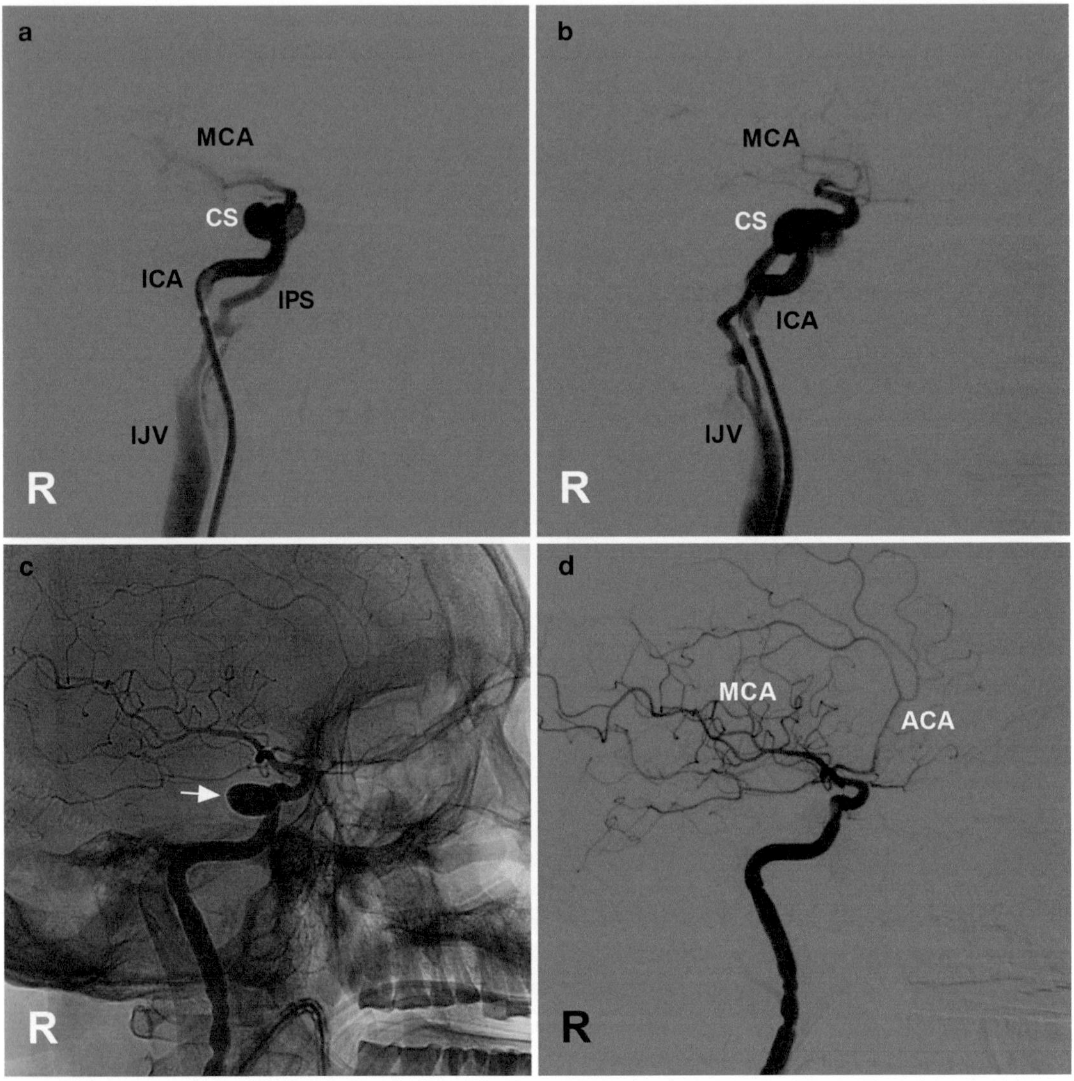

Fig. 5.3 TAE of the TICCF with the detachable balloon. (**a**, **b**) An early arterial phase DSA of the right ICA showed the TICCF drained into the IPS, and the MCA was unclear, (**a**) was anterior posterior view, (**b**) was the lateral view. (**c**) A unsubtracted DSA showed that the balloon (arrow) was deployed into the CS. (**d**) After the detachable balloon was deployed, the DSA showed that the TICCF was cured, and the ACA and MCA were shown clearly in the arterial phase. *Abbreviations*: *ACA* anterior cerebral artery, *CS* cavernous sinus, *DSA* digital subtracted angiography, *ICA* internal carotid artery, *IJV* internal jugular vein, *IPS* inferior petrous sinus, *MCA* middle cerebral artery, *R* right, *TAE* transarterial embolization, *TICCF* traumatic internal carotid cavernous fistula

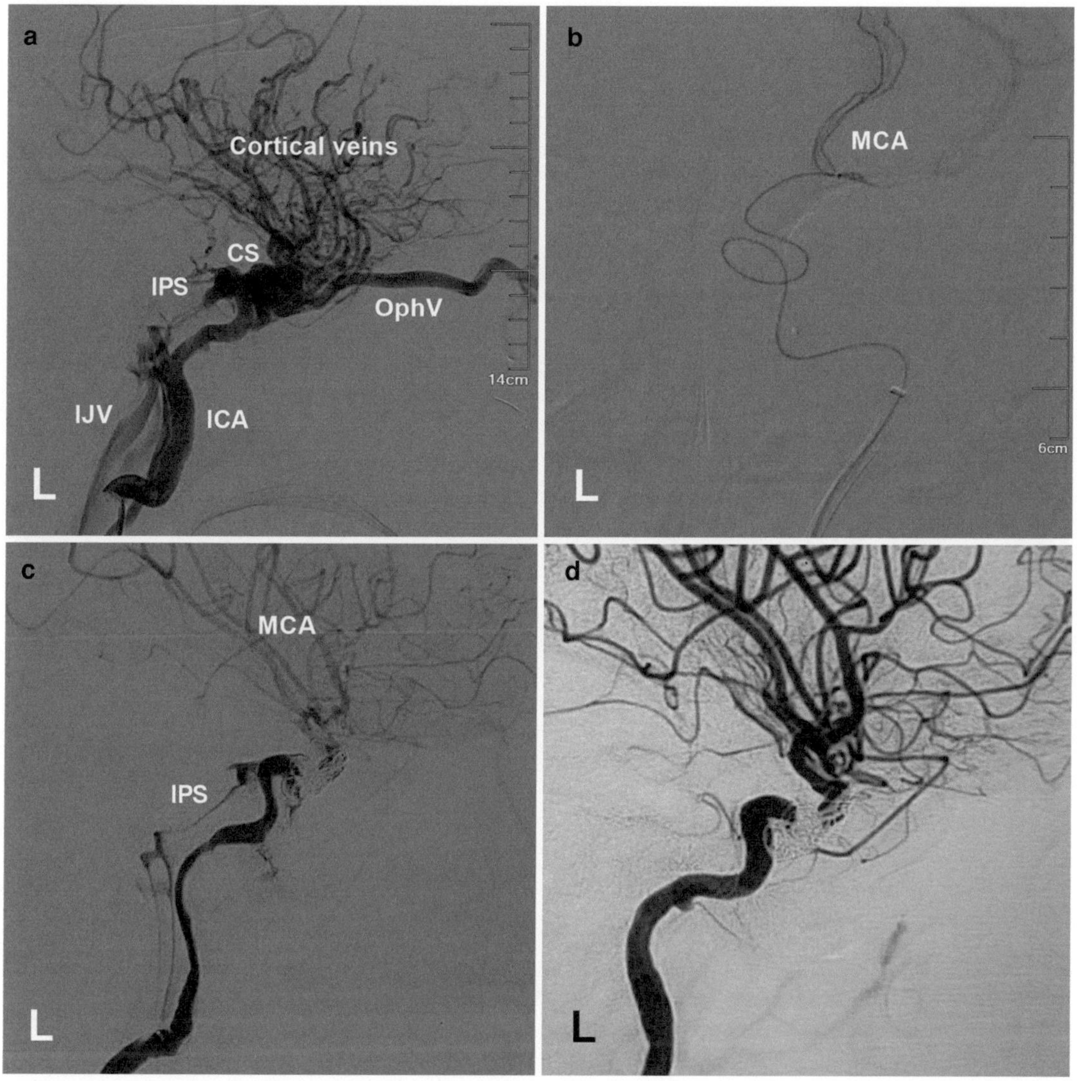

Fig. 5.4 TAE of TICCF with stent-assisted coiling. (**a**, **b**) An early arterial phase DSA of the lateral view of the left ICA showed that the TICCF drained into the OphV, IPS and cortical veins, and the MCA was not seen. (**b**) After a microcatheter was passed through the fistula into the MCA, the selective angiogram confirmed the microcatheter position. (**c**) After stent-assisted coiling for the TICCF, the OphV and cortical veins were not seen, but IPS drainage was left in the late arterial phase. (**d**) Follow-up DSA of the lateral view of the left ICA showed that the TICCF was cured. *Abbreviations*: *CS* cavernous sinus, *DSA* digital subtracted angiography, *ICA* internal carotid artery, *IJV* internal jugular vein, *IPS* inferior petrous sinus, *L* left, *MCA* middle cerebral artery, *OphV* ophthalmic vein, *TAE* transarterial embolization, *TICCF* traumatic internal carotid cavernous fistula

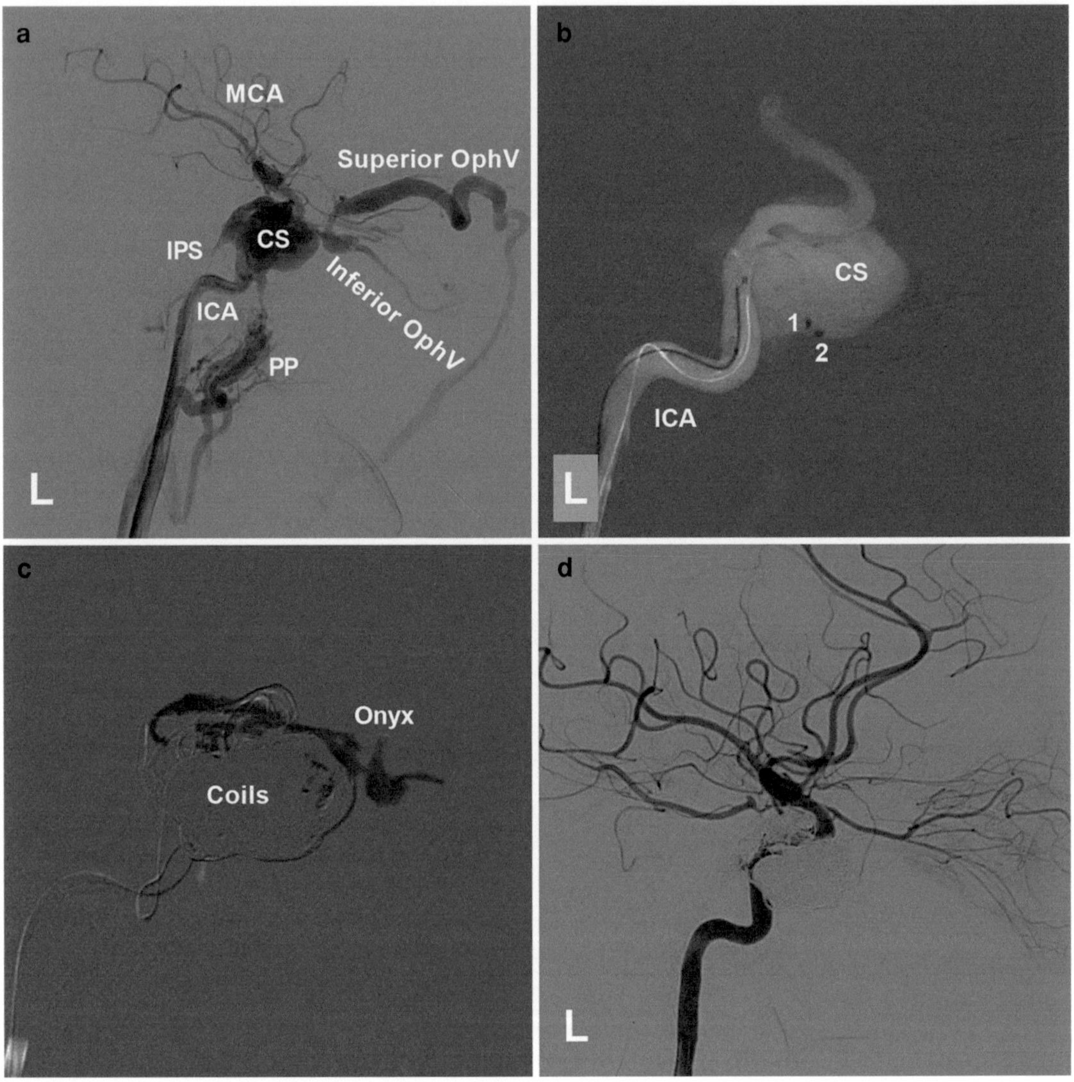

Fig. 5.5 TAE of TICCF with the combination of coiling and Onyx. (**a**, **b**) An early arterial phase DSA of the lateral view of the left ICA showed that the TICCF drained into the superior and inferior OphVs, IPS and PP, and the MCA could be seen. (**b**) The roadmap shows that the two microcatheters (numbers 1 and 2) were put into the CS. (**c**) The roadmap shows that after the coiling had finished framing, Onyx was cast. (**d**) DSA of the left ICA showed that TICCF was cured. *Abbreviations*: *CS* cavernous sinus, *DSA* digital subtracted angiography, *ICA* internal carotid artery, *IPS* inferior petrous sinus, *L* left, *MCA* middle cerebral artery, *OphV* ophthalmic vein, *PP* pterygoid plexus, *TICCF* traumatic internal carotid cavernous fistula

5.4.2 Reconstructive with Covered Stent and FD

5.4.2.1 Covered Stent

For the treatment of TICCFs, covered stent deployment can be an alternative [57]. After successful deployment of the covered stent, the TICCFs can be immediately cured [42]. The deployment of covered stents in the high cavernous segment of the ICA is challenging due to its stiffness. The covered stent is easily applied to the lower petrous segment of the ICA (Fig. 5.6).

To deliver the covered stent, a good support system is necessary. A Penumbra Neuron guiding catheter (Penumbra Inc., San Leandro, California, USA)

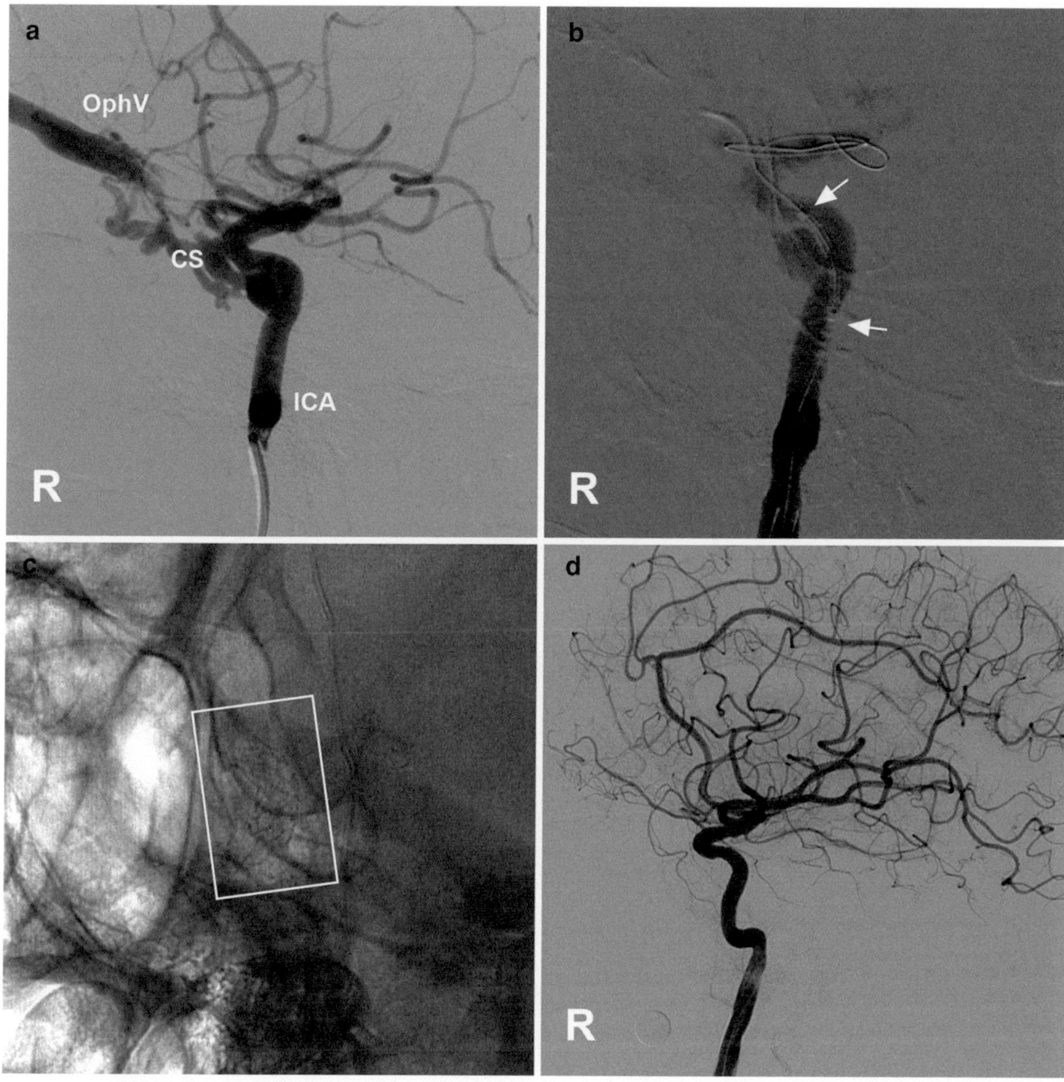

Fig. 5.6 TAE of TICCF with the covered stent deployment. (**a**) An early arterial phase DSA of the lateral view of the right ICA showed that the TICCF drained into the superior OphV. (**b**) The covered stent crossed the fistula, and the arrows show its tip and the end of the stent. (**c**) The X-ray film showed that the stent was released (frame). (**d**) A DSA of the right ICA showed that the TICCF was cured. *Abbreviations*: *CS* cavernous sinus, *DSA* digital subtracted angiography, *ICA* internal carotid artery, *OphV* ophthalmic vein, *R* right, *TICCF* traumatic internal carotid cavernous fistula

associated with a 5F Navien intermediate catheter (Medtronic, Irvine, California, USA) is helpful for this technique. A Navien intermediate catheter can pass through or can pass close to the fistula, and then it is easy to deliver the covered stent.

However, the covered stent has other drawbacks, and it is quite thrombogenic, thus further exposing the patient to risks of distal emboli and strokes. Moreover, it necessitates the need for dual antiplatelet therapy, which can be hazardous and even contraindicated in the setting of acute brain trauma. In addition, endoleaks are not uncommon.

5.4.2.2 Flow Diversion

Recently, FD has become an option, especially for low-flow TICCFs, by reducing arteriovenous shunts to induce thrombosis in the CS [58–60]. FD can also serve as a scaffold and enables endothelial overgrowth of the lacerated ICA. TICCF can be cured by the sole use of an FD [61]. However, FD deployment will be associated with endoleak. Therefore, assisted coiling is recommended [62]. FD deployment will reduce the need for extensive coil packing in the CS and thus will minimize the mass effect. To reduce endoleaks, multiple FD overlaps have also been suggested [59, 60, 63].

However, FD has drawbacks, and FD deployment requires long-term antiaggregation, which slows the complete occlusion of a TICCF. In addition, multiple FDs increase the risk of distal emboli and stent occlusion [63].

5.4.3 Deconstruction with ICA Trapping

In extensive ICA damage with good collateral circulation, if reconstructive EVT is difficult or impossible, an ICA sacrifice can be performed (Fig. 5.7). To trap the ICA, both the proximal and distal segments of the ICA across the TICCF should be occluded using a detachable balloon coiled with/without liquid embolic agents and a Micro Vascular Plug System (MVP) (Medtronic, Irvine, California, USA) [64]. When casting the liquid embolic agents, the embolization of unwanted territory must be avoided.

Sometimes, ipsilateral ICA trapping is not easy because the high-flow shunt results in the inability to visualize the distal ICA or due to the difficulty navigating into the distal ICA. The dis-

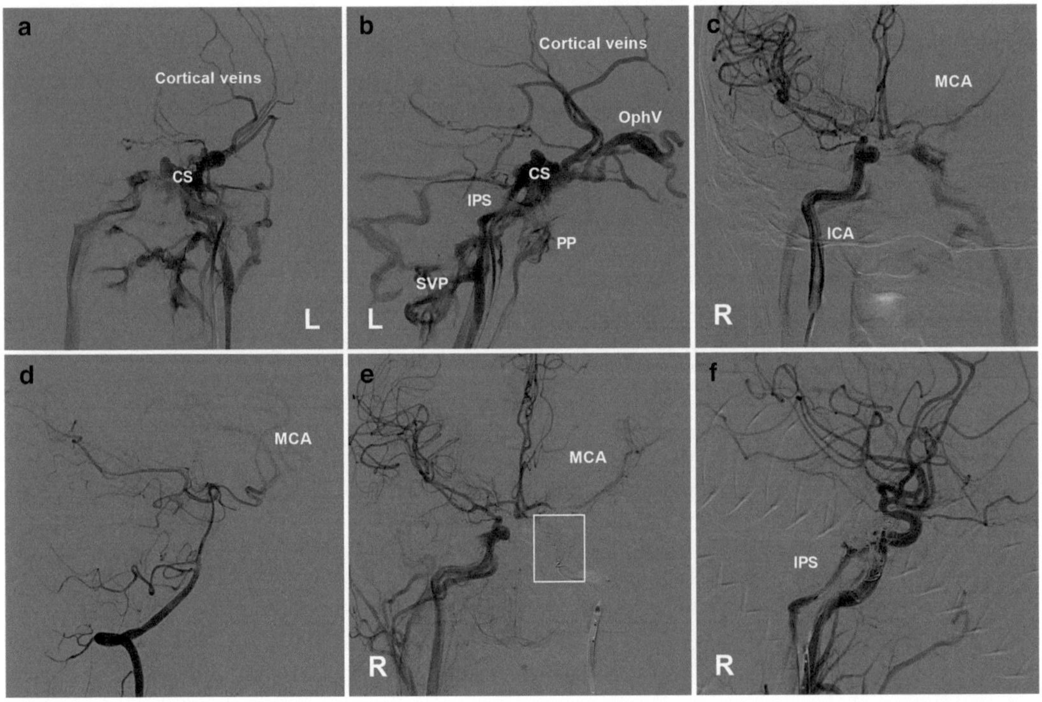

Fig. 5.7 Transarterial trapping for the TICCF. (**a**, **b**) Early arterial phase DSA of the left ICA showed that the TICCF drained into the OphV, IPS, PP and cortical veins, (**a**) was anterior posterior view, (**b**) was the lateral view. (**c**) DSA of the right ICA showed that the left MCA was compensated via the AcomA from the right ICA system, and a right TICCF was also found. (**d**) A DSA of the VA showed that the left MCA was compensated via the posterior circulation via the PcomA. (**e**, **f**) A DSA of the right ICA showed that the left MCA had good compensation from the right ICA after ICA trapping, and the right TICCA was not treated. (**e**) Shows the anterior posterior view, (**f**) shows the lateral view, (**e**) shows the location of the trapping, and (**f**) shows the right low-flow CCF. *Abbreviations*: *AcomA* anterior communicating artery, *CCF* carotid cavernous fistula, *CS* cavernous sinus, *DSA* digital subtracted angiography, *ICA* internal carotid artery, *IJV* internal jugular vein, *IPS* inferior petrous sinus, *MCA* middle cerebral artery, *OphV* ophthalmic vein, *PcomA* posterior communicating artery, *PP* pterygoid plexus, *R* right, *SVP* suboccipital venous plexus, *TICCF* traumatic internal carotid cavernous fistula

tal ICA is difficult to be occluded. At this time, the retrograde path through the contralateral AcomA and ipsilateral PcomA can be a treatment choice, even if it is the only way [65–67]. In addition, when the TICCF was associated with an ipsilateral ICA occlusion due to traumatic dissection, the retrograde path was the only way [65, 66].

5.5 Transvenous or Combined Transarterial EVT Techniques

The need for a transvenous approach is uncommon, especially when TAE is hampered. Alternatively, after incomplete TAE of the fistula, further canulation of the fistula was not possible via the arterial route. In addition, TVE combined with TAE can be a good choice [68]. Under high pressure, the CS and its tributaries become very thick, and it is not difficult to reach the CS. The transvenous routes included the IPS, SPS, OphV, facial vein, pterygoid plexus, etc., and the most common path was the IPS [69]. Other transvenous strategies, such as the OphV, facial vein and pterygoid plexus, are difficult and are less reproducible [70, 71].

During TVE, the protective balloon may be inflated in the ICA during coiling or when casting the liquid embolic agents (Fig. 5.8). In addi-

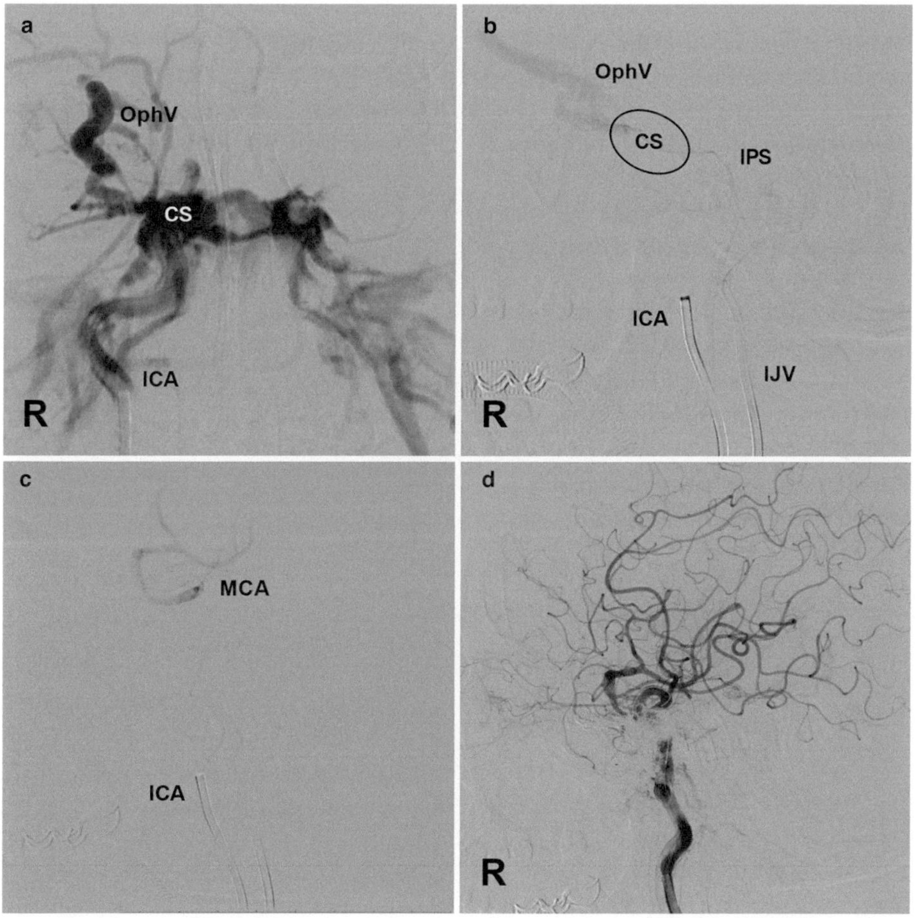

Fig. 5.8 Combined transarterial and transvenous EVT for the TICCF. (**a**) Early arterial phase DSA of the right ICA showed that the TICCF mainly drained into the OphV. (**b**) After a microcatheter was navigated into the CS via IPS, a superselective angiogram showed the OphV drainage. (**c**) After the balloon microcatheter crossed the TICCF, the superselective angiogram showed the MCA. (**d**) After balloon protection in the ICA, coiling was performed via the transvenous path. The DSA of the right ICA showed the TICCF was cured. *Abbreviations*: *CS* cavernous sinus, *DSA* digital subtracted angiography, *ICA* internal carotid artery, *IJV* internal jugular vein, *IPS* inferior petrous sinus, *MCA* middle cerebral artery, *OphV* ophthalmic vein, *R* right, *TICCF* traumatic internal carotid cavernous fistula

tion, when FD is deployed, the combined transvenous path to pack the CS with coiling is a good choice [59].

5.6 Special Types of TICCF

5.6.1 Bilateral TICCFs

Bilateral TICCFs occur in approximately 1–2% of TICCFs cases (Fig. 5.7) [72]. They often have severe symptoms; the arterial steal phenomenon is not uncommon [73]. Bilateral TICCFs are not necessarily followed by bilateral symptoms, and they may also present with unilateral or contralateral symptoms [74]. EVT is challenging for bilateral TICCFs because sacrificing the ICAs on both sides is likely to cause cerebral hypoperfusion [75].

Compromised flow in the ICA due to therapeutic occlusion may sufficiently increase the intravascular pressure on the contralateral side to expand the shunt. Therefore, bilateral TCCFs should be treated simultaneously [76, 77]. However, if the first fistular anatomy is complex or is difficult to approach and the procedure is long time and associated with potential risk, treatment of the second fistula at another session is also acceptable [73].

For bilateral TICCFs and for patients who accept treated with TAE, sometimes the unilateral venous approach can finish the EVT of the contralateral or bilateral TICCFs by crossing the midline via the anterior or posterior circular sinuses [78].

5.6.2 Recurrent TICCF

After EVT, TICCFs have a substantial 10–28% recurrence rate [79]. Detachable balloons are prone to recurrence compared with detachable coils in the treatment of TICCFs [51, 80]. Recurrent TICCFs require a more difficult and complex EVT [79, 81]. When the recurrence symptoms are mild, the patient's vision is not immediately at risk, or if the shunt flow is small and slow, conservative follow-up care should be attempted first. In addition, an aggressive EVT is needed.

In recurrent TICCF, if the first EVT was the detachable balloon, the navigation of additional balloons into the fistula is often unsuccessful because a prematurely deflated or migrated balloon may partially block the orifice of the fistula; coiling is a good choice for these types of lesions [51]. When the ipsilateral ICA approach is difficult, the retrograde path through the AcomA and PcomA can be performed [65, 66]. In addition, the transvenous approach is an alternative method. A covered stent can be tried.

5.7 Complications

The percentage of patients experiencing morbidity associated with EVT of TICCFs has ranged from 10% to 40% [82]. Most of the complications have been mild and have resolved spontaneously [19].

5.7.1 Technique Complication

This type of complication included coil loops protruding into the ICA, balloon displacement, and unintended distal embolization of liquid embolic agents. Careful manipulation and good therapeutic strategies are necessary.

5.7.2 Cranial Nerve Palsy

The complication was mainly from the compression of the coil mass. Cranial nerves III and VI are believed to be vulnerable to injury in distinct and anatomically separate areas of the CS. These injuries can be divided into immediate and delayed palsies. Late cranial nerve palsies may be due to chronic ischemia and delayed inflammation created by EVT materials [26]. To reduce the mass effect of the coils, targeted occlusion of the fistulous compartment of the CS becomes an option.

5.7.3 Ischemic Complication

Ischemic complications can be mainly from ICA trapping [83]. In general, ICA sacrifice is associated with a 1.4–1.9% annual risk of new neurological deficits due to ischemia [84]. Therefore, a balloon occlusion test (BOT) of the ICA should be carried out before permanent occlusion of the ICA. Even if patients have good tolerance to BOT, the ischemic complication rates range from 5% to 22% [85].

5.7.4 Trigeminocardiac Reflex

This reaction is a trigeminal depressor response, and patients can present with bradycardia and hypotension, which occurs as a consequence of acute stretching of the lateral wall of the CS, where the ophthalmic nerve runs and is innervated [86]. In the EVT of TICCFs, the rapid injection of liquid embolic materials, the injection of dimethyl sulfoxide, and even balloon embolization can result in the trigeminocardiac reflex [87].

5.8 Prognosis

The overall success rates of EVT have been reported to be 85% and 99% [61]. In a report by Chi et al. of 172 TICCFs, fistula occlusion under EVT was 94% with preservation of the ICA in 70% of patients with TICCFs [19]. In the study by Higashida et al. which was a report of more than 200 TICCFs, a complete occlusion was achieved in 99% of TICCFs and a preservation of the ICA was achieved in 88% of TICCFs [82]. The reported success rates to date of detachable balloons, FDs and covered stents for occlusion of TCCF as the primary treatment modality were 55–98%, 71%, and 75–100%, respectively [85].

Successful embolization of TICCF will result in immediate resolution of proptosis, chemosis, and bruits. The visual outcomes vary widely depending on the etiology, severity, and duration of the visual impairment, which may take 4 months to resolve. Cranial nerve palsy may resolve 1–2 months after treatment.

5.9 Summary

TICCF is uncommon, and EVT is the first-line treatment for most TICCF cases. A complete understanding of the EVT techniques is necessary, and the angioarchitecture of TICCF, EVT principle, transarterial EVT technique, the transvenous or combined transarterial EVT techniques, the EVT of the bilateral and recurrent TICCFs, and the complications and prognosis of the EVT should all be understood. We believe that a deep understanding of the EVT strategy for TICCF is necessary and that a good prognosis could be obtained.

References

1. Barrow DL, Spector RH, Braun IF, Landman JA, Tindall SC, Tindall GT. Classification and treatment of spontaneous carotid-cavernous sinus fistulas. J Neurosurg. 1985;62:248–56.
2. Nguyen T, Cho YH, Jang YJ, Park MC, Shin SJ. Long delayed traumatic carotid-cavernous sinus fistula. J Craniofac Surg. 2013;24:e237–9.
3. Ellis JA, Goldstein H, Connolly ES Jr, Meyers PM. Carotid-cavernous fistulas. Neurosurg Focus. 2012;32:E9.
4. Wu Z, Wang C, Yang X, Sun Y, Zhang Y, Li Y, et al. Endovascular embolization of traumatic carotid cavernous fistulas. Chin Med J (Engl). 1999;112:433–7.
5. Lang M, Habboub G, Mullin JP, Rasmussen PA. A brief history of carotid-cavernous fistula. J Neurosurg. 2017;126:1995–2001.
6. Albuquerque FC, Heinz GW, McDougall CG. Reversal of blindness after transvenous embolization of a carotid-cavernous fistula: case report. Neurosurgery. 2003;52:233–6; discussion 6–7.
7. Iampreechakul P, Tirakotai W, Tanpun A, Wattanasen Y, Lertbusayanukul P, Siriwimonmas S. Spontaneous resolution of direct carotid-cavernous fistulas: case series and literature review. Interv Neuroradiol. 2019;25:71–89.
8. Alkhani A, Willinsky R, TerBrugge K. Spontaneous resolution of bilateral traumatic carotid cavernous fistulas and development of trans-sellar intercarotid vascular communication: case report. Surg Neurol. 1999;52:627–9.

9. Fattahi TT, Brandt MT, Jenkins WS, Steinberg B. Traumatic carotid-cavernous fistula: pathophysiology and treatment. J Craniofac Surg. 2003;14:240–6.
10. Debrun G, Lacour P, Vinuela F, Fox A, Drake CG, Caron JP. Treatment of 54 traumatic carotid-cavernous fistulas. J Neurosurg. 1981;55:678–92.
11. Malan J, Lefeuvre D, Mngomezulu V, Taylor A. Angioarchitecture and treatment modalities in posttraumatic carotid cavernous fistulae. Interv Neuroradiol. 2012;18:178–86.
12. Chae SW, Choi G, Lee HM, Song JJ, Choi JO, Seol HY. Intrasaccular detachable platinum coil embolization for traumatic pseudoaneurysm treatment of a cavernous carotid artery. Otolaryngol Head Neck Surg. 2001;124:230–1.
13. Lo D, Vallee JN, Bitar A, Guillevin R, Lejean L, Van Effenterre R, et al. Endovascular management of carotid-cavernous fistula combined with ipsilateral internal carotid artery occlusion due to gunshot: contra-lateral arterial approach. Acta Neurochir. 2004;146:403–6; discussion 6.
14. Gao BL, Zhao W, Xu GP. The development of a de novo indirect carotid-cavernous fistula after successful occlusion of bilateral direct carotid-cavernous fistulas. J Trauma. 2009;66:E28–31.
15. Yoshino H, Ishihara H, Oka F, Kato S, Suzuki M. Development of indirect cavernous dural arteriovenous fistula after trapping for direct carotid cavernous fistula. A case report. Interv Neuroradiol. 2011;17:104–7.
16. Parkinson D. Lateral sellar compartment: history and anatomy. J Craniofac Surg. 1995;6:55–68.
17. Parkinson D. Extradural neural axis compartment. J Neurosurg. 2000;92:585–8.
18. van Rooij WJ, Sluzewski M, Beute GN. Ruptured cavernous sinus aneurysms causing carotid cavernous fistula: incidence, clinical presentation, treatment, and outcome. AJNR Am J Neuroradiol. 2006;27:185–9.
19. Chi CT, Nguyen D, Duc VT, Chau HH, Son VT. Direct traumatic carotid cavernous fistula: angiographic classification and treatment strategies. Study of 172 cases. Interv Neuroradiol. 2014;20:461–75.
20. Jeong DE, Kim JW, Kim BM, Hwang W, Kim DJ. Impact of balloon-guiding catheter location on recanalization in patients with acute stroke treated by mechanical thrombectomy. AJNR Am J Neuroradiol. 2019;40:840–4.
21. Luo CB, Chang FC, Teng MM, Lirrng JF, Chen SS. Endovascular embolization of carotid-cavernous fistula using the posterior communicating artery approach: a case report. Kaohsiung J Med Sci. 2001;17:112–5.
22. Hayashi K, Suyama K, Nagata I. Traumatic carotid cavernous fistula complicated with intracerebral hemorrhage: case report. Neurol Med Chir (Tokyo). 2011;51:214–6.
23. Chavan RG, Kamble RB, Bonde V. Endovascular treatment in an unusual case of direct carotid cavernous fistula. Neuroradiol J. 2014;27:207–12.
24. Kasturi N, Kumari P, Nagarajan G, Krishnan N. Post-traumatic carotid-cavernous fistula with bilateral proptosis simulating cavernous sinus thrombosis. BMJ Case Rep. 2019;12:e227757.
25. Zenteno M, Santos-Franco J, Rodriguez-Parra V, Balderrama J, Aburto-Murrieta Y, Vega-Montesinos S, et al. Management of direct carotid-cavernous sinus fistulas with the use of ethylene-vinyl alcohol (Onyx) only: preliminary results. J Neurosurg. 2010;112:595–602.
26. Bou Ghannam A, Subramanian PS. Delayed onset cranial nerve palsies after endovascular coil embolization of direct carotid-cavernous fistulas. J Neuroophthalmol. 2018;38:156–9.
27. Peng TJ, Stretz C, Mageid R, Mac Grory B, Yaghi S, Matouk C, et al. Carotid-cavernous fistula presenting with bilateral abducens palsy. Stroke. 2020;51:e107–10.
28. Krishnan V, Searls DE, Haussen DC, Henninger N, Thomas A. Venous ischemia secondary to drainage constriction in a carotid-cavernous arteriovenous fistula. Clin Neurol Neurosurg. 2013;115:1476–8.
29. Klevtsova E, Nguyen-Min C, Lalani T, Carlan SJ, Madruga M. Posttraumatic carotid cavernous fistula that presented as seizure and focal neurological deficits with symptom resolution after therapeutic coil embolization. J Emerg Med. 2015;48:186–90.
30. Koekkoek JA, Lycklama à Nijeholt GJ, Jellema K, Walchenbach R. Traumatic carotid-cavernous fistula combined with pseudoaneurysm requires immediate treatment. BMJ Case Rep. 2013;2013. https://doi.org/10.1136/bcr-2013-009013.
31. Ko JK, Lee SW, Lee TH, Choi CH. Traumatic carotid cavernous fistula with a connection between the supraclinoid internal carotid artery and cavernous sinus via a pseudoaneurysm presenting with delayed life-threatening epistaxis. NMC Case Rep J. 2017;4:43–6.
32. Iida K, Kurisu K, Arita K, Ohba S, Shibukawa M, Ohtani M, et al. Critical cerebral ischemia revealed by magnetic resonance imaging in a traumatic carotid-cavernous fistula without high-risk patterns on angiograms: a case report. J Trauma. 2002;53:109–11.
33. Yu J, Guo Y, Zhao S, Xu K. Brainstem edema caused by traumatic carotid-cavernous fistula: a case report and review of the literature. Exp Ther Med. 2015;10:445–50.
34. Bussiere M, Lownie SP, Pelz DM, Nicolle D. Direct carotid-cavernous fistula causing brainstem venous congestion. J Neuroophthalmol. 2009;29:21–5.
35. Ract I, Drier A, Leclercq D, Sourour N, Gabrieli J, Yger M, et al. Extensive basal ganglia edema caused by a traumatic carotid-cavernous fistula: a rare presentation related to a basal vein of Rosenthal anatomical variation. J Neurosurg. 2014;121:63–6.
36. Iampreechakul P, Tanpun A, Lertbusayanukul P, Siriwimonmas S. Contralateral extensive cerebral hemorrhagic venous infarction caused by retrograde venous reflux into the opposite basal vein of Rosenthal in posttraumatic carotid-cavernous fistula:

a case report and literature review. Interv Neuroradiol. 2018;24:546–58.
37. Herrera DA, Vargas SA, Dublin AB. Traumatic carotid-cavernous fistula with pontomesencephalic and cervical cord venous drainage presenting as tetraparesis. J Neuroimaging. 2011;21:73–5.
38. Hou K, Li G, Qu L, Liu H, Xu K, Yu J. Intracranial dural arteriovenous fistulas with brainstem engorgement: an under-recognized entity in diagnosis and treatment. Front Neurol. 2020;11:526550.
39. Halbach VV, Hieshima GB, Higashida RT, Reicher M. Carotid cavernous fistulae: indications for urgent treatment. AJR Am J Roentgenol. 1987;149:587–93.
40. Holland LJ, Mitchell Ranzcr K, Harrison JD, Brauchli D, Wong Y, Sullivan TJ. Endovascular treatment of carotid-cavernous sinus fistulas: ophthalmic and visual outcomes. Orbit. 2019;38:290–9.
41. Vitek JJ, Smith MJ. The myth of the Brooks method of embolization: a brief history of the endovascular treatment of carotid-cavernous sinus fistula. J Neurointerv Surg. 2009;1:108–11.
42. Tiewei Q, Ali A, Shaolei G, Feng L, Zhongsong S, Xuesong L, et al. Carotid cavernous fistulas treated by endovascular covered stent grafts with follow-up results. Br J Neurosurg. 2010;24:435–40.
43. Pradeep N, Nottingham R, Kam A, Gandhi D, Razack N. Treatment of post-traumatic carotid-cavernous fistulas using pipeline embolization device assistance. BMJ Case Rep. 2015;2015. https://doi.org/10.1136/bcr-2015-011786.
44. Archondakis E, Pero G, Valvassori L, Boccardi E, Scialfa G. Angiographic follow-up of traumatic carotid cavernous fistulas treated with endovascular stent graft placement. AJNR Am J Neuroradiol. 2007;28:342–7.
45. Li J, Lan ZG, Xie XD, You C, He M. Traumatic carotid-cavernous fistulas treated with covered stents: experience of 12 cases. World Neurosurg. 2010;73:514–9.
46. Ahn JY, Lee BH, Joo JY. Stent-assisted Guglielmi detachable coils embolisation for the treatment of a traumatic carotid cavernous fistula. J Clin Neurosci. 2003;10:96–8.
47. Yu Y, Huang Q, Xu Y, Hong B, Zhao W, Deng B, et al. Use of onyx for transarterial balloon-assisted embolization of traumatic carotid cavernous fistulas: a report of 23 cases. AJNR Am J Neuroradiol. 2012;33:1305–9.
48. Zhang X, Guo W, Shen R, Sun J, Yin J, Chen X, et al. Combined use of Onyx and coils for transarterial balloon-assisted embolization of traumatic carotid-cavernous fistulas: a report of 16 cases with 17 fistulas. J Neurointerv Surg. 2016;8:1264–7.
49. Ryu J, Chang S, Choi SK, Lee SH, Chung Y. Radial artery graft bypass with endovascular trapping of the internal carotid artery for recurrent carotid cavernous fistula: different surgical fields, different surgical considerations. World Neurosurg. 2017;98(884):e7–e12.
50. Tu YK, Liu HM, Hu SC. Direct surgery of carotid cavernous fistulae and dural arteriovenous malformations of the cavernous sinus. Neurosurgery. 1997;41:798–805; discussion 805–6.
51. Wang W, Li YD, Li MH, Tan HQ, Gu BX, Wang J, et al. Endovascular treatment of post-traumatic direct carotid-cavernous fistulas: a single-center experience. J Clin Neurosci. 2011;18:24–8.
52. De Renzis A, Nappini S, Consoli A, Renieri L, Limbucci N, Rosi A, et al. Balloon-assisted coiling of the cavernous sinus to treat direct carotid cavernous fistula. A single center experience of 13 consecutive patients. Interv Neuroradiol. 2013;19:344–52.
53. Andrade G, Ponte De Souza ML, Marques R, Silva JL, Abath C, Azevedo-Filho HR. Endovascular treatment of traumatic carotid cavernous fistula with balloon-assisted sinus coiling. A technical description and initial results. Interv Neuroradiol. 2013;19:445–54.
54. Fatih Nas O, Buyukkaya R, Kacar E, Erdogan C, Hakyemez B. Use of Solitaire retrievable stent-assisted coiling technique for endovascular treatment of post-traumatic direct carotid cavernous fistula. Diagn Interv Imaging. 2016;97:1193–5.
55. Yu Y, Li Q, Huang Q, Zhang Y, Fang Y, Xu Y, et al. Embolization of direct carotid cavernous fistula with Onyx and coils under transarterial balloon protection. Cardiovasc Intervent Radiol. 2014;37:679–85.
56. Troffkin NA, Given CA 2nd. Combined transarterial N-butyl cyanoacrylate and coil embolization of direct carotid-cavernous fistulas. Report of two cases. J Neurosurg. 2007;106:903–6.
57. Wang YL, Ma J, Ding PX, Li YD, Han XW, Wu G. Treatment of post-traumatic carotid-cavernous fistulas with the Willis covered stent. A preliminary prospective study. Interv Neuroradiol. 2012;18:172–7.
58. Wendl CM, Henkes H, Martinez Moreno R, Ganslandt O, Bazner H, Aguilar PM. Direct carotid cavernous sinus fistulae: vessel reconstruction using flow-diverting implants. Clin Neuroradiol. 2017;27:493–501.
59. Huseyinoglu Z, Oppong MD, Griffin AS, Hauck E. Treatment of direct carotid-cavernous fistulas with flow diversion—does it work? Interv Neuroradiol. 2019;25:135–8.
60. Ghorbani M, Lafta G, Rahbarian F, Mortazavi A. Treatment of post-traumatic direct carotid-cavernous fistulas using flow diverting stents: Is it alone satisfactory? J Clin Neurosci. 2021;86:230–4.
61. Nadarajah M, Power M, Barry B, Wenderoth J. Treatment of a traumatic carotid-cavernous fistula by the sole use of a flow diverting stent. J Neurointerv Surg. 2012;4:e1.
62. Nossek E, Zumofen D, Nelson E, Raz E, Potts MB, Desousa KG, et al. Use of Pipeline Embolization Devices for treatment of a direct carotid-cavernous fistula. Acta Neurochir (Wien). 2015;157:1125–9; discussion 30.
63. Baranoski JF, Ducruet AF, Przbylowski CJ, Almefty RO, Ding D, Catapano JS, et al. Flow diverters as a scaffold for treating direct carotid cavernous fistulas. J Neurointerv Surg. 2019;11:1129–34.

64. Beaty NB, Jindal G, Gandhi D. Micro Vascular Plug (MVP)-assisted vessel occlusion in neurovascular pathologies: technical results and initial clinical experience. J Neurointerv Surg. 2015;7:758–61.
65. Wilms G, Demaerel P, Lagae L, Casteels I, Mombaerts I. Direct caroticocavernous fistula and traumatic dissection of the ipsilateral internal carotid artery: endovascular treatment. Neuroradiology. 2000;42:62–5.
66. Pagiola I, Amaral B, Saito C, Nalli D, Junior HC, Frudit M. Is the retrograde access for endovascular treatment of a traumatic carotid cavernous fistula associated with dissection of the ipsilateral carotid possible? J Cerebrovasc Endovasc Neurosurg. 2021;23:54–9.
67. Coley SC, Pandya H, Hodgson TJ, Jeffree MA, Deasy NP. Endovascular trapping of traumatic carotid-cavernous fistulae. AJNR Am J Neuroradiol. 2003;24:1785–8.
68. Lin CJ, Luo CB, Chang FC, Teng MM, Wang KL, Chu SH. Combined transarterial, transvenous, and direct puncture of the cavernous sinus to cure a traumatic carotid cavernous fistula. J Clin Neurosci. 2009;16:1663–5.
69. Lee KA, Kim JW, Sun H, Kang SJ, Jung JH. New aesthetic approach to carotid cavernous sinus fistula for coil embolization. J Craniofac Surg. 2012;23:e238–41.
70. Bulsara KR, Vasudevan R, Erdem E. Superior ophthalmic vein approach to carotid-cavernous fistulas. Technical note. Neurosurg Focus. 2005;18:ECP3.
71. Ou CH, Chen TY, Lin PL, Lee CL, Lin WC. Transvenous embolization of a direct carotid-cavernous fistula through the pterygoid plexus approach. Radiol Case Rep. 2021;16:1806–9.
72. Gemmete JJ, Ansari SA, Gandhi D. Endovascular treatment of carotid cavernous fistulas. Neuroimaging Clin N Am. 2009;19:241–55. Table of Contents.
73. Luo CB, Teng MM, Chang FC, Sheu MH, Guo WY, Chang CY. Bilateral traumatic carotid-cavernous fistulae: strategies for endovascular treatment. Acta Neurochir (Wien). 2007;149:675–80; discussion 80.
74. Gapsis BC, Ranjit RU, Malavade S, Carey A, Murtagh R, Drucker MD, et al. Spontaneous resolution of ophthalmologic symptoms following bilateral traumatic carotid cavernous fistulae. Digit J Ophthalmol. 2013;19:33–8.
75. Liang W, Xiaofeng Y, Weiguo L, Desheng P, Gang S, Xuesheng Z, et al. Bilateral traumatic carotid cavernous fistula: the manifestations, transvascular embolization and prevention of the vascular complications after therapeutic embolization. J Craniofac Surg. 2007;18:74–7.
76. Chiriac A, Iliescu BF, Dobrin N, Poeata I. One-step endovascular treatment of bilateral traumatic carotid-cavernous fistulae with atypical clinical course. Turk Neurosurg. 2014;24:422–6.
77. Kamel HA, Choudhari KA, Gillespie JS. Bilateral traumatic caroticocavernous fistulae: total resolution following unilateral occlusion. Neuroradiology. 2000;42:462–5.
78. Nossek E, Lombardo K, Schneider JR, Kwan K, Chalif DJ, Setton A. Unilateral venous approach to contralateral or bilateral carotid cavernous shunts. World Neurosurg. 2020;133:e479–86.
79. Gao BL, Wang ZL, Li TX, Xu B. Recurrence risk factors in detachable balloon embolization of traumatic direct carotid cavernous fistulas in 188 patients. J Neurointerv Surg. 2018;10:704–7.
80. Lin TC, Mao SH, Chen CH, Chen YL, Wong HF, Chang CJ, et al. Systematic analysis of the risk factors affecting the recurrence of traumatic carotid-cavernous sinus fistula. World Neurosurg. 2016;90:539–45.e1.
81. Dang NV, Hai NT, Cuong TC. Recurrent caroticocavernous fistula after internal carotid artery ligation: a case with embolization of the fistula via contralateral internal carotid artery approach. Interv Neuroradiol. 2014;20:482–6.
82. Higashida RT, Halbach VV, Tsai FY, Norman D, Pribram HF, Mehringer CM, et al. Interventional neurovascular treatment of traumatic carotid and vertebral artery lesions: results in 234 cases. AJR Am J Roentgenol. 1989;153:577–82.
83. Dai RQ, Bai WX, Gao BL, Li TX, Zhang K. Internal carotid artery occlusion may affect long-term quality of life in patients with high-flow carotid cavernous fistulas. Interv Neuroradiol. 2020;26:83–9.
84. Roski RA, Spetzler RF, Nulsen FE. Late complications of carotid ligation in the treatment of intracranial aneurysms. J Neurosurg. 1981;54:583–7.
85. Jeong SH, Lee JH, Choi HJ, Kim BC, Yu SH, Lee JI. First line treatment of traumatic carotid cavernous fistulas using covered stents at level 1 regional trauma center. J Korean Neurosurg Soc. 2021;64:818–26.
86. Lv X, Li Y, Jiang C, Wu Z. The incidence of trigeminocardiac reflex in endovascular treatment of dural arteriovenous fistula with onyx. Interv Neuroradiol. 2010;16:59–63.
87. Varadharajan S, Ramalingaiah AH, Saini J, Gupta AK, Swaminathan A. Sustained trigeminocardiac reflex following balloon embolization of caroticocavernous fistula. Interv Neuroradiol. 2016;22:577–8.

6 Angioarchitecture of Dural Arteriovenous Fistula

Karthik Kulanthaivelu, Sriharish Vankayalapati, Chandrajit Prasad, and Dwarakanath Srinivas

Abstract

The understanding of angioarchitecture of dAVFs is important since endovascular therapy frequently becomes non-targeted, thereby resulting in percolation of vascular structures not immediately relevant to the pathogenic shunt. A multitude of concepts with nomenclature of "parallel venous channel," "venous septation/pouch" and "common arterial collector" at the fistulous point of dural arteriovenous fistulas (dAVF) exist. A "shunted pouch" (SP) that is independent and outside the lumen of the sinus proper is the bottom-line to patho-anatomy. Discrete shunting domains exist between this vessel and the lumen proper of the sinus. Superselective embolization and exclusion of such a common collector are desirable to minimize hazards of collateral/non-target embolization and preserve sinus patency and function. The arterial feeders and venous drainage reflect the anatomic disposition of the vasculature in a location-specific manner.

Keywords

Angioarchitecture · Venous pouch · Parallel collector · Venous compartment

Learning Objectives

At the end of the chapter, the reader should be able to

- Understand the need for thoroughly appreciating angioarchitecture of dural arteriovenous fistulae (dAVF).
- Comprehend the various theories posited to explain the shunting zone.
- Have an overview of classification systems related to venous drainage.
- Identify location-specific angioarchitectural attributes of dAVF.

6.1 Introduction

The angioarchitecture of dAVFs begs a deeper understanding since endovascular therapy (via either the arterial or venous route) frequently becomes non-targeted, lacking specificity, ending in (avoidable) percolation of vascular structures not immediately relevant to the pathogenic shunt. Varied notions of a "parallel venous channel," "venous septation/pouch" and "common arterial collector" at the fistulous point of dural arteriove-

K. Kulanthaivelu · S. Vankayalapati · C. Prasad
Department of Neuroimaging and Interventional Radiology, National Institute of Mental Health and Neurosciences, Bengaluru, Karnataka, India

D. Srinivas (✉)
Department of Neurosurgery, National Institute of Mental Health and Neurosciences, Bengaluru, Karnataka, India

X. Lv (ed.), *Intracranial and Spinal Dural Arteriovenous Fistulas*,
https://doi.org/10.1007/978-981-19-5767-3_6

nous fistulas (dAVF) are proof that the pathologic angioarchitecture and pathoanatomy have not been well agreed upon [1, 2]. Knowledge gaps do exist about the identity of the various vascular constituents (arterial/venous), the exact topography of vascular shunts concerning the dural sinus walls, and drivers of the natural history of the disease.

Before delving into pathological angioarchitecture, the anatomic fact that arterial channels normally lie on the walls of the dural sinuses has been well accepted [3–5]. A rich and connected arterial network is formed around dural sinus walls by the dural branches of the anterior (ethmoidal, AEA), middle (MMA), posterior meningeal (PMA), ascending pharyngeal (APhA), and occipital arteries (OA), meningohypophyseal (MHT) and inferolateral trunks (ILT) of the internal carotid artery (based on the location and proximity). Rarely visible on normal angiograms, they may enlarge in dimensions under pathologic conditions as dAVF to be visible angiographically. Evidence that disease morbidity consistently scales alongside the severity of dAVF-driven cerebral venous congestion is acknowledged, however [6, 7]. Of the angioarchitectural characteristics, the most important prognosticator of clinical course and outcome related to the venous drainage [8]. The classification scheme related to the (all-important) venous drainage is discussed at length in other sections of this text and only briefly discussed in this chapter.

The broader scope of this chapter resides in other angioarchitectural aspects of dAVFs, especially with an emphasis on "where" exactly the fistula is. Interchangeably and vaguely used terms for this shunting domain of dAVF include venous recipients, accessory sinuses, septations, parallel channels/sinus, and common collector. Suffice to say that a "shunted pouch" (SP) that is independent and outside the lumen of the sinus proper is the bottom-line to pathoanatomy [9]. This interesting concept is discussed at length to begin the chapter below before the venous angioarchitecture and location-specific observations.

6.2 Understanding dAVF Angioarchitecture from a Pathogenetic Point of View

dAVFs are known to form and progress through a three-stage evolution [10]. Stage 1: Venous sinus thrombosis. Stage 2: Enlargement of nascent/preexistent microscopic fistulas in the venous sinus' walls with the build-up of venous backpressure. Stage 3: Partial recanalization of thrombosed, the degree of which determines the extent of cortical venous drainage (CVD). Evidence exists for the presence of microscopic fistulas amidst meningeal arteries and under normal conditions, veins are normal and present throughout the dura [11]. It is then not unreasonable to assume that the dural sinus wall is the most relevant as the site of the arteriovenous shunting in dAVF. Further expanding this notion are theories of dural venous sinus "compartment," parallel venous channel and common arterial collector detailed below.

6.2.1 The Dural Venous Sinus "Compartment" as the Site of the Fistula

Piske et al. remarked that in a few instances of dAVFs, the shunt involves only a single (or a few) compartments of the venous sinus. This compartment may be either within the sinus ("septation"), or outside ("accessory sinus"). Identification of such a compartment facilitates curative therapy by selective exclusion/embolization and still preserving sinus patency [12]. Transvenous superselective cannulation and embolization of such a shunted pouch (SP) confer the benefits of excluding the DAVF with preservation of sinus drainage (Fig. 6.1). While a formal description of such compartments was not available before the work by Piske et al., a few "selective" transvenous approaches in the literature to treat dAVF indeed targeted these structures [13]. The existence of DAVF fistula point not exactly into the sinus proper but rather in the vicinity has been noted

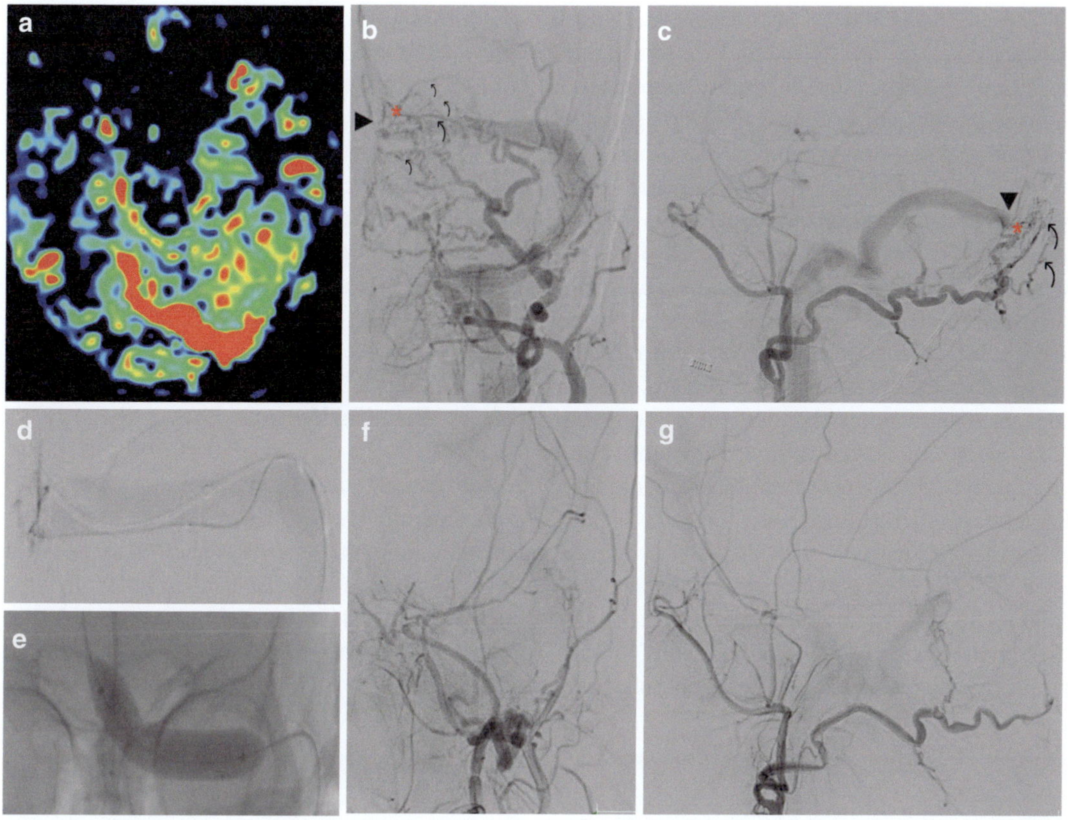

Fig. 6.1 (**a**) Diagnostic MRI with Arterial Spin Labelling reveals shunting of labelled spins in the torcula and left TS system raising possibility of a DAVF. (**b**) Frontal and (**c**) lateral projection of left ECA reveal Cognard type IIa + b DAVF at the torcula with numerous minute feeders (arrows) from MMA and occipital artery. Multiple arterial feeders (arrows) converging on the fistula common venous compartment (red*) at the fistulous site before draining into torcula (solid arrows). (**d**) Lateral projection of microcatheter injection via transvenous route after reaching the fistulous site. (**e**) post balloon inflation in the left transverse sinus. (**f**) Frontal and (**g**) lateral projection of left ECA injections reveal no residual fistula

across multiple studies in the literature that has delved into the angioarchitecture of the lesions [14–16]. Such compartments are not a rarity and may indeed be noted in one-third of the cases. It seems reasonable that newer techniques of transvenous embolization of dAVF such as the Onyx tunnel technique exploit this anatomic disposition. The Onyx tunnel is a reconstructive technique wherein using transvenous balloon-assistance liquid embolic material is injected to permeate the wall of the fistula across the entire 360° circumference of the recipient sinus, thereby preserving sinus patency [17].

The mechanism of SP genesis is only speculated. The "septation" partly seems related to partial thrombosis of the sinus with subsequent recanalization, thereby forming a double channel. Such a septated area can present trabeculae, making catheterization difficult. Fistula points outside the sinus are similar to those occurring in the tentorial edge where a preexistent embryologic sinus is available [18]. An ontogenic background to these observations does exist in dural sinus development. Primitive dural venous plexii (formed from veins) in the base of the dural folds result in the formation of the major dural venous sinuses [19]. Incomplete/aberrant fusion can compartmentalize the venous system which may be recruited during dAVF genesis.

Three-dimensional C-arm-based flat-panel detector-cone-beam CT (Dyna CT) has been proposed as a technique that elaborates more angioarchitectural information on dAVFs compared to conventional two-dimensional digital subtraction angiography (DSA) [20]. The fistulous point apart, retrograde leptomeningeal venous drainage (RLVD), venous anatomy is well depicted. Where the risk of over packing-induced cranial nerve palsy exists [e.g. cavernous sinus (CS) dAVF], selective-targeted embolization close to the fistulous points is desirable. Dyna CT facilitates the identification of such fistulous points. In their work on dAVF angioarchitecture using multiplanar-reformatted rotational-angiography Kiyosue et al. identified the "shunted pouch" using imaging markers such as (1) convergence of the arterial feeders, (2) distinction/separation from the lumen proper of the dural sinus. The SP was demarcated from the dural sinus' lumen proper by a hypoattenuating linear non-enhancing structure (septation), and/or a protrusion from the sinus. (3) Transition in Caliber, being larger than feeders, (4) transition/gradient in contrast opacification. Also, the SP location has a consistent association with their arterial feeders: those abutting the transverse-sigmoid junction and sigmoid sinus are fed by the petrosal division of the middle meningeal artery (MMA) and jugular twig of ascending pharyngeal artery (APhA) respectively.

6.2.2 Parallel Venous Channel

A substantial body of literature is devoted to understanding the fistula site in terms of a recipient venous channel that stays parallel to the dural (major) sinuses (transverse/sigmoid in the majority) [1, 21] (Fig. 6.2). The idea 2 has accrued importance from work by Caragine et al. (2003) although earlier descriptions date to the

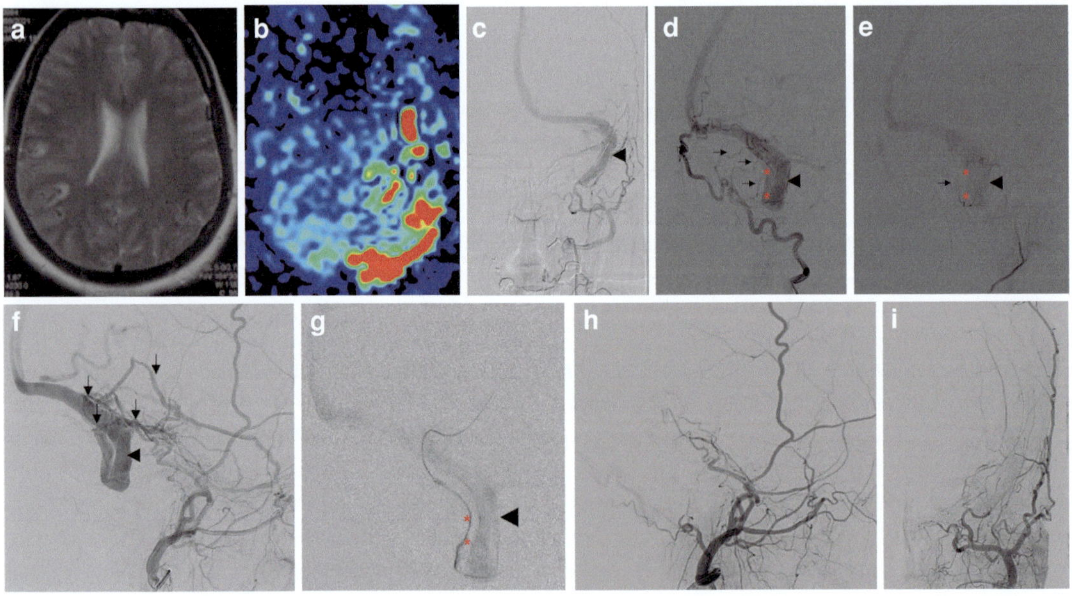

Fig. 6.2 (**a**) Axial T2 image shows serpiginous extra-axial flow voids the bilateral parietal region—suggestive of ectatic venous channels. (**b**) ASL reveals shunting of labelled spins in the left TS system raising DAVF possibility. (**c**) Frontal and lateral projection of left IMA injection reveal Cognard type IIa + b DAVF at the left transverse sigmoid junction with numerous minute feeders (arrows) from the hypertrophied MMA. (**d**) Lateral projection of left occipital artery, (**e**) left APA injection, (**f**) left MMA shows multiple feeders (arrows) to fistulous site. Multiple arterial feeders (arrows) converging on the fistula at a common parallel venous collector (red* in **d**–**f**) at the fistulous site before draining into left transverse sigmoid sinus (solid arrows). (**g**) Lateral projection of micro catheter injection after reaching the fistulous site via petrous squamous branch of left MMA shows common parallel venous collector (red*). Post embolization lateral projection (**h**) and frontal projection (**i**) of left ECA injections reveal no residual fistula

1990s [22]. Prompt identification of such a channel (should it exist), selective cannulation and embolization can be of value in fistula obliteration with minimal use of embolic material. More importantly, should the sinus be inadvertently embolized with patency of the pouch, redirection of venous outflow to cortical veins with potential catastrophic haemorrhage is imminent. It should be noted that the concept of the "parallel channel" is independent of the classification of dAVF according to the system by Borden/Cognard et al. Thus, endovascular management algorithms need not be further modified. The plexiform nature of the primitive embryonic dural venous system that determines venous variations is a plausible explanation for the development of such channels. dAVFs may manifest when elevated sinovenous pressure recruits such preexisting partly regressed embryonic remnants of dural venous plexus [23].

6.2.3 The Common Arterial Collector

Shapiro et al. (2018) present a radical and diagonal view of the fistulous point in dAVF [2]. Most TSS dAVFs are single holes or limited to a few connections. According to them, the angioarchitecture represents a multitude of arterioarterial connections, eventually converging on a common collector within the wall of the dural sinus. They differ in their opinion that this collector is indeed "arterial" in its nature (Fig. 6.3). Targeted transarterial embolization of this collector can mitigate the chances of inadvertent collateral embolization and its concomitant costs. This arrangement is best delineated in lower grade fistulas. This proposition borrows heavily from the earlier discussed ideas of the "arterial network" that resides on the dural sinus walls. Given this proximity of these arteries to the dural venous sinus, it is cogent that

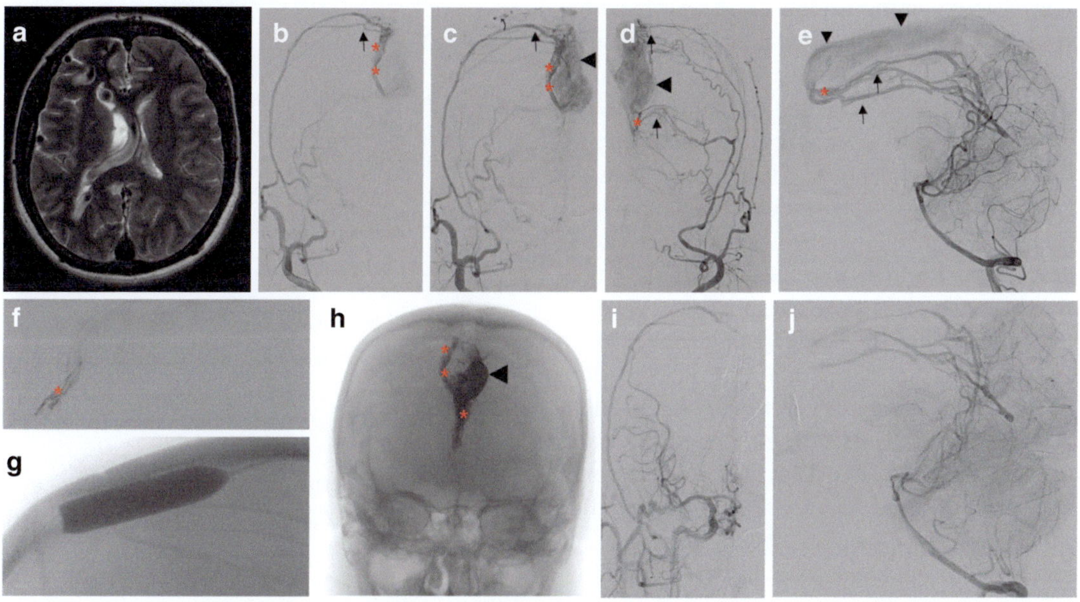

Fig. 6.3 (**a**) Diagnostic Axial T2 image shows serpiginous extra-axial flow voids in the right frontal region and dilated superior sagittal sinus raising DAVF possibility. (**b**, **c**) Frontal projection of right IMA injection and (**d**) frontal projection of left IMA injection reveal Cognard type IIa + b DAVF at the mid superior sagittal sinus with numerous minute feeders (arrows) from the anterior division of bilateral hypertrophied MMA. (**e**) Lateral projection of vertebral artery shows feeders (arrows) from artery of Davidoff and Schechter. Multiple arterial feeders (arrows) converging on the fistula common arterial collector (red*) at the fistulous site before draining into superior sagittal sinus (solid arrows). Associated cortical venous reflux noted on right side (curved arrow). (**f**) Lateral projection of microcatheter injection after reaching the fistulous site. (**g**) Post balloon inflation in the mid superior sagittal sinus. (**h**) Post embolization cast in situ. Post embolization frontal projection of (**i**) right ECA and (**j**) lateral projections of vertebral artery injections reveal no residual fistula

common arterial conduit may be central to the evolution of dAVF angioarchitecture. In the usual TSS dAVF scenario, this collector is located inferior to the plane of the true sinus. It implies that despite the angiographic ramification and intricacy, the true shunting zone may not be all that extensive and can be strategically tackled with better understanding. The idea goes on to have a reductionist view of a few communications of this collector to the sinus rather than the apparent involvement of entire lengths of sinuses.

Although it seems antithetical to call this collector arterial in nature, this overture by Shapiro et al. is like the above-discussed concepts of "shunted pouch/septation/parallel channel" in that it localises the site of the shunting domain to an extra-sinus common collector. They discuss similarities with works by Mironov et al., Piske et al., Kiyosue et al., Caragine et al. and Baik et al. and how they differ in calling it arterial.

Neuroendovascular interventional observations do support the common collector hypothesis that is being deliberated here. Fistulas never get obliterated, no matter the volume of embolizing material deposited on the sinus, unless a "critical/strategic" location is reached when a dramatic closure happens. This likely reflects the collector's continued patency and eventual arrest. Should such a collector be a vein, rather than an artery, one might even expect a rediversion of flow into the cortical veins rather than a fistula cure. The theory of dAVF pathogenesis which invokes sinus thrombosis and lysis would be congruent with aberrant arteriovenous connections on the sinus wall, rather than a parallel venous channel. This at least in part challenges the parallel venous channel theory. It is hypothesized that the recurrence of dAVF following proximal and partial arterial embolization is due to the non-percolation of the common arterial collector and its communication with the sinus. There's the compatibility of this common arterial collector hypothesis with the success of either transvenous and transarterial approaches. Importantly, it underscores the need for meticulousness in the approach in the identification and super-selective cannulation of the collector. The benefits: reduced risk to regional cranial nerves, saving the sinus lumen proper and cost on embolic material.

Criticisms do exist for the common collector conjecture. From the histopathologic understanding of dAVFs, numerous ultrastructural arteriovenous connections reside in the sinus wall, communicating with the lumen [24, 25]. But Hamada et al. do mention that the eventual opening of these fistulae into the lumen of the sinus occurs via a common channel. Angiographically specifying and defining this so-called "arterial common conduit" with digital subtraction angiography amidst its challenges with temporal resolution is a difficult task, especially with competing inflows in high-grade lesions. Despite sounding counterintuitive, radical and reductionistic the common arterial collector theory does give a perspective—it is not free from refutation, modification, and exceptions.

6.3 Classification Schemes That Detail Venous Aspects of the Angioarchitecture of dAVF

Widely adopted schemes that elaborate on the venous end of angioarchitecture of DAVF include those by Borden et al. and Cognard et al. [6, 7]. Briefly, the Borden-Shucart classification uses cortical venous drainage (CVD) to stratify dAVF into [26]

- Type I (absence of CVD)
- Type II (presence of CVD with antegrade into the dural sinus)
- Type III (exclusive drainage into cortical veins)

The Cognard scheme classification is predicated on venous outflow angioarchitecture apart from shunt location:

- Type I dAVF lesions drain antegrade into a dural venous sinus
- Type IIa lesions drain retrogradely to a venous sinus
- Type IIb lesions drain antegrade into the dural sinus and have CVD
- Type IIa + b lesions drain retrograde into the dural sinus and have CVD
- Type III dAVFs have only CVD as drainage pathways

Type IV fistulae demonstrate CVD along with venous ectasia

Type V lesions drain exclusively to the spinal perimedullary veins

Lesions named type IIb–V have an aggressive clinical course [26].

6.4 Location-Specific Angioarchitecture

By far, the transverse-sigmoid sinus region is the most common location for intracranial dAVF. The angioarchitecture is summarized thus. The arterial feeders are petrosal/petrosquamosal branches of the MMA, posterior meningeal artery (PMA), and neuromeningeal trunk of the APhA, transosseous meningeal branches of the occipital artery (OA) [27]. Infrequently, the artery of the falx cerebelli, tentorial branches of the meningohypophyseal trunk (MHT) may hypertrophy and perfuse the fistula. Fistula points may be multiple and expansive in cross-sectional areas. Venous hypertension may be reflected in TSS, superior sagittal sinus (SSS), superior petrosal sinus (SPS), a basal vein of Rosenthal (BVR), and anastomotic vein of Labbé, and brainstem and medulla veins. The arterial steal phenomenon, although rare, is possible [17] (Figs. 6.2 and 6.4).

Tentorial dAVF (TDAVF) and those located in the region of the superior petrosal sinus (SPS) are among the next most common group of dAVF (except for caroticocavernous fistula, classification discussed elsewhere) [28]. TDAVF may have feeders from tentorial branches of the ICA (MHT or inferolateral trunk), MMA, OA, occipital artery, APhA, PMA, cerebellar arteries (PICA, AICA),

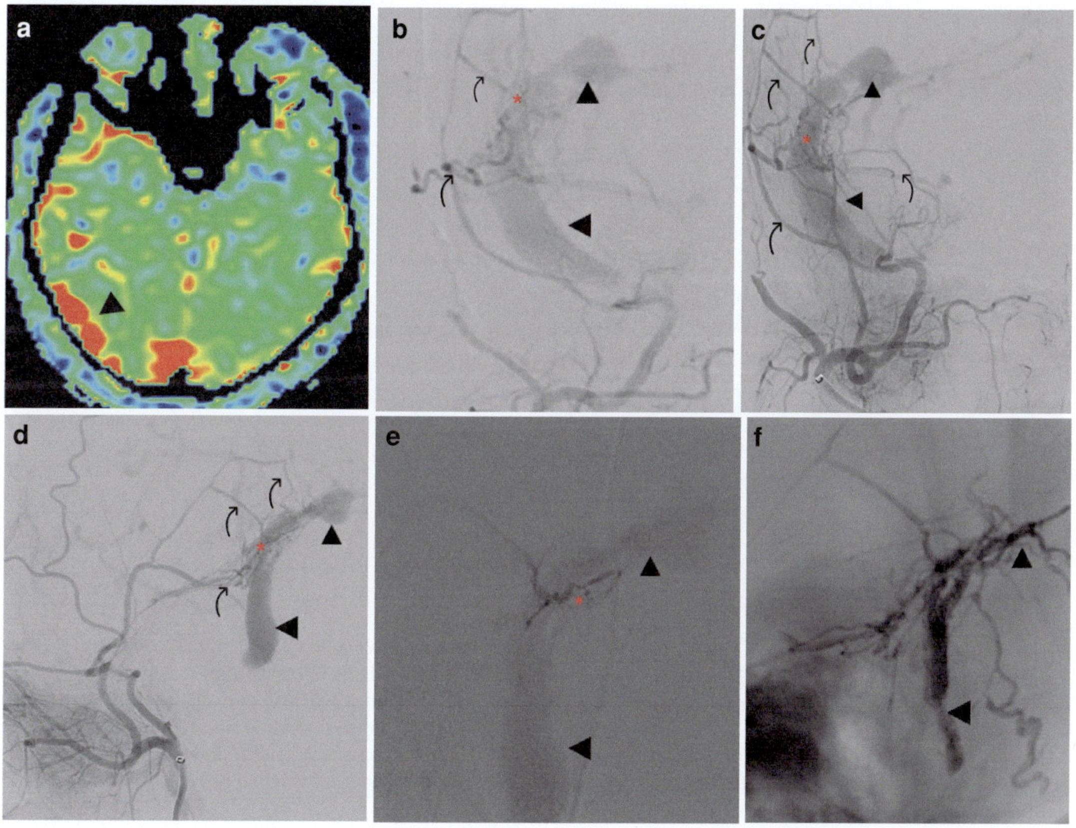

Fig. 6.4 (**a**) Diagnostic MRI with ASL reveals shunting of labelled spins in the right TS system raising DAVF possibility. (**b**, **c**) Frontal and (**d**) lateral projection of right IMA injection reveal Cognard type IIa + b DAVF at the right transverse sigmoid junction with numerous minute feeders (arrows) from the hypertrophied MMA. Multiple arterial feeders (arrows) converging on the fistula (red*) at the fistulous site before draining into right transverse sigmoid sinus (solid arrows). (**e**) Lateral projection of microcatheter injection after reaching the fistulous site via petrous squamous branch of left MMA. Post embolization (**f**) lateral projection shows onyx cast in situ

medial dural-tentorial branch of the SCA or pial branches from the posterior cerebellar artery. The point of transition may be sited in (1) falx cerebelli, (2) torcular (Fig. 6.1), and (3) petrotentorial location (in that order of frequency). Venous drainage (Cognard 3 or above) is both supratentorial and infratentorial [29–32] (Fig. 6.4).

Anterior Cranial Fossa base (ACF) dAVF are rare and pernicious. The arterial feeders were from the anterior ethmoidal branches (AEA) of the ophthalmic artery, frontal branches of the MMA, infraorbital/sphenopalatine/grater palatine divisions of the internal maxillary artery. Venous drainage is usually into a cortical vein (viz., frontal, either frontopolar or orbitofrontal) and eventually into the SSS. These are intrinsically high-grade lesions (Cognard 3 above) [33] (Fig. 6.5).

6.5 Summary

Meticulous evaluation of angiography frequently allows identification of a common vascular channel in relation to the wall of the sinus (that is debatably arterial or venous in lineage). Discrete shunting domains exist between this vessel and the lumen proper of the sinus. Superselective embolization and exclusion of such a common collector are desirable to minimize hazards of collateral/non-target embolization and preserve sinus patency and function. The locoregional angioarchitecture of dAVF is variable, depending on the location of the fistula. The arterial feeders and venous drainage reflect the anatomic disposition of the vasculature in a location-specific manner.

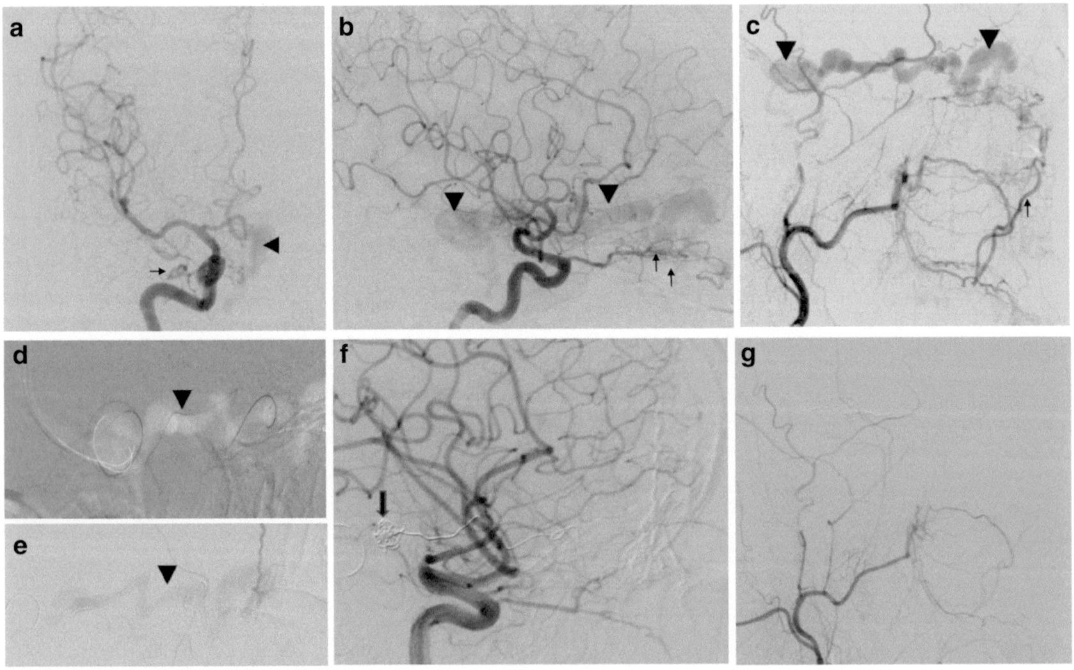

Fig. 6.5 (**a**) Frontal and (**b**) lateral projection of right ICA injection reveal Cognard type I DAVF at the anterior cranial fossa base with numerous minute feeders (arrows) from the anterior ethmoidal branches of the right ophthalmic artery. (**c**) lateral projections of right ECA injection reveal a dominant feeder from the frontal branch of the right MMA converging on the fistula, (**d**, **e**) lateral projection of micro catheter injection after reaching the fistulous site via BVR (arrow heads in **a**–**c**, **e**) and coils were (solid arrow in **f**) deployed into the venous side. Post embolization (**f**) lateral projection of ICA and (**g**) lateral projection of left ECA injections reveal no residual fistula

References

1. Caragine LP, Halbach VV, Dowd CF, Ng PP, Higashida RT. Parallel venous channel as the recipient pouch in transverse/sigmoid sinus dural fistulae. Neurosurgery. 2003;53(6):1261–6; discussion 1266–7.
2. Shapiro M, Raz E, Litao M, Becske T, Riina H, Nelson PK. Toward a better understanding of dural arteriovenous fistula angioarchitecture: superselective transvenous embolization of a sigmoid common arterial collector. AJNR Am J Neuroradiol. 2018;39(9):1682–8.
3. Geibprasert S, Pereira V, Krings T, Jiarakongmun P, Toulgoat F, Pongpech S, et al. Dural arteriovenous shunts. Stroke. 2008;39(10):2783–94.
4. Berenstein A, Choi IS. Surgical neuroangiography of intracranial lesions. Radiol Clin N Am. 1988;26(5):1143–51.
5. Lasjaunias P. Surgical neuroangiography, Endovascular treatment of craniofacial lesions, vol. 2. Berlin: Springer; 1987. [cited 2021 Sept 2]. Available from: https://ci.nii.ac.jp/naid/10019221011/.
6. Borden JA, Wu JK, Shucart WA. A proposed classification for spinal and cranial dural arteriovenous fistulous malformations and implications for treatment. J Neurosurg. 1995;82(2):166–79.
7. Cognard C, Gobin YP, Pierot L, Bailly AL, Houdart E, Casasco A, et al. Cerebral dural arteriovenous fistulas: clinical and angiographic correlation with a revised classification of venous drainage. Radiology. 1995;194(3):671–80.
8. Li C, Wang Y, Li Y, Jiang C, Yang X, Wu Z. Clinical and angioarchitectural risk factors associated with intracranial hemorrhage in dural arteriovenous fistulas: a single-center retrospective study. PLoS One. 2015;10(6):e0131235.
9. Kiyosue H, Tanoue S, Okahara M, Hori Y, Kashiwagi J, Sagara Y, et al. Angioarchitecture of transverse-sigmoid sinus dural arteriovenous fistulas: evaluation of shunted pouches by multiplanar reformatted images of rotational angiography. Am J Neuroradiol. 2013;34(8):1612–20.
10. Mullan S. Reflections upon the nature and management of intracranial and intraspinal vascular malformations and fistulae. J Neurosurg. 1994;80(4):606–16.
11. Kerber CW, Newton TH. The macro and microvasculature of the dura mater. Neuroradiology. 1973;6(4):175–9.
12. Piske RL, Campos CMS, Chaves JBL, Abicalaf R, Dabus G, Batista LL, et al. Dural sinus compartment in dural arteriovenous shunts: a new angioarchitectural feature allowing superselective transvenous dural sinus occlusion treatment. Am J Neuroradiol. 2005;26(7):1715–22.
13. Mironov A. Selective transvenous embolization of dural fistulas without occlusion of the dural sinus. Am J Neuroradiol. 1998;19(2):389–91.
14. Eftekhar B, Morgan MK. Surgical management of dural arteriovenous fistulas of the transverse-sigmoid sinus in 42 patients. J Clin Neurosci. 2013;20(4):532–5.
15. Carlson AP, Alaraj A, Amin-Hanjani S, Charbel FT, Aletich V. Endovascular approach and technique for treatment of transverse-sigmoid dural arteriovenous fistula with cortical reflux: the importance of venous sinus sacrifice. J Neurointerv Surg. 2013;5(6):566–72.
16. Kirsch M, Liebig T, Kühne D, Henkes H. Endovascular management of dural arteriovenous fistulas of the transverse and sigmoid sinus in 150 patients. Neuroradiology. 2009;51(7):477–83.
17. Kerolus MG, Chung J, Munich SA, Matsuda Y, Okada H, Lopes DK. An Onyx tunnel: reconstructive transvenous balloon-assisted Onyx embolization for dural arteriovenous fistula of the transverse-sigmoid sinus. J Neurosurg. 2018;129(4):922–7.
18. Piske RL, Lasjaunias P. Extrasinusal dural arteriovenous malformations. Neuroradiology. 1988;30(5):426–32.
19. Padget DH. The cranial venous system in man in reference to development, adult configuration, and relation to the arteries. Am J Anat. 1956;98(3):307–55.
20. Hiu T, Kitagawa N, Morikawa M, Hayashi K, Horie N, Morofuji Y, et al. Efficacy of DynaCT digital angiography in the detection of the fistulous point of dural arteriovenous fistulas. Am J Neuroradiol. 2009;30(3):487–91.
21. de Paula LC, Prandini MN, Spelle L, Piotin M, Mounayer C, Moret J. Parallel transverse-sigmoid sinus harboring dural arteriovenous malformation. How to differentiate the pathological and normal sinus in order to treat and preserve patency and function. Acta Neurochir (Wien). 2010;152(3):523–7.
22. Barnwell SL, Halbach VV, Dowd CF, Higashida RT, Hieshima GB, Wilson CB. A variant of arteriovenous fistulas within the wall of dural sinuses. Results of combined surgical and endovascular therapy. J Neurosurg. 1991;74(2):199–204.
23. Lasjaunias P, Berenstein A, Brugge KG. Clinical vascular anatomy and variations. Berlin: Springer; 2001. [cited 2021 Aug 30]. Available from: http://public.ebookcentral.proquest.com/choice/publicfullrecord.aspx?p=3098872.
24. Hamada Y, Goto K, Inoue T, Iwaki T, Matsuno H, Suzuki S, et al. Histopathological aspects of dural arteriovenous fistulas in the transverse-sigmoid sinus region in nine patients. Neurosurgery. 1997;40(3):452–8.
25. Nishijima M, Takaku A, Endo S, Kuwayama N, Koizumi F, Sato H, et al. Etiological evaluation of dural arteriovenous malformations of the lateral and sigmoid sinuses based on histopathological examinations. J Neurosurg. 1992;76(4):600–6.
26. Reynolds MR, Lanzino G, Zipfel GJ. Intracranial dural arteriovenous fistulae. Stroke. 2017;48(5):1424–31.
27. Xu K, Yang X, Li C, Yu J. Current status of endovascular treatment for dural arteriovenous fistula of the transverse-sigmoid sinus: a literature review. Int J Med Sci. 2018;15(14):1600–10.

28. Harrigan MR, Deveikis JP. Handbook of cerebrovascular disease and neurointerventional technique, Contemporary medical imaging. 3rd ed. Cham: Humana Press; 2018. [cited 2021 Sept 2]. Available from: https://www.springer.com/gp/book/9783319667775.
29. Byrne JV, Garcia M. Tentorial dural fistulas: endovascular management and description of the medial dural-tentorial branch of the superior cerebellar artery. Am J Neuroradiol. 2013;34(9):1798–804.
30. Kortman H, Boukrab I, Bloemsma G, Peluso J, Sluzewski M, van der Pol B, et al. Tentorial dural arteriovenous fistulas: a single-center cohort of 12 patients. J Cerebrovasc Endovasc Neurosurg. 2017;19(4):284–90.
31. Kim H-J, Yang J-H, Lee H-J, Lee H-J. Tentorial dural arteriovenous fistula treated using transarterial onyx embolization. J Korean Neurosurg Soc. 2015;58(3):276–80.
32. Rezende MTS, Trivelato FP, de Castro-Afonso LH, Nakiri GS, Silva CCM, Abud TG, et al. Endovascular treatment of tentorial dural arteriovenous fistulas using the transarterial approach as a first-line strategy. Oper Neurosurg. 2021;20(5):484–92.
33. Kulanthaivelu K, Pendharkar H, Prasad C, Kumar Gupta A, Hanumanthapura Ramalingaiah A, Saini J, et al. Anterior cranial fossa dural arteriovenous fistulae—angioarchitecture and intervention. Clin Neuroradiol. 2021;31:661–9.

7 The Clinical Value of SWI in Dural Arteriovenous Fistula: Detection of Extensive Parenchymal Pathology

Youle Su and Xianli Lv

Abstract

A 51-year-old man with an otherwise unremarkable previous medical history presented with the first episode of seizure 2 weeks ago. Susceptibility weighted magnetic resonance imaging sequence revealed extensive findings consistent with dysplastic venous vessels and parenchymal necrosis chiefly localizing to the right cerebral and cerebellar hemispheres, discovered on conventional magnetic resonance imaging. Transfemoral transaortic digital subtracted angiography examination revealed a dural arteriovenous fistula chiefly residing within the region of the right transverse-sigmoid sinus evidencing transverse-sigmoid sinus thrombosis and retrograde pial venous reflux. We successfully obliterated the dural arteriovenous fistula using transarterial Onyx embolization. The present case indicates susceptibility weighted magnetic resonance imaging sequences may be successfully exploited to evaluate the angioarchitectural features of dural arteriovenous fistulas.

Y. Su
Neurosurgery Department, The Affiliated Hospital of Inner Mongolia Medical University, Hohhot, Inner Mongolia, China

X. Lv (✉)
Department of Neurosurgery, Beijing Tsinghua Changgung Hospital, School of Clinical Medicine, Tsinghua University, Beijing, China

Keywords

Dural arteriovenous fistula · Susceptibility weighted imaging · Malformed venous vessels · Cerebrum · Cerebellum

Key Message

- Susceptibility weighted magnetic resonance imaging sequences proved superior compared with conventional (T1-, T2-, and proton density-weighted) MRI and digital subtraction cerebral angiograms in detecting abnormal dilated veins within the cerebral parenchyma.

Recent advances in neuroendovascular surgery have inspired a more intimate appreciation of the clinical symptomatology, distinguishing radiological features, and treatment of dural arteriovenous fistulas (DAVFs) [1, 2]. Though conventional magnetic resonance imaging (MRI) is commonly used in clinical and research settings [3], modifications of imaging technique and parameters may permit more detailed evaluation of complex vascular malformations. Susceptibility weighted imaging (SWI) can detect microhemorrhage and microvasculature with enhanced fidelity by exploiting the differential resonance properties of protons relaxing from their excited spins in oxyhemoglobin, deoxyhemoglobin, and methemo-

X. Lv (ed.), *Intracranial and Spinal Dural Arteriovenous Fistulas*,
https://doi.org/10.1007/978-981-19-5767-3_7

globin [4–6]. During the past several years, SWI may illustrate the fistulous point between the arterial inflow and venous egress, cortical venous reflux, and magnitude of arteriovenous shunt in DAVF, thus providing a unique noninvasive modality by which to evaluate hemodynamic modifications induced by the presence of congener lesions [6–9]. We describe an exceptional instance of a patient presenting with seizures in whom SWI successfully characterized the parenchymal pathology of DAVF, putatively constituting a noninvasive modality adjunct to digital subtraction angiography (DSA).

7.1 Case Report

A 51-year-old man presented with the first episode of epileptic fits generalized tonic-clonic seizure 2 weeks ago. The patient underwent MRI evaluation of the head via a conventional 3.0-T MRI unit (Magnetom Verio; Siemens, Erlangen, Germany). T1-, T2-, and SWI sequences were obtained. Conventional MRI revealed a small lesion restricted to the right cerebellum without other lesions in the cerebral hemispheres. However, SWI revealed extensive atrophy and multiple hypointense lesions consistent with flow voids signifying the likely presence of dilated parenchymal veins in the right cerebrum and cerebellum (Fig. 7.1). The brain stem was also of abnormality. Selective DSA of the external and internal carotid arteries and vertebral arteries revealed a Borden type II DAVF with venous egress into the right transverse-sigmoid sinus with arterial supply from branches of the external carotid artery. Premature venous filling was mostly restricted to lateral extents of the right transverse-sigmoid sinus junction and internal jugular vein, with prominent interval retrograde reflux into the vein of Labbé (Fig. 7.2). The patient underwent transarterial Onyx embolization coordinately through the right middle meningeal artery and ascending pharyngeal artery. Digital subtraction cerebral angiography following therapy revealed complete obliteration of arteriovenous shunting (Fig. 7.3). The patient was fortunately discharged without any neurological deficits.

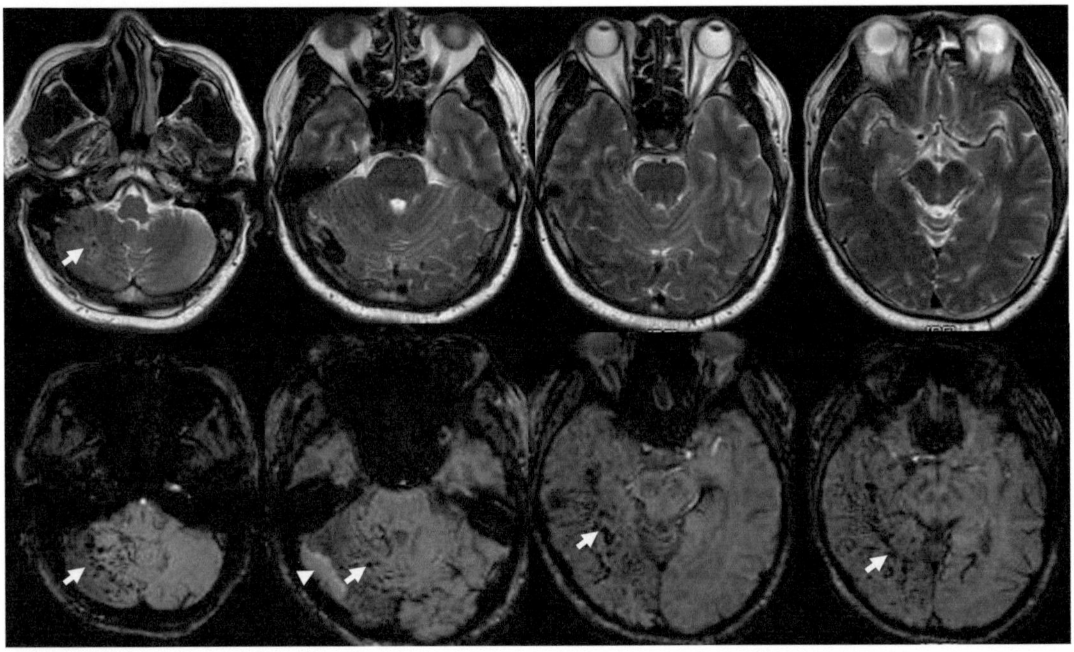

Fig. 7.1 Upper, axial MR images, T2-weighted, showing a small hypertensity and flow void in the right cerebellum. Lower, SWI images showing extensive distribution of abnormal venous vessels (arrows) in the brain. The vessels are extremely numerous in the right cerebellum and cerebrum

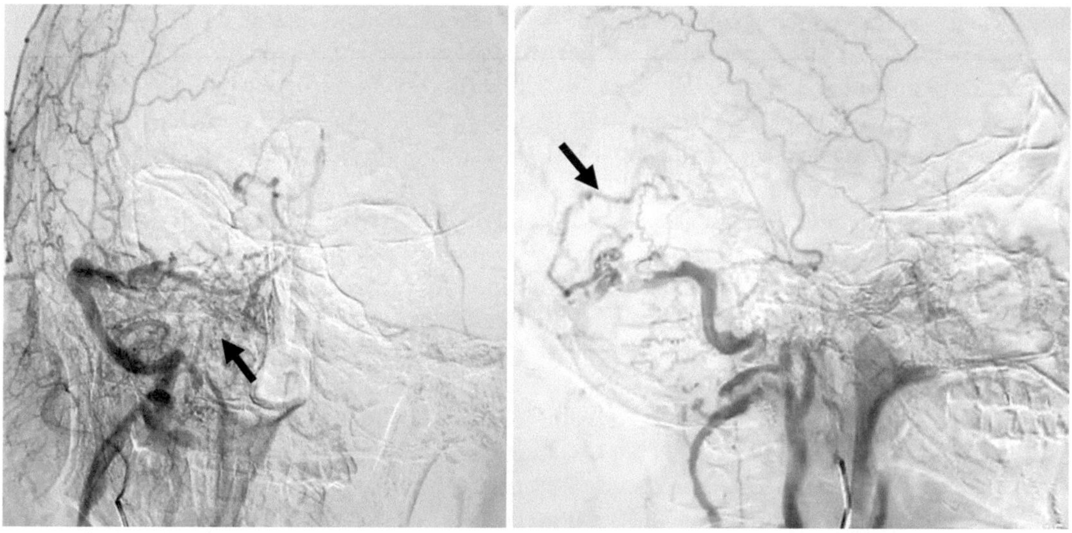

Fig. 7.2 Right external carotid artery arteriograms, antero-posterior (left) and lateral (right) views, arterial phase. Branches of right external carotid artery directly fill the right transverse-sigmoid sinus with retrograde filling of Labbe vein. Right transverse sinus is opacified only in the lateral portion

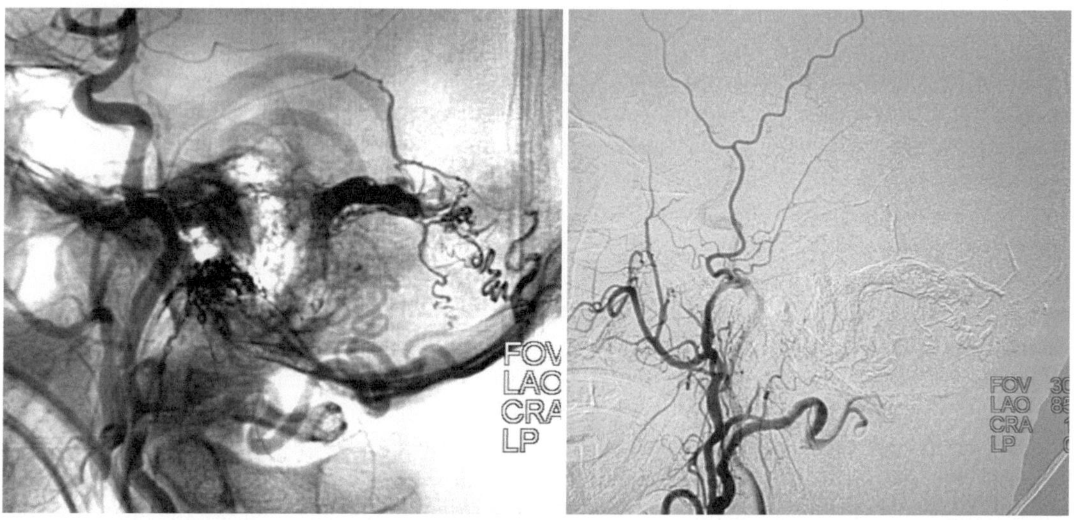

Fig. 7.3 Unsubtracted image, lateral (left) view, showing the Onyx cast. Right external carotid artery arteriogram, lateral (right) view, arterial phase, showing complete occlusion of the dural fistula

7.2 Discussion

Intracranial arteriovenous fistulas are complex vascular malformations whereby sequential thrombosis and recanalization of a dural venous induces the elaboration of vascular endothelial growth factor promoting local angiogenesis and fistula formation, constituting among the chief theories explaining the development of these lesions. Arterial feeders to the venous egress may derive from pial and/or dural arteries, roughly classifying these lesions and allowing us to predict their clinical behavior. The most conspicuous finding on SWI was the presence of extensive, dilated veins throughout right cerebral and cerebellar hemispheres. High flow through arteriovenous shunts promotes retrograde reflux into cortical veins. Remarkable density and extensive distribution of abnormal venous vessels indicates the presence of our case of DAVF may insidiously cause cytotoxic damage to locoregional parenchyma.

SWI constitutes a three dimensional gradient-recalled echo (GRE) sequence originally developed to enhance image quality obtained using magnetic resonance venography by using the blood oxygen level-dependent (BOLD) effect and refined phase information for contrast enhancement in MRI [5, 6]. SWI may be obtained with magnetic field strengths of 1.5, 3, and 7 T [7, 8]. Higher strength magnetic fields enhances visualization of fine details in brain structures, with ultrahigh field strengths exceeding 7 T putatively distorting the size of brain structures in zones characterized by high iron concentrations [9].

SWI may be more sensitive in detecting parenchymal venous anomalies compared with other imaging modalities, including T1, contrast-enhanced T1, T2* and FLAIR [7]. Authors have made similar observation regarding the use of SWI MRI in the setting of cortical venous outflow obstruction typifying Sturge-Weber syndrome [4], a finding congruous with previous reports describing use of SWI to depict venous congestion secondary to dural arteriovenous fistula [8, 9]. Nakagawa et al. reduced the prominence of these abnormally dilated cortical veins by treating culprit DAVF in a wonderfully conducted series of 17 patients [7].

The confluence of multiple mechanisms increases the prominence of the venous elements directly draining and/or mediating collateral drainage of otherwise normal cerebral parenchyma. Dilated hypointense flow voids identified by SWI engorged by retrograde venous reflux from DAVF may represent enlarged tortuous collateral veins rerouting venous blood away from obstructed and/or hypertensive venous drainage pathways. Venous hypertension resulting from DAVF leads to hypoperfusion and may enhance oxygen extraction in ischemic tissue, which may successively augment deoxyhemoglobin concentration and increased susceptibility effects [5]. A hemodynamic study of DAVF has identified raised intravenous pressures [1, 2]. Positron-emission tomography studies effectively identify increased oxygen extraction fraction has in a subset of DAVF, resulting from reduced cerebral blood flow and impairment of venous drainage with oxygen metabolism preserved [7, 9]. Increased deoxyhemoglobin mass within dilated veins may explain the notable conspicuity of the venous elements locoregionally related to DAVF on SWI. Borden type I and Cognard types I and IIa DAVF are accompanied by arteriovenous shunting within dural sinuses [1, 2]. In these circumstance, SWI may effectively demonstrate engorged parenchymal veins and the characteristically hyperintense fistulous point, with presence or absence of venous reflux dictating benignity of the fistula.

Successive thrombosis or thrombophlebitis and recanalization in the dural sinus or vein followed by fistulization of a proximate artery with the inflamed venous wall constitutes the prevailing hypothesis explaining the ontogenic development of DAVF [1, 2]. Arteriomural and/or venomural inflammation putatively explains the presence of contrast enhancement of the venous wall in a subset of patients with various intracranial various malformations. Dedicated angiographic evaluation of our patient revealed a DAVF and intraluminal thrombosis in the right transverse sinus coursing within leaflets deriving from the free convex edge of the tentorium cerebelli separating the tentorial surface of the right occipital lobe from the tentorial surface of the right cerebellar hemisphere. Our patient manifested occlusion restricted chiefly to the medial transverse sinus and high arterial flow into the dural venous sinuses. The presentation of blood flow under arterial pressure to the venous elements may cause prominent intracranial venous hypertension and consequent edema and/or infarction of drained parenchyma, most prominent in the parenchymal contents of the posterior and middle fossa in our patients, putatively exacerbating degeneration of the venous vessels. Parenchymal necrosis in our patient may result from enhanced ischemia and intracranial venous hypertension. In previous reports, patients harboring DAVF of the transverse sinuses experienced severe neurological deficits or expired from consequences of high rates of arterial blood flow into the arteriovenous fistula and retrograde propagation of venous hypertension from the transverse and sigmoid sinuses [10]. The parenchymal changes experienced by the patient presented in our present case supports these mechanistic conjectures.

7.3 Conclusion

SWI may constitute a useful noninvasive modality in evaluating and characterizing intracranial vascular malformations in patients harboring DAVF. Exquisite sensitivity to susceptibility effects of SWI may provide unparalleled illustration of venous congestion, though parenchymal venous reflux may be underestimated using this imaging technique. Our findings may be generalized to indicate SWI may be quite effective in characterizing intracranial arteriovenous malformations with a prominent venous component.

References

1. Freeman CW, Lazor JW, Loevner LA, Nabavizadeh SA. Variations of the CNS venous system mimicking pathology: spectrum of imaging findings. J Neuroimaging. 2019;29(6):673–88.
2. Lv X, Jiang C, Li Y, Liu L, Liu J, et al. Transverse-sigmoid sinus dural arteriovenous fistulae. World Neurosurg. 2010;74:297–305.
3. Kitajima M, Hirai T, Korogi Y, Yamura M, Kawanaka K, Ikushima I, et al. Retrograde cortical and deep venous drainage in patients with intracranial dural arteriovenous fistulas: comparison of MR imaging and angiographic findings. AJNR Am J Neuroradiol. 2005;26(6):1532–8.
4. Di Ieva A, Lam T, Alcaide-Leon P, Bharatha A, Montanera W, Cusimano MD. Magnetic resonance susceptibility weighted imaging in neurosurgery: current applications and future perspectives. J Neurosurg. 2015;123(6):1463–75.
5. Schwarz D, Bendszus M, Breckwoldt MO. Clinical value of susceptibility weighted imaging of brain metastases. Front Neurol. 2020;11:55.
6. Wiest R, Beisteiner R. Recent developments in imaging of epilepsy. Curr Opin Neurol. 2019;32(4):530–8.
7. Nakagawa I, Taoka T, Wada T, Nakagawa H, Sakamoto M, Kichikawa K, et al. The use of susceptibility-weighted imaging as an indicator of retrograde leptomeningeal venous drainage and venous congestion with dural arteriovenous fistula: diagnosis and follow-up after treatment. Neurosurgery. 2013;72(1):47–55.
8. Noguchi K, Kuwayama N, Kubo M, Kamisaki Y, Kameda K, Tomizawa G, et al. Intracranial dural arteriovenous fistula with retrograde cortical venous drainage: use of susceptibility-weighted imaging in combination with dynamic susceptibility contrast imaging. AJNR Am J Neuroradiol. 2010;31(10):1903–10.
9. Letourneau-Guillon L, Krings T. Simultaneous arteriovenous shunting and venous congestion identification in dural arteriovenous fistulas using susceptibility-weighted imaging: initial experience. AJNR Am J Neuroradiol. 2012;33(2):301–7.
10. Hinokuma K, Ohama E, Ikuta F, Tanimura K, Kameyama S. Dural arteriovenous malformation with abnormal parenchymal vessels: an autopsy study. Acta Neuropathol. 1990;80(6):656–9.

Transvenous Embolization of Dural Arteriovenous Fistulas

8

Huachen Zhang and Xianli Lv

Abstract

The goal of embolization of dural arteriovenous fistulas (DAVFs) is total fistula occlusion without interfering with the normal dural venous drains. Embolization can be performed by transarterial and/or transvenous routes or direct puncture of the affected dural sinus. Selection of embolic materials depends on angioarchitecture of the fistula and access route. When the DAVF is supplied by many small tortuous artery, the transvenous approach is preferred because of the lack of transarterial access. When the DAVF is only supplied by the branch directly from the internal carotid artery or the vertebral artery, when the DAVF is supplied by the dangerous extracranial to intracranial anastomosed artery, or when the DAVF is supplied by the nutrient arteries of the cranial nerve, the transvenous embolization should be considered. In the transvenous method, the catheters are retrogradely navigated into the affected sinus or the affected pial vein to occlude them using a microcoils, liquid embolic agent, or a combination of them. For the transvenous approach, appropriate patient selection is essential to achieve complete occlusion and avoid complications. The selected sinus or pial vein should fully participate in fistula drainage, not in normal cerebral venous drainage, and the venous access should be accessable.

Keywords

Dural arteriovenous fistula · Embolization
Inferior petrosal sinus

8.1 Introduction

Intracranial dural arteriovenous fistulas (DAVFs) are acquired abnormal epidural arteriovenous shunts, particularly at the sinus wall [1]. Most of the DAVFs are associated with progressive sinus occlusion. They are located in the cavernous sinus, lateral (transverse-sigmoid) sinus, superior-sagittal sinus, anterior condylar confluence, tentorial sinus, craniocervical junction, and anterior skull base (ethmoidal sinus) [1]. The treatment strategy differs based on the etiology and drainage pattern of DAVFs [2]. The most effective treatment for DAVFs at the sinus wall is transvenous embolization (TVE) with coils and Onyx [2]. This technique is valid as long as the diseased dural sinus is completely occluded or does not participate in normal venous drainage [3]. Embolization of affected sinus by direct puncture of cavernous sinus via transorbital [4] or via craniotomy (e.g., lateral, superior sagittal

H. Zhang · X. Lv (✉)
Department of Neurosurgery, Beijing Tsinghua Changgung Hospital, School of Clinical Medicine, Tsinghua University, Beijing, China

X. Lv (ed.), *Intracranial and Spinal Dural Arteriovenous Fistulas*,
https://doi.org/10.1007/978-981-19-5767-3_8

sinus, or sinus confluence) [2] has been reported successfully. Because of the procedure's inherent invasiveness, it has only been considered when endovascular routes are not accessible based on angioarchitecture analysis. In this article, we will discuss the method of TVE, with emphasis on the access routes, embolic arterials, and individual selection.

8.2 Transvenous Methods

The TVE procedures are performed with the patient under general anesthesia. A 5-Fr diagnostic catheter is placed in the ipsilateral or contralateral common carotid artery via the left transfemoral puncture for control arteriography. Various approaches are used to achieve transvenous access. A transvenous access can be established through the femoral vein, the internal jugular vein, or directly puncture the draining venous pouch under the guidance of drilling, craniotomy, or ultrasound [2]. In the case of a thrombotic sinus, the transvenous approach can be achieved by recanalization of the closed venous segment, such as traversing the ipsilateral occluded inferior petrosal sinus to access the trapped cavernous sinus or traversing the occluded sigmoid sinus to access an isolated transverse sinus [5]. In this method, neurointerventionists need to carefully manipulate the catheter and guide wire to avoid the risk of thrombosis sinus or vein perforation. Sometimes the contralateral approach can also be used, such as the contralateral jugular vein can be used to pass through torcula to the sigmoid sinus. The trapped sinus can also be directly punctured by drilling or craniotomy [2]. The direct access to the trapped cavernous sinus in the indirect carotid-cavernous fistula can be achieved by a transforaminal approach via foramen ovale or transorbital puncture [6, 7]. The hybrid angio-operating room is the ideal choice for this type of combined endovascular surgical method.

8.3 Selection of Embolic Materials

Different embolic materials have been used, including *n*-butyl-2-cyanoacrylate (NBCA; Codman, Raynham, MA, USA), particles (polyvinyl alcohol; PVA), Onyx (eV3; Neurovascular Inc., Irvine, CA, USA) or detachable coils [8, 9]. In current practice, Onyx-18 was used commonly with or without additional coils in TVEs (Fig. 8.1). Onyx embolization is very effective for filling and occluding affected sinuses or venous pouch, especially an isolated transverse sinuses [3]. Sometimes it is necessary to select coils to decrease the shunt flow [8]. The "dual catheter technique" can be used, one is a proximal microcatheter used to deploy the coils, and the other is a distal microcatheter used to inject Onyx after coiling. Onyx provides advantages by the ability to perform a slow, controlled injection. Injection of larger amounts of Onyx can result in filling of the venous compartment in a single embolization. However, there are some disadvantages of Onyx. Onyx has been thought to cause significant inflammation within the cavernous sinus resulting in various cranial nerve palsies, which are reversible during 3–4 months follow-up [10]. Prior to the advent of Onyx, NBCA was also used in TVE [9]. NBCA is a cheap, fast embolic material. This procedure requires a highly experienced operator with the ability to determine the appropriate concentration of NBCA (about 20–25%) because NBCA is a liquid adhesive.

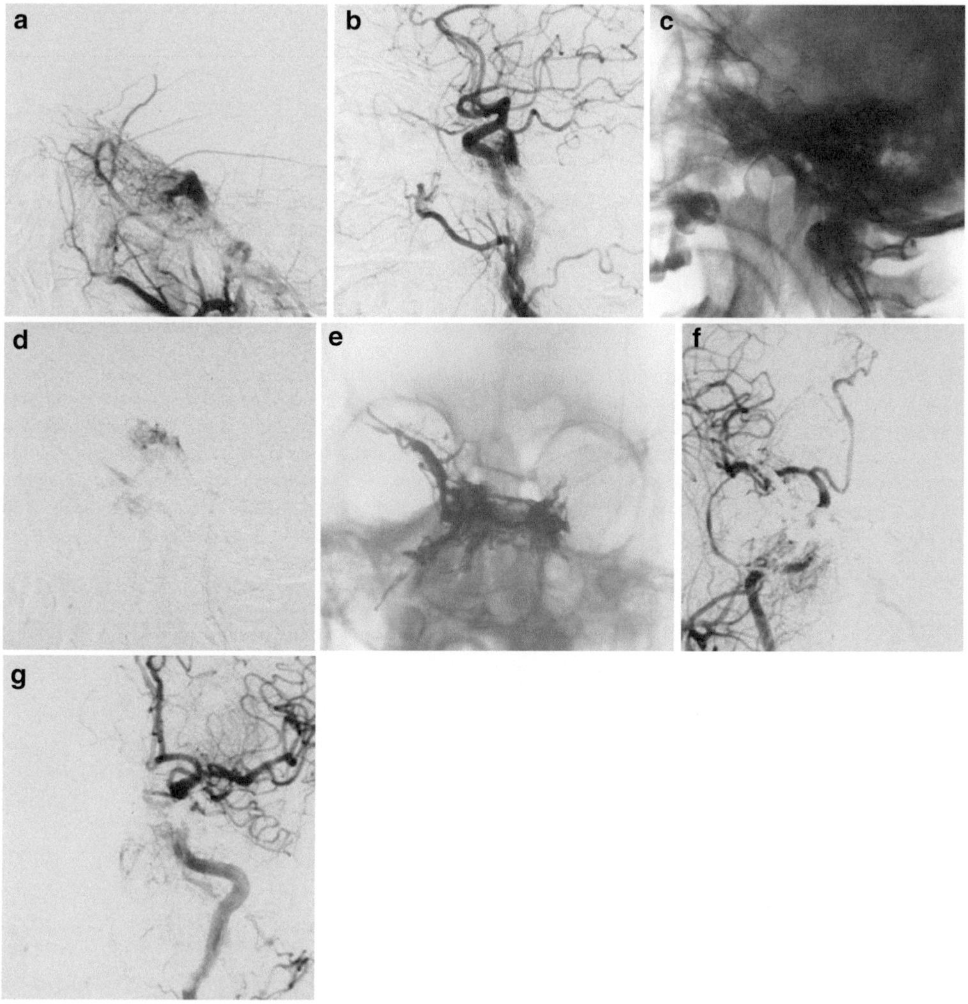

Fig. 8.1 A 71-year-old woman presented with oculomotor nerve palsy of the right eye. (**a**) Lateral view of the right external carotid artery angiography showing a cavernous sinus DAVF was supplied by multiple dural branches of the external carotid artery. (**b**) Lateral view of the left carotid artery angiography showing the cavernous sinus DAVF was supplied by multiple dural branches of the carotid artery. (**c**) During the procedure, lateral view of the fluoroscopic image showing the cavernous sinus was accessed through the right inferior petrosal sinus. (**d**) During the procedure, lateral view of the selective angiography showing the cavernous sinus was accessed through the inferior petrosal sinus. (**e**) Frontal view of the fluoroscopic image showing the Onyx cast after embolization. (**f**) Frontal view of the right carotid artery angiography showing the fistula was completely occluded. (**g**) Frontal view of the left carotid artery angiography showing the fistula was completely occluded

8.4 Carotid-Cavernous Fistulas (CCFs)

The TVE is the first-line treatment for indirect CCF, in which dangerous anastomosis, arteries supplying cranial nerves, and very small supply arteries supplying fistulas are very likely to be involved [11]. The cure rate varied from 80% to 100% [11]. There are many transvenous routes to reach the cavernous sinus (CS), and these include the inferior petrosal sinus (IPS) (Fig. 8.1), basilar plexus, facial vein (FV) (Figs. 8.2, 8.3 and 8.4), angular vein, and superior petrosal sinus (Fig. 8.5), or through the pterygoid plexus [12]. These veins are accessable by transfemoral or transjugular approach, by direct puncture or surgical exposure. In treatment of direct CCF, it is necessary to temporarily block the internal carotid artery using a

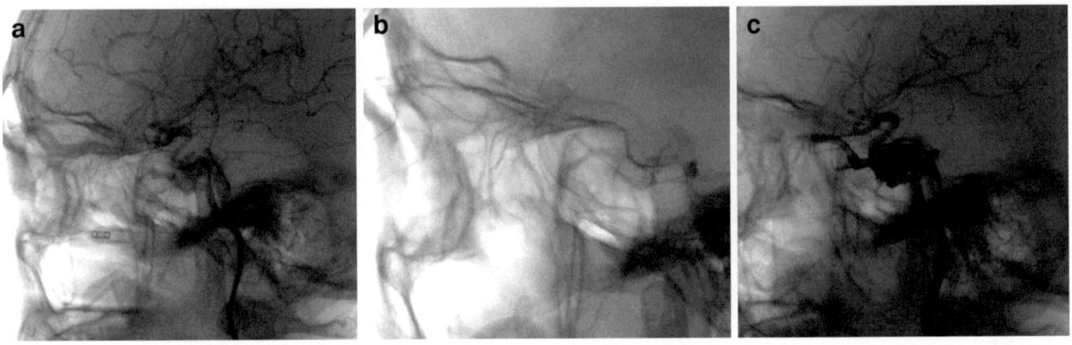

Fig. 8.2 A 47-year-old man presented with blindness of the right eye for 1 week. (**a**) Lateral view of the unsubtracted image of the right carotid artery injection showing a cavernous sinus DAVF was supplied by multiple dural branches of the carotid artery with ipsilateral-IPS occlusion and main venous drainage of the superior ophthalmic vein. (**b**) During the procedure, lateral view of the unsubtracted image of the selective angiography showing the cavernous sinus was accessed through the right facial vein and superior ophthalmic vein. (**c**) Lateral view of the unsubtracted image of the right carotid artery injection showing the Onyx cast after embolization and complete obliteration of the fistula. The patient's vision improved remarkably on the next day of treatment

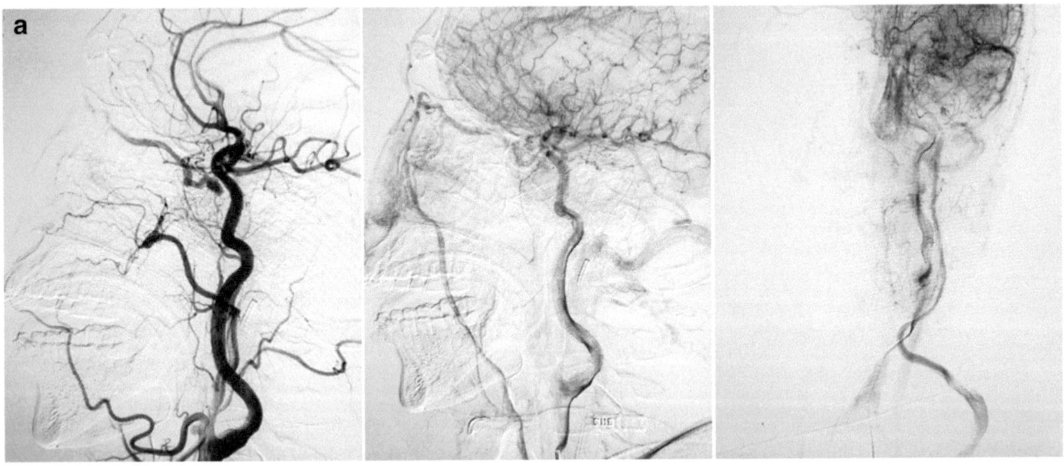

Fig. 8.3 Representative case showing the transvenous embolization of cavernous DAVF through facial vein. (**a**) The left carotid artery angiography (left, early phase; middle, late phase; right, late phase of frontal view) Showing a cavernous sinus DAVF was supplied by multiple dural branches of the carotid artery with ipsilateral-IPS occlusion and main venous drainage of the superior ophthalmic vein to the facial vein and external jugular vein. (**b**) A 5-Fr diagnostic catheter was placed in the ipsilateral carotid artery via a left transfemoral approach for control arteriography. Another 5-Fr guiding catheter was placed in the ipsilateral external jugular vein via a right transfemoral approach for navigation of the microcatheter (left). The use of a loop at the tip of 0.014 in. microguidewire within the facial vein was helpful to avoid getting stuck in the irregular, trabeculated venous walls (middle). The microguidewire was advanced into the superior ophthalmic vein (right). (**c**) The microguidewire was advanced into the cavernous sinus (right). The selective angiography showing the tip of the microcatheter was in the cavernous sinus (middle). Onyx-18 was injected through the microcatheter under negative roadmap (right). (**d**) Lateral view of the left carotid artery angiography showing the fistula was completely occluded (left). Unsubtracted image showing the Onyx-18 cast (right)

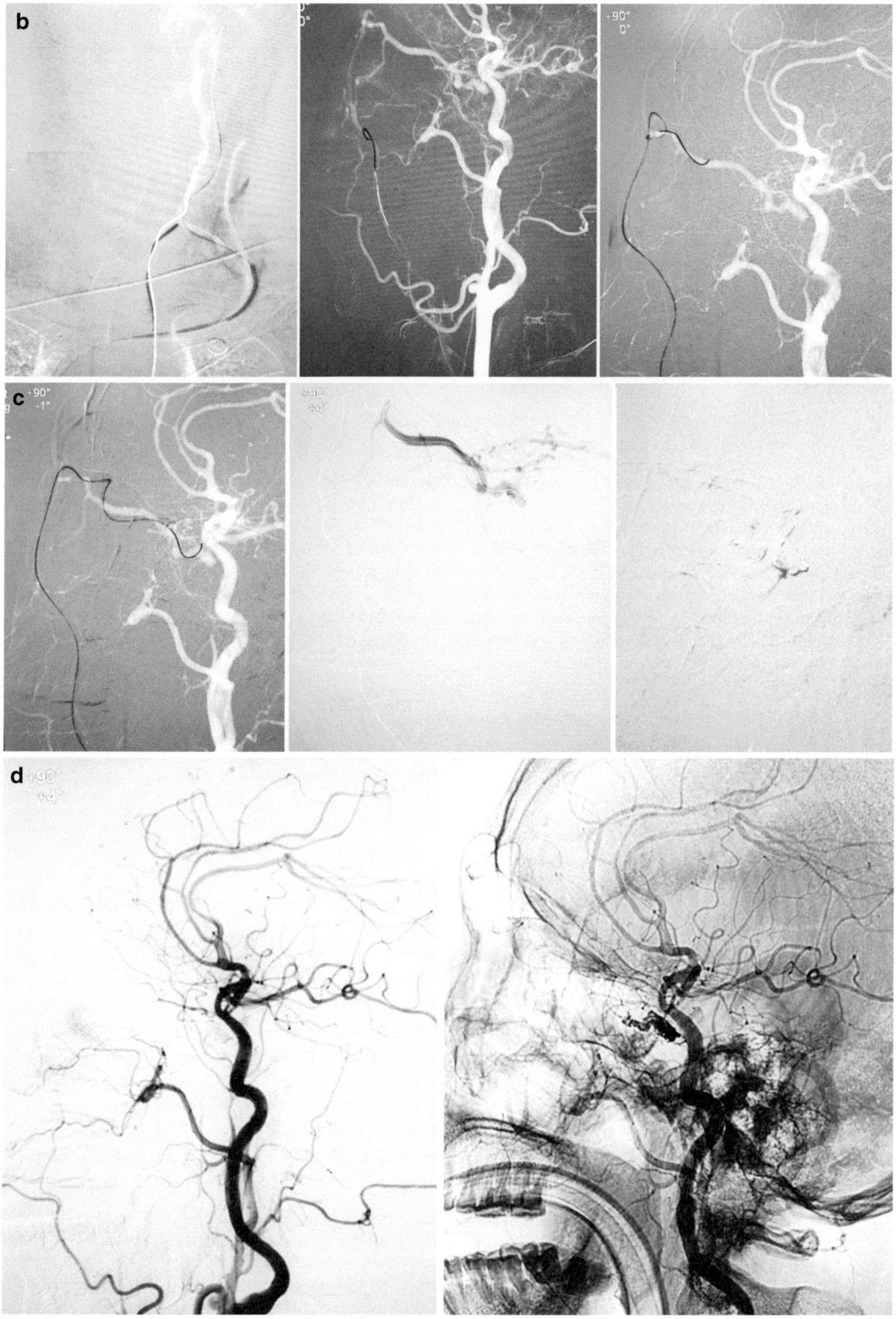

Fig. 8.3 (continued)

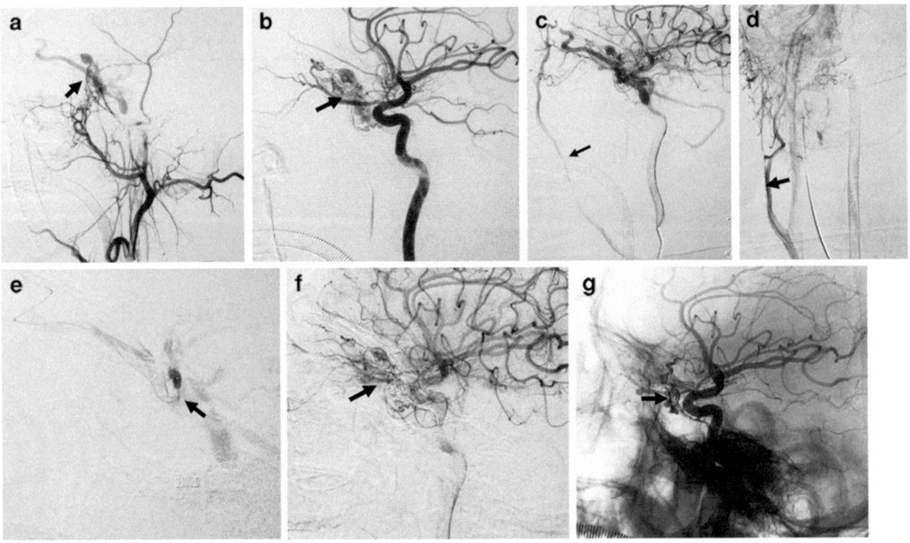

Fig. 8.4 A 24-year-old woman presented with exophthalmos of the right eye. (**a**) Lateral view the right external carotid artery angiography. (**b**) Lateral view the right internal carotid artery angiography. Showing a intra-orbital AVF was supplied by multiple dural branches of the carotid artery and main venous drainage of the superior ophthalmic vein (arrows). (**c**) Lateral view the right internal carotid artery angiography showing the venous drainage to the facial vein and external jugular vein (arrow). (**d**) Frontal view the right internal carotid artery angiography showing the facial vein drained into the external jugular vein (arrow). (**e**) The selective angiography showing the tip of the microcatheter was at the fistula (arrow) through the facial vein to the superior ophthalmic vein. (**f**) Lateral view of the left carotid artery angiography showing the fistula was completely occluded using Onyx-18 (arrow). (**g**) Unsubtracted image showing the Onyx-18 cast (arrow)

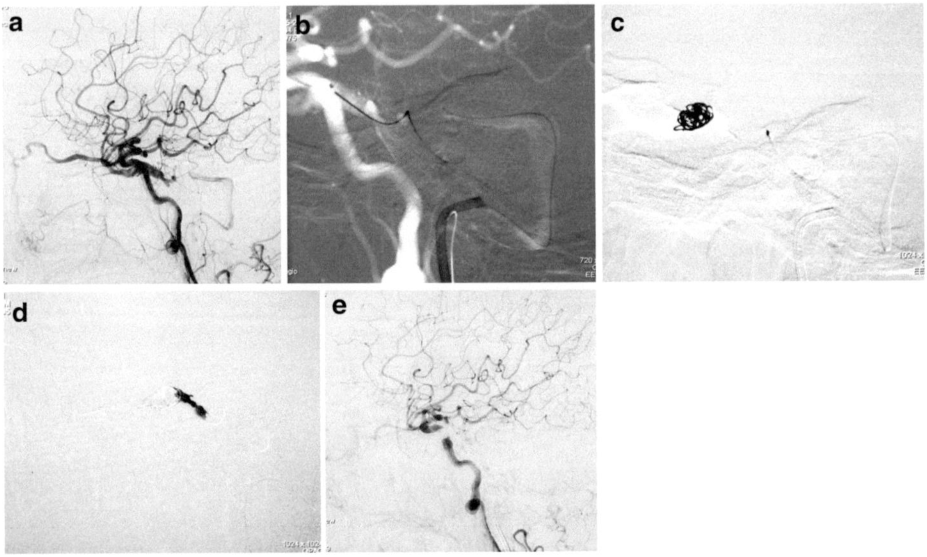

Fig. 8.5 Representative case showing the transvenous embolization of cavernous DAVF through the superior petrosal sinus. (**a**) Lateral view of the left carotid artery angiography showing a cavernous sinus DAVF drained into the superior ophthalmic vein to the hypoplastic facial vein and the superior petrosal sinus. (**b**) Showing a microcatheter was advanced into the cavernous sinus via a right transfemoral approach under roadmap. (**c**) Showing several coils were inserted into the cavernous sinus under roadmap to decrease the shunting flow. (**d**) Showing Onyx-18 was injected under negative roadmap to seal the DAVF. (**e**) Lateral view of the left carotid artery angiography showing the fistula was completely occluded

balloon catheter during the Onyx embolization of the fistula venous pouch [13].

The most commonly transvenous approach to obliterate the CCF is the IPS, which provides a relatively direct and shortest route from the internal jugular vein (IJV) to the CS [14]. Even the IPS does not serve as a venous outflow on angiograms due to its thrombosis, this does not exclude it as a reasonable choice for reaching the CS [15]. The successful rate of catheterization of angiographically invisible IPS has been reported 50–80% by some authors [15]. Lv et al. suggested a new method for detecting the invisible origin of the IPS [16]. In the Lv et al. study, when the microguidewire showed an angle of about 117° on the lateral projection, which is the IPS (Figs. 8.6, 8.7 and 8.8). The microcatheter is advanced into the orifice of the IPS, and then continue to open the IPS using the microguidewire in this direction. The angle of microguidewire is useful for confirming the orifice of thrombosed IPS to save time and avoid unnecessary irradiation. To avoid any risk of perforation, only 0.0140 in. wire is used. If there is substantial resistance when advancing the microcatheter, switching to a Transend14 or an Avigo14 microguidewire is a sensible alternative for their higher support. While advancing the wire within the thrombosed IPS, the use of a loop at the tip was found to be helpful. Advancing a loop of a 0.014 hydrophilic wire is much less traumatic than the tip, particularly if the catheter is already wedged. The softness of the 0.014 loop allows it to avoid getting stuck in the irregular, trabeculated venous walls and to conform to the specific anatomy of the IPS. Microguidewires and microcatheters minimize the risk of venous perforation. The angulate theory is found to be useful in thrombosed IPS route and to be associated with a higher technical successful rate. The thrombosed IPS approach avoids the necessity of more aggressive procedures in so-called intractable indirect CCFs.

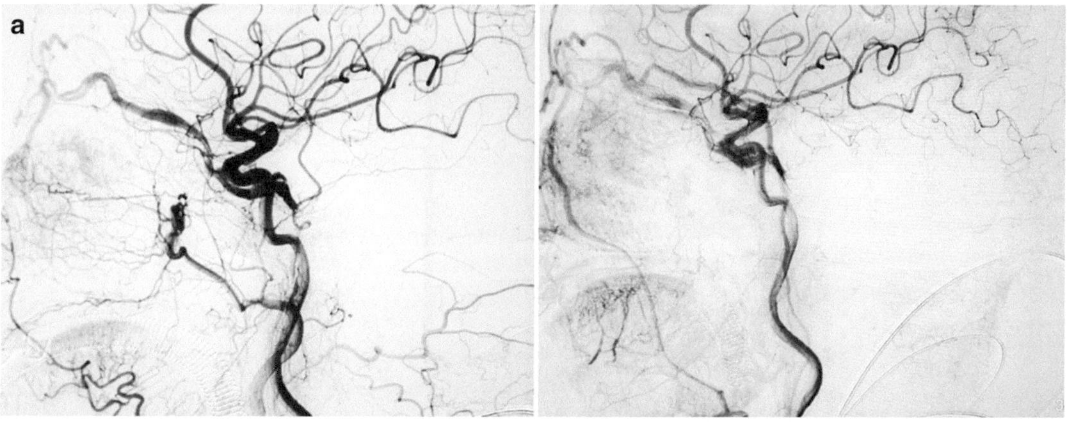

Fig. 8.6 Representative case showing the transvenous embolization of cavernous DAVF through the invisible inferior petrosal sinus. (**a**) Lateral view of the left carotid artery angiography (left, early phase; right, late phase) showing ipsilateral inferior petrosal sinus occlusion and main venous drainage of the superior ophthalmic vein. (**b**) During the procedure, attempt to find the orifice of the inferior petrosal sinus using microguidewire, which showed a nearly 110° angle under roadmap. (**c**) Images showing the microcatheter was advanced into the cavernous sinus and the fistula was complete occluded using a combination of coils and Onyx

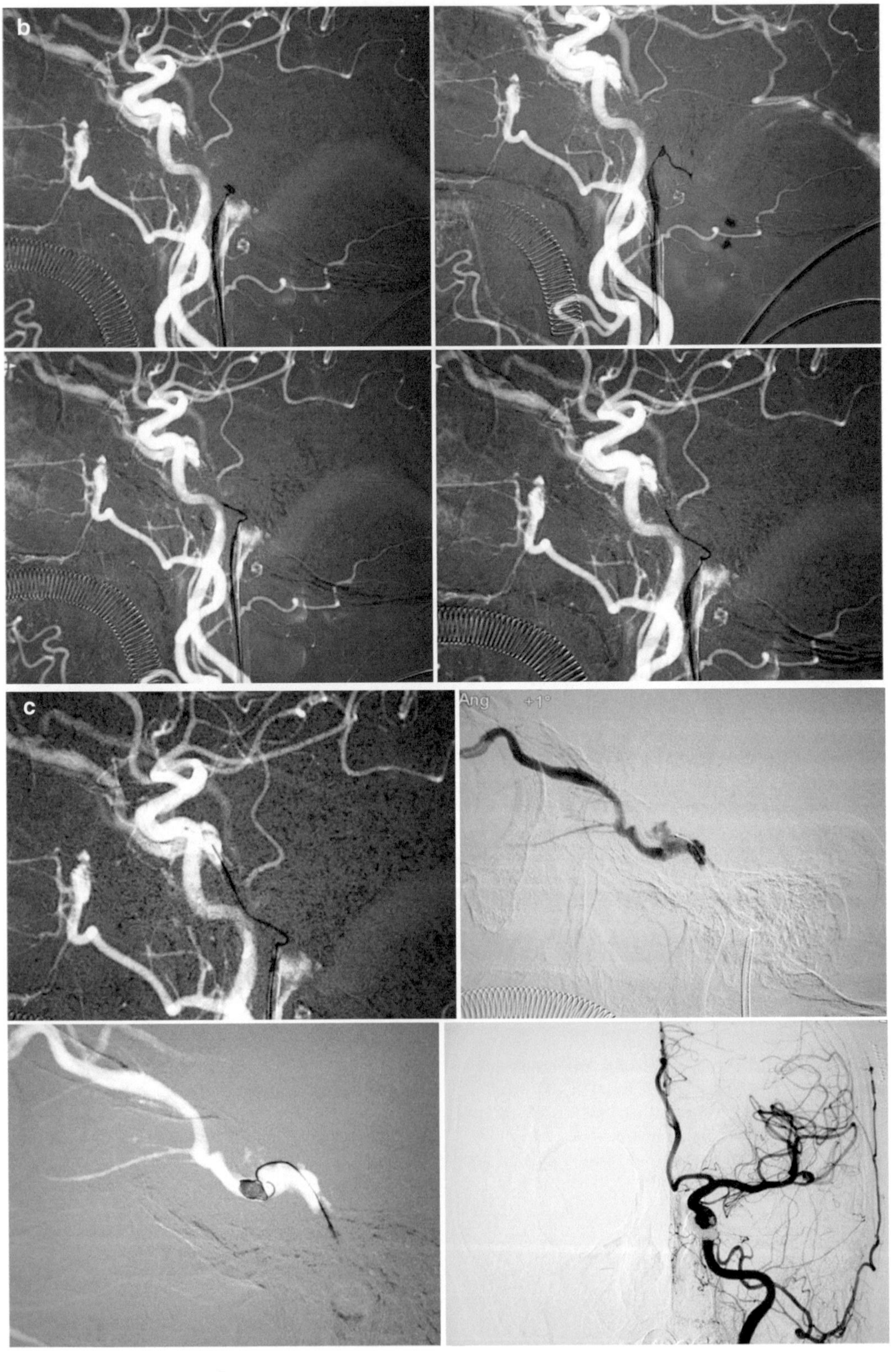

Fig. 8.6 (continued)

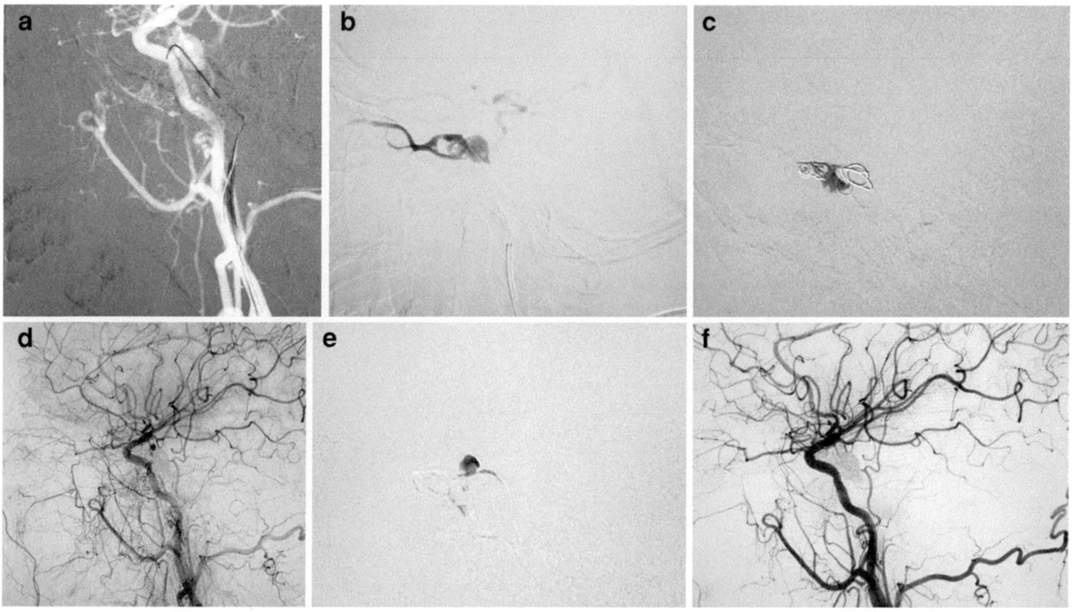

Fig. 8.7 Representative case showing the transvenous embolization of cavernous DAVF through the invisible inferior petrosal sinus. (**a**) During the procedure, the cavernous sinus was accessed through the occluded inferior petrosal sinus using a microguidewire, which showed a nearly 120° angle under roadmap. (**b**) Selective angiography showing the microcatheter was advanced into the cavernous sinus. (**c**) Showing the fistula was occluded using a combination of coils and Onyx. (**d**) Lateral view of the carotid artery angiography showing the residual fistula superior to the cavernous sinus. (**e**) Showing Onyx injection under negative roadmap and the residual fistula was occluded. (**f**) Lateral view of the carotid artery angiography showing the fistula was completely occluded

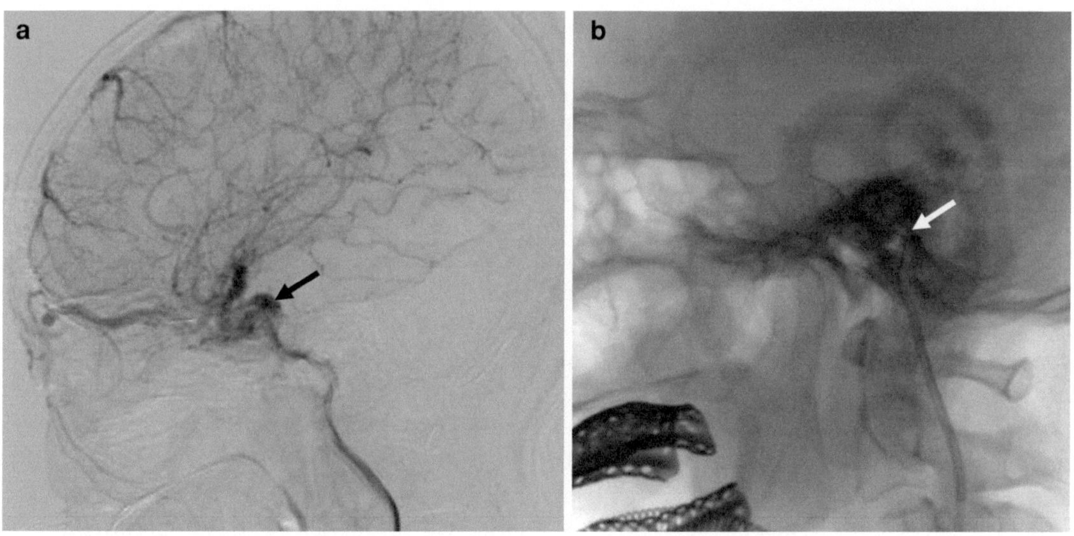

Fig. 8.8 A 61-year-old woman presented with chemosis and proptosis of the left eye. (**a**) Lateral view of the left internal carotid artery angiography showing ipsilateral inferior petrosal sinus occlusion and main venous drainage of the superior ophthalmic vein (arrow). The CSDAVF was supplied by multiple dural branches of the internal carotid artery. (**b**) During the procedure, microguidewire showed a 109° angle under fluoroscopic image, meaning it's the orifice of the IPS. (**c**) Fluoroscopic image showing the fistula was occluded using a combination of coils and Onyx (arrow) on the lateral projection. (**d**) Lateral view of the left carotid artery angiography showing the fistula was completely occluded

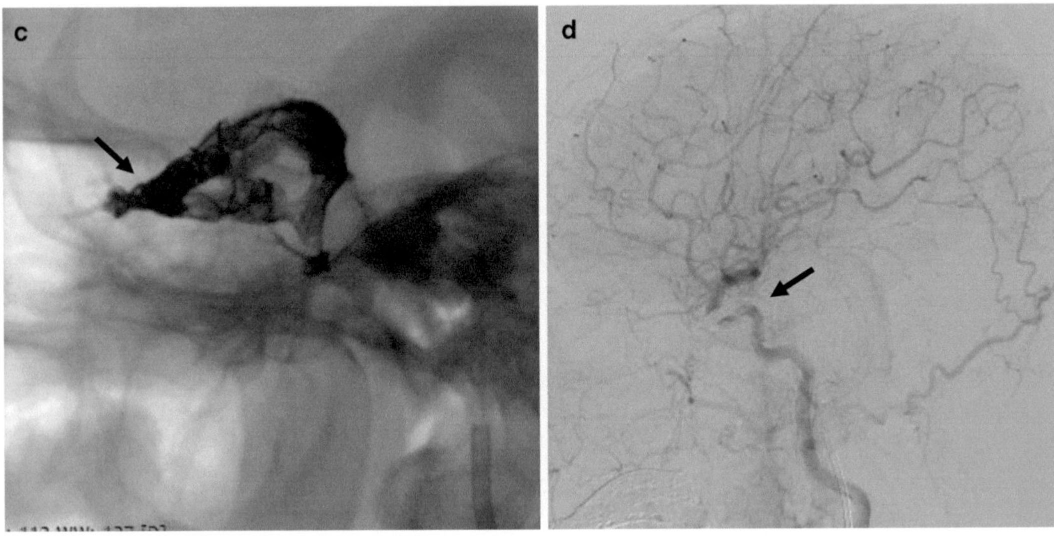

Fig. 8.8 (continued)

8.5 Transverse-Sigmoid Sinus DAVFs

Transvenous embolization is effective if the affected TSS does not participate in normal venous drainage. Angiographic cure can be achieved in 80–100% of patients [17]. This procedure requires sacrifice of dural sinus flow avoiding occlusion of the nearby normal antegrade cortical venous drainage. The rate of permanent complications is approximately 4% [18]. Another option for managing DAVFs with high-grade stenosis or occlusion of TSS is transvenous angioplasty and stenting. When the venous drainage of the brain depends on the transverse sinus of the fistula, the use of a stent to reconstruct the transverse sinus, with or without transarterial Onyx embolization may be a good choice [2]. Recanalization, angioplasty, and stenting of stenosis/occlusive TSS can restore antegrade sinus flow and close shunts within the sinus wall, and a few successful cases have been reported [2]. Further investigation of the effectiveness of TSS angioplasty in the treatment of DAVFs is necessary.

When a DAVF flows directly into the TSS and there is no venous pouch, the possibility of Onyx diffusing into the normal sinus is high in TVE. A large amount of reflux to the normal sinuses can cause pulmonary embolism or inadvertent sinus thrombosis. In these cases, reconstructive transvenous balloon-assisted embolization was introduced as an option. For this technique, a microcatheter and a DMSO-compliant balloon are simultaneously guided to the affected transverse sigmoid sinus. After the balloon is inflated, Onyx 18 is injected around the balloon and slowly penetrates into the blood suppliers resulting in complete occlusion of DAVFs. In this technique, the preservation of normal cortical veins, such as Labbé vein and normal bridging vein, is essential to prevent complications such as venous infarction and cerebral or cerebellar hemorrhage [19]. Transvenous Onyx embolization for the treatment of high-risk transverse sigmoid sinus DAVF, in which a microcatheter is passed through the sinus into the venous pouch and positioned to the arterial ostium. In these cases, Onyx penetrates into multiple arterial suppliers, and a small amount of reflux enters the venous pouch. According to this report, this technique is safe when there is a venous pouch or an isolated sinus.

8.6 Tentorial DAVFs

TVE with coils was preferred when the lesion was anatomically suited. In some cases, transvenous coil or Onyx embolization may be safe when there is an uncurved draining vein that allows the catheter to enter the venous pouch [20].

8.7 Superior Sagittal Sinus DAVFs

TVE with coil packing of affected SSS can be a choice if the SSS is not functional for normal cortical vein drainage [2]. Nevertheless, SSS DAVFs are usually associated with SSS occlusion or stenosis; the TVE is often difficult.

8.8 Anterior Cranial Fossa DAVFs

For ethmoidal or anterior cranial fossa DAVF, the blood supply arteries are usually small and very tortuous, making it difficult or impossible to perform a safe superselective transarterial catheterization [21]. A few anterior fossa DAVFs have been reported safely treated with TVE. This approach is complicated and rarely used when treating this type of DAVF because the anterior fossa DAVF is often associated with venous aneurysm and the transvenous route is tortuous.

8.9 Other DAVFs

DAVFs can also occur at the marginal sinus, inferior and superior petrosal sinuses, and hypoglossal canal [2]. Coil packing of these minor dural sinuses is preferred because these affected sinus is nonfunctional and does not participate the normal venous drains.

8.10 Conclusions

Embolization of DAVF via intravenous route is a very useful treatment. This method should be frequently applied in the treatment of DAVF. In the treatment process, attention should be paid to the choice of cases and the grasp of indications to avoid complications.

References

1. Cognard C, Gobin YP, Pierot L, Bailly AL, Houdart E, Casasco A, Chiras J, Merland JJ. Cerebral dural arteriovenous fistulas: clinical and angiographic correlation with a revised classification of venous drainage. Radiology. 1995;194(3):671–80.
2. Luo CB, Chang FC, Teng MM. Update of embolization of intracranial dural arteriovenous fistula. J Chin Med Assoc. 2014;77(12):610–7.
3. Jiang C, Lv X, Li Y, Wu Z. Transarterial Onyx packing of the transverse–sigmoid sinus for dural arteriovenous fistulas. Eur J Radiol. 2011;80:767–70.
4. Lv X. Direct trans-orbit puncture for embolization of the intra-orbital or cavernous arteriovenous fistula. In: Lv X, editor. An eBook on vascular diseases. Reno, NV: MedDocs Publishers LLC; 2020. p. 67–83. http://meddocsonline.org/.
5. Yamauchi S, Nishio A, Takahashi Y, Kondo K, Kawakami T, Terakawa Y, Mitsuhashi Y, Ohata K. An innovative technique for detecting the caudal end of occluded inferior petrosal sinus in cavernous arteriovenous fistula using intravascular ultrasonography—technical note. Neuroradiology. 2015;57(8):799–804.
6. Matsumoto A, Okauchi M, Shindo A, Kawanishi M, Tamiya T. Cavernous sinus dural arteriovenous fistula treated by facial vein direct puncture: case report and review of the literature. Interv Neuroradiol. 2017;23(3):301–6.
7. Jiang C, Lv X, Li Y, Wu Z, Shi J. Surgical access on the superior ophthalmic vein to the cavernous sinus dural fistula for embolization. J Neurointerv Surg. 2013;5(3):e13.
8. Jiang C, Lv X, Li Y, Liu A, Lv M, Jiang P, Wu Z. Transvenous embolization of cavernous sinus dural arteriovenous fistula with Onyx-18 and platinum coils: technical note. Neuroradiol J 2007;20(3):47-52.
9. Benndorf G, Bender A, Lehmann R, Lanksch W. Transvenous occlusion of dural cavernous sinus fistulas through the thrombosed inferior petrosal sinus: report of four cases and review of the literature. Surg Neurol. 2000;54(1):42–54.
10. Lv X, Jiang C, Li Y, Yang X, Wu Z. Recovery of opthalmoplegia associated with cavernous sinus dural arteriovenous fistulas after transvenous cavernous sinus packing. Eur J Radiol. 2010;75:139–42.
11. Lv X, Jiang C, Li Y, Wu Z. Percutaneous transvenous packing of cavernous sinus with Onyx for cavernous dural arteriovenous fistula. Eur J Radiol. 2009;71:356–62.
12. Rhim JK, Cho YD, Park JJ, Jeon JP, Kang HS, Kim JE, Cho WS, Han MH. Endovascular treatment of cavernous sinus dural arteriovenous fistula with

ipsilateral inferior petrosal sinus occlusion: a single-center experience. Neurosurgery. 2015;77(2):192–9.
13. Lv X, Wang G, Wang J. Craniospinal vascular diseases and endovascular neurosurgery. New York: Nova Science; 2021.
14. Kawamura Y, Takigawa T, Hyodo A, Suzuki K. Transvenous embolisation via an occluded inferior petrosal sinus for cavernous sinus dural arteriovenous fistulas. Neurol Neurochir Pol. 2020;54(6):585–8.
15. Luo CB, Chang FC, Teng MM, Guo WY, Ting TW. Transvenous embolization of cavernous sinus dural arteriovenous fistula via angiographic occlusive inferior petrous sinus. J Chin Med Assoc. 2015;78(9):526–32.
16. Lv X. The angle of the microguidwire on the lateral projection: a prediction of cannulation of the occluded inferior petrosal sinuses for the transvenous embolization of cavernous sinus dural arteriovenous fistulas (unpublished).
17. Lv X, Jiang C, Li Y, Yang X, Wu Z. Intraarterial and intravenous treatment of transverse/sigmoid sinus dural arteriovenous fistulas. Interv Neuroradiol. 2009;15:291–300.
18. Duvvuri M, Caton MT, Narsinh K, Amans MR. Balloon-backstop technique: Preserving physiologic venous drainage during transvenous coil embolization of sigmoid sinus dural arteriovenous fistulas. Neuroradiol J. 2022;35(3):412–17.
19. Lv X, Jiang C, Liang S, Wang J. The variant with the absence of the superior petrosal venous and sinus: A potential pitfall of transvenous balloon-assisted embolisation of Borden type II transverse-sigmoid dural arteriovenous fistula. Interv Neuroradiol. 2019;25(4):474–7.
20. Jiang C, Lv X, Li Y, Wu Z. Transarterial and transvenous embolization for tentorial dural arteriovenous fistula: case report. Neuroradiol J. 2007;20(6):726–9.
21. Lv X, Li Y, Liu A, Lv M, Jiang C, Wu Z. Endovascular embolization of dural arteriovenous fistulas of the anterior cranial fossa: three case reports. Neurol Res. 2008;30(8):852–9.

Dural Carotid-Cavernous Fistula Treatment

9

Anchalee Churojana, Ekawut Chankaew, and Ittichai Sakarunchai

Abstract

The aggressive characteristic of dural carotid-cavernous fistula (dCCF) is characterized by elevated intraocular pressure or the presentation of leptomeningeal venous drainage. It is necessary to treat an aggressive dCCF to prevent permanent secondary glaucoma and intracerebral sequelae. The endovascular approach is the treatment modality for dramatic improvement after fistula obliteration. Transvenous catheterizations are performed through the inferior petrosal sinus (IPS) and selection of coil packing within each of the venous drainage channel, such as cavernous sinus (CS)-superior orbital vein (SOV) junction, the connection between the CS and the leptomeningeal vein if there is presence of leptomeningeal drainage. An alternative to the CS and SOV approach can be performed using the transfemoral transvenous or percutaneous approach if cannulation of the IPS fails. Coils are mainly used as the embolic material rather than liquid embolic materials to prevent intracerebral complications and cranial nerve dysfunction. The angiographic endpoint of the endovascular procedure is either subtotal or complete occlusion of the fistula. Any small residual non-aggressive angiographic characteristic can be completely obliterated in a future surgery after routine clinical and radiological follow-up. The results are excellent with a low rate of complications. However, dCCF treatment requires experienced operators with a good understanding of the angiographic architecture and the appropriate skills in endovascular techniques.

Keywords

Dural carotid-cavernous fistula
Endovascular treatment · Transvenous catheterization · Coil embolization · IPS cannulation

A. Churojana (✉)
Department of Radiology, Siriraj Hospital, Mahidol University, Bangkok, Thailand
e-mail: unchalee.cho@mahido.ac.th

E. Chankaew
Division of Neurosurgery, Department of Surgery, Siriraj Hospital, Mahidol University, Bangkok, Thailand

I. Sakarunchai
Division of Neurosurgery, Brain and Cerebrovascular Center, Taksin Hospital, Bangkok, Thailand

9.1 Introduction

Dural carotid-cavernous fistulas (dCCFs) or indirect carotid-cavernous fistulas are defined as an abnormal connection between the dural branches of either the external or internal carotid artery and the cavernous sinus (CS) [1]. Bilateral dCCFs are not uncommon [2].

X. Lv (ed.), *Intracranial and Spinal Dural Arteriovenous Fistulas*,
https://doi.org/10.1007/978-981-19-5767-3_9

A dCCF is the most frequent dural arteriovenous shunt, and the incidence is more common in Asian populations than in Western countries [3]. Although the exact etiology is unknown, dCCFs are considered to be an acquired disease following different triggers such as venous thrombosis, trauma, or infection [4].

Clinical presentations depend on the pattern of venous drainage of the shunts. Most dCCFs have orbital venous congestion symptoms such as chemosis, exophthalmos, bruit, or visual acuity impairment [5–7]. However, dCCFs with cortical venous reflux are associated with the potential risk of neurological deficits or even intracranial hemorrhage (Fig. 9.1) [4–7].

Nevertheless, arteriovenous fistulas or dural arteriovenous shunts in other locations may drain toward the CS and ophthalmic vein (Figs. 9.2 and 9.3) [8]. Furthermore, cerebral venous drainage may convert into the cavernous sinuses as a rerouting pathway in the presence of venous hyperpressure from an intracranial dural venous thrombosis or venous obstruction (Fig. 9.4) [7]. These conditions may have clinical presentations mimicking a dCCF.

The current classifications for dural arteriovenous fistulas are from Borden, Cognard, and the Bicetre group. They are helpful in understanding the morphology and predicting the natural history or prognosis leading to proper options and timing for treatment (Table 9.1) [7, 9, 10]. However, in the case of dCCFs, these existing classifications are not applicable for practical use in planning treatment. They do not incorporate the special characteristics of dCCFs, such as unilateral or bilateral shunt location, ipsilateral, contralateral or bilateral venous drainage, and the relevant antegrade drainage of the inferior petrosal sinus (IPS). Even the modified Cognard classification, which attempted to describe the morphology and characteristics of shunts and venous drainage [11], does not satisfactorily decide on the proper treatment of fistulas.

In our therapeutic strategy, dCCFs are classified into two groups according to presentation and the pattern of venous drainage.

1. The benign group shows antegrade drainage to the IPS or only retrograde drainage into the superior ophthalmic vein (SOV). Clinically the orbital symptoms of congestion are minimal, and intraocular pressure can be controlled medically. In this group, according to the natural history, spontaneous regression can be expected. In particular, if the SOV is not visualized during manual compression, delayed SOV thrombosis can be anticipated. Patients are then advised to perform this maneuver. Usually, invasive treatment is not required (Fig. 9.5) [7].
2. The aggressive group includes dCCFs with the presence of cortical venous reflux, or even dCCFs with SOV drainage only but uncontrolled elevated intraocular pressure. It is necessary to treat aggressive dCCFs to prevent permanent brain damage, intracranial hemorrhage, or secondary glaucoma (Figs. 9.1 and 9.6).

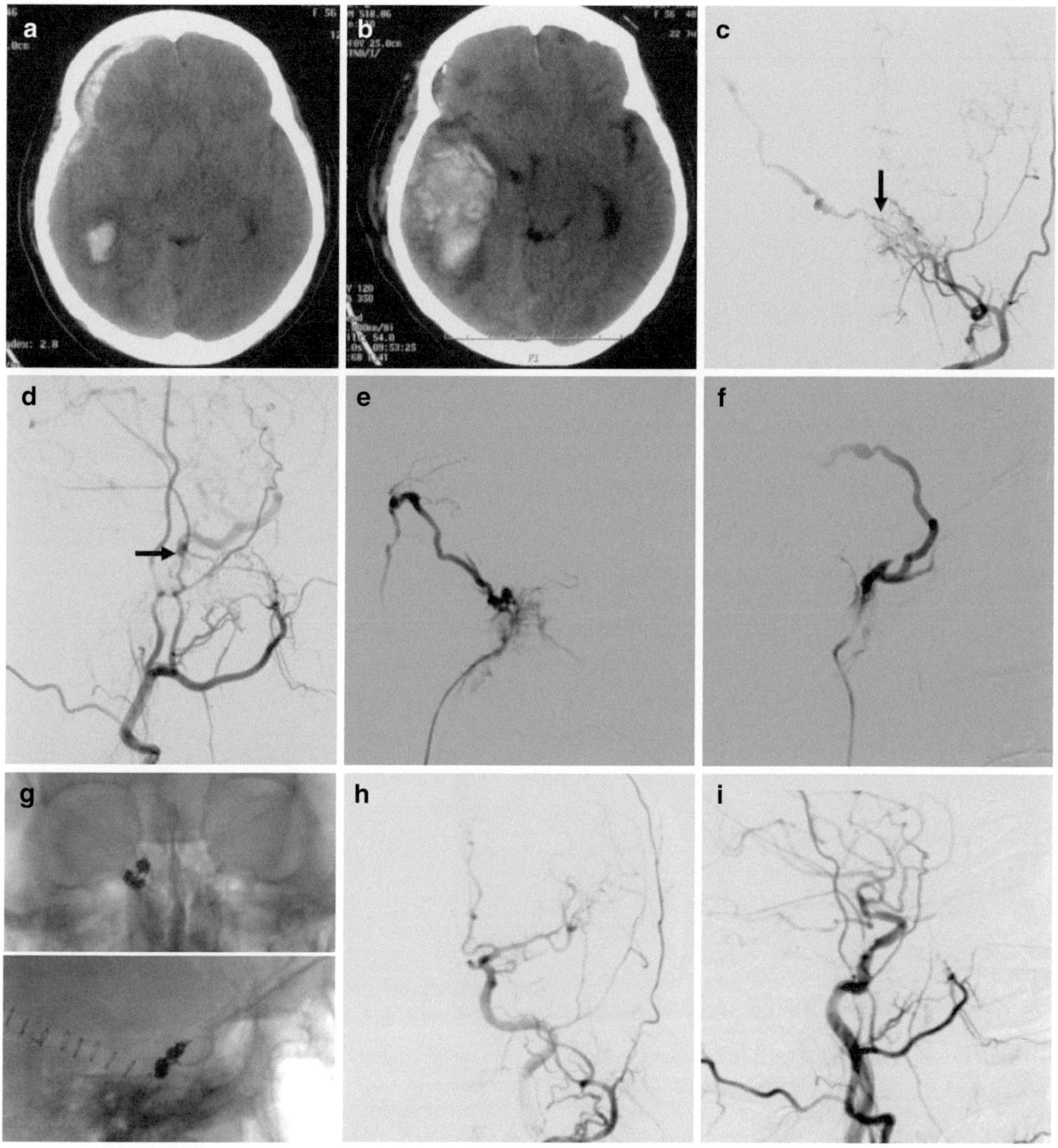

Fig. 9.1 Hemorrhagic presentation of an aggressive dCCF. (**a**) A 56-year-old male with nontraumatic right subdural hematoma and right temporal hemorrhage. (**b**) Expansion of right intraparenchymal hemorrhage after subdural hematoma removal. (**c**, **d**) AP and lateral projection of a left external carotid angiogram showing right dCCF (arrow) supplied from the contralateral middle meningeal artery and the artery of the foramen rotundum, draining into the right superficial middle cerebral vein with subsequent cortical reflux. (**e**, **f**) Blind recanalization of the right inferior petrosal sinus on AP and lateral views. (**g**) Fibered coil deposition in the right cavernous sinus on AP and lateral views. (**h**, **i**) AP and lateral views of controlled left common carotid angiogram revealing complete cure of right dCCF

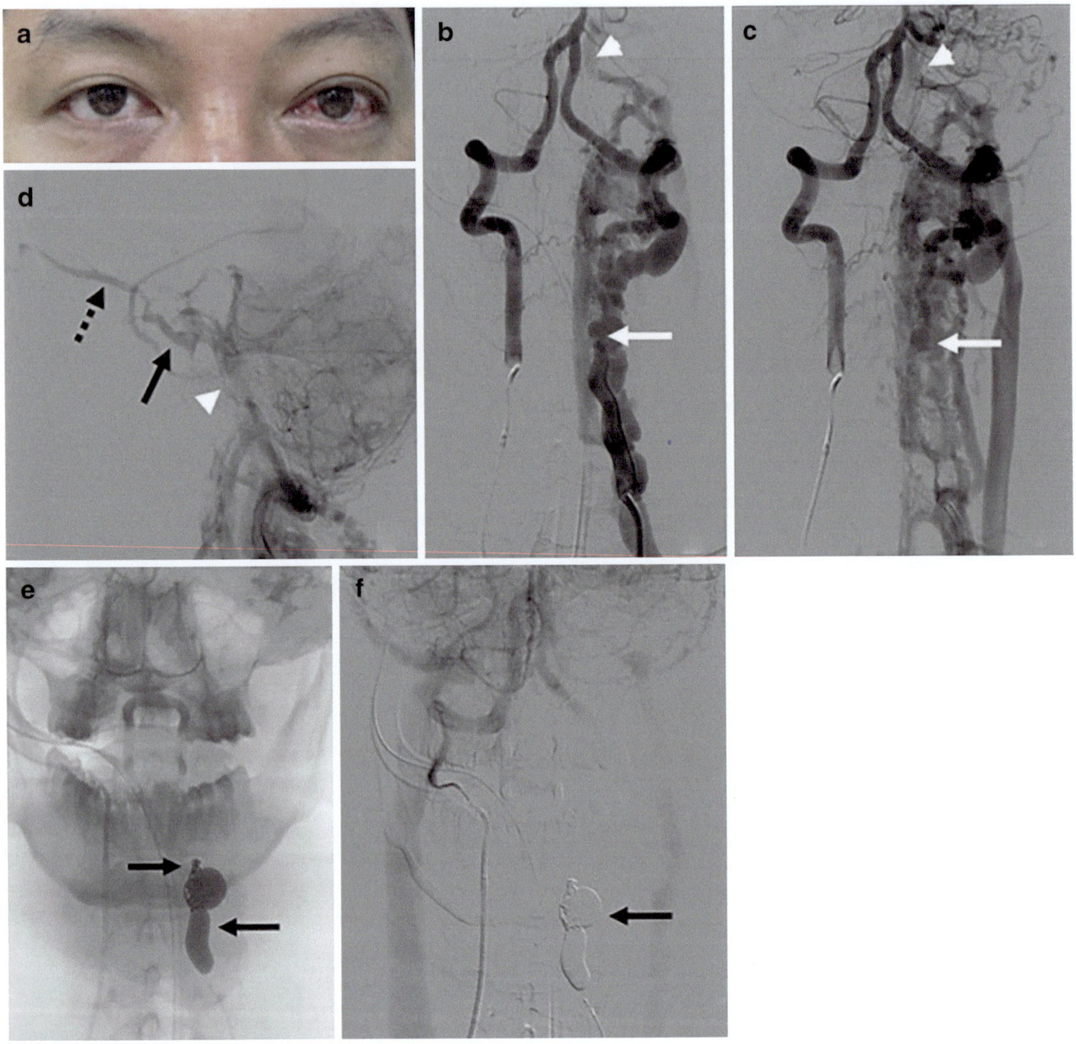

Fig. 9.2 Vertebro-vertebral fistula (VVF) with retrograde IPS drainage. (**a**) A 42-year-old male presented with left eye proptosis for 4 months. (**b**, **c**) AP and (**d**) lateral views of simultaneous injection of bilateral vertebral arteries revealing a VVF at V2 segment of left vertebral artery (white arrows) with drainage into the vertebral venous plexus and retrograde into the left inferior petrosal sinus (white arrowheads), cavernous sinus (black arrow), and superior ophthalmic vein (black dashed arrow) consequently. (**e**) Detachable balloons and coils were used to occlude the fistula and sacrifice the left vertebral artery (black arrows). (**f**) Controlled right vertebral artery injection demonstrating complete closure of the VVF

Fig. 9.3 Bilateral condylar dural AV shunts with retrograde IPS drainage. (**a**, **b**) TOF MRI of a 50-year-old female who had bilateral tinnitus for 5 months, right eye chemosis for 10 days, and diplopia for 4 days, demonstrating AV shunts at bilateral anterior condylar confluences (white arrow) with abnormal flow at the bilateral cavernous sinuses (white dashed arrow). (**c**, **d**) AP and lateral views of right ECA angiography showing dural AV shunt at right anterior condylar confluence (ACC) with retrograde drainage into the CS and consequently into the intercavernous sinus and left SMCV. White arrow = shunt location at right ACC, white arrowhead = right IPS, white dashed arrow = CS. Note two discrete vessels of right IPS. (**e**, **f**) AP and lateral views of left ECA angiography, white arrow = shunt location at left ACC with drainage into vertebral venous plexuses. (**g**) Coil deposition at right IPS and left ACC via transvenous access (not shown). (**h**, **i**) AP view of right ECA and left ECA injection to demonstrate total obliteration of bilateral shunts at 1-year follow-up. (**j**, **k**) Venous phase of the same right ECA and left ECA injection as in (**h**, **i**) showing visualization and function of left CS (white dash arrow) and IPS (white arrowhead)

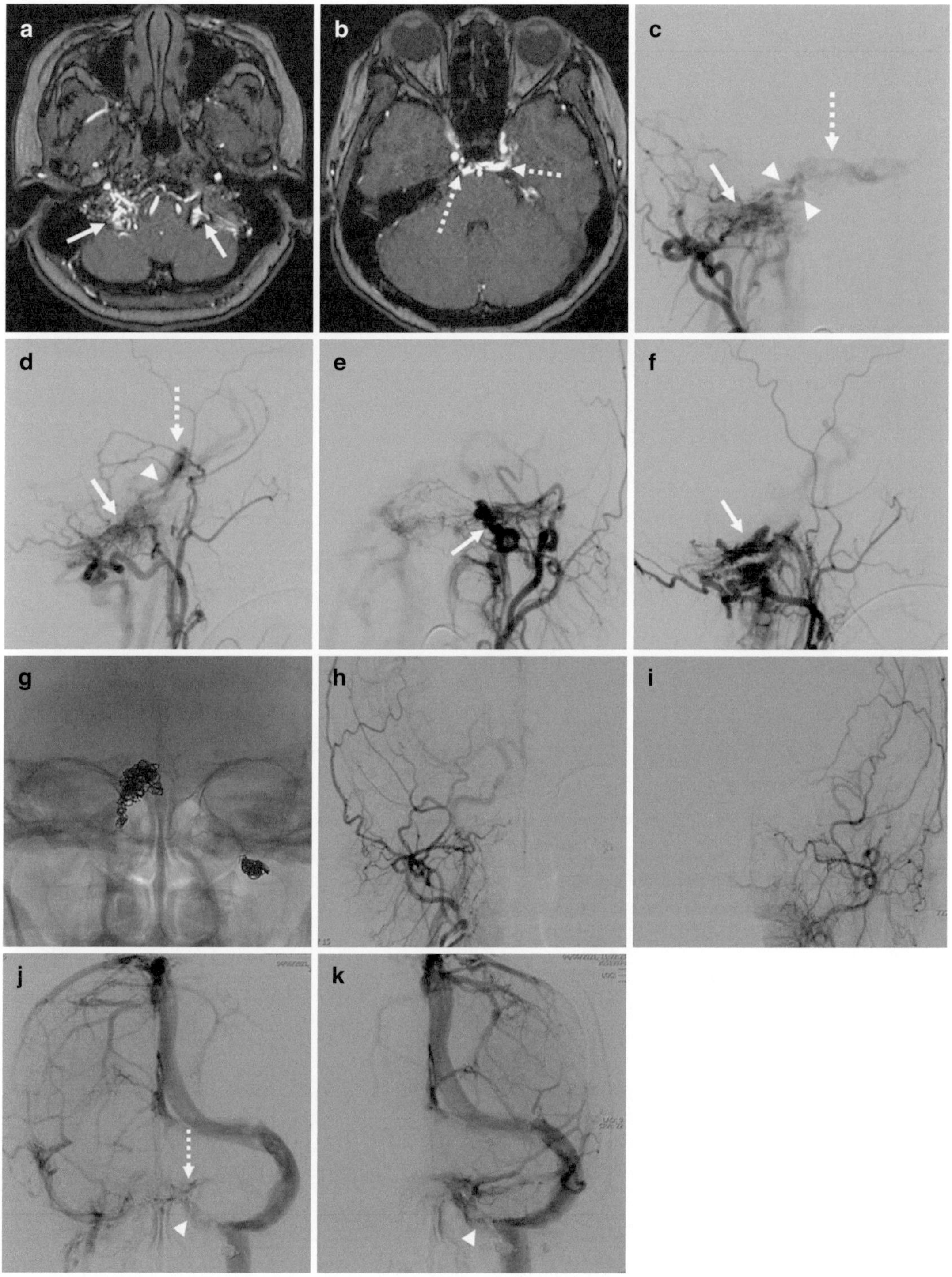
a
b
c
d
e
f
g
h
i
j
k

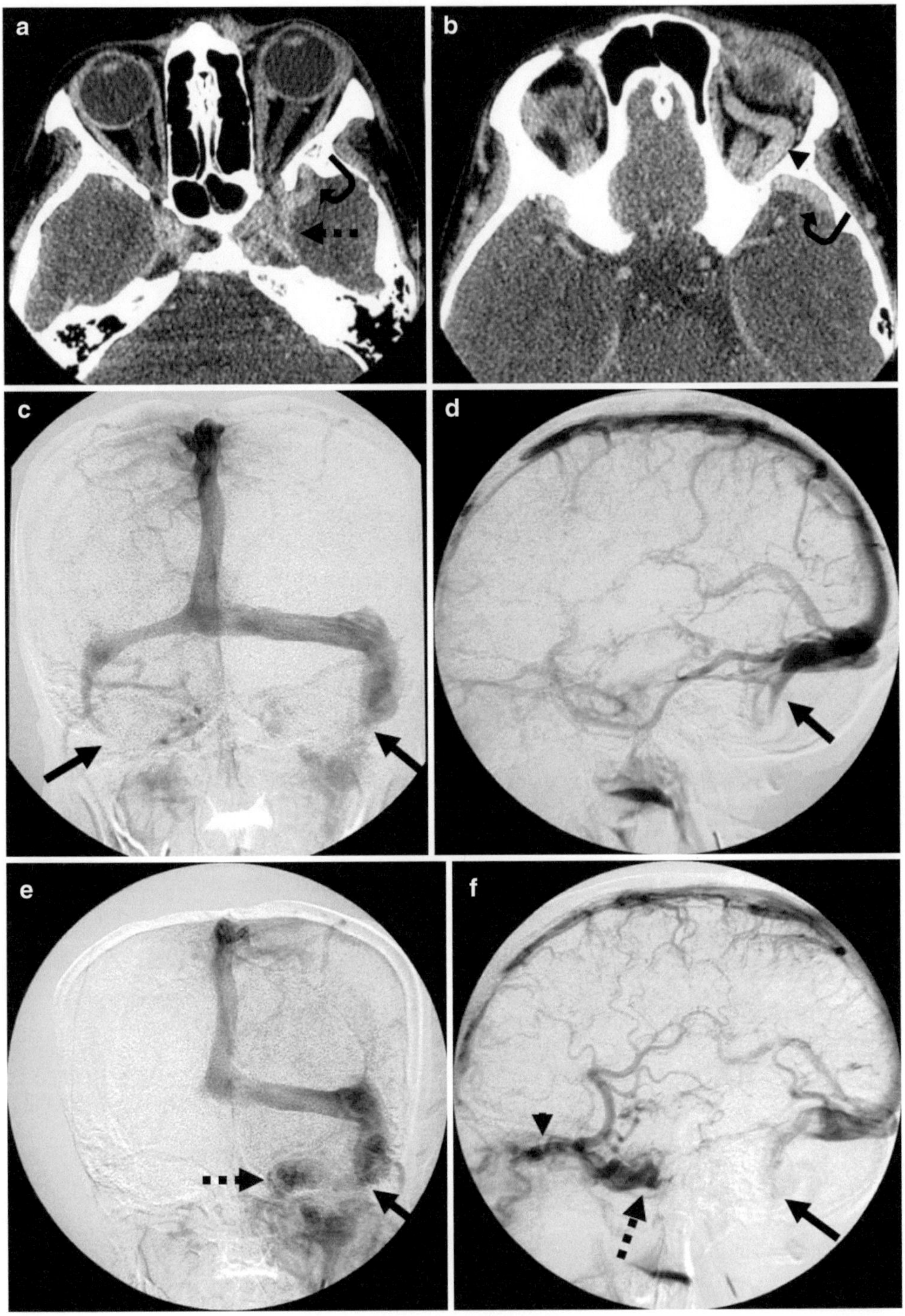

Fig. 9.4 Congenital jugular stenosis with rerouting of drainage pathway via the SOV. (**a**, **b**) Axial contrast CT scan of a 7-year-old girl who presented with mild proptosis and compressible mass at the medial canthus of the left eye, no chemosis, no limitation of eye movement, no history of trauma, revealing enlarged left cavernous sinus (dashed arrow), with dilatation of left SMCV (curved arrow) and SOV (arrowhead). Venous phase of right ICA (**c**, **d**) and left ICA (**e**, **f**) injection demonstrating rerouting of cerebral venous drainage to left CS (dashed arrow) and left SOV (arrowhead) as the consequences of jugular bulb occlusion on the right and severe stenosis on the left (arrows)

Table 9.1 Comparison between Borden and Cognard classifications according to venous drainage of intracranial dural arteriovenous fistulas

Borden classification	Cognard classification
Type I: DVS drainage or meningeal vein	Type I: DVS drainage with antegrade flow
Type II: DVS drainage with CVR	Type IIA: DVS drainage with retrograde flow
	Type IIB: DVS drainage with antegrade flow and CVR
	Type IIA + B: DVS drainage with retrograde flow and CVR
Type III: CVR only	Type III: CVR only (no venous ectasia)
	Type IV: CVR only (venous ectasia)
	Type V: CVR and drainage into spinal vein

DVS dural venous sinus, *CVR* cortical venous reflux

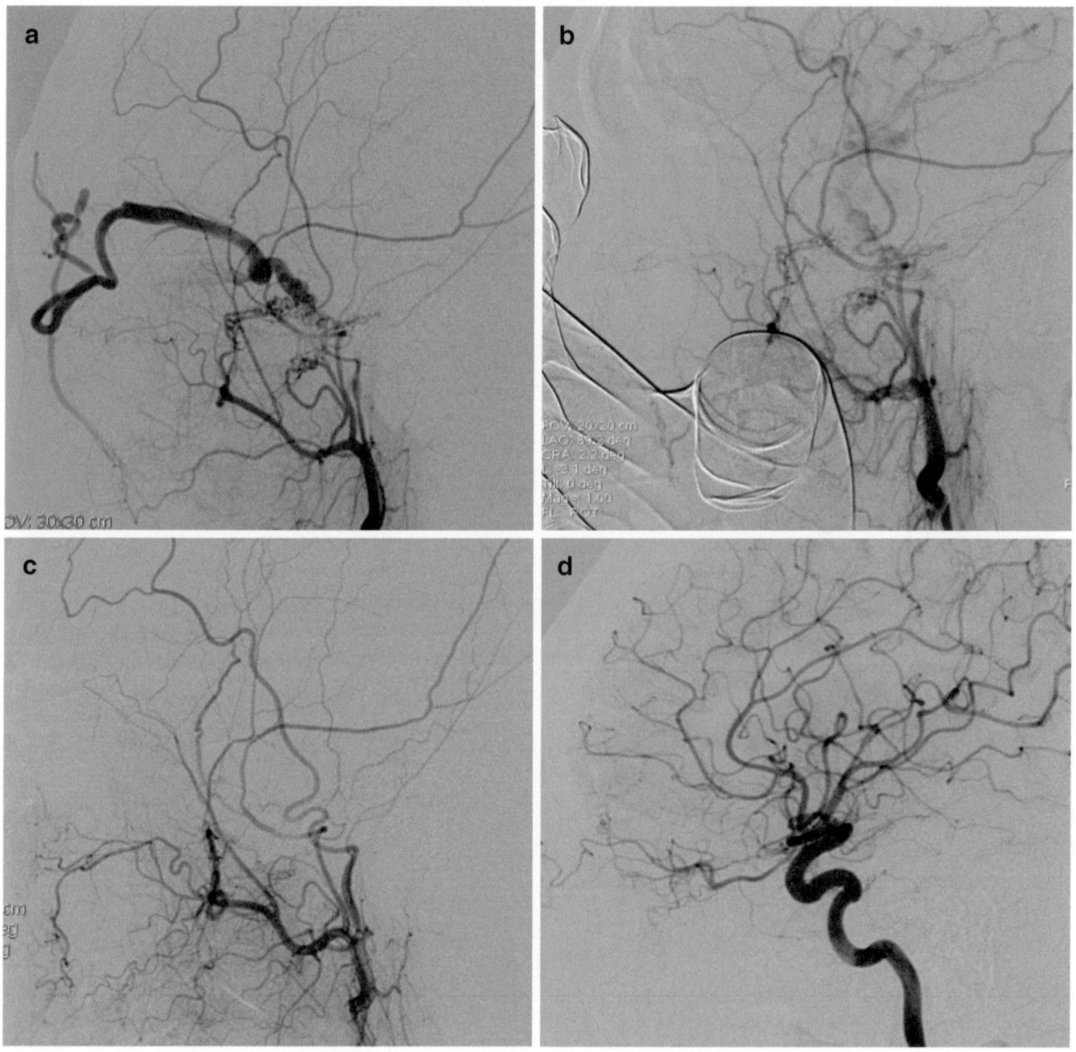

Fig. 9.5 Benign dCCF with spontaneous cure. (**a**) Right ECA angiography, lateral view of a 24-year-old woman who had right eye redness and proptosis for 2 months, showing a dCCF at the anterior cavernous sinus with sole drainage into the right SOV with no connection to the IPS. (**b**) No visualization of the SOV during manual compression at the right medial canthus. (**c**) Right ECA and (**d**) right ICA angiograms at 6-month follow-up after advice to do self-compression of SOV showing complete cure of the right dCCF

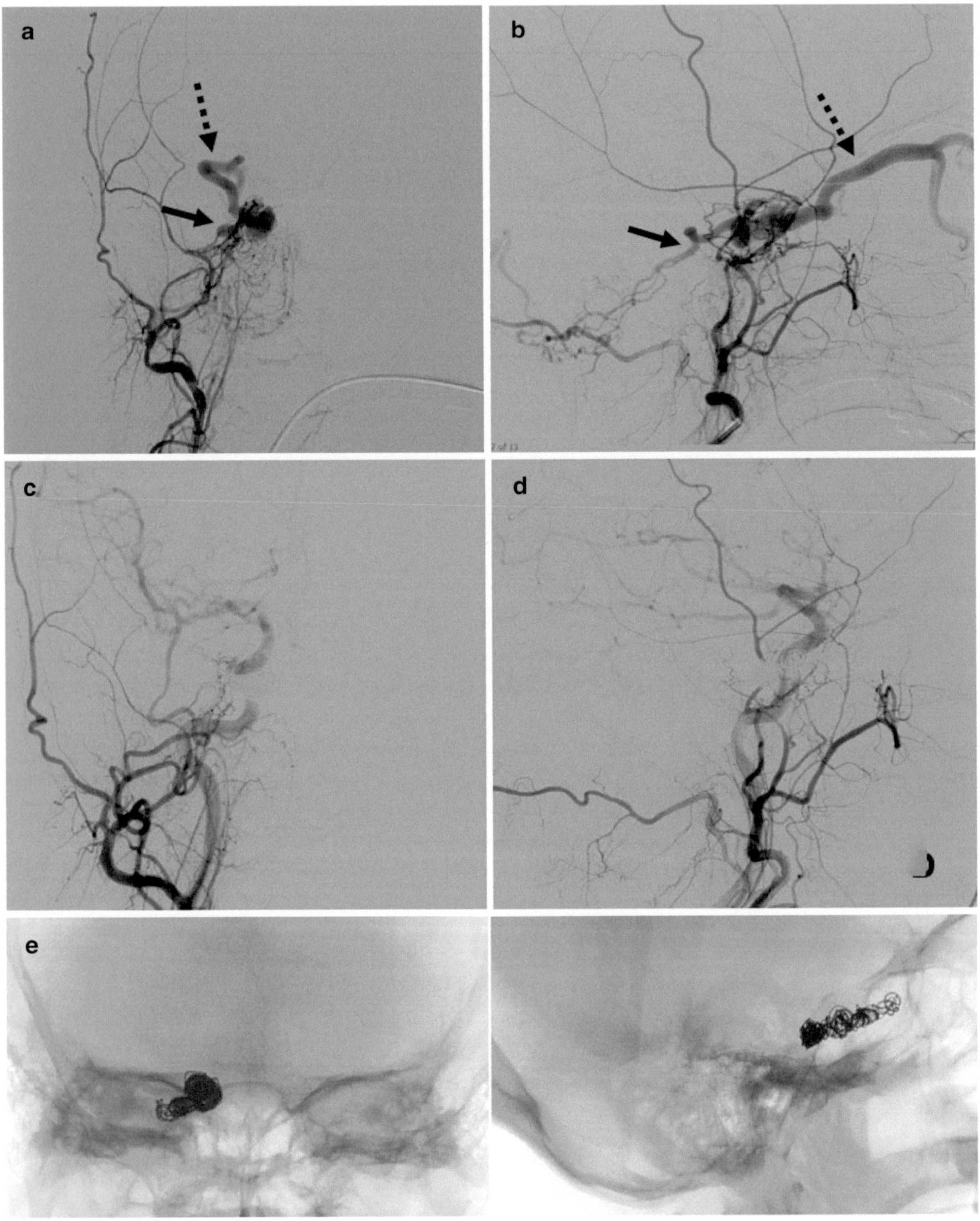

Fig. 9.6 Asymptomatic posterior fossa drainage of a dCCF. (**a**, **b**) Right ECA angiogram demonstrating right dCCF with drainage into the right SOV (dash arrow) with retrograde reflux into the right petrosal vein (arrow) and also into the cerebellar veins. (**c**, **d**) Controlled right ECA angiogram after coil embolization at the CS via blind recanalization of the IPS (not shown) revealing complete occlusion of the dCCF and no further filling of the right SOV and petrosal vein. (**e**) Coil deposition at the right CS

9.2 Cavernous Sinus Anatomy

To facilitate safety and effective treatment of dCCFs, it is essential to understand and recognize the morphology and functional anatomy of those afferent and efferent venous channels around the CS. The CS is a complex venous sinus with different embryological origins of its venous channels. It plays a major role in the contribution to venous drainage from both the cranial and extracranial structures, including the brain, orbit, pituitary gland, adjacent cranial vault, and nasopharynx.

Mitsuhashi et al. demonstrated the concept of CS anatomy in the patterns of longitudinal venous axes and their communication, which are separated into three axes [12].

1. The medial venous axis is a channel medial to the internal carotid artery and is the primary sinus for the chondrocranium and hypophysis that connects with the contralateral side through the anterior and posterior intercavernous sinuses.
2. The lateral venous axis is a venous channel situated lateral to the cranial nerves for venous drainage from the brain via the superficial middle cerebral vein (SMCV). The posterolateral part drains the superior petrosal sinus and also serves as bridging veins from the brainstem.
3. The intermediate venous axis is the remaining venous channel between the internal carotid artery (ICA) and cranial nerves that connects with the SOV and superficial petrosal vein and drains into the pterygoid plexus through emissary veins in the middle cranial fossa.

The medial and lateral venous axes drain posteriorly into the IPS, which also receives venous drainage from the labyrinth, brainstem, and inferior cerebellar surface through bridging veins (Figs. 9.7, 9.8, and 9.9).

According to this concept of cavernous sinus anatomy, if occlusion of the dCCF shunt is incomplete, the residual shunt flow may be redistributed into the cerebral or ocular venous drainage routes leading to focal brain congestion, hemorrhage, or the deterioration of ocular symptoms [13, 14].

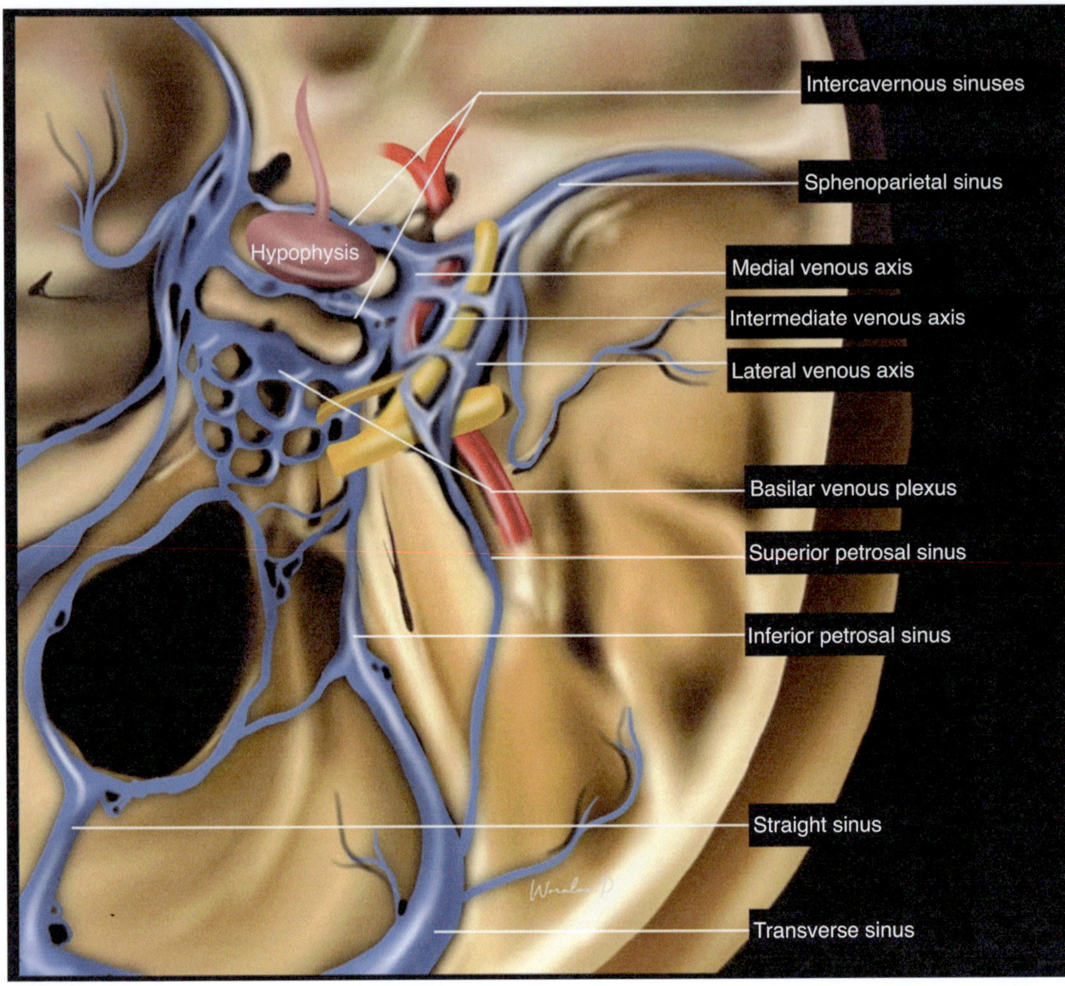

Fig. 9.7 Diagram illustrating the cavernous sinus anatomy and longitudinal venous axes

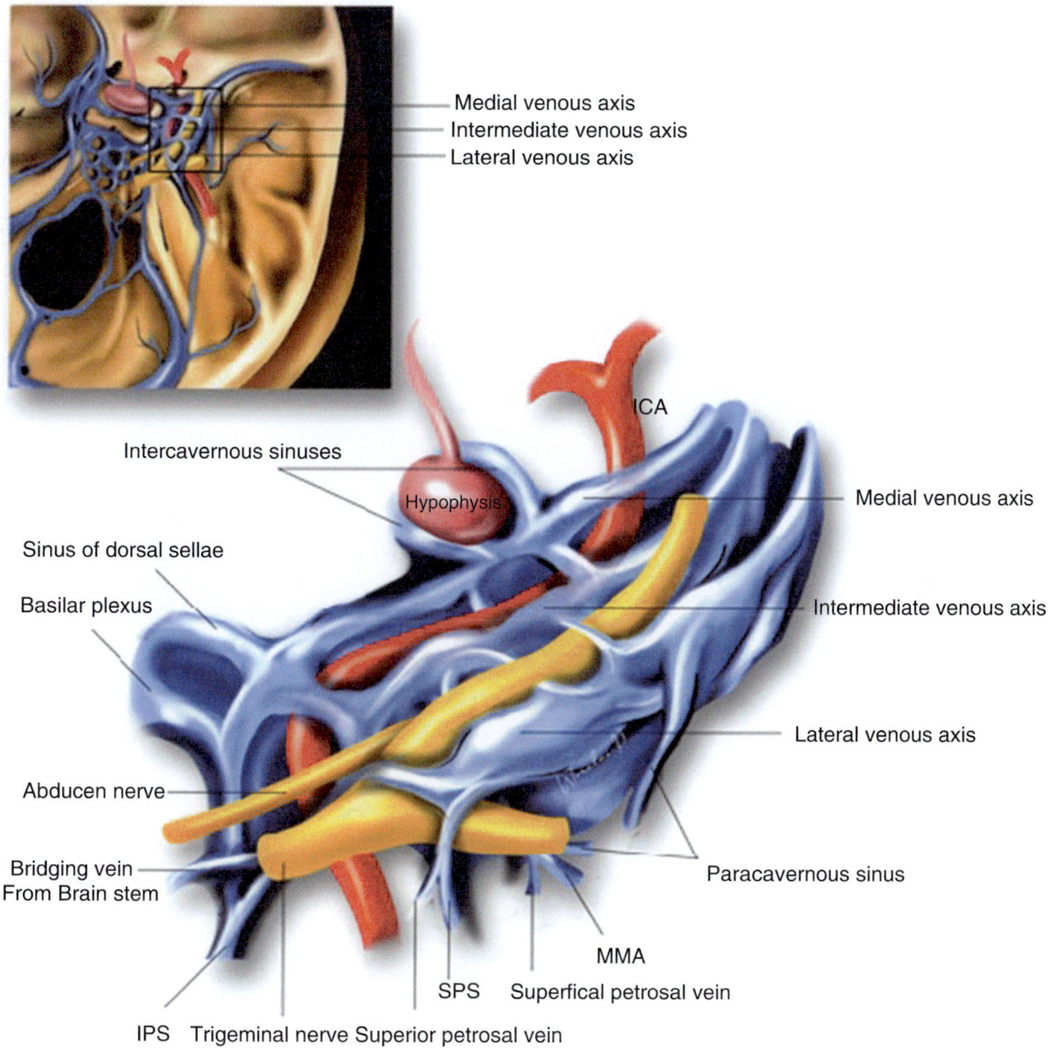

Fig. 9.8 Diagram illustrating the longitudinal venous axes and their communication

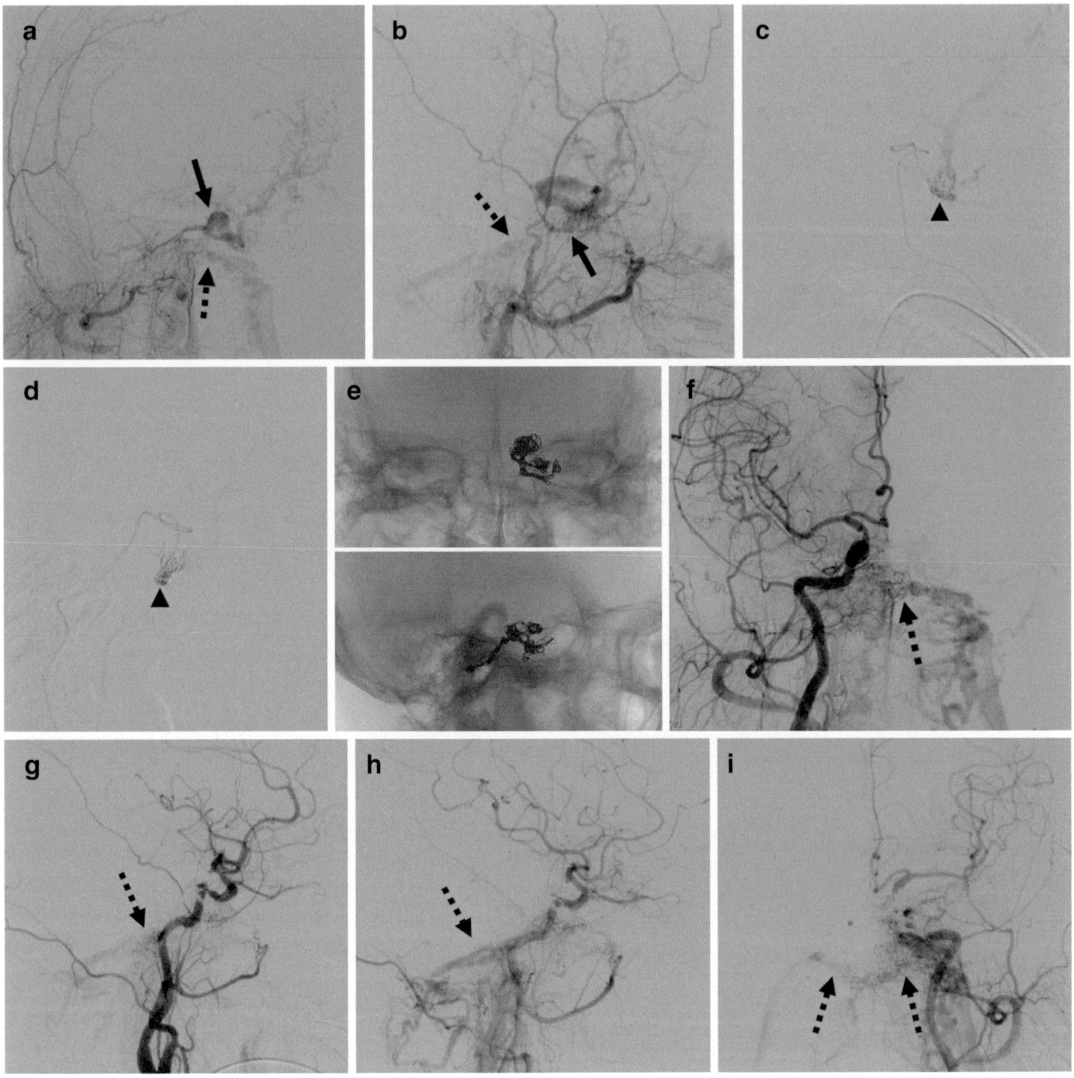

Fig. 9.9 dCCFs at different venous axes. (**a**, **b**) Right ECA injection of a 73-year-old female who had vision impairment of the left eye showing two locations of dCCFs. One at the left lateral venous axis with direct retrograde drainage into the SMCV (arrow) and the other at the basilar plexus of the medial venous axis (dashed arrow) with antegrade drainage to the left internal jugular vein. (**c**) AP and (**d**) lateral views of superselective injection of the left SMCV via transvenous access through the left IPS (arrowhead = tip of microcatheter). (**e**) Coil mass at lateral venous axis and IPS, post transvenous access for embolization. (**f**, **g**) Controlled right CCA angiograms showing complete obliteration of the dangerous reflux. Note the remaining benign shunts at the basilar venous plexus (dashed arrow). (**h**, **i**) Controlled left CCA angiograms also demonstrating shunts at the left basilar plexus connecting to the right side then eventual antegrade drainage to the bilateral internal jugular veins (IJV)

9.3 Arterial Supply to a dCCF

A dCCF usually acquires arterial feeders from meningeal arteries of the external carotid artery (ECA) and/or from the ICA around the CS, which can be ipsilateral, contralateral, or bilateral supply to the shunt.

The most consistent meningeal branches of the cavernous ICA are the meningohypophyseal trunk (MHT) and inferolateral trunk (ILT). There are four major pathways of anastomosis between the ICA and ECA: (1) lateral clival branch of the MHT and clival branch of the ascending pharyngeal artery at the foramen lacerum; (2) anterolateral branch of the ILT and artery of the foramen rotundum at the foramen rotundum; (3) posteromedial branch of the ILT and accessory meningeal artery at the foramen ovale; and (4) posterolateral branch of the ILT and middle meningeal artery at the foramen spinosum [4]. These anastomosis groups should always be kept in mind whenever transarterial embolization is desirable (Fig. 9.10).

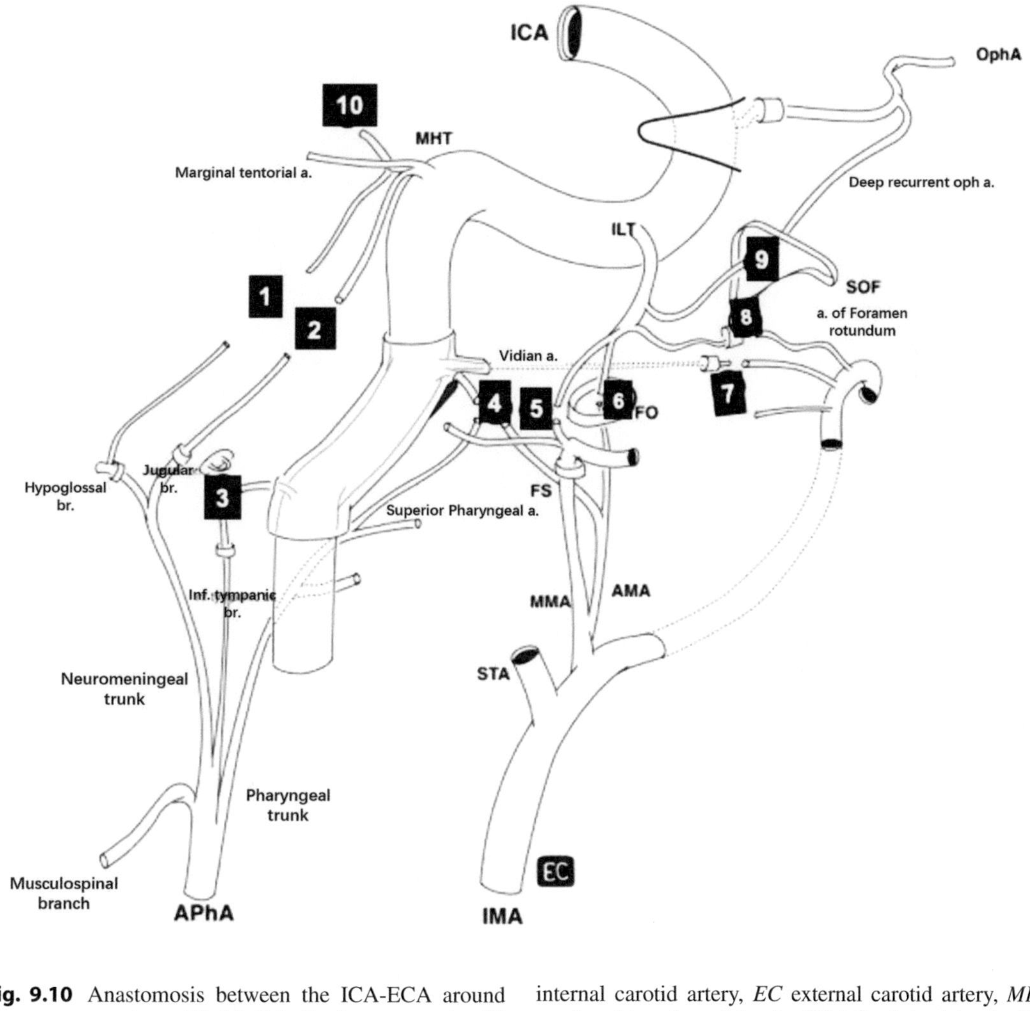

Fig. 9.10 Anastomosis between the ICA-ECA around the cavernous sinus. (1) Medial clival anastomosis. (2) Lateral clival anastomosis. (3) Tympanic anastomosis. (4) Eustachian tube anastomosis. (5) ILT-MMA anastomosis. (6) ILT-AMA anastomosis (at F. ovale). (7) Vidian anastomosis (at vidian canal). (8) ILT-A. of F. rotundum anastomosis. (9) ILT-deep recurrent ophthalmic A. anastomosis. (10) Contralateral clival anastomosis. *Abbreviations*: *ICA* internal carotid artery, *EC* external carotid artery, *MHT* meningohypophyseal trunk, *ILT* inferolateral trunk, *Oph A* ophthalmic artery, *MMA* middle meningeal artery, *AMA* accessory meningeal artery, *STA* superficial temporal artery, *IMA* internal maxillary artery, *APhA* ascending pharyngeal artery, *SOF* superior orbital fissure, *FO* foramen ovale, *FS* foramen spinosum

9.4 Endovascular Treatment of a dCCF

Any dCCF should be considered for endovascular treatment if there is at least one of the following reasons.

1. Cortical venous reflux into the SMCV or posterior fossa despite no clinical symptoms of venous congestion (Figs. 9.6 and 9.9).
2. A benign type with uncontrolled orbital symptom(s) such as severe proptosis, chemosis, and especially increased intraocular pressure (IOP) because it may lead to secondary glaucoma or impaired visual function (Fig. 9.11).

The goal of treatment is to obliterate the affected shunt compartment. If it is not feasible, the alternate goal is to achieve complete occlusion of the

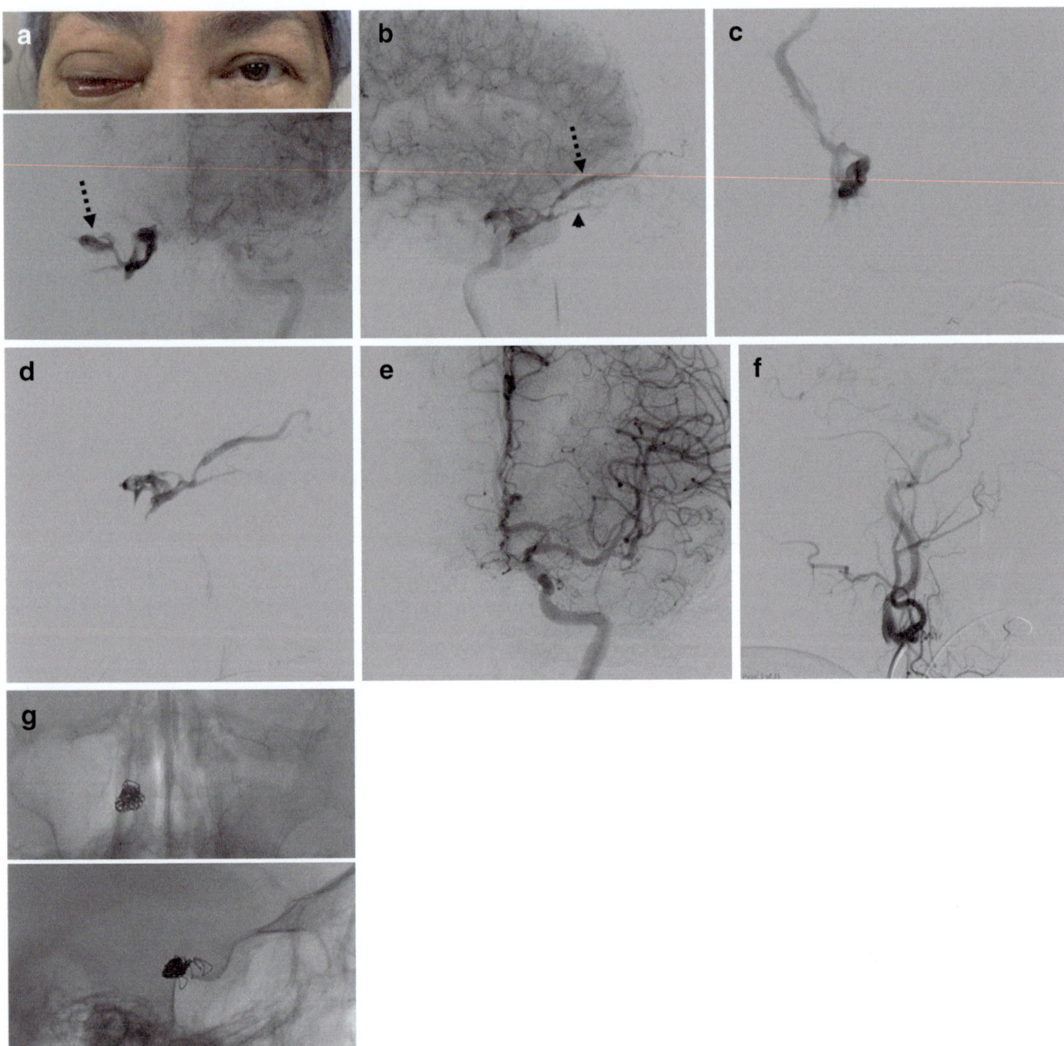

Fig. 9.11 Benign dCCF with uncontrolled eye symptoms. (**a**, **b**) Left ICA angiography of a 65-year-old woman who presented with proptosis, tenderness, and increased IOP of the right eye revealing right dCCF supplied from cavernous branches of the left ICA, right accessory meningeal artery, and C5 branches of the right ICA (not shown), draining into both the superior (dashed arrow) and inferior ophthalmic veins (arrow head) without visualization of the IPS. (**c**) Frontal and (**d**) lateral projections of CS venography, which was performed through blind recanalization of the right IPS showing the venous channel draining the dCCF. (**e**, **f**) Controlled angiogram after coiling via trans-IPS access exhibiting complete obliteration of the right dCCF. (**g**) Coil deposition in the CS

outflow of cortical reflux. Once partial closure of a dCCF is obtained, a follow-up angiogram is required to confirm there is no new acquired dangerous venous drainage.

By reason of the existence of anastomosis between the external and internal carotid systems, a transvenous approach to reach the shunt location of a dCCF is safer when the risk-benefit ratio is a concern. Usually, the embolic material using the transvenous route is a detachable coil; however, a combination of liquid embolic materials, such as n-butyl cyanoacrylate (NBCA) or dimethyl sulfoxide (DMSO) based products, can help to enhance the efficacy of the coil mass or eradicate the residual venous space. Although incomplete occlusion may initially occur, delayed thrombosis after complete curing can be expected (Fig. 9.12).

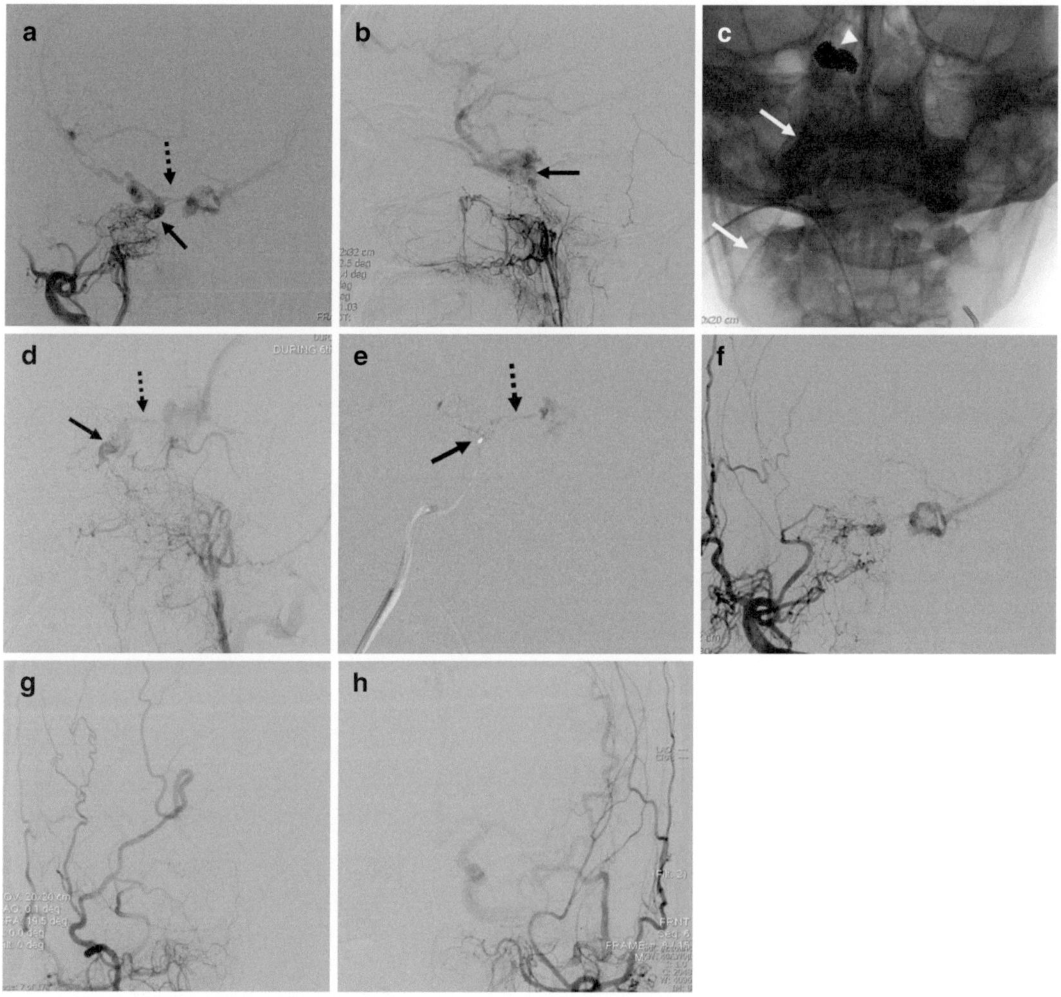

Fig. 9.12 Combined transvenous coil and NBCA embolization. (**a**, **b**) AP view of the right ECA and (**b**) lateral view of the left ascending pharyngeal (APA) angiogram of a 50-year-old woman who had right eye proptosis and ptosis for 8 months showing a right dCCF (arrow) supplied from the right ECA and bilateral APAs, draining into the right SOV with reflux into the right SMCV as well as through the intercavernous sinus (dashed arrow) to the left SMCV. (**c**) Transvenous access (arrows) via right IPS with coil embolization at the right CS (arrowhead). (**d**) Left APA injection showing residual right dCCF (arrow) with intercavernous drainage (dashed arrow) to the left SMCV. (**e**) Decision to use NBCA or glue (NBCA:Lipiodol = 1:3) injection through the same microcatheter to obliterate residual venous space, arrow = tip of microcatheter, dashed arrow = glue passing to intercavernous sinus. (**f**) Residual shunt draining to intercavernous sinus and left SMCV on right ECA controlled angiogram. (**g**) Right ECA and (**h**) left ECA follow-up angiogram at 3 months demonstrating further complete obliteration of the shunt and cortical reflux

Much more caution is required when using liquid embolic materials, even when injected into the venous channels, because these materials can penetrate into a dangerous anastomosis.

A suggested decision-making algorithm for treatment of a dCCF is illustrated in Fig. 9.13.

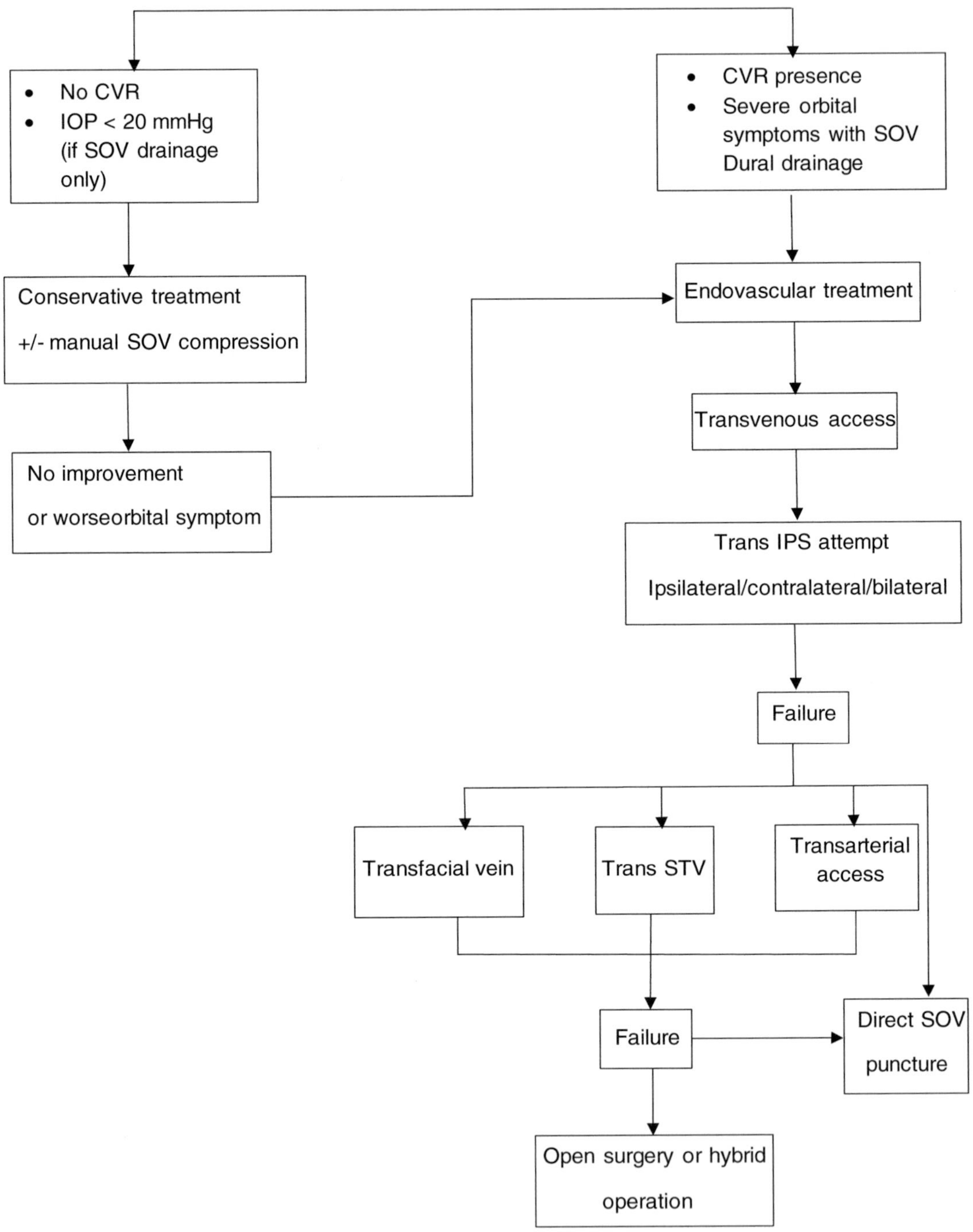

Fig. 9.13 Algorithm flow diagram for the treatment of dCCFs

9.5 Transvenous Access

Several venous pathways are available to reach the CS. The shortest and easiest route is the IPS because it can be navigated retrogradely via the internal jugular vein (IJV) without difficulty if it presents. The alternative routes include the anterior facial vein and middle temporal vein to gain access via the SOV. However, the superior petrosal sinus can be reached via the sigmoid sinus is some cases.

9.5.1 Inferior Petrosal Sinus Approach

If the IPS can be visualized as a drainage from the shunt, it is the perfect direct pathway to reach the shunt at the CS. Nevertheless, if it is thrombosed, we can perform blind recanalization without much fear on the basis of anatomy of the IPS which is the tract along the osseous structure (Figs. 9.1, 9.6, and 9.9). In our experience, the trans-IPS is the initial attempt to access the shunts with an 80% success rate of treatment.

9.5.1.1 Ipsilateral IPS Approach

Both arterial and venous femoral punctures are prepared. Once the venous guiding catheter (5F is preferable) reaches the jugular bulb, biplane roadmap fluoroscopy is achieved by injection into the arterial catheter to demonstrate the dCCF and IPS. The working projection of the frontal X-ray tube is recommended to move some degree caudally in Water's view or semi-Water's view projection. Using a 038 guidewire to select the IPS, the guiding catheter is then moved forward to keep stability at the IPS. A microcatheter can now easily navigate into the CS for selection of the targeted venous channel or shunting site. A test injection via the microcatheter is necessary to confirm the exact venous channel to be embolized (Fig. 9.14). Selection for coil packing at different positions may be needed depending on the morphology and appearance of the venous drainage outlet from the shunts (Fig. 9.15). In general, coil deployment is suggested from the anterior to posterior while carefully preventing inadvertent coil placement or catheter kickback. If one of these events occurs and it is not possible to reselect the SOV or CS, the contralateral IPS or another route of access must be tried.

If the IPS is not demonstrated, blind recanalization of the IPS should be attempted initially using a 038 guidewire to search for the IPS outlet in the antero-medial direction. If successful, a 5F guiding catheter can be advanced forward at least to the IPS-IJV junction. Then a microcatheter can be advanced over a microguidewire using the "drilling" manipulation gently through the thrombus. A test contrast injection should be repeated every time the microcatheter tip changes position. In our experience, this technique has been successfully used in 70% of cases on average in reaching the posterior part of the CS. Once the posterior CS is reached, it is possible to advance the microcatheter into the anterior compartment of the CS and the outlet of the SOV. Initial packing should be started at the SOV-CS junction. Occlusion at the outlet of the SMCV is also necessary in those cases with cortical reflux (Fig. 9.16). However, in some patients with unfavorable anatomy it is impossible to reach the SOV outlet.

9.5.1.2 Contralateral IPS Approach

This approach is usually desired when the dCCF drainage is contralateral or when ipsilateral IPS access has failed. Using a microcatheter over the microguidewire it is essential to pass through the intercavernous sinus under roadmap fluoroscopy. Upon entering the contralateral CS, a test venogram is suggested. If it is similar to the shunt drainage, superselection is then pursued into each targeted venous channel for coil packing in the same manner as mentioned earlier (Fig. 9.17). The obstacle of this technique is non-visualization of the intercavernous sinus on angiogram. If that is the case, another alternative route of access is required.

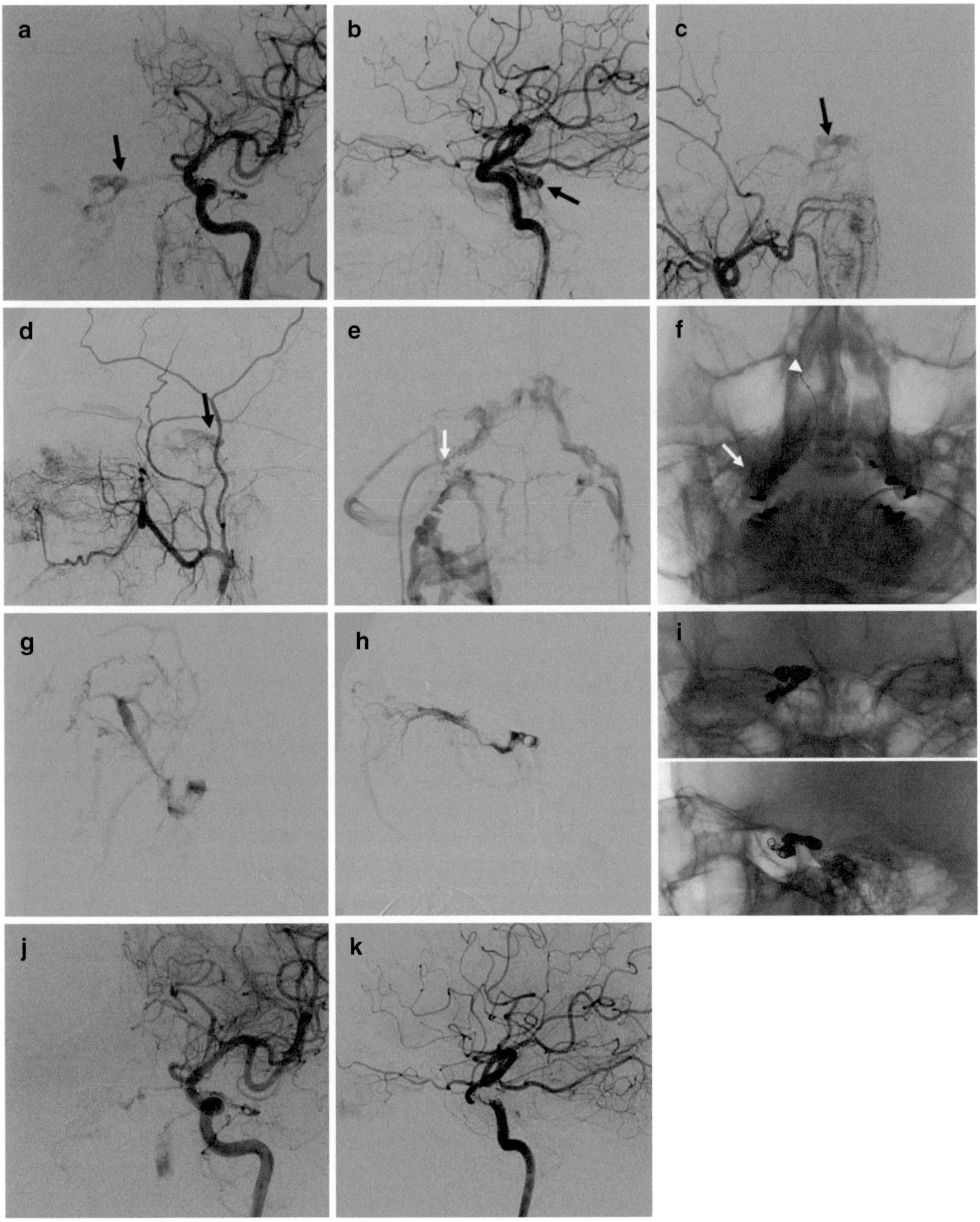

Fig. 9.14 Ipsilateral IPS approach with selection into the SOV. (**a**, **b**) Right dCCF supplied from cavernous branches of the left ICA. (**c**, **d**) Small pedicles of the right middle meningeal artery and artery of the foramen rotundum with drainage into the right SOV. Note the thrombosis of the right IPS. (**e**) Blind recanalization of the right IPS; however, the right SOV is not visualized. White arrow = tip of guiding catheter in the right IPS. (**f**) Further superselection using a microcatheter with successful entry to the SOV outlet, white arrowhead = tip of microcatheter. (**g**) AP and (**h**) lateral views of injection through the microcatheter in (**f**) confirming the SOV outlet, prior to coil embolization. (**i**) Coil mass at anterior CS and SOV outlet. (**j**, **k**) Controlled left ICA angiogram showing complete occlusion of the right dCCF

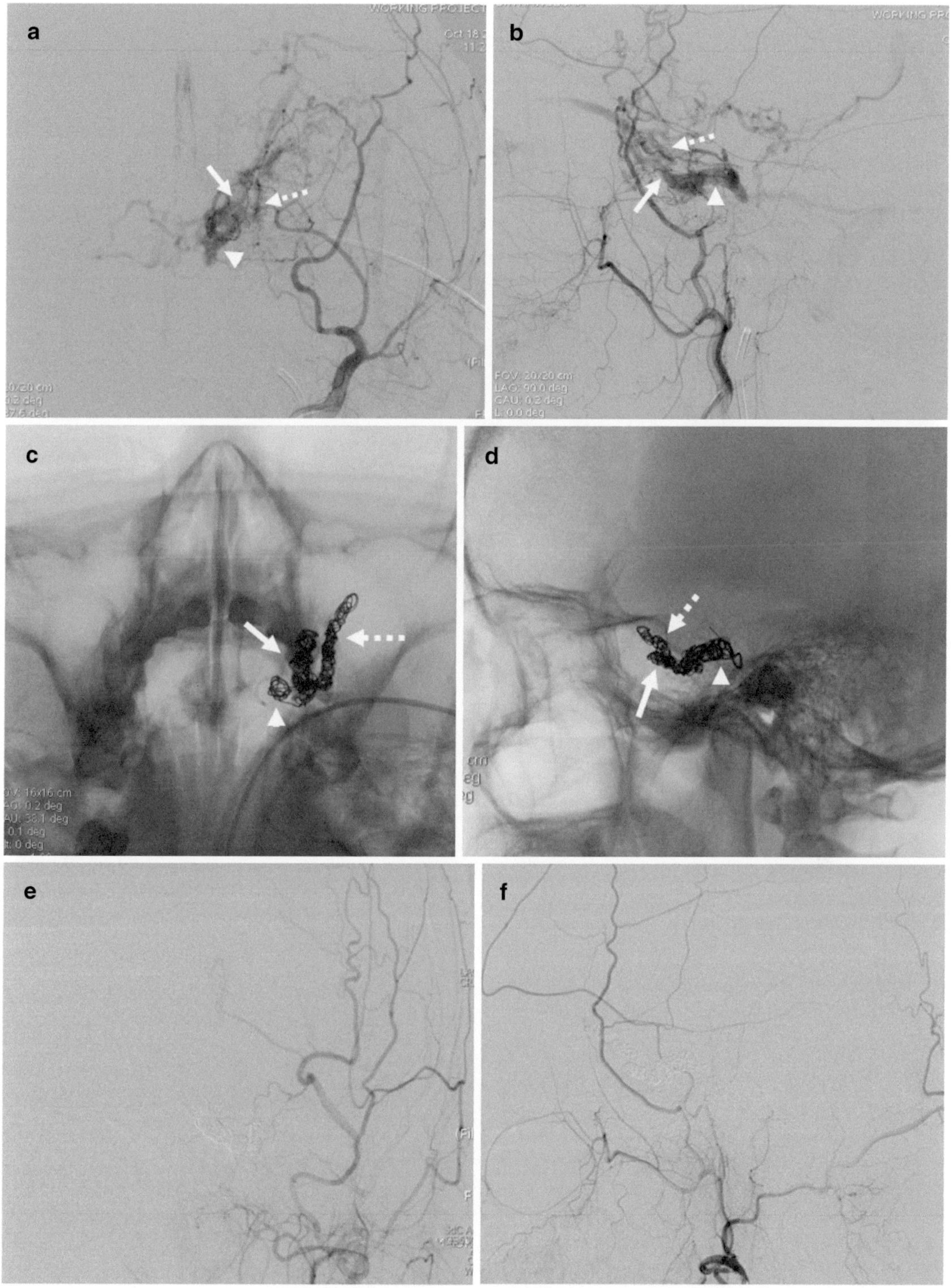

Fig. 9.15 Selective venous channel embolization. (**a**, **b**) Left ECA angiogram showing left dCCF (arrowhead) with drainage to the left SOV (arrow) and left SMCV (dashed arrow) with thrombosis of the IPS. (**c**, **d**) Demonstration of coil deposition from selective embolization in each venous channel, arrowhead = CS, arrow = SOV, dash arrow = SMCV. (**e**, **f**) Controlled left ECA injection showing total occlusion of the left dCCF

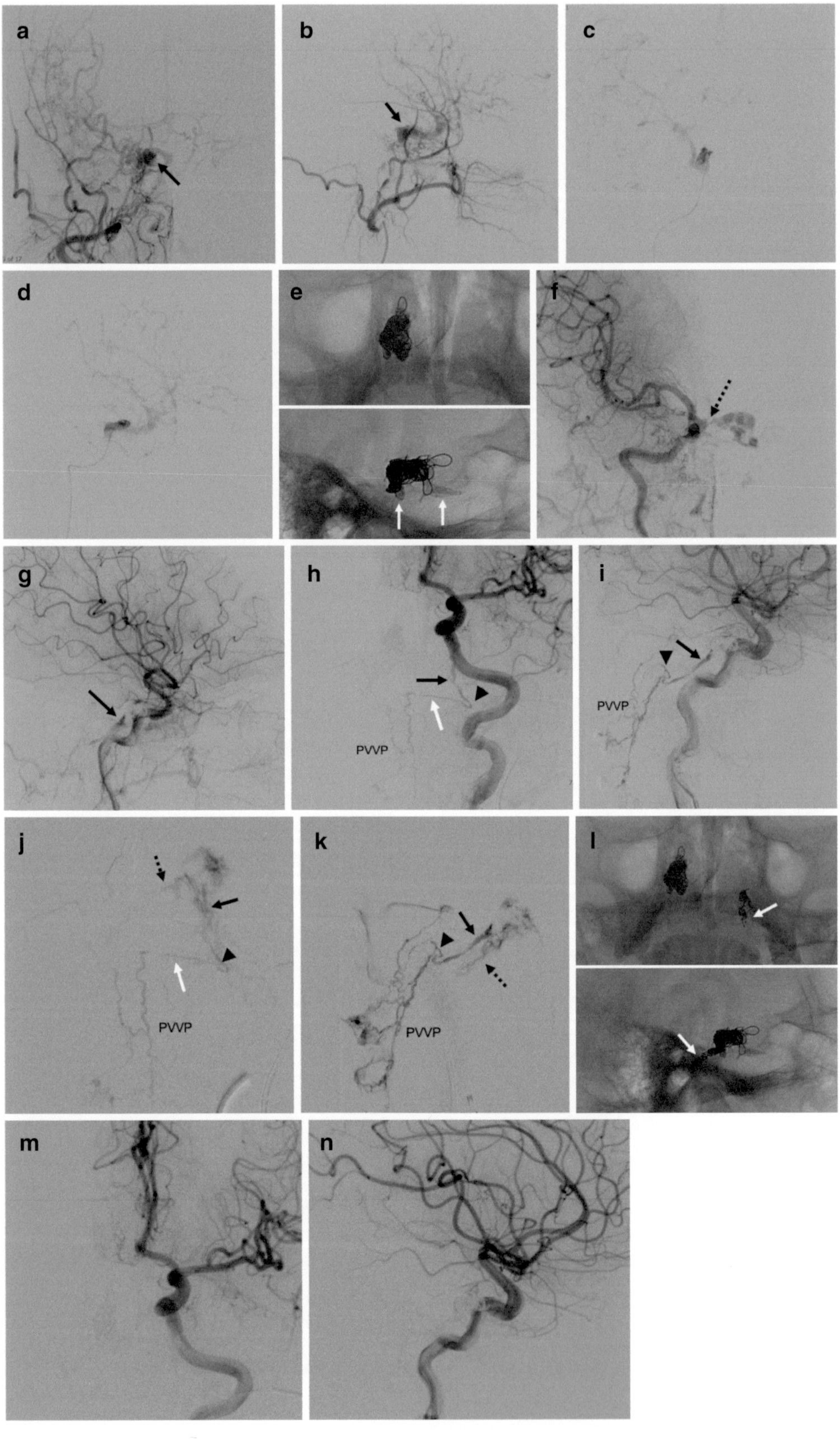
a
b
c
d
e
f
g
h
PVVP
i
PVVP
j
PVVP
k
PVVP
l
m
n

Fig. 9.16 Aggressive dCCF and IPS dural AVF. (**a**, **b**) Right ECA angiogram demonstrating right dCCF (arrow) with direct drainage to the right SMCV and intercavernous sinus. The SOV and IPS are not visualized. (**c**, **d**) Superselection of lateral venous axis of the right CS via the recanalized IPS. (**e**) Combined coil and Onyx embolization via transvenous access in (**c**, **d**), white arrows = Onyx cast in the right CS. (**f**, **g**) Right ICA controlled angiogram revealing complete obliteration of SMCV reflux with residual antegrade intercavernous drainage (dashed arrow) into the left IPS (arrow). (**h**, **i**) Follow-up left ICA angiogram at 3 months showing progression of dural AV shunt at left IPS with reflux into the anterior condylar confluence (ACC) and posterior vertebral venous plexus (PVVP). Note thrombosis at the IPS-IJV junction, black arrow = IPS, arrowhead = ACC, white arrow = marginal sinus (**j**) AP and (**k**) lateral views of left IPS venogram via a microcatheter that was navigated through a recanalized IPS-IJV thrombosis showing similar venous channels as shown on (**h**, **i**). Note opacification of basilar venous plexus (dashed arrow) connected to the cranial end of the IPS, black arrow = IPS, arrowhead = ACC, white arrow = marginal sinus, dash arrow = basilar venous plexus. (**l**) Transvenous coil embolization in the left IPS (white arrow). (**m**, **n**) Controlled left ICA showing complete obliteration of shunt and abnormal venous drainage. Note: Three difference venous channels drained the dural shunts in this patient: (1) CCF drained the lateral venous axis to the SMCV; (2) CCF drained the medial venous axis to the intercavernous sinus; and (3) proximal IPS shunt drained into the anterior condylar confluence, marginal sinus, and posterior vertebral venous plexus

9.5.1.3 Approach for Bilateral Dural CCFs

The definition of bilateral dCCFs is shunts at the bilateral cavernous sinuses where each side has separate feeding arteries and each has its own venous drainage. The disease is not uncommon. It was reported in 26% of patients with dCCFs in our series [2]. The concept of endovascular treatment is not different from the unilateral shunt. The trans-IPS approach is still the initial choice of access. If the intercavernous sinus is recognized from an angiogram, the success of embolization of bilateral shunts through the single IPS approach can be expected with side-by-side embolization. The dangerous venous outlet should be accomplished first, followed by the symptomatic venous outlet. Then shunt occlusion will be obtained lastly in the sequence. If bilateral IPSs are available, we usually choose to access the contralateral IPS of the more aggressive side. Under roadmap fluoroscopy, a microcatheter is navigated across the intercavernous sinus to select each targeted venous channel for coil packing. It is then withdrawn back into the ipsilateral CS and followed by the same steps of the maneuver. Coil deployment at the intercavernous sinus may not be needed (Figs. 9.18 and 9.19).

9.5.2 Facial Vein Approach

The superior ophthalmic vein communicates with the angular vein via the nasofrontal vein. The angular vein continues as the anterior facial vein (AFV) and then joins the anterior branch of the retromandibular vein to form the common facial vein which empties into the internal jugular vein at about its mid-cervical segment. However, in the case of an undivided retromandibular vein, the AFV drains directly into the IJV (Fig. 9.20).

Retrograde catheterization along the course of the AFV should be tried under roadmap fluoroscopy by catching an image at late venous phase of the shunt drainage. The guiding catheter should be placed in the AFV as far as possible. A microcatheter is then navigated over the microguidewire to access the angular vein, SOV, and CS in that order. Usually, the most difficulty is at the angular vein and SOV junction due to much angulation and tortuosity. Once the CS is reached, coil deployment should be started as close as possible to the shunt location at the CS to CS-SOV junction until complete occlusion of the dCCF is achieved from the test angiogram.

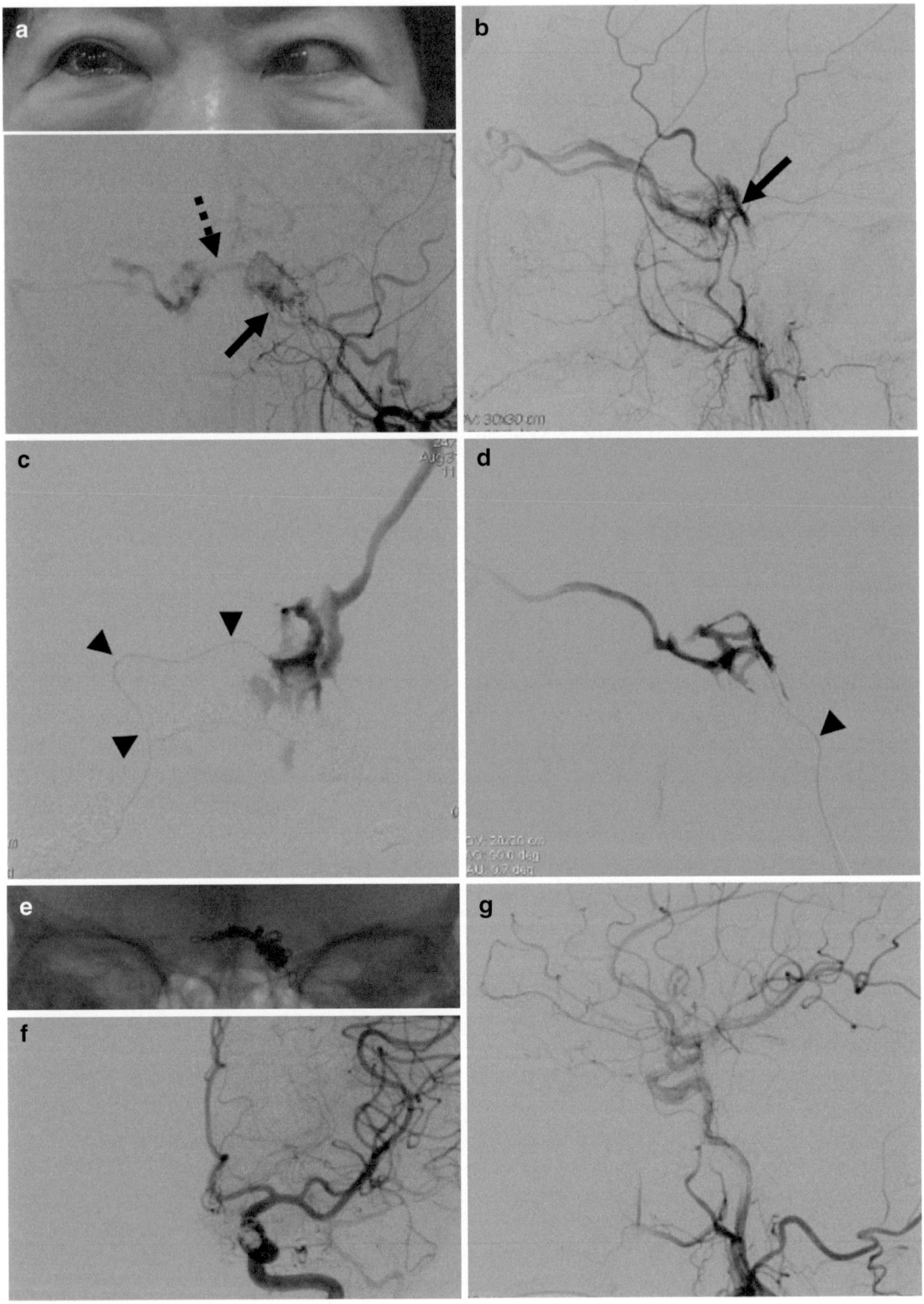

Fig. 9.17 Contralateral IPS approach. (**a**, **b**) Left dCCF of a 69-year-old female with injection of the right eye, limitation of right lateral rectus movement, and increased intraocular pressure of both eyes (29 mmHg on the right and 20 mmHg on the left) showing drainage into the SOV and intercavernous sinus with eventual drainage into the contralateral SOV. Note the thrombosis of the bilateral IPS. (**c**, **d**) Catheterization via the right IPS passing the intercavernous sinus to the left SOV, arrowheads = course of catheter. (**e**) Post-coil embolization in the left CS and intercavernous sinus. (**f**, **g**) Controlled angiogram showing cure of the dCCF

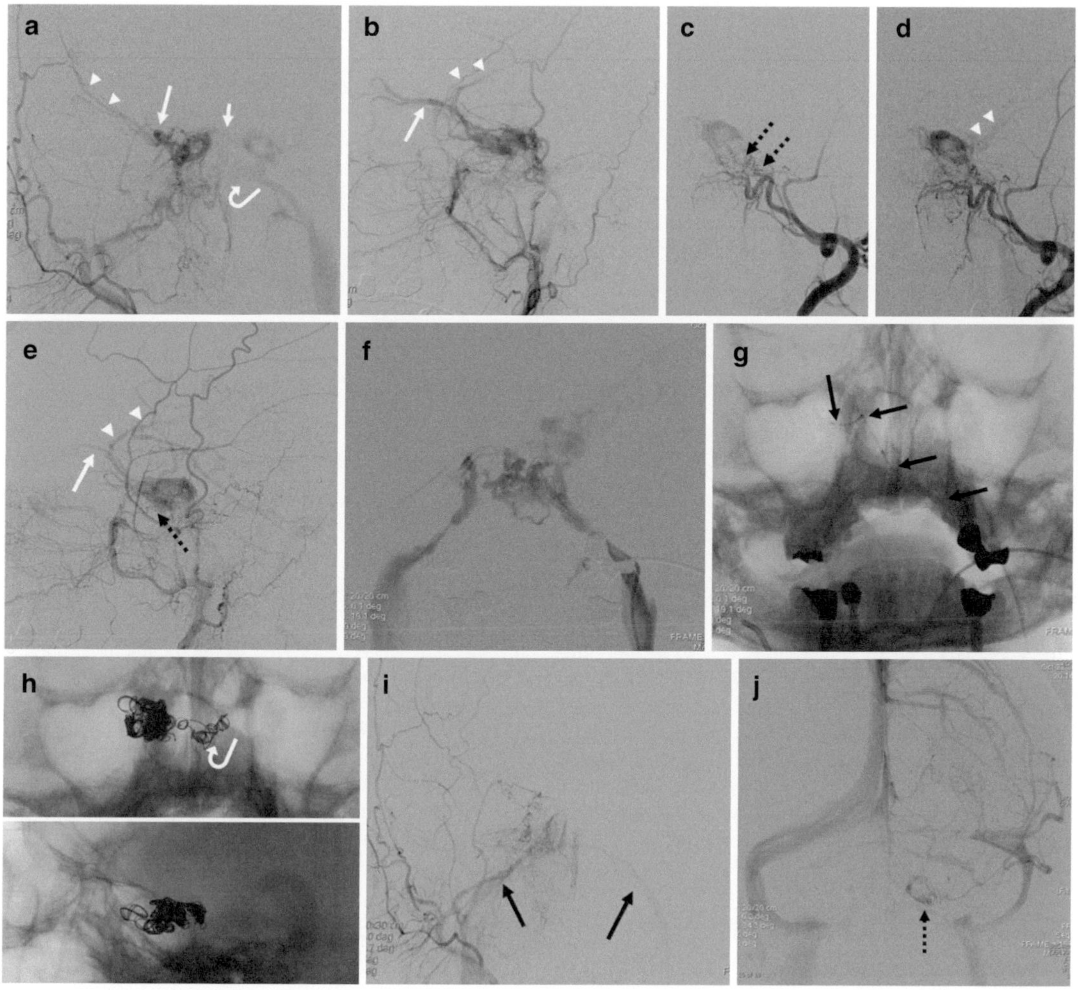

Fig. 9.18 Bilateral dCCFs. Bilateral dCCFs in a 52-year-old female. (**a**, **b**) Right ECA and (**c–e**) left ECA angiograms. The right dCCF had retrograde drainage to the SOV (white arrows) and SMCV (white arrowhead) including contralateral drainage via both anterior (white short arrow) and posterior (white curve arrow) intercavernous sinuses, then consequently retrograde to the left SOV. Note the left shunt supply from the artery of the foramen rotundum and middle meningeal artery at the inferior-medial aspect of the left cavernous sinus (dashed arrow). Transvenous access was planned via the visualized left IPS to pass the intercavernous sinus to occlude the right SMCV and SOV outlets as the first priority. (**f**) Venography of the CS as the roadmap for coil embolization. (**g**) Microcatheter (arrows) superselection to the right SOV. (**h**) Coil deposition at the right CS, left inferomedial CS, and partially posterior intercavernous sinus (curve arrow). (**i**) Controlled right ECA angiogram revealing small residual right dCCF with bilateral IPS drainage. (**j**) Venous phase of left ICA injection demonstrating return of normal venous drainage to the left CS (dashed arrow)

This alternative route is usually applied after failure of IPS recanalization or failure of a forward microcatheter from the posterior CS to the anterior compartment. Either AFV should be demonstrated to be large enough for retrograde catheterization (Fig. 9.21).

9.5.3 Superficial and Middle Temporal Vein Approach

The supraorbital vein connects to the angular vein and communicates to the middle temporal vein (MTV). The MTV joins the superficial tem-

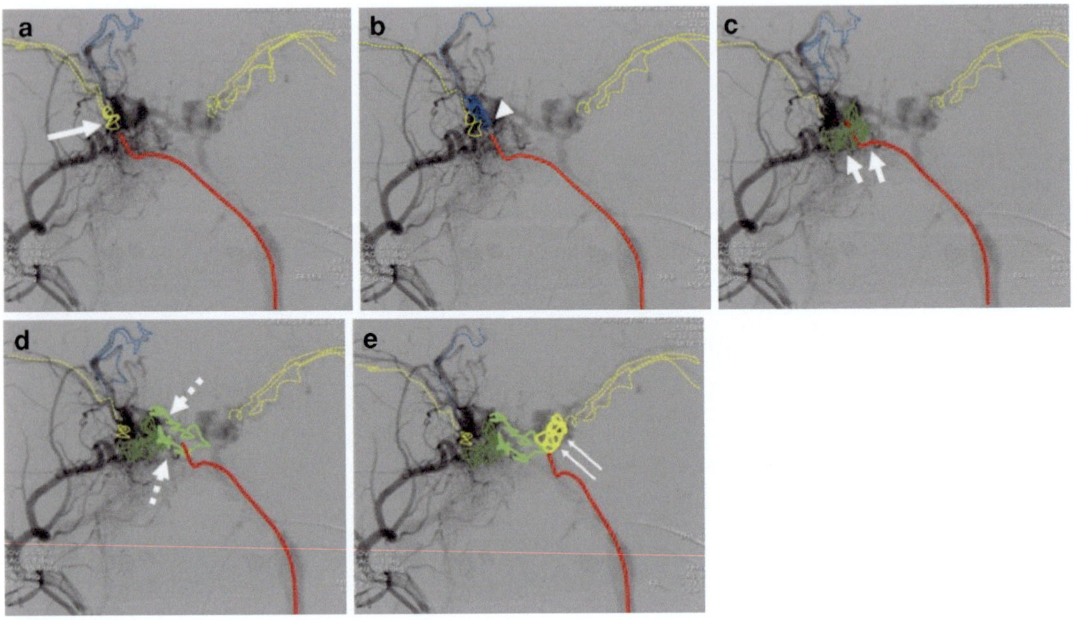

Fig. 9.19 Diagram of transvenous access to embolize bilateral dCCFs (same case as in Fig. 9.17). (**a**) From visualized or dominant IPS access, superselection was done passing the intercavernous sinus to the contralateral SMCV for the first target to embolize the most dangerous venous outlet. (**b**) Moving then toward the SOV outlet which was the symptomatic drainage. (**c**) Closing right dCCF shunt location. (**d**) Superselection of the IC. (**e**) Coiling at the ipsilateral SOV outlet and partially at the ipsilateral dCCF. Red = course of microcatheter along left IPS where its tip in each target, yellow = SMCV and cortical reflux, blue = SOV, arrow in (**a**) = coil mass at right SMCV outlet, arrowhead in (**b**) = coil deposition at right SOV outlet, double short arrows in (**c**) = coil packing at right CS, dashed arrows in (**d**) = coil at anterior and posterior IC, double thin arrows in (**e**) = last coil mass embolized at left SOV outlet and CS

poral vein (STV). At the level of the parotid gland, the STV is joined by the maxillary vein to form the retromandibular vein. The retromandibular vein divides into the anterior and posterior branches. The anterior branch anastomoses with the AFV, and the posterior branch anastomoses with the posterior auricular vein to be the external jugular vein. In some circumstances, the retromandibular vein is undivided and continues as the external jugular vein.

This is another alternative route to access the SOV. An angiogram in delayed venous phase with projection at the neck is the key to understand the venous outlet and plan for retrograde catheterization. The guiding catheter should be placed as far as possible in the MTV to facilitate movement of the microcatheter to reach the CS (Figs. 9.22 and 9.23).

9.5.4 Superior Petrosal Sinus (SPS) Approach

The SPS approach is considered if the IPS fails recanalization and it is not possible to reach the SOV via the AFV or MTV. The SPS originates in the posterior and superior portion of the CS at the petrous apex, and runs posteriorly and laterally in

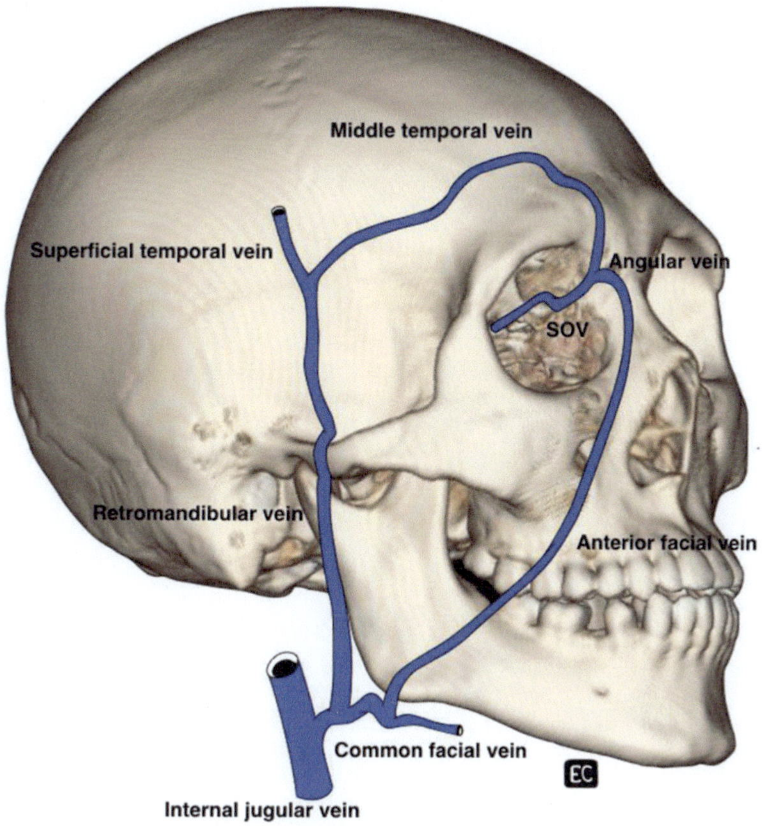

Fig. 9.20 Diagram of the connections between the superficial veins and SOV

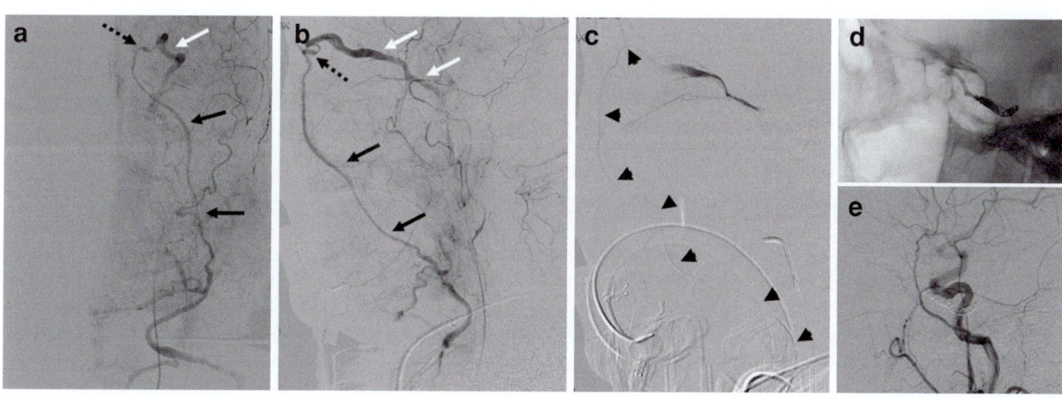

Fig. 9.21 Trans-anterior facial vein approach. A benign left dCCF of a 72-year-old female who had left eye proptosis, conjunctival injection, and increased intraocular pressure up to 22 mmHg for 2 months with failed attempts to recanalized the IPS (not shown). (**a**, **b**) Left ECA angiogram at neck level to identify facial vein for route of access. White arrow = SOV, white arrow head = middle temporal vein, black arrow = superficial temporal vein, curved arrow = retromandibular vein, dashed arrow = angular vein, black arrows = facial vein. (**c**) Retrograde catheterization via the external jugular vein into the facial vein, SOV, and then the CS. (**d**) Coil deposition at the CS and proximal SOV. (**e**) Post-embolization showing complete dCCF occlusion

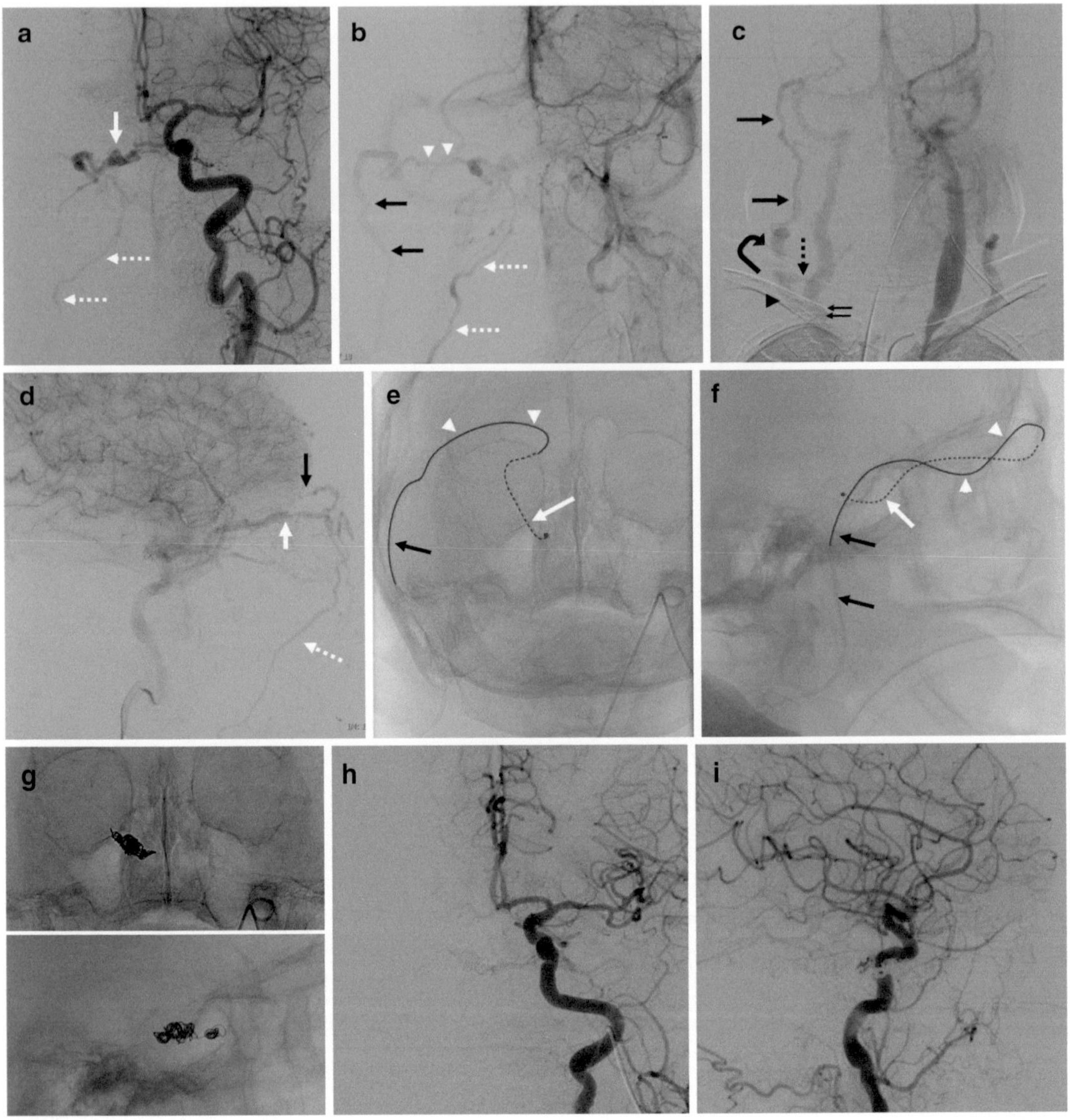

Fig. 9.22 Trans-middle temporal vein access. A right dCCF of an 83-year-old female with failed attempt to recanalize the IPS. (**a–d**) Left ICA angiogram for determination of venous route access. Note more prominent right STV and lesser angulation compared to the right facial vein. White arrow = SOV, dashed white arrow = anterior facial vein, dashed black arrow = common facial vein, white arrowhead = MTV, black arrow = STV, curved black arrow = retromandibular vein, black arrowhead = right external jugular vein, double arrows = IJV. (**e**, **f**) Course of the microcatheter. (**g**) Coil mass in the right CS and SOV outlet. (**h**, **i**) Complete occlusion of the right dCCF

the superior petrosal sulcus and empties into the distal transverse sinus or transverse-sigmoid junction.

In this maneuver, the guiding catheter is placed in the sigmoid sinus. The SPV is then catheterized with a microcatheter over a microguidewire to the CS. Special consideration is needed, particularly at the acute angle between the sigmoid sinus and the small size of the SPV. Injury during catheterization may lead to subarachnoid hemorrhage. Therefore, a soft microwire with gently manipulation is required.

9.5.5 Direct SOV Puncture

This procedure should be the last option whenever the other routes fail to access the SOV. The procedure is performed under general anesthesia in the hybrid operating room (if available) by an experi-

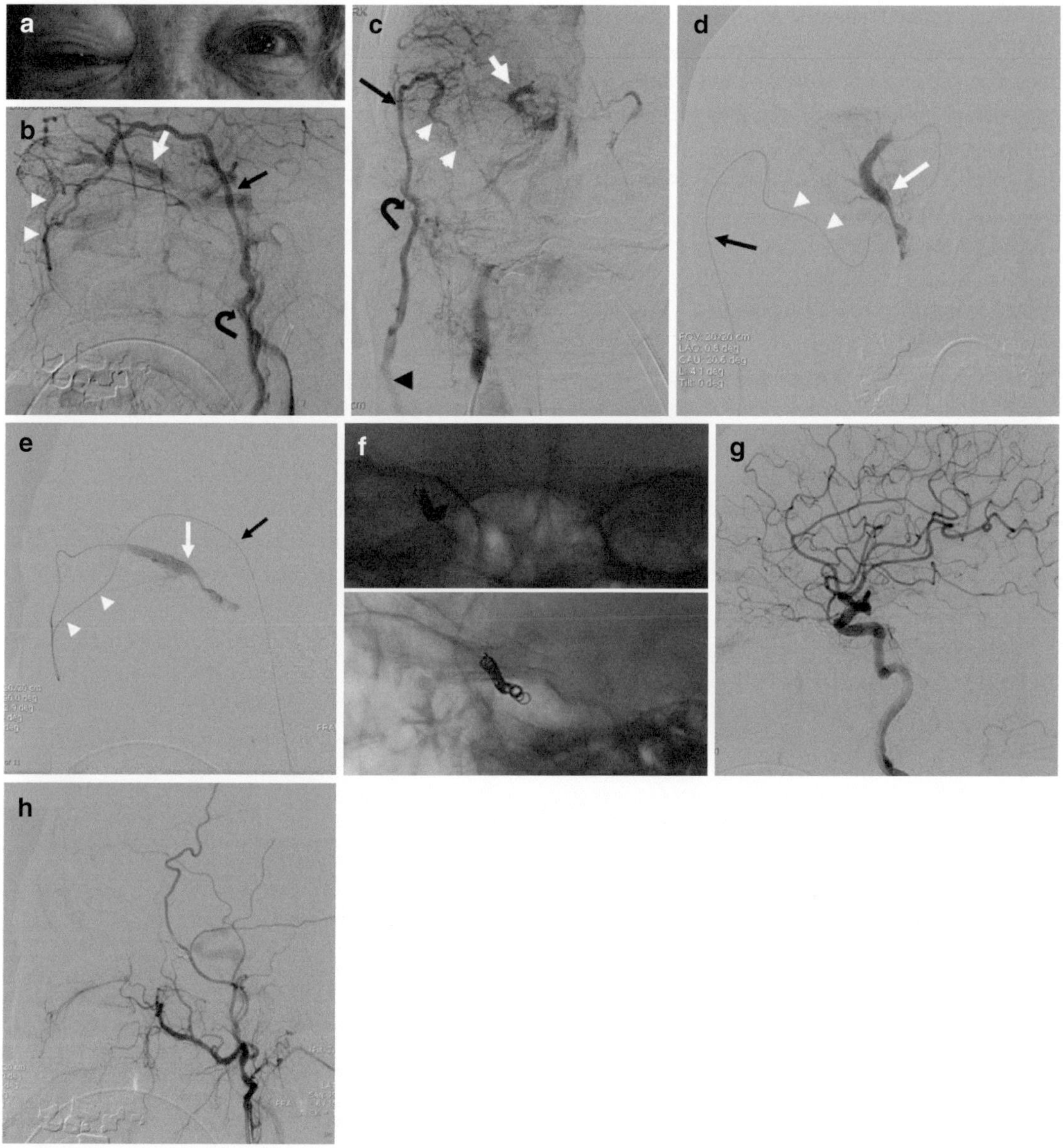

Fig. 9.23 Trans-middle temporal vein access. (**a**) A 72-year-old female presented with progressive right eye redness and diplopia for 2 months. (**b**, **c**) Right CCA angiogram demonstrating right dCCF with drainage into the right SOV, angular vein, MTV, STV, and retromandibular vein. Note the retromandibular vein continues to be the external jugular vein, the small facial vein, and no visualization of the IPS in this case. White arrow = SOV, white arrow head = MTV vein, black arrow = STV, curved arrow = retromandibular vein, black arrowhead = right external jugular vein. (**d**, **e**) Retrograde catheterization via right external jugular vein to the MTV, SOV, and CS. (**f**) Coil deposition at the anterior CS and SOV junction. (**g**, **h**) Complete occlusion of the right dCCF

enced surgeon. The incision is performed at the upper lid or sub-eyebrow to mobilize the angular vein. Using blunt dissection, the SOV is located just below the superior orbital rim. Ultrasound may be useful to identify the SOV. Once SOV is exposed, this vessel is then gently held with a suture and cannulated with a 21G needle. A micropuncture wire is then introduced through the needle into the CS under live fluoroscopy. The SOV runs medial to lateral. A small microguidewire and a microcatheter are then carefully navigated into the dilated SOV. The suture material should be stabilized with a plastic tube during the procedure. Once catherization of the CS is achieved, coil embolization is carried out in the same manner of selection through the SOV as in other pathways. However, if a hybrid operating room is not available, the patient should be transferred to the angiosuite after proper fixation of the introducer sheath. After finishing the procedure, the SOV is manually compressed and followed by suturing (Fig. 9.24).

9.5.6 Transarterial Access

Transarterial embolization is preserved only in dCCF when venous access fails (Fig. 9.25). Much attention and awareness of anastomosis with the ICA must be considered (Fig. 9.7). Liquid embolic materials, such as NBCA and ethylene vinyl alcohol (EVOH), are always the embolic agents of choice. To prevent penetration of the embolic material through the anastomosis, consider using balloon protection at the cavernous ICA when injecting EVOH. In any case, in some particular dCCFs which have a single dilated arterial feeder, the transarterial coil embolization technique can be applied with occlusion at the cavernous inlet and distal artery (Fig. 9.26).

9.5.7 Open Surgery

Open surgery exposure for CS occlusion should be considered as the last option only in cases with cortical reflux when all routes of access to reach the CS by catheterization have failed. A pterional craniotomy and intradural approach to the lateral wall of the CS is performed for the purpose of surgically disconnecting the dangerous venous outlet (Fig. 9.27).

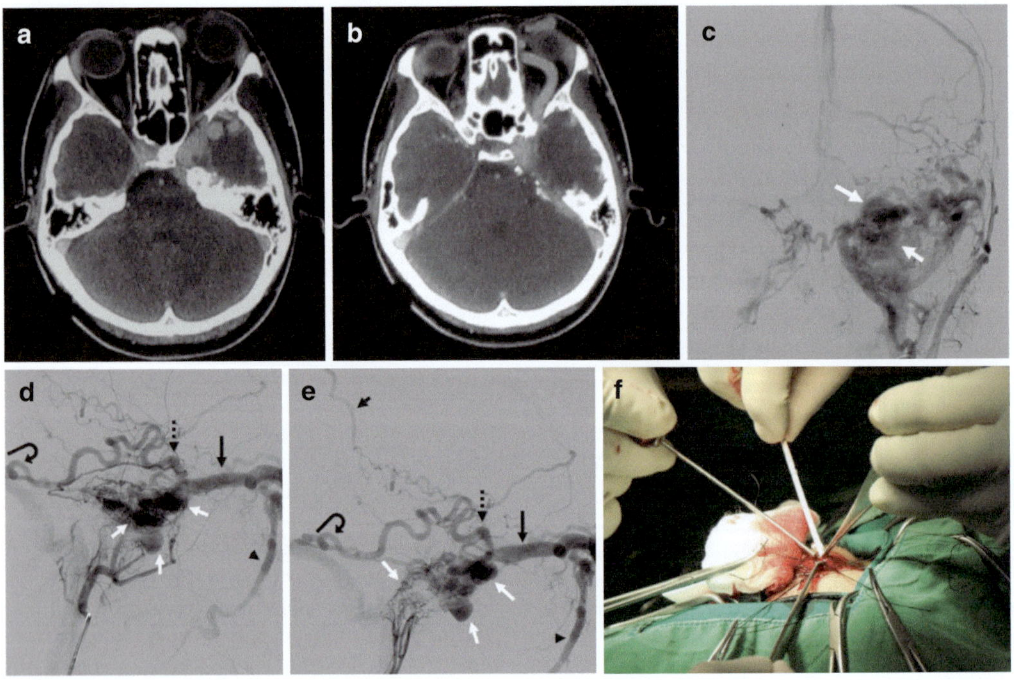

Fig. 9.24 Direct SOV puncture. (**a**, **b**) Axial contrasted CT of a 20-year-old female who presented with left eye proptosis and bruit without a history of trauma revealing enlarged left CS, dilated left SOV, and SMCV. (**c**–**e**) Left ECA angiogram showing huge left dCCF (white arrow) supplied from all meningeal arteries, especially the ascending pharyngeal branches with drainage to the left SOV (black arrow) and significant cortical reflux from the SMCV (dashed arrow) to Labbe's vein (curve arrow) and Trolard vein (short black arrow), arrowhead = facial vein. Note no demonstrable IPS. (**f**, **g**) Decision was made to puncture directly into the left SOV using a 5F introducer sheath. (**h**, **i**) Coil embolization in the enlarged left CS via direct puncture of the SOV. (**j**) During injection of transarterial glue (NBCA) into the residual pouch posteriorly via the ascending pharyngeal branch. (**k**, **l**) Post-embolization revealing significant diminished size and flow of the huge dCCF (white arrows); however, dural supply remained from the left middle meningeal artery (black arrows) and cortical reflux (dash arrows). (**m**) Onyx cast (white dash arrows) after repeated transarterial embolization via accessory meningeal artery using Onyx during inflation of a protection balloon in the cavernous ICA. (**n**, **o**) Follow-up angiogram showing minimal staining at left CS without abnormal venous drainage

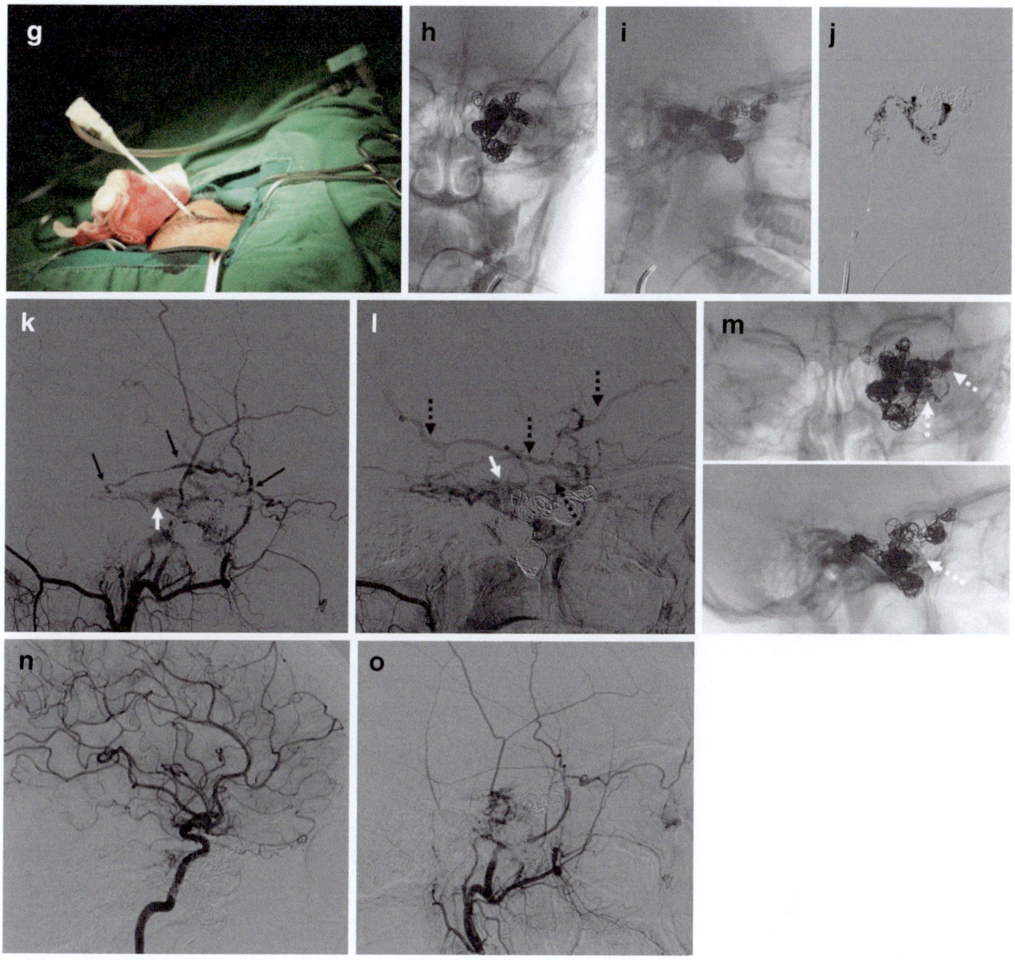

Fig. 9.24 (continued)

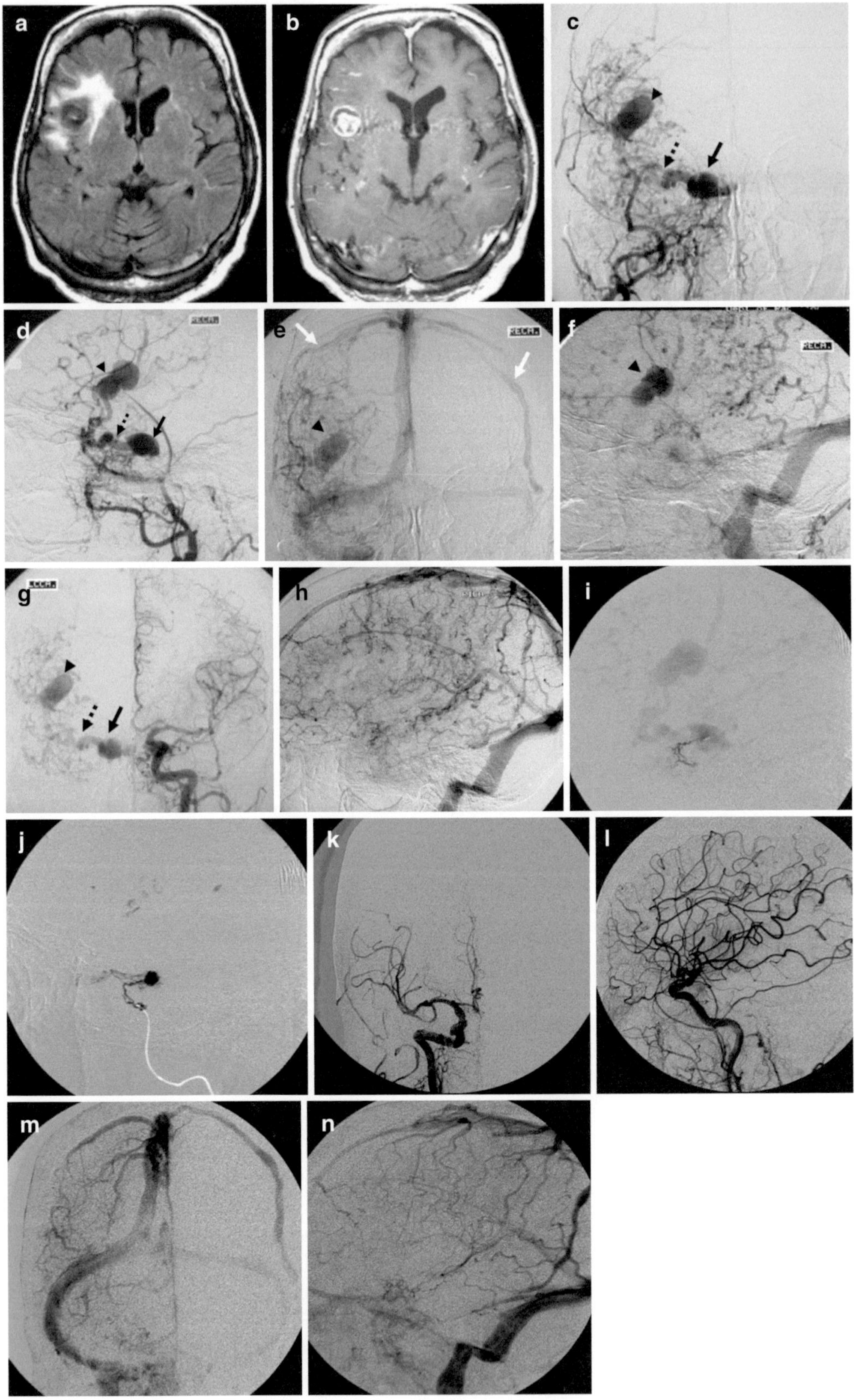
a
b
c
d
e
f
g
h
i
j
k
l
m
n

Fig. 9.25 Transarterial glue embolization. (**a**, **b**) MRI of a 78-year-old female who presented with headache, diplopia, and right lateral rectus palsy showing a partial thrombosed aneurysmal mass with perifocal edema at the right frontal operculum. (**c**, **d**) Right ECA angiogram revealing right dCCF (arrow) with SMCV (dashed arrow) drainage only, causing significant cortical reflux with dilated venous pouch (arrowhead). Note no visualization of the SOV or IPS. (**e**, **f**) Same injection as in (**c**, **d**) showing stagnation of venous pouch (arrowhead) with retrograde cortical reflux draining into the superior sagittal sinus and epidural veins (white arrows). (**g**) Supply of the right dCCF from the dural arteries of the left ICA and ECA with the same venous drainage as in (**c**, **d**). (**h**) Significant venous congestion of the right hemisphere. Note no drainage of normal brain into the right SMCV. (**i**) Superselective injection of the right artery of foramen rotundum which is a supplying pedicle. (**j**) During glue injection at the same position as in (**i**) showing glue cast in the right CS with some spillage into the SMCV. (**k**, **l**) Complete obliteration of the dCCF and SMCV on right CCA angiogram at 1-month follow-up. (**m**, **n**) Significant resolution of venous congestion compared to (**h**)

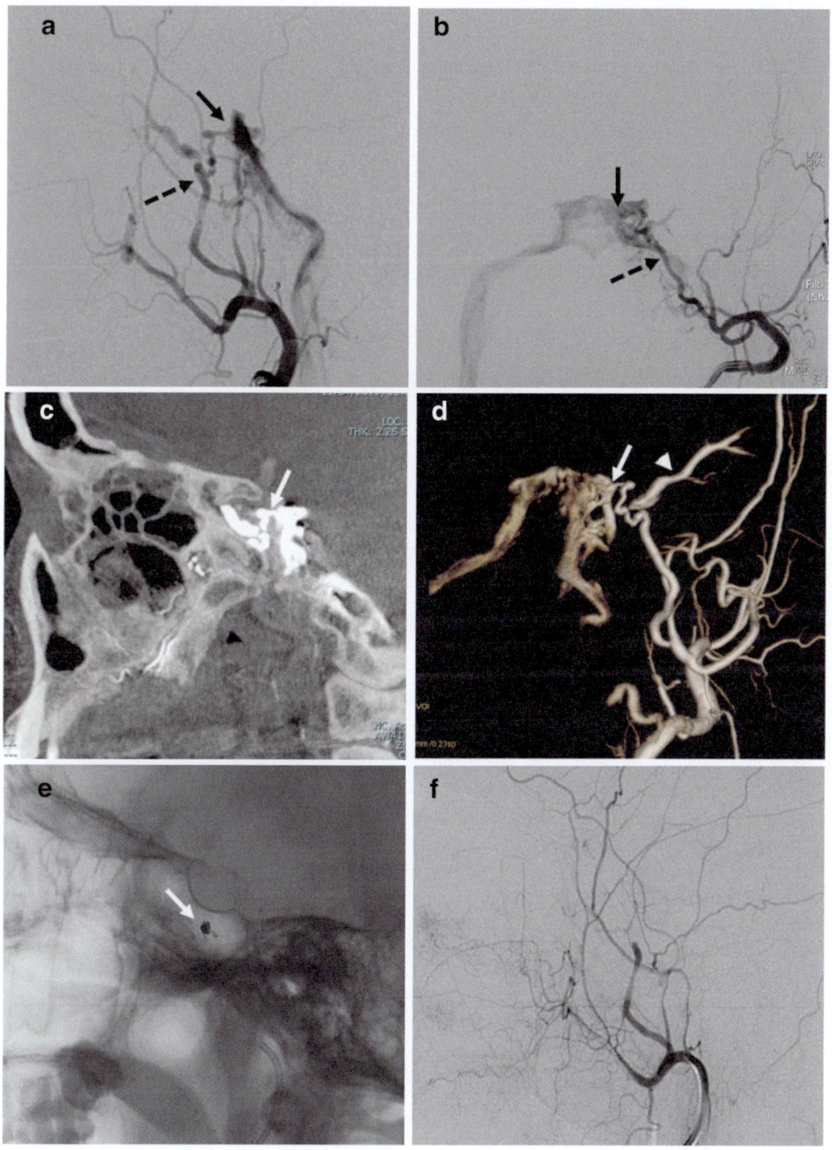

Fig. 9.26 Transarterial coil embolization. (**a**, **b**) Left dCCF showing single supply from accessory meningeal artery (dashed arrow) to medial venous axis with drainage into the posterior IC and contralateral IPS. Also note retrograde flow into the left SOV. (**c**, **d**) 3D angiogram demonstrating fistulous point (arrow), arrowhead = left SOV. (**e**, **f**) Post-coil embolization via left accessory meningeal artery with complete cure

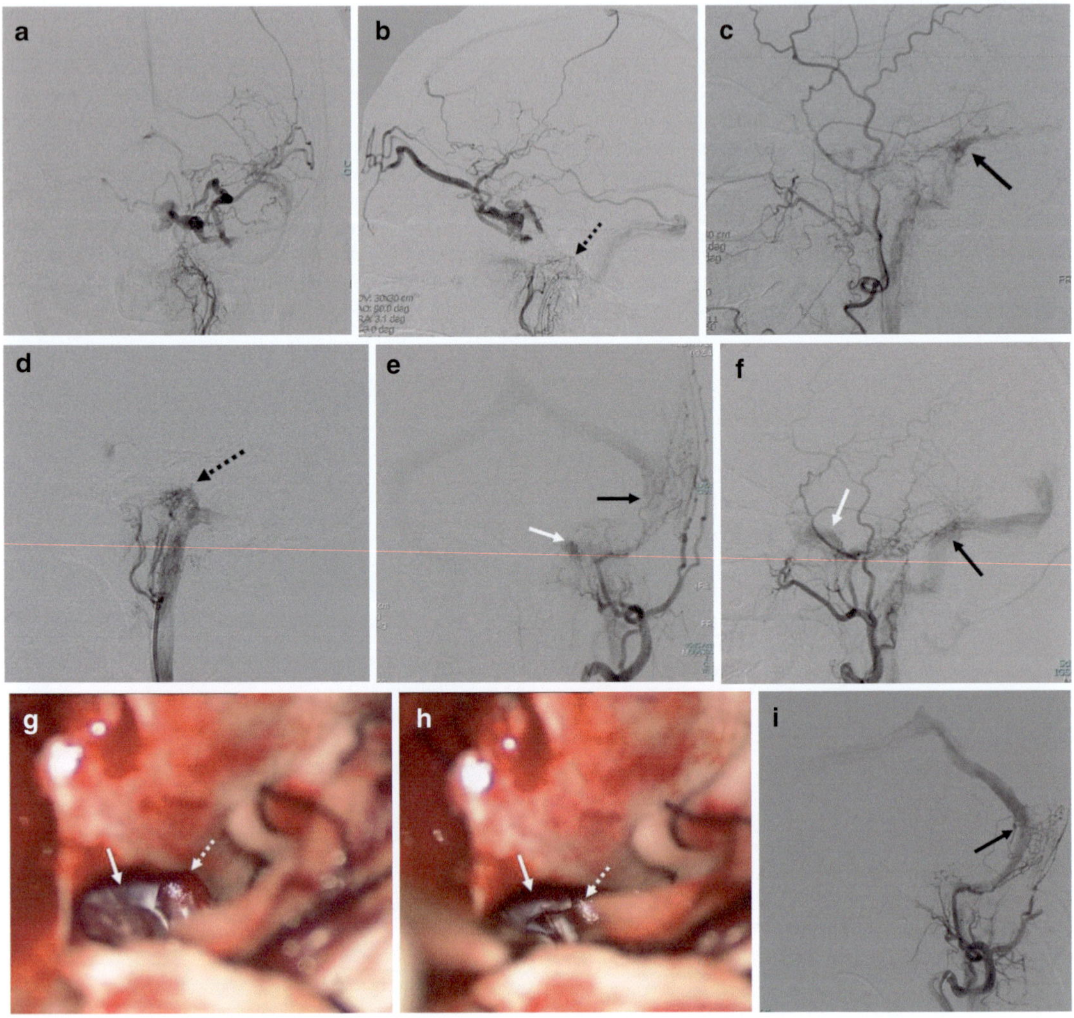

Fig. 9.27 Open surgery for cavernous sinus. (**a**, **b**) Left ECA angiogram of a 64-year-old female who presented with proptosis and chemosis of left eye showing left dCCF with ipsilateral SOV and SMCV drainage. Note occlusion of the IPS and another benign dural shunt at left sigmoid-jugular junction (dashed arrow). The patient had failure of recanalized IPS and access to the CS. (**c**, **d**) Left ECA angiogram at 3 months with planning to retry embolization, revealing unexpected spontaneous occlusion of the SOV and dangerous drainage; however, persistence of the shunt at the sigmoid-jugular junction (dashed arrow) with a new acquired shunt at left sigmoid sinus (arrow). (**e**, **f**) Re-appearance of the left dCCF with SMCV drainage (white arrow) and persistence of the left sigmoid dural shunt (arrow) on follow-up angiogram at 1 year 6 months. After a failed attempt to access the CS again, surgical disconnection of the SMCV was planned. (**g**) Intraoperative pictures of the left frontotemporal approach of a craniectomy. (**h**) Post-coagulation of the sphenoparietal sinus white arrow = sphenoparietal sinus, dashed white arrow = SMCV. (**i**, **j**) Immediate post-surgical angiogram showing complete obliteration of the dCCF; however, increased retrograde sinus drainage of the left sigmoid dural shunt occurred, which would receive endovascular treatment in the next session. During the hospital stay, the patient had progressive left eye chemosis during the next 2 days. (**k**, **l**) Left ECA angiogram revealing rerouting of drainage of the left dCCF (white arrow) via the SOV (white dashed arrow). Surgical CS exposure was again performed in the hybrid operating room for direct puncture at the SOV outlet for coil embolization. (**m**, **n**) Intraoperative pictures. Arrow = SOV. (**o**) Needle puncture at the SOV (arrow). (**p**) Direct catheterization via the SOV for coiling at the CS. Dashed arrow = microcatheter. (**q**) Coil deposition at the CS and SOV outlet. (**r**) Controlled angiogram showing complete obliteration of the left dCCF. The dural AV shunt at the left sigmoid sinus was scheduled for embolization later with complete cure (not shown)

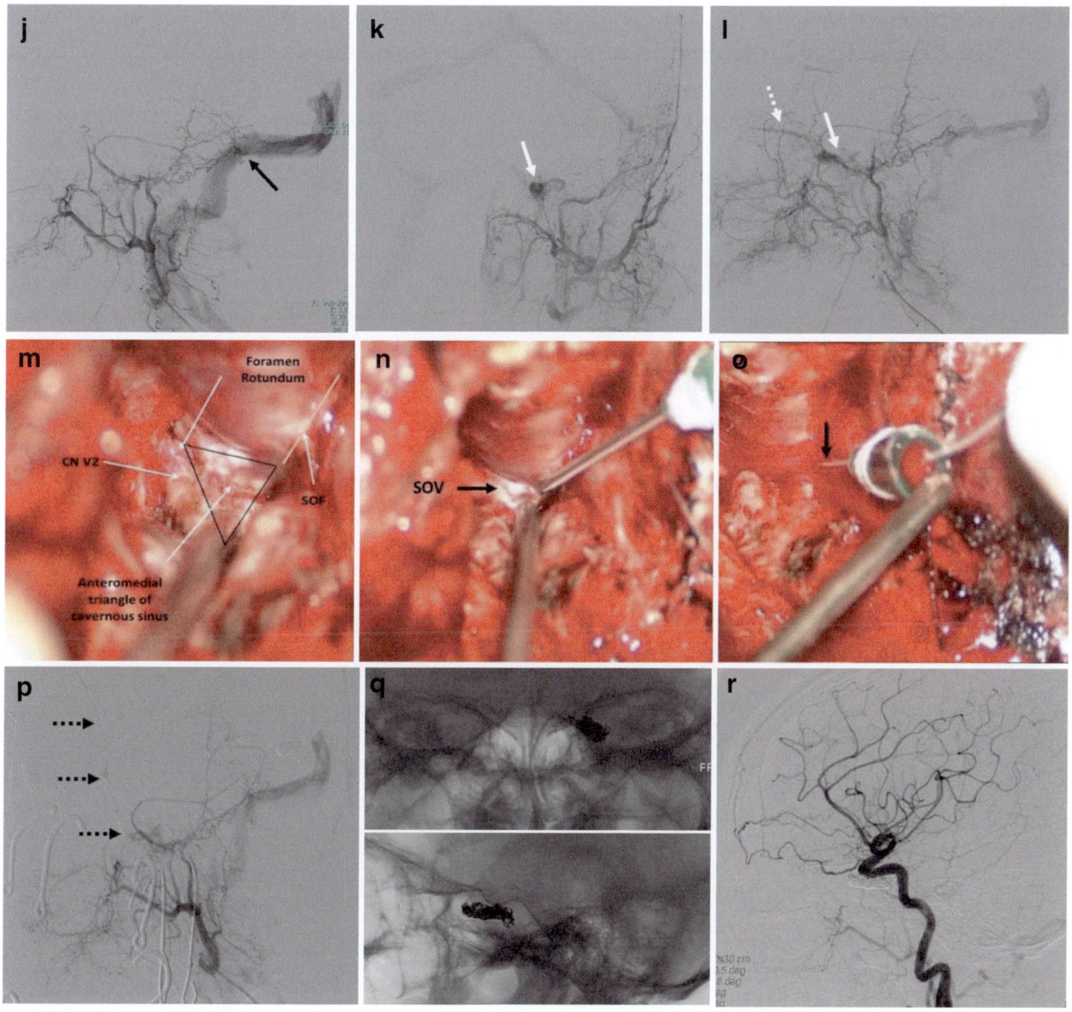

Fig. 9.27 (continued)

9.6 Complications of Endovascular Embolization

Complications need to be considered in endovascular treatment of dCCFs.

1. Cranial nerve palsy: The coil mass in the CS may cause mass effect to cranial nerves III, IV, and VI resulting in ptosis or ophthalmoplegia [15, 16], particularly when combined with liquid embolization. Nevertheless, most of those ocular symptoms from mass effect will recover within 6 months. Conversely, toxicity of DMSO was reported to cause cranial nerve damage with permanent deficit [17]. Thus, selective coil packing only in the affected venous channel is essential to avoid this undesirable consequence.
2. Iatrogenic vascular injury during blind catheterization through the occluded IPS: Hemorrhaging can occur as a subdural hematoma, direct carotid-cavernous fistula, or subarachnoid hemorrhage, or even intraparenchymal hemorrhage depending on the location of vessel injury (Fig. 9.28).
3. Neurological deficit from arterial occlusion: This is the most dangerous sequela from transarterial embolization using liquid embolic materials. They may easily reflux through the anastomosis between the ECA and ICA that may lead to cerebral infarction or permanent cranial nerve palsy [18].
4. Rerouting drainage into the deep venous system of the brainstem or spinal cord veins after incomplete closure of a dCCF: A follow-up angiogram with planning for complete treatment at least within a few months is recommended in patients with residual venous drainage in the aggressive type of dCCF.

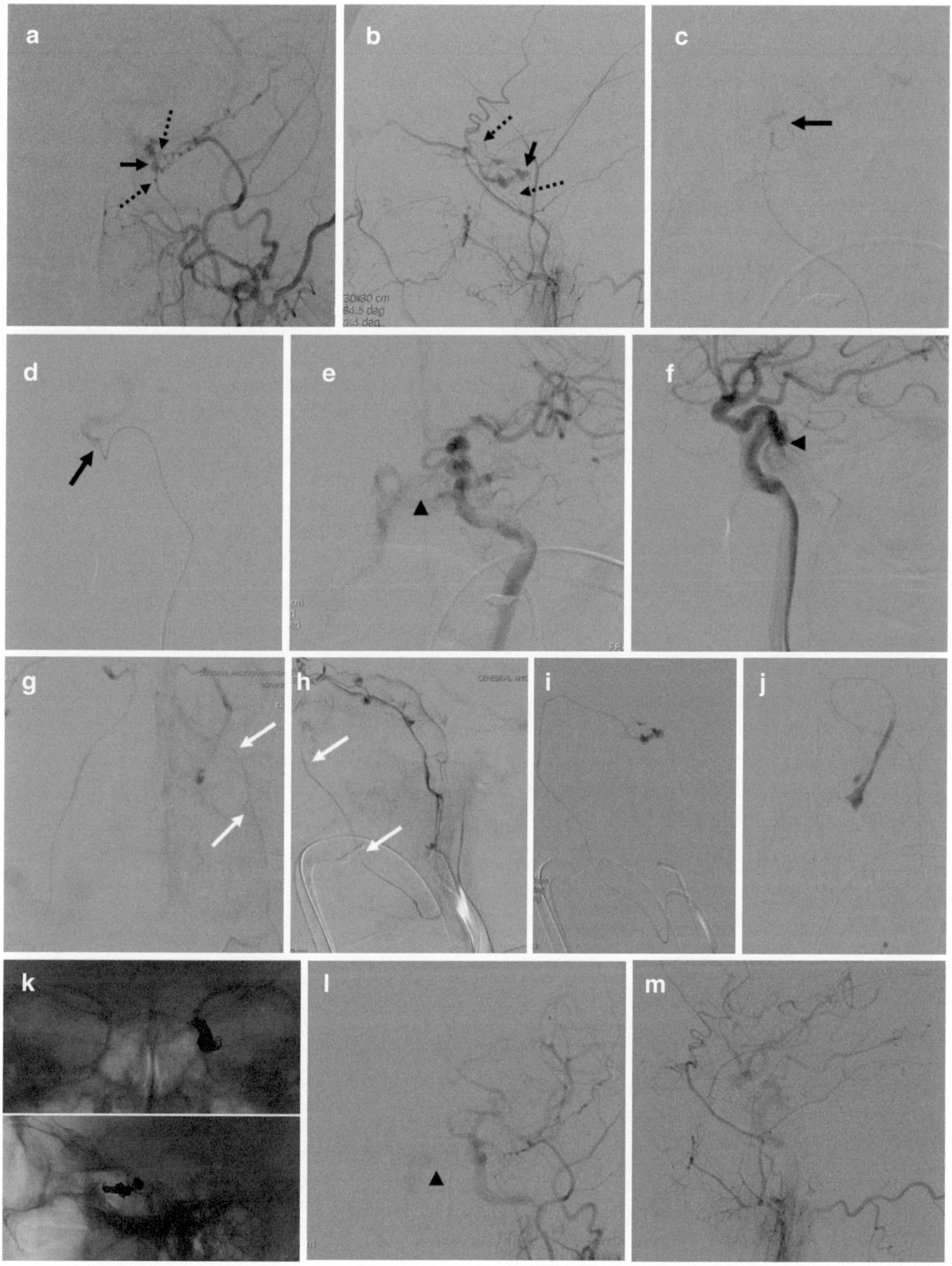

Fig. 9.28 Perforation complication. (**a**, **b**) Left dCCF (arrow) supplied from tiny pedicles from the middle meningeal and accessory meningeal arteries (dashed arrows) with drainage to the SOV. Note no visualization of the IPS. (**c**, **d**) Transvenous catherization via blind recanalized left IPS. The catheter tip (arrow) indwelling in the CS. Test injection showing perforation into the cavernous ICA. (**e**, **f**) Injection of the left ICA subsequently demonstrating direct CCF (arrowhead) with intercavernous drainage. (**g**, **h**) Left ECA angiogram at neck level to identify left facial vein (white arrows) for an alternate route of access. (**i**, **j**) Retrograde navigation of the microcatheter in the facial vein to the SOV and CS. (**k**) Coil deposition in the CS. Compare the morphology in (**a**–**b**). (**l**, **m**) Controlled angiogram revealing complete obliteration of left dCCF; however, persistent iatrogenic direct CCF (arrowhead). On 3-month angiogram follow-up, this direct CCF demonstrated spontaneous healing (not shown)

9.7 Conclusion

The aggressive type of dCCF requires treatment with the goal of curing or at least obliterating the dangerous venous outlet and/or symptomatic venous outlet. The transvenous approach to access the CS for coil embolization is a more favorable treatment method to achieve this goal with safety and effectiveness. Selective embolization at the affected venous channel of the CS is feasible. The IPS is suggested as the initial route of access, even though it is not visualized. The other alternative pathways include the anterior facial vein and middle temporal vein as routes to access the SOV. If transarterial embolization is desired, a dangerous anastomosis between the ECA and ICA along with the risk of complications should always be kept in mind. Direct puncture of the SOV and surgery is the option in a dCCF when it is not safely accessible by the endovascular approach.

References

1. Reynolds MR, Lanzino G, Zipfel GJ. Intracranial dural arteriovenous fistulae. Stroke. 2017;48(5):1424–31.
2. Churojana A, Sakarunchai I, Aurboonyawat T, et al. Efficiency of endovascular therapy for bilateral cavernous sinus dural arteriovenous fistula. World Neurosurg. 2020; https://doi.org/10.1016/j.wneu.2020.10.001.
3. Cho YD, Rhim JK, Yoo DH, et al. Transvenous microguide wire looping technique for breach of ipsilateral inferior petrosal sinus occlusions en route to cavernous sinus dural arteriovenous fistulas. Interv Neuroradiol. 2016;22:590–5.
4. Berenstein A, Lasjaunias PL, TerBrugge KG. Surgical neuroangiography, vol. 2. 2nd ed. Heidelberg: Springer; 2004.
5. Geibprasert S, Krings T, Pereira V, Pongpech S, Piske R, Lasjaunias P. Clinical characteristics of dural arteriovenous shunts in 446 patients of three different ethnicities. Interv Neuroradiol. 2009;15:395–400.
6. Suh DC, Lee JH, Kim SJ, Chung SJ, Choi CG, Kim HJ, et al. New concept in cavernous sinus dural arteriovenous fistula: correlation with presenting symptom and venous drainage patterns. Stroke. 2005;36:1134–9.
7. Cognard C, Gobin YP, Pierot L, Bailly AL, Houdart E, Casasco A, et al. Cerebral dural arteriovenous fistulas: clinical and angiographic correlation with a revised classification of venous drainage. Radiology. 1995;194:671–80.
8. Kobkitsuksakul C, Jiarakongmun P, Chanthanaphak E, Pongpech S. Noncavernous arteriovenous shunts mimicking carotid cavernous fistulae. Diagn Interv Radiol. 2016;22(6):555–9.
9. Borden JA, Wu JK, Shucart WA. A proposed classification for spinal and cranial dural arteriovenous fistulous malformations and implications for treatment. J Neurosurg. 1995;82:166–79.
10. Geibprasert S, Pereira V, Krings T, et al. Dural arteriovenous shunts: a new classification of craniospinal epidural venous anatomical bases and clinical correlations. Stroke. 2008;39:2783–94.
11. Wenderoth J. Novel approaches to access and treatment of cavernous sinus dural arteriovenous fistula (CS-DAVF): case series and review of the literature. J Neuro Interv Surg. 2017;9:290–6.
12. Mitsuhashi Y, et al. Dural venous system in the cavernous sinus: a literature review and embryological, functional, and endovascular clinical considerations. Neurol Med Chir (Tokyo). 2016;56:326–39.
13. Nakagawa I, Wada T, Nakagawa H, Hironaka Y, Kichikawa K, Nakase H. A rare brainstem hemorrhage during transvenous embolization of a cavernous dural arteriovenous fistula. J Clin Neurosci. 2012;19:589–92.
14. Lee RJ, Chen CF, Hsu SW, Lui CC, Kuo YL. Cerebellar hemorrhage and subsequent venous infarction followed by incomplete transvenous embolization of dural carotid cavernous fistulas: a rare complication: case report. J Neurosurg. 2008;108:1245–8.
15. Kim DJ, Kim DI, Suh SH, Kim J, Lee SK, Kim EY, Chung TS. Results of transvenous embolization of cavernous dural arteriovenous fistula: a single-center experience with emphasis on complications and management. AJNR Am J Neuroradiol. 2006;27:2078–82.
16. Lee SH, Cho WS, Kang HS, Kim JE, Cho YD, Yoo DH, Han MH. Newly occurring cranial nerve palsy after endovascular treatment of cavernous sinus dural arteriovenous fistulas. J Neurointerv Surg. 2019;11:1168–72.
17. Lee JM, Whang K, Cho SM, Kim JY, Oh JW, Koo YM, Hu C, Pyen J, Choi JW. Cranial nerve palsy after onyx embolization as a treatment for cerebral vascular malformation. J Cerebrovasc Endovasc Neurosurg. 2017;19:189–95.
18. Ashour R, Chavali R. Neuromeningeal access for transarterial intravenous carotid-cavernous fistula embolization. Interv Neuroradiol. 2015;21:234–9.

10 Cavernous Dural Arteriovenous Fistulas: Transorbital Cavernous Sinus Direct Puncture

Luciano Bambini Manzato, José Ricardo Vanzin,
Felipe Padovani Trivelato,
Alexandre Cordeiro Ulhôa,
and Marco Túlio Salles Rezende

Abstract

Cavernous sinus dural arteriovenous fistulas (CSDAVFs) are abnormal connections between the meningeal branches of the external and/or internal carotid artery and the walls of the cavernous sinus. The most common clinical presentation of CSDAVFs are symptoms resulting from venous hypertension, such as exophthalmos, chemosis, painful eyeball, and visual loss. Progressive visual impairment, elevated intraocular pressure, debilitating ocular symptoms, and leptomeningeal venous drainage are indications for invasive therapy. Endovascular management is currently the treatment of choice and aims to occlude the arteriovenous shunting point, which is most often achieved by obliterating the involved segment of the cavernous sinus. In most cases, transvenous access through the inferior petrosal sinus is the approach of choice. However, this strategy is not always feasible, and alternative approaches can be used, such as direct transorbital puncture. This chapter aims to describe this technique in detail.

Keywords

Cavernous sinus · Dural arteriovenous fistula
Embolization · Endovascular

10.1 Introduction

Intracranial arteriovenous fistulas (AVFs) in the carotid-cavernous region are connections between the carotid artery, and the cavernous sinus. They communicate a high-pressure arterial system to a low-pressure venous system. These lesions are usually classified as direct or indirect. Direct fistulas are caused by trauma, ruptured intracranial aneurysms, collagen deficiency, arterial dissection, or iatrogenic causes (eg. surgical trauma). Indirect fistulas are typically low-flow lesions and are also called dural fistulas [1].

Carotid sinus dural arteriovenous fistulas (CSDAVFs) result from an abnormal communication between the meningeal branches of the internal carotid artery, the external carotid artery or both, to the cavernous sinus. CSDAVFs have an incidence ranging from 0.16 to 0.29 per 100,000 adults per year. They occur mainly in the fifth and sixth decades of life and women are more commonly affected than men [2].

L. B. Manzato · J. R. Vanzin
Neurology and Neurosurgery Service,
Passo Fundo, RS, Brazil

F. P. Trivelato · A. C. Ulhôa · M. T. S. Rezende (✉)
Neurovascular Institute, Belo Horizonte, MG, Brazil

X. Lv (ed.), *Intracranial and Spinal Dural Arteriovenous Fistulas*,
https://doi.org/10.1007/978-981-19-5767-3_10

Classically, the endovascular transvenous approach is the treatment of choice. However, in some cases, transvenous and/or transarterial accesses fails to occlude CSDAVFs [3].

The purpose of this chapter is to address the anatomical relationships of the structures of the cavernous sinus, show the current limitations of the endovascular treatment, and discuss the indications for direct transorbital puncture and its technique for the treatment of CSDAVFs.

10.2 Anatomy

The term 'cavernous sinus' was first used by Winslow in 1732 and cited by Bedford in 1966 [4], describing the presence of numerous filaments and trabeculations that gave the interior of the sinus a plexiform appearance. This appearance allowed Winslow to compare the interior of the sinus to that of the corpus cavernosum of the penis, thus coining the term 'cavernous sinus.'

10.2.1 Venous Connections

The cavernous sinus is composed of a network of trabeculated venous channels in the extradural parasellar space [5] and is connected to some venous structures of the brain, skull, face, and eyes [6]. The anterior portion of the cavernous sinus receives drainage from the superior (SOV) and inferior ophthalmic vein (IOV) through the common ophthalmic vein (trunk). The SOV is located superomedial and the IOV is located inferolateral to the venous trunk, and both veins enter the superior orbital fissure (SOF). The facial vein, angular vein and frontal vein join medially and connect to the cavernous sinus through the SOV or IOV. The anterior portion of the cavernous sinus, in a superolateral position, is the point of junction with the superficial middle cerebral vein. The superior petrosal sinus is connected to the superolateral portion of the cavernous sinus, and drain into the junction of the transverse and sigmoid sinuses. The inferior petrosal sinus, joins the cavernous sinus in an inferolateral position, draining posteriorly into the jugular bulb. The anterior and posterior intercavernous sinus connects both cavernous sinuses, which are separated by the sella turcica. The pterygoid plexus is located in the pterygoid fossa and connects to the cavernous sinus via emissary veins in the middle third in an inferolateral position and also to the inferior ophthalmic vein (IOV) more anteriorly. These venous connections are shown in Fig. 10.1. Given the absence of venous valves inside the cavernous sinus, blood flow direction can be easily reversed, especially in the presence of arterial flow inside it [6]. The numerous possible anatomic variations reported in the literature are not being considered [6, 7].

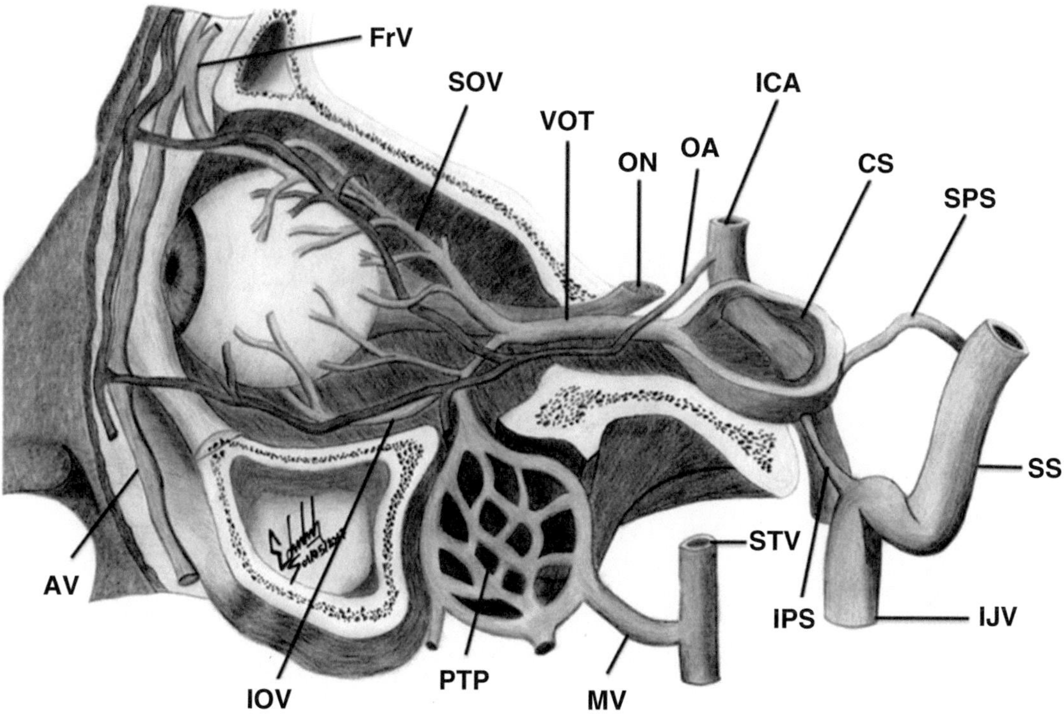

Fig. 10.1 The orbit, lateral view. *FrV* frontal vein, *SOV* superior ophthalmic vein, *VOT* venous ophthalmic trunk, *ON* optic nerve, *OA* ophthalmic artery, *ICA* internal carotid artery, *CS* cavernous sinus, *SPS* superior petrosal sinus, *SS* sigmoid sinus, *IJV* internal jugular vein, *IPS* inferior petrosal sinus, *STV* superficial temporal vein, *MV* maxilar vein, *PTP* pterygoid plexus, *IOV* inferior ophthalmic vein, *AV* angular vein

10.2.2 Cranial Nerves, Optic Canal and Orbital Fissures

In addition to the complex venous circulation, the cavernous sinus is closely related to several cranial nerves, the optic canal, the SOF, and the inferior orbital fissure (IOF). The oculomotor nerve (III), trochlear nerve (IV), and first and second branches of the trigeminal nerve (V1 and V2) are located between the two dural leaflets on the lateral wall of each cavernous sinus and distributed from top to bottom in the following order: III, IV, V1, and V2. The abducens nerve (VI) is located internally in the trabeculae of the cavernous sinus. Figure 10.2 shows the connection of structures within the cavernous sinus, which, together with the orbital structures, are particularly important for direct transorbital approach. The orbit connects to intracranial structures through the optic canal, SOF, and IOF. The optic nerve and ophthalmic artery traverse the optic canal, and the cranial nerves III, IV, V1, and VI reach the orbit through the SOF. Less important structures run within the IOF, such as the emissary veins, the zygomatic branch of V2, and the infraorbital branch of V2 (Fig. 10.3). These anatomical considerations are important when planning an approach to CSDAVFs.

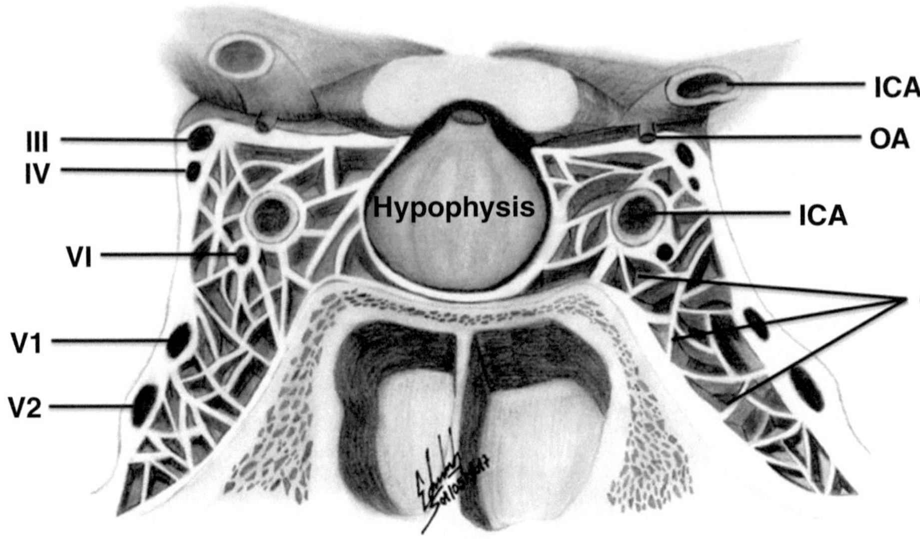

Fig. 10.2 Cavernous sinus, anterior view. ICA—internal carotid artery, OA—ophthalmic artery, CS—cavernous sinus, III—oculomotor nerve, IV—trochlear nerve, VI—abducens nerve, V1—ophtalmic nerve, V2—maxilar nerve (trigeminal roots)

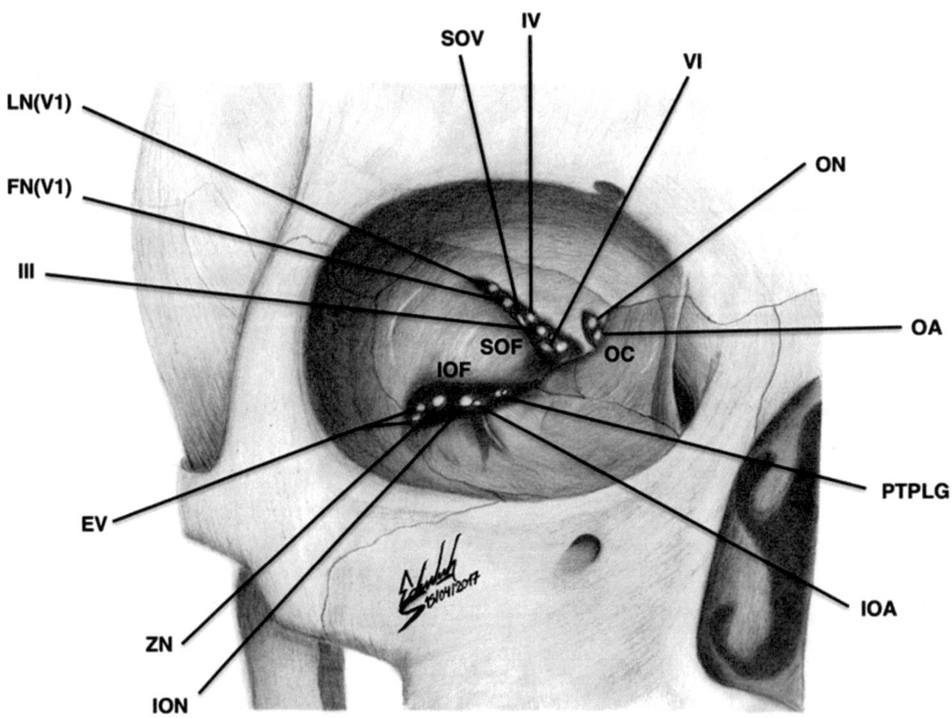

Fig. 10.3 The orbit, anterior view. Optic canal (OC) and its content: ON—optic nerve, OA—ophthalmic artery. Inferior orbital fissure (IOF) and its content: PTPLG—pterygopalatine ganglion (sensitive portion), IOA—inferior orbital artery, ION—inferior orbital nerve, ZN—zygomathic nerve, EV—emissary vein. Superior orbital fissure (SOF) and its content: FN—frontal nerve, LN—lacrimal nerve, SOV—superior ophthalmic vein, IV—trochlear nerve, III—oculomotor nerve (superior branch), VI—abducens nerve

10.3 Classification

Initially, cavernous sinus fistulas were classified according to three criteria: pathogenetically as spontaneous or traumatic fistulas, hemodynamically as high-flow or low-flow fistulas, and angiographically as direct or dural fistulas. These classifications, which are based on the presence or absence of trauma, overlook anatomic and hemodynamic aspects of the fistulas, characteristics that have important prognostic and therapeutic implications. Unfortunately, there are no objective criteria to differentiate high-flow from low-flow lesions. This is a subjective distinction based on angiographic findings and the severity of clinical symptoms. In view of these uncertainties, Barrow et al. [8], in 1985, proposed an angiographic classification that would provide an objective method for grouping all cavernous sinus fistulas, determining prognosis, and planning treatment. It is based on the arterial supply of the fistula in the cavernous sinus.

According to Barrow's classification, the fistulas are type A, B, C, or D. Type A fistulas are direct shunts between the ICA and the cavernous sinus. Types B, C, and D are dural fistulas. Type B fistulas are supplied by meningeal branches of the ICA, type C are dural shunts between the cavernous sinus and meningeal branches of the external carotid artery (ECA), and type D are those supplied by the meningeal branches of both the ICA and ECA (Fig. 10.4).

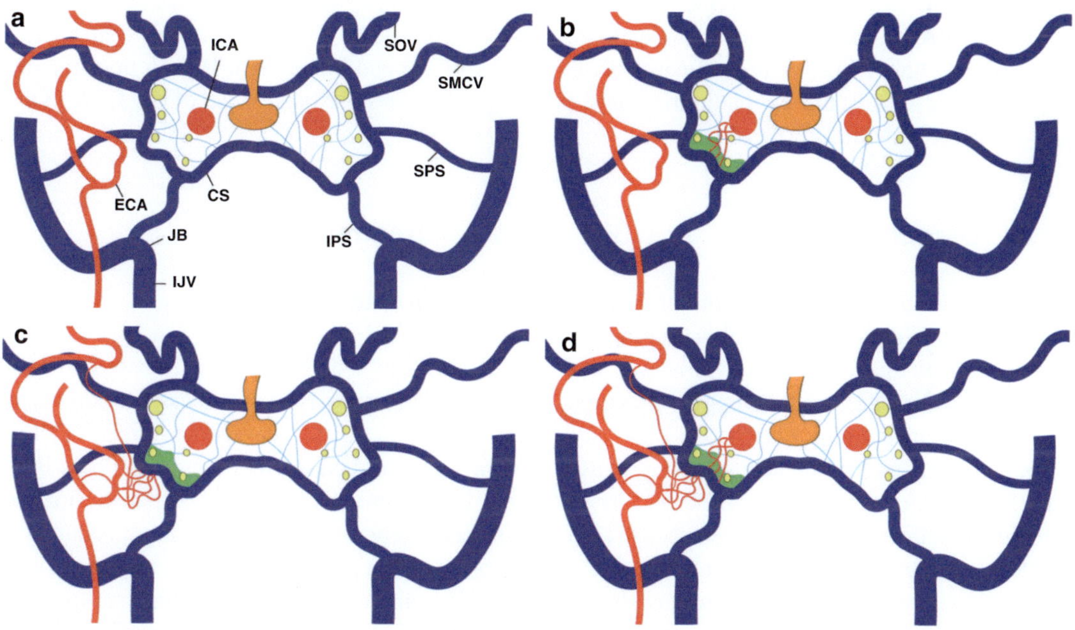

Fig. 10.4 Cavernous sinus region and Barrow classification of cavernous sinus fistulas (B, C and D types). (**a**) Cavernous sinus (CS), inferior petrosal sinus (IPS), superior petrosal sinus (SPS), superficial middle cerebral vein (SMCV), superior ophthalmic vein (SOV), jugular bulb (JB), internal jugular vein (IJV), external carted artery (ECA), cavernous segment of the internal carotid artery (ICA). (**b**) Type B, connection between meningeal branches of the internal carotid and the cavernous sinus. Culprit chamber (free shadow). (**c**) Type C, connection between meningeal branches of the external carotid artery and the cavernous sinus. (**d**) Type D, connection between meningeal branches from the internal and external carotid arteries with the cavernous sinus

10.4 Clinical Manifestations

The onset of symptoms of CSDAVFs is more insidious compared with direct fistulas and clinical presentation is mainly determined by the venous drainage pattern.

Clinical manifestations appear after venous hypertension has reached critical levels, which may take weeks to occur. Intracavernous pressure can be transmitted to the contralateral cavernous sinus through the intercavernous sinuses, resulting in contralateral or bilateral ocular deficits. CSDAVFs are responsible for a high degree of visual impairment, with complete visual loss in 25% of patients and any degree of visual impairment in an additional 20% of patients. The duration of symptoms is an important prognostic factor. The classic triad of CSDAVFs results from venous hypertension, which leads to engorgement of the ophthalmic veins, causing ocular bruit, chemosis, pulsatile exophthalmos, and is present in approximately 60% of cases [9].

10.5 Diagnosis

Several neuroimaging tests are helpful in the diagnosis of CSDAVFs. Cerebral angiography is still considered the gold standard. However, noninvasive tests, such as orbital Doppler ultrasound and brain computed tomography (CT), CT angiography, magnetic resonance imaging (MRI), and MRI angiography, are useful and reveal direct and indirect imaging findings.

Doppler ultrasound shows an inversion of venous flow direction and spectrography shows a low-resistance arterial flow pattern, compatible with an artery, that is, the SOV arterialized [10]. Another possible finding is the presence of SOV thrombosis [11].

Brain CT can identify a dilated or thrombotic SOV, proptosis, early contrast enhancement of the cavernous sinus, extraocular muscle thickening, and bulging periorbital fat pads. An ectatic SOV on post-contrast images is identified in 86–100% of cases [11].

MRI can easily detect a minimally dilated SOV, mild proptosis, and slight thickening of the extraocular muscles. MRI sensitivity improves with intravenous paramagnetic contrast administration, T2-weighted sequences, and SWI sequences. MRI can detect an ectatic SOV, both on T2-weighted and post-contrast images, in 75–100% of patients [12].

The use of angiography is essential for diagnostic confirmation, anatomic assessment, and classification of CSDAVFs. Angiography can detect the fistula and the "culprit" chamber, identify the meningeal branches supplying the CSDAVFs, and assess blood flow of the cavernous sinus and other venous sinuses, thus identifying possible thrombosis or reflux to cortical veins and other sinuses.

Treatment planning is based on the analysis of the angiographic data obtained. Complete bilateral angiography should always be performed. It will be necessary to acquire selective images of the cervical and intracranial ICA in posteroanterior and lateral views and also of the ECA in the same views.

10.6 Treatment

10.6.1 Treatment Options

The treatment is defined primarily based on their type, according to Barrow's classification. Type A, which are direct cavernous sinus fistulas, always require invasive intervention. Types B, C and D, which are dural fistulas, can be treated conservatively, such as by repeated manual compression of the common carotid artery at the cervical level. When associated with intractable symptoms, elevated intraocular pressure, progressive vision loss or high-risk cortical venous drainage, interventional therapy is warranted.

Invasive treatment includes surgery, radiosurgery, and embolization. Conventional surgery has fallen into disuse due to difficulty in accessing the cavernous sinus and high morbidity rates. Radiosurgery has occlusion rates ranging from 44% to 87%, but the major limiting factor is the time required for fistula occlusion, 6–12 months, which can determine worsening of symptoms in this interval [12]. Therefore, endovascular management is currently the treatment of choice for CSDAVFs [13, 14].

10.6.2 Endovascular Treatment: Results and Limitations

Endovascular treatment aims to occlude the arteriovenous shunting point, which is most often achieved by obliterating the involved segment of the cavernous sinus. Kirsch et al. [15] reported a large series of 141 patients treated in 161 sessions of transvenous embolization, with a complete occlusion rate of 81%. Meyers et al. [16] reported a series of 133 patients who underwent endovascular treatment with a mean follow-up of 56 months, a cure rate of 90%, a favorable clinical outcome in 97% of the cases, and a complication rate of only 2.3%.

Endovascular treatment can be carried out through the arterial or venous routes. The difficulty of transarterial access lies in the fact that the meningeal branches originating from both the ECA and ICA are often extremely tortuous and short, thus hindering safe navigation and injection of embolic agents. Furthermore, they may supply some cranial nerves, and anastomose with pial branches, thus making the injection of embolic material dangerous [17]. Transvenous access is the preferred approach to treat most of CSDAVFs, because it is faster, easier, and safer than transarterial approach. The most used venous route, and currently the first option, is through the inferior petrosal sinus, with access via the transfemoral route, or direct internal jugular vein puncture. In many cases, the IPS is occluded or just cannot be visualized on an angiogram, but its recanalization can be achieved in most cases [18]. However, in some circumstances IPS approach fails and other routes have to be used.

Another commonly used access is through the facial vein [19], which is usually dilated and allows access to the fistula through the angular vein and the SOV. There are some limitations to use this approach. The SOV course is often tortuous and delicate, navigation can be quite difficult, and the risk of dissection and venous rupture is not negligible. Anyway, according to Meyers et al., CSDAVFs were treated using IPS or SOV access in 76% of cases [15].

In a series of 63 patients harboring CSDAVFs, 92% were accessed through an endovascular route. Among patients treated by the endovascular approach, the IPS was the main route accessed (65% of cases), and its recanalization was obtained in 20.6% of cases [20]. Venous approach (IPS, SOV or superior petrosal sinus) was performed in 60 (95.2%), venous and arterial embolization was performed in one (1.5%), and arterial approach was performed in two patients (3.1%). For a minority (8%) of cases, access to the CSDAVF could not be achieved by the endovascular approach.

10.6.3 Alternative Approaches

Some fistulas cannot be treated by conventional endovascular approaches; in these cases, several alternative access can be used. The choice of approach should be based on the angioarchitecture of the fistula and mainly on the venous drainage pattern. They can be divided into: (1) surgical approach and (2) direct percutaneous approach.

Often, fistulas that cannot be accessed through usual routes are those with isolated venous drainage to a non-functioning part of the cavernous sinus, which does not participate in cerebral venous drainage. Therefore, the choice of an alternative approach will depend on the drainage of the fistula, as this will be the route to be chosen for treatment.

For example, there are reports of a surgical approach for catheterization of the facial vein, superficial sylvian vein, and SOV [21]. The rationale behind the treatment is the same: reaching the point of drainage of the arteriovenous shunt for occlusion. Once the access vein has been chosen, it is microsurgically dissected, isolated, and catheterized directly, and the remainder of the treatment follows the course of a conventional approach.

When the draining vein has a smaller caliber, this can make dissection difficult and, when it is too deep, surgical approach is not possible. If the operator prefers, direct percutaneous access to these fistulas can be used. The draining vein itself can be punctured directly, guided by radioscopy or ultrasound.

When access through the vein is not possible, an alternative is to perform direct puncture of the cavernous sinus. Importantly, this technique is reserved only for cases where the fistula cannot be accessed through conventional routes. Some reports in the literature suggest a direct approach through the foramen ovale and the orbit [22]. Some authors advocate direct puncture of the cavernous sinus instead of dissection of the superior orbital vein when it is not dilated. Possible advantages of a direct percutaneous approach include better esthetic results, no need for skin incisions, and lower infection rates. Trivelato et al. [23] reported a series of 8 cases of transorbital cavernous sinus direct puncture, with a cure rate of 87%. Only one procedure-related complication occurred by inadvertent ICA puncture, but without clinical complications. The main indications for direct puncture were (1) inability to recanalize the IPS, (2) impossibility to navigate through the IPS with multiple small channels, (3) ophthalmic veins not visualized on angiography, (4) pattern of very small connections between angular vein and ophthalmic veins, (5) intercavernous sinus with multiple channels not allowing navigation from one side to another, (6) insufficient cavernous sinus packing with coils and/or liquid embolic agents via venous approach and (7) liquid embolic agent did not reach the fistulous zone.

Figure 10.5 shows a Barrow-type D cavernous DAVF, with venous drainage into the SOV, which was not dilated. Access through the IPS was attempted bilaterally, without success. Then, it was decided to directly puncture the sinus due to the impossibility of accessing the ophthalmic vein. A needle was inserted, followed by contrast injection that confirmed the position inside the

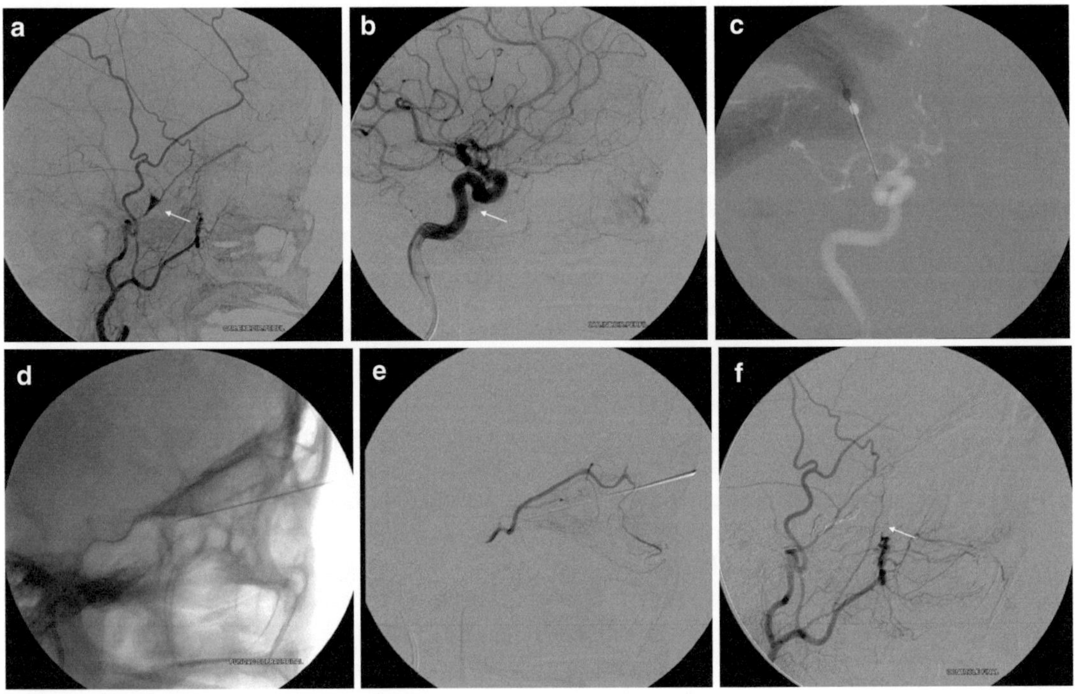

Fig. 10.5 Right external carotid (**a**) and internal carotid (**b**) angiogram, lateral view, showing a type D cavernous fistula (white arrows). The culprit chamber is isolated. Superomedial direct puncture under road mapping (**c**), and fluoroscopy, lateral view (**d**). Selective injection from the needle confirms its correct location (**e**). Right external carotid artery, lateral view. Final control demonstrating total occlusion of the fistula and the cast of coils filling the culprit chamber (white arrow) (**f**)

fistulous part of the sinus, which was embolized with coils. The final result was complete occlusion. There were no complications during or after the procedure.

Transorbital cavernous sinus puncture has some potential risks. Ocular complications of direct access include orbital cellulitis, puncture of the globe, cranial nerve damage, and injury to arterial structures along the needle trajectory, which could lead to an intraorbital hematoma [24, 25]. Additionally, there is a risk of puncture of the carotid artery with subarachnoid hemorrhage or intracerebral hemorrhage. Fu et al. [26] described the technique of cone-beam CT-guided puncture in three patients, with 100% cure and no complications, which proved to be a valid and safe option.

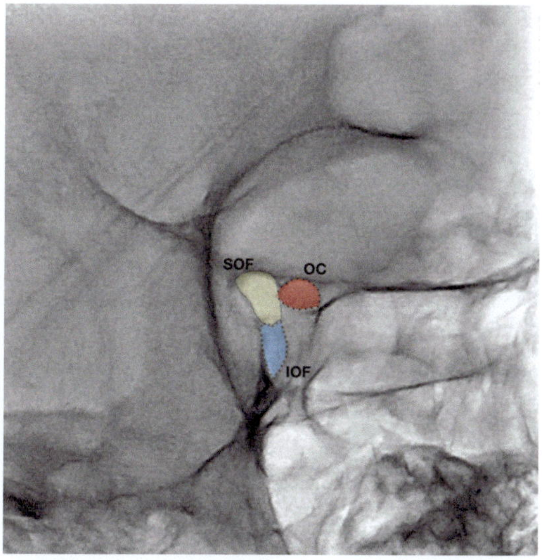

Fig. 10.6 Fluoroscopy in right oblique view demonstrating the superior orbital fissure (SOF—yellow shadow), the optic canal (OC—red shadow) and the inferior orbital fissure (IOF—blue shadow)

10.6.4 Cavernous Sinus Direct Puncture: Technique

The transorbital cavernous sinus direct puncture procedure should be performed in the interventional neuroradiology room with the patient in the supine position under general anesthesia. Skin preparation should include antisepsis of the periorbital and inguinal regions. Arterial access is usually achieved via the right common femoral artery using the Seldinger technique with a 5F sheath, a diagnostic catheter, and a 0.035 in. hydrophilic guidewire. Complete cerebral angiography should always be performed, including the ICA, ECA, and vertebral arteries, which should be studied prior to treatment in order to determine the angioarchitecture of the CSDAVFs. The diagnostic catheter is kept in the artery that best identifies the fistula under perfusion of a 0.9% saline solution. No heparin is used during the procedure. With the patient's head in a neutral position, the eye region should be sterilized with an aqueous solution, avoiding any type of alcoholic solution in this region.

The target of direct puncture is the SOF on the affected side. The best way to identify the SOF in the ipsilateral oblique view at approximately 30° with a submentovertex inclination (Hirtz view) of 20°. These angles may vary, and their correction is performed under fluoroscopy until a good visualization of the SOF is achieved (Fig. 10.6). Its radiological identification is essential to separate the SOF from the optic canal, thus preventing damage to the optic nerve. The target point is at the lowest part of the SOF at the junction with the IOF (Fig. 10.7). Because this region does not have any vascular structure passing through the orbital fissure, it is considered the safest point of access to the cavernous sinus. After antisepsis and placement of sterile drapes, direct access to the cavernous sinus is gained using a number 22 lumbar puncture needle. The needle is slowly advanced under fluoroscopic guidance in the projection that best identifies the junction of the SOF and IOF. At this point, a road map is created via the arterial route to visualize the venous drainage of the fistula. This process should be performed slowly and progressively under fluoroscopic guidance in both the posteroanterior and lateral views. The target will always be the lower third of the SOF or the point of junction of the SOF with the IOF. Once the target has been reached, there is loss of needle residence. At this point, we are close to the cavernous sinus. Note that, from this point onward, we can reach the intracranial structures. After

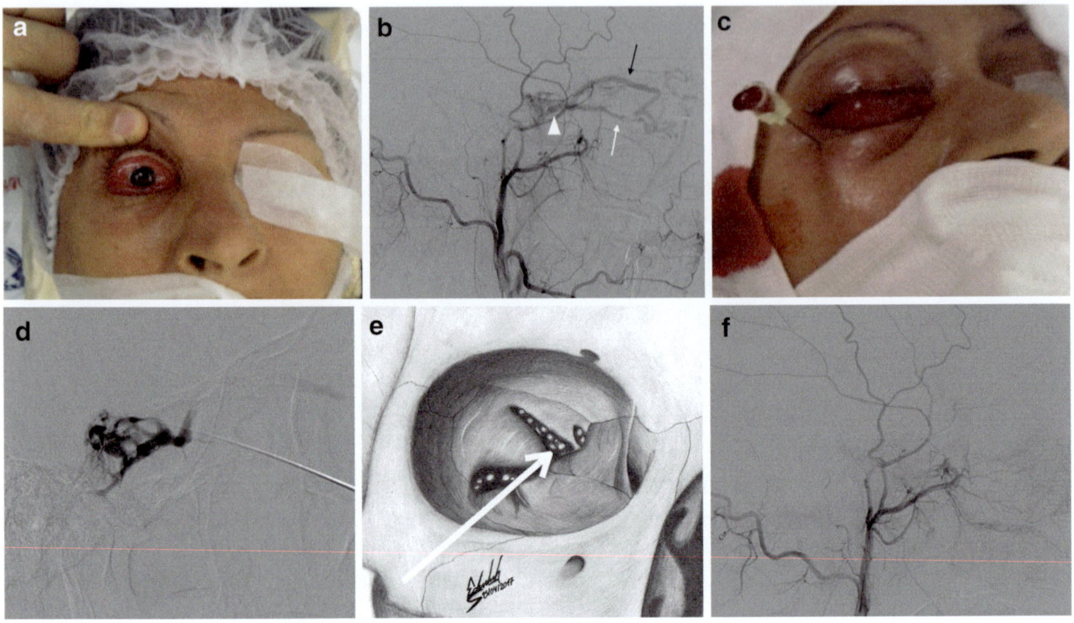

Fig. 10.7 Patient with proptosis, chemosis and conjunctival hyperemia in the right eye (**a**). Angiogram of the right external carotid artery in the lateral view showing a cavernous sinus dural arteriovenous fistula draining to the ophtalmic venous trunk (white arrowhead), superior (black arrow) and inferior ophthalmic (white arrow) veins (**b**). Inferolateral percutaneous puncture (**c**), Needle injection confirms its position in the fistulous point of the cavernous sinus (**d**). Intended trajectory of the needle in the infero-lateral access aiming the inferior part of the superior orbital fissure (white arrow) (**e**). Final control angiogram showing total occlusion of the fistula (**f**)

small advances of the needle, the stylet is removed to observe blood reflux. Presence of reflux means that we have probably reached the cavernous sinus. Depending on anatomic variations of the ophthalmic venous trunk, if the segment is long, we sometimes puncture the trunk before directly reaching the cavernous sinus. We confirm the correct positioning of the needle by performing venous angiography with a 3-mL syringe directly connected to the needle. After confirming the intracavernous position, a 0.014 in. microguidewire is passed. The microguidewire should make one or two loops inside the cavernous sinus to provide stability to the microguidewire in order to advance the microcatheter into the cavernous sinus (Fig. 10.8). A small skin incision can be made with a number 11 scalpel blade before passing an 18-gauge Abbocath over the microguidewire, which serves as a sheath inside the orbit, thus facilitating the passage of the microcatheter while keeping it more stable during treatment. A microcatheter compatible with non-adhesive liquid embolic agents (NALEAs) can be passed, which should also allow passing platinum coils. Selective microcatheterization of the fistulous point should be performed once the microcatheter is inside the cavernous sinus. Caution is needed as there is little support for bolder maneuvers, which can lead to excessive pressure on the microcatheter, pushing it outward. Ideally, the fistulous point should be punctured directly with the needle, but this is not always possible, as the space for maneuvering inside the orbit is very limited and repeated attempts can render the procedure dangerous. Once correct positioning has been confirmed, embolization is performed with coils and/or liquid embolic agents. As they are low-flow fistulas, in most cases using only coils is curative. Liquid agents are used when the use of coils alone cannot occlude the fistula, or when the microcatheter does not reach a sufficiently distal point of the fistula for treatment with coils alone. If NALEA is not available, another option is the use of cianoacrylates.

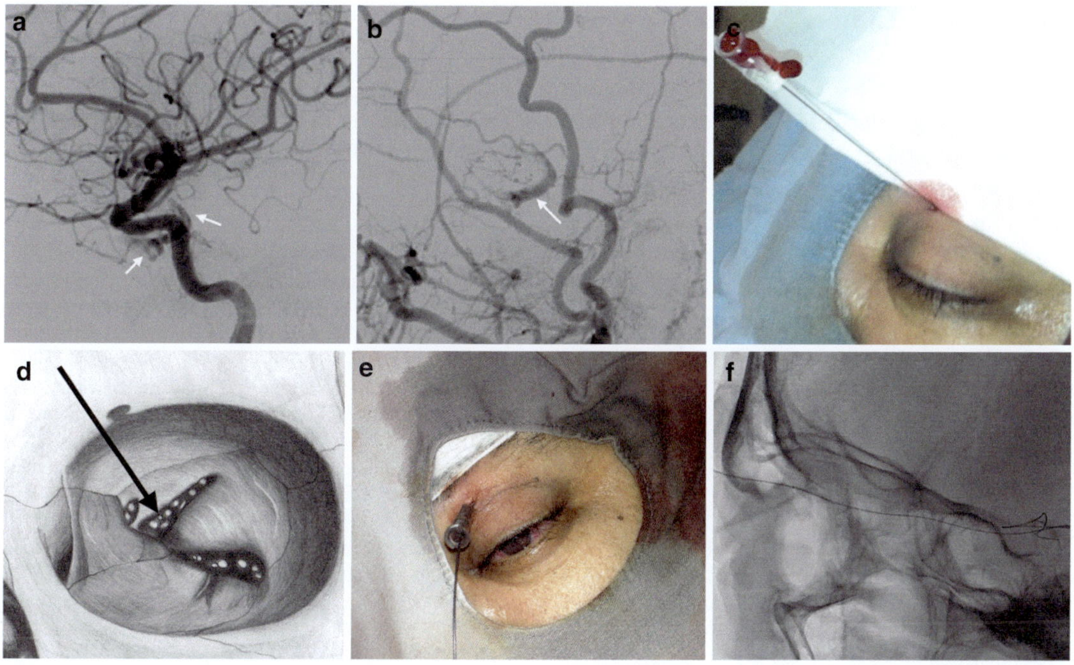

Fig. 10.8 Angiogram in lateral view with internal (**a**) and external (**b**) carotid artery injection, showing cavernous sinus dural fistula (white arrows), the sinus is isolated. Superomedial transorbital puncture in the left eye (**c**). Programmed path for the insertion of the needle in the inferior portion of the superior orbital fissure (black arrow) (**d**). Abbocath inserted into the skin to give support the microcatheter navigation (**e**). Radioscopy in profile showing the microguidewire with some loops inside de cavernous sinus (**f**)

In rare cases, in the presence of orbital hypertension due to venous congestion of the CSDAVF or after repeated needle punctures (due to failed attempts to access the cavernous sinus), the Abbocath and/or microcatheter may not advance along the orbital path. Whenever navigating the microcatheter to the fistulous point is not possible, an alternative is to inject the NALEA directly through the lumbar puncture needle. Control angiograms are obtained, and, after confirming fistula occlusion, the material is removed and local hemostasis is achieved by gentle digital compression.

Two different access routes have been reported for a direct approach, the inferolateral and superomedial access routes.

10.6.4.1 Inferolateral Access

The entry point is the lateral third of the lower eyelid (Fig. 10.7). With the thumb, the operator elevates the globe superiorly. The needle is advanced along the lower edge of the orbital rim under fluoroscopic guidance in the projection that best identifies the SOF. The needle is directed anteroposteriorly with the necessary inclination to advance along the floor of the orbit toward the orbital apex. Some bone resistance is commonly found during this maneuver, which must be corrected with the angulation of the needle as it advances through the floor of the orbit.

10.6.4.2 Superomedial Access

The entry point is the medial third of the upper eyelid, and, with the thumb, the operator depresses the globe inferiorly (Fig. 10.8). Likewise, the needle is advanced under fluoroscopic guidance in the projection that best identifies the SOF. The needle is directed along the roof of the orbit toward its apex. As with the inferolateral access, bone resistance can also be found, and maneuvers to correct the needle direction will be necessary. Fluoroscopic monitoring in posteroanterior and lateral views is often performed.

10.7 Conclusion

The treatment of CSDAVFs is still challenging, but it has been associated with excellent cure rates and several approaches to be chosen. A well-done prior vascular study of these lesions, as well as an early treatment planning, are mandatory in the treatment of this condition. If the usual approaches are deemed not possible, transorbital direct puncture of the cavernous sinus can be a safe and effective alternative for selected cases.

References

1. Satomi J, Satoh K. Epidemiology and etiology of dural arteriovenous fistula. Brain Nerve. 2008;60:883–6.
2. Soderman M, Pavic L, Edner G, Holmin S, Andersson T. Natural history of dural arteriovenous shunts. Stroke. 2008;39:1735–9.
3. Klisch J, Huppertz HJ, Spetzger U, Hetzel A, Seeger W, Schumacher M. Transvenous treatment of carotid cavernous and dural arteriovenous fistulae: results for 31 patients and review of the literature. Neurosurgery. 2003;53:836–56.
4. Bedford MA. The "cavernous" sinus. Br J Ophthalmol. 1966;50:41–6.
5. Parkinson D. A surgical approach to the cavernous portion of the carotid artery. Anatomical studies and case report. J Neurosurg. 1965;23:474–83.
6. Rhoton AL Jr, Hardy DG, Chambers SM. Microsurgical anatomy and dissection of the sphenoid bone, cavernous sinus and sellar region. Surg Neurol. 1979;12:63–104.
7. Dolenc V. Direct microsurgical repair of intracavernous vascular lesions. J Neurosurg. 1983;58:824–31.
8. Barrow DL, Spector RH, Braun IF, Landman JA, Tindall SC, Tindall GT. Classification and treatment of spontaneous carotid-cavernous sinus fistulas. J Neurosurg. 1985;62(2):248–56.
9. Hamby WB, Dohn DF. Carotid-cavernous fistulas: report of thirty-six cases and discussion of their management. Clin Neurosurg. 1964;11:150–70.
10. Berges O. Colour Doppler flow imaging of the orbital veins. Acta Ophthalmol Suppl. 1992;204:55–8.
11. Dos Santos D, Monsignore LM, Nakiri GS, Velasco e Cruz AA, Colli BO, Abud DG. Imaging diagnosis of dural and direct cavernous carotid fistulae. Radiol Bras. 2014;47(4):251–5.
12. Hirabuki N, Hliura T, Mitomo M, et al. MR imaging of dural arteriovenous malformations with ocular signs. Neuroradiology. 1988;30(5):390–4.
13. O'Leary S, Hodgson TJ, Coley SC, Kemeny AA, Radatz MW. Intracranial dural arteriovenous malformations: results of stereotactic radiosurgery in 17 patients. Clin Oncol (R Coll Radiol). 2002;14:97–102.
14. Zhang J, Lv X, Jiang C, et al. Transarterial and transvenous embolization for cavernous sinus dural arteriovenous fistulae. Interv Neuroradiol. 2010;16(3):269–77.
15. Kirsch M, Henkes H, Liebig T, Weber W, Esser J, Golik S, et al. Endo-vascular management of dural carotid-cavernous sinus fistulas in 141 patients. Neuroradiology. 2006;48:486–90.
16. Meyers PM, Halbach VV, Dowd CF, Lempert TE, Malek AM, Phatouros CC, et al. Dural carotid cavernous fistula: definitive endovascular management and long-term follow-up. Am J Ophthalmol. 2002;134:85–92.
17. Lekkhong E, Pongpech S, Ter Brugge K, Jiarakongmun P, Willinsky R, Geibprasert S, et al. Transvenous embolization of intracranial dural arteriovenous shunts through occluded venous segments: experience in 51 patients. AJNR Am J Neuroradiol. 2011;32:1738–44.
18. Théaudin M, Saint-Maurice JP, Chapot R, Vahedi K, Mazighi M, Vignal C, Saliou G, Stapf C, Bousser MG, Houdart E. Diagnosis and treatment of dural carotid-cavernous stulas: a consecutive series of 27 patients. J Neurol Neurosurg Psychiatry. 2007;78:174–9.
19. Biondi A, Milea D, Cognard C, et al. Cavernous sinus dural fistulae treated by transvenous approach through the facial vein: report of seven cases and review of the literature. Am J Neuroradiol. 2003;24:1240–6.
20. Castro-Afonso LH, Trivelato FP, Rezende MT, Ulhôa AC, Nakiri GS, Monsignore LM, Abud DG. The routes for embolization of dural carotid cavernous fistulas when the endovascular approach is indicated as a first-line strategy. Interv Neuroradiol. 2019;25(1):66–70. https://doi.org/10.1177/1591019918796493. Epub 2018 Aug 30.
21. Berlis A, Klisch J, Spetzger U, et al. Carotid cavernous fistula: embolization via a bilateral superior ophthalmic vein approach. Am J Neuroradiol. 2002;23:1736–8.
22. Andrade GC, Alves HP, Parente R, Salvarani CP, Clímico VM, Pereira ER. Spontaneous isolated dural arteriovenous fistula of the cavernous sinus: endovascular approach via the foramen ovale. Interv Neuroradiol. 2012;18:458–62.
23. Trivelato FP, Manzato LB, Filho PMM, Ulhôa AC, Vanzin JR, Abud DG, Rezende MTS. Transorbital cavernous sinus direct puncture: alternative to treat dural arteriovenous fistula. Clin Neuroradiol. 2018;28(1):55–61. https://doi.org/10.1007/s00062-016-0534-z. Epub 2016 Aug 9.
24. Dashti SR, Fiorella D, Spetzler RF, Albuquerque FC, McDougall CG. Transorbital endovascular embolization of dural carotid cavernous fistula: access to cavernous sinus through direct puncture: case examples and technical report. Neurosurgery. 2011;68(ONS Suppl 1):ons75–83.
25. Puffer RC, Lanzino G, Cloft HJ. Using Xperguide planning software to safely guide catheter access to

the cavernous sinus via transorbital puncture: a case report. Oper Neurosurg. 2014;10:E370–3.
26. Fu ZY, Feng Y, Ma C, Chen JC, Krings T, Zhao WY. Endovascular treatment of cavernous sinus dural arteriovenous fistulas via direct transorbital puncture using cone-beam computed tomography image guidance: report of 3 cases. World Neurosurg. 2019;130:306–12.

11 Cranial Dural Arteriovenous Fistulas: The Role of Transarterial and Transvenous Balloon-Assisted Embolization

Felipe Padovani Trivelato,
Alexandre Cordeiro Ulhôa,
and Marco Túlio Salles Rezende

Abstract

The treatment of dural arteriovenous fistulas (DAVFs) consists of occluding the venous component related to the fistula. The arterial route, the venous route or a combination of both can be used. The great challenge of endovascular treatment, especially through the arterial route, is to control the progression of the liquid embolic agent. It should reach the fistulous point and the draining vein but without excessive reflux on the arterial side. Additionally, extensive occlusion of the draining vein or inadvertent occlusion of a venous sinus should be avoided. To obtain a better control of the liquid embolic agent progression, transarterial double-lumen balloon catheters have been used with or without transvenous balloon catheters to protect the dural sinus. Transarterial treatment of DAVFs assisted by double-lumen balloon catheters is safe and effective. The use of the balloon makes the occipital artery an excellent access route, since the problem of excessive reflux and greater resistance of the transosseous branches is overcome. This route presents results as good as when the middle meningeal artery is used. The transvenous balloon catheter is also safe and can prevent inadvertent occlusion of the dural venous sinus. Complications related to temporary sinus occlusion are rare. The association of transvenous and transarterial balloon catheters is very effective, determining high rates of total occlusion of DAVFs. The introduction of two balloons simultaneously, through the middle meningeal artery and the occipital artery, seems to be a very promising approach, since it provides greater control over the flow toward the fistula.

Keywords

Dural arteriovenous fistula · Balloon Embolization · Endovascular

F. P. Trivelato (✉) · A. C. Ulhôa · M. T. S. Rezende
Division of Interventional Neuroradiology,
Felício Rocho Hospital,
Belo Horizonte, Minas Gerais, Brazil

Division of Interventional Neuroradiology,
Rede Mater Dei Saúde,
Belo Horizonte, Minas Gerais, Brazil

Neurovascular Institute,
Belo Horizonte, Minas Gerais, Brazil

X. Lv (ed.), *Intracranial and Spinal Dural Arteriovenous Fistulas*,
https://doi.org/10.1007/978-981-19-5767-3_11

Key Points

- DAVFs can be treated by transarterial or transvenous approaches.
- The transarterial approach is the first choice for treating most DAVFs with direct leptomeningeal venous drainage.
- Transarterial balloon-assisted embolization improves the rate of cure in high-grade DAVFs.
- Dural sinus occlusion is associated with higher rates of angiographic cure for sinus wall DAVFs.
- Occlusion of a dural sinus might lead to a substantial risk of complications.
- Dural sinus preservation with a transvenous balloon catheter is safe and very effective.
- The association of transvenous and transarterial balloon catheters offers flow/pressure control in the treatment of DAVFs.

11.1 Introduction

The first authors to correlate the clinical behavior of cranial dural arteriovenous fistulas (DAVFs) with the pattern of venous drainage and to propose a classification based on this drainage were Djindjian and Merland in 1978 [1, 2]. The classifications currently used, especially those of Cognard and Borden, are based on this same concept, and they allow an accurate comparison between clinical manifestations and radiological patterns [1, 3].

The endovascular treatment of DAVFs consists of occluding the venous component related to the fistula [3]. The drainage pattern guides the therapeutic management of these lesions. Therefore, DAVFs with direct drainage to a leptomeningeal vein should be treated by occluding the draining vein at the point closest to the fistulous zone, called the "foot of the vein" [2, 4, 5]. On the other hand, the treatment of DAVFs draining to a dural sinus wall should be treated by occluding the lumen of this sinus or the fistulous point located in the wall of the sinus [2, 6].

The arterial route, the venous route or a combination of both can be used [3]. However, the great challenge of endovascular treatment, especially through the arterial route, is to control the progression of the liquid embolic agent. It should reach the fistulous point and the draining vein but without excessive reflux on the arterial side. Additionally, extensive occlusion of the draining vein or inadvertent occlusion of a venous sinus should be avoided [2, 3, 6].

To order to obtain a better control of the liquid embolic agent progression, transarterial double lumen balloon catheters have been used with or without transvenous balloon catheters to protect the dural sinus [7–15]. This strategy allows the injection of the embolic agent through the arterial route without extensive reflux, since the retrograde flow is blocked by the inflated balloon inside the arterial feeder. The risk of inadvertent venous sinus occlusion is minimized, as the inflated balloon inside the sinus protects its lumen.

11.2 Pros and Cons of Transarterial and Transvenous Approaches

11.2.1 Transarterial Approach

Most DAVFs can be treated through an arterial approach [2, 6]. This route has been successfully used to treat DAVFs with direct leptomeningeal drainage [4, 5].

In the pre-ethylene vinyl alcohol (EVOH) copolymer era, with the use of polyvinyl alcohol (PVA) particles and glue, the results of transarterial treatment were disappointing. PVA particles were associated with a high chance of recanalization. Similarly, there was great difficulty in controlling the anterograde progression of the glue in such a way that it reached the venous side, but without migration too distally inside the drainage vein [4].

Since the introduction of EVOH in 2006, for the treatment of DAVFs, this scenario has changed [4]. Because of the better control of embolic agent progression, high cure rates have been reported [2, 5].

The failures are mainly related to the impossibility of obtaining adequate arterial access. A position close to the fistulous zone, which allows the injection of the embolic agent, especially through the middle meningeal artery, provides a better progression of EVOH.

Another limiting factor is reflux inside the arterial feeder. This reflux is expected to occur, as it is part of the EVOH injection technique, allowing the formation of a proximal plug that will favor the anterograde progression of the liquid embolic agent [7].

However, depending on the position of the microcatheter, a delicate balance must be respected between the anterograde progression of the embolic agent and reflux. Usually, the more extensive the reflux is, the greater the chance that the embolic agent will reach the draining vein and the more likely it is to obtain angiographic cure of the lesion. On the other hand, the more extensive the reflux is, the greater the rate of complications, especially those related to the filling of dangerous anastomoses of the external carotid artery and those related to the occlusion of cranial nerve feeders [7–9].

11.2.2 Transvenous Approach

Transvenous access has been classically used to treat DAVFs located in the wall of a sinus. Sinus occlusion is associated with a higher chance of complete obliteration of the fistula compared to selective treatment by the transarterial access. However, complete obliteration of a dural sinus can lead to a substantial risk of complications if the occluded sinus impairs normal brain drainage [3].

Thus, when the involved dural sinus participates in normal venous drainage, transvenous access is quite limited. It has been used when an accessory dural sinus or a compartmentalized sinus are present [3, 6]. In these cases, venous access can still be used to selectively occlude the involved compartment, preserving the main sinus [3, 6].

Another limitation of the venous route for treating dural sinus wall fistulas is the isolated sinuses. In such cases, there is some obstacle, most often a thrombus inside the dural sinus, which obstructs the sinus lumen both proximal and distal to the fistulous zone [6, 10]. Thus, access to the involved segment of the sinus cannot be reached directly. It is necessary to recanalize the sinus lumen or even perform direct access to the sinus through a craniotomy.

Regarding DAVFs with direct leptomeningeal venous drainage, transvenous access is usually not preferred [2, 4]. This has been avoided in this type of fistula since venous navigation within a leptomeningeal vein is usually challenging from a technical point of view and has considerable risks [2, 4, 5]. Exceptions would be fistulas in the anterior cranial base and fistulas in the hypoglossal canal region.

11.3 Dural Sinus Sacrifice Versus Dural Sinus Preservation

Dural fistulas located in the wall of a sinus can be treated in two completely different ways, either by occluding the segment of the dural sinus involved, or by preserving the sinus lumen [3]. Sinus occlusion can be performed via a venous approach, using coils with or without the association of liquid embolic agents, or via an arterial approach, through the injection of liquid embolic agents that will migrate to the venous side [3, 6].

The strategy of preserving the lumen of the dural sinus is associated with a lower risk of complications, especially those related to the impairment of venous drainage. However, lower rates of total occlusion of the fistulas are expected in the selective treatment [3, 4].

A major controversy occurs when the sinus is not functioning, whether there is a reason to still preserve its patency. The sinus may be nonfunctioning because of a hemodynamic competition, rather than anatomical disruption, a true occlusion [7, 11].

Based on the pathophysiological origin of DAVFs, multiple abnormal arteriovenous connections are present in the dural venous sinus wall and not within the sinus [7]. Consequently, occlusion of connections in the venous sinus wall seems to be more reasonable than occlusion of the entire lumen of the dural sinus, especially if the sinus is being used for normal venous drainage [3, 7, 11].

11.4 Specific Challenges While Treating DAVFs

11.4.1 DAVFs with Direct Leptomeningeal Venous Drainage

DAVFs with direct leptomeningeal venous drainage are preferentially treated through a transarterial approach because of the technical difficulty in navigating inside dilated and tortuous leptomeningeal veins. The middle meningeal artery is the access of choice for the treatment of most lesions, including fistulas of the tentorium, transverse and sigmoid sinuses, torcula and convexity [2, 4, 5].

In the best scenario, the microcatheter should be navigated to a position close to the fistulous zone. Thus, the migration of the liquid embolic agent toward the draining vein will occur earlier, before the occurrence of excessive reflux [5].

In most cases, with a single session through the middle meningeal artery, it is possible to treat most DAVFs with direct leptomeningeal drainage. However, very tortuous and thin arterial access may prevent the microcatheter from reaching a position close to the fistulous zone [2, 4, 5]. In this situation, excessive reflux may occur before the embolic agent reaches the draining vein. Complications related to excessive reflux include cranial nerve ischemia and microcatheter entrapment [5]. The advent of detachable tip microcatheters has partially solved this problem.

In some cases, the middle meningeal artery is not the main supply of the fistula, or it has been previously occluded, or navigation within this vessel is not possible. In these scenarios, the occipital artery tends to be an important supplier of the fistula. This artery is usually quite large and tortuous. Thus, it is difficult to navigate the microcatheter distally and specially to form the proximal plug after the initial reflux of the embolic agent, which will determine the anterograde migration of the EVOH [7, 12].

Another complicating factor is that the occipital artery supplies DAVFs through transosseous branches, which have greater resistance [7]. The liquid embolic agent tends to preferentially penetrate into scalp branches instead of branches directly supplying the fistulous zone. Thus, long reflux of the embolic agent inside the occipital artery and excessive filling of scalp branches are necessary before EVOH reaches the fistula [12]. Numerous dangerous anastomoses exist in the most proximal portion of the occipital artery, which limits the amount of acceptable reflux.

The duration of the procedure and the radiation dose used are also limiting factors [12]. Therefore, access through the occipital artery is considered not ideal.

11.4.2 DAVFs Draining to a Dural Sinus

The treatment of DAVFs located in the sinus wall through the venous approach is technically easy. The sinus can be occluded with liquid agents, coils, or both [3]. We have adopted the strategy of using two microcatheters. One of these compounds, compatible with dimethyl sulfoxide (DMSO), is kept distally. Through a second microcatheter, coils are placed throughout the involved sinus segment until reaching the most proximal portion of the fistulous zone. If angiographic control still shows residual filling of the fistula, the first microcatheter, positioned in the most distal portion of the cast of coils, is used for the injection of a liquid embolic agent.

This two-microcatheter technique ensures that, after coil implantation, if there is still residual filling of the fistula, it is not necessary to gain new access to the fistulous point across the cast of coils.

The arterial route is commonly used when it is decided to preserve the sinus lumen [2, 3, 6]. In this situation, the aim is that the liquid embolic agent penetrates into the wall of the venous sinus, between the sheets of the dura mater without migrating into the sinus. Some migration is inevitable and occurs in most cases. Care must be taken to ensure that the amount of embolic agent that crosses to the venous side is minimal, avoiding dural sinus occlusion or distal embolism.

In most cases, it is possible to treat the fistula and to preserve the lumen of the dural sinus via an arterial approach. However, this technique requires a long fluoroscopy time, and the reflux inside the arterial feeder can be excessive [2, 6]. Multiple arterial accesses in multiple sessions may be necessary. Controlling the migration of the liquid embolic agent becomes very challenging in lesions with very high flow.

11.5 Rationale for the Use of Balloon Catheters in DAVF Treatment

11.5.1 Transarterial Double-Lumen Balloon

To order to improve the penetration of the liquid embolic agent inside the fistulous zone during the treatment of DAVFs, some strategies have been used, including the pressure cooker technique with coils or glue and the use of a balloon in parallel with a microcatheter to avoid reflux [16, 17]. When double-lumen balloon catheters are used, instead of these techniques, the navigation of a single device for each arterial access is sufficient.

The use of a double-lumen balloon catheter for the injection of liquid embolic agents was described for the first time in 2013 [13]. When the balloon is inflated, it is able to create a barrier, which will favor the anterograde migration of the embolic agent.

The balloon catheter allows more aggressive embolization, with a longer injection and larger volumes, without any reflux. Thus, the procedure becomes safer [9, 10].

11.5.2 Transvenous "Protective" Balloon

Although the double-lumen balloon catheter is an innovative solution for managing reflux, it does not provide any protection for the dural sinuses. In contrast, the balloon inflated in the arterial feeder tends to increase the migration of the embolic agent into the sinus at an early stage.

This unintentional migration of the liquid embolic agent into the sinus must be avoided. The use of a balloon inside the sinus to protect its lumen facilitates the management of these DAVFs. Without the presence of any barrier inside the sinus, the distal embolism of the liquid agent can only be controlled by stopping the injection [11, 15, 18].

The transvenous balloon catheter allows the embolic agent to penetrate the sinus wall, where multiple arteriovenous connections are located [11, 15, 18]. Once the sinus lumen is protected by the inflated balloon, the migration of the embolic agent occurs along the entire sinus wall circumferentially, occluding the fistulous zone.

In some cases, the use of a transvenous balloon catheter is impossible or unnecessary, including isolated sinuses, sinuses containing a thrombus causing partial occlusion, severe stenosis (>80%), or a very ectatic sinus [19]. In other cases, especially in fistulas involving the torcula, the dural sinus may be extremely dilated. The Copernic RC balloon catheter diameter is not sufficient to occlude the sinus; thus, it does not offer sufficient protection. In this situation, it is possible to use two balloons in parallel [19].

11.6 Technical Nuances for the Use of Transarterial and Transvenous Balloon Catheters

11.6.1 DAVFs with Direct Leptomeningeal Venous Drainage

There are several double-lumen balloon catheters available on the market, including Scepter (Microvention, Tustin, USA), Copernic 2L (Balt

Extrusion, Montmorency, France), Eclipse 2L (Balt Extrusion, Montmorency, France) and Ascent (Cerenovus, Irvine, USA) [20–25]. Such balloons have two lumens: the first is dedicated to the introduction of the guidewire (usually 0.014 in.), and the second lumen is used to inflate the balloon. Thus, after removing the guidewire, it is possible to inject the embolic agent through the lumen of the wire without deflating the balloon [9, 22] (Fig. 11.1a).

The balloon can be navigated through a 6F guiding catheter that will usually be positioned in the external carotid artery inside feeding branches of the DAVF. If the anatomy is complex, with very tortuous vessels and the need for very distal navigation, a triaxial system with a long sheath and a guide catheter with a flexible tip can be used [19] (Fig. 11.1b).

The middle meningeal artery should be used as the preferred access whenever possible. Usually, in the presence of DAVFs, the middle meningeal artery is the main supplying artery, and it has an increased caliber and a straighter path embedded in the dura mater [12, 19]. The

a

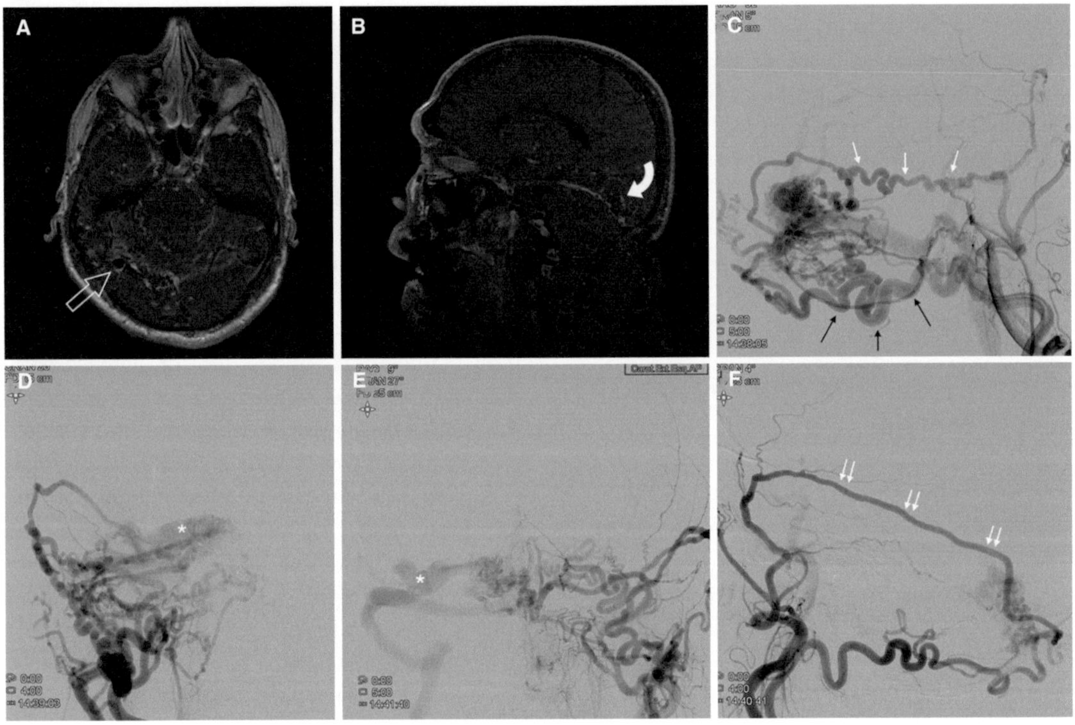

Fig. 11.1 (**a**) (A) MRI shows an ectatic vein (open arrow) and multiple arterial feeders. (B) Note the tentorial location (curved arrow) of the lesion. (C) Right external carotid artery angiogram (lateral view) demonstrates a lateral tentorial DAVF supplied by a very tortuous MMA (white arrows) and a large occipital artery (black arrows). (D) Note the "foot" of the draining vein (asterisk). (E, F) Left external carotid artery angiograms (AP and lateral views) demonstrate a right tentorial DAVF supplied by a straight left MMA draining directly to an occipital vein (asterisk). (**b**) (A) Road mapping image shows a double-lumen balloon (open arrow) placed in the origin of the mastoid branch (black arrow) of the occipital artery. (B) Note the double-lumen balloon inflated (open arrow) and the position of the guide catheter with a flexible tip (large arrow). (C) Lateral fluoroscopy demonstrates two guide catheters inside the MMA and occipital arteries (large arrows). The tip of the balloon catheter (black arrow) is inside the mastoid branch and the tip of a standard microcatheter (white arrow) is in the MMA. (D) Double-injection through the microcatheter (whiter arrow) and balloon catheter (black arrow) shows the fistulous zone and the draining vein (asterisk). (**c**) (A) Control angiography (bilateral injection) after embolization reveals total occlusion of the DAVF. (B) Venous phase shows a patent right transverse sinus (double-arrows), with no migration of EVOH. (C) Note the cast of EVOH inside the draining vein (asterisk) of the fistula. (D) MRI after 6 months demonstrates total occlusion of the DAVF

b

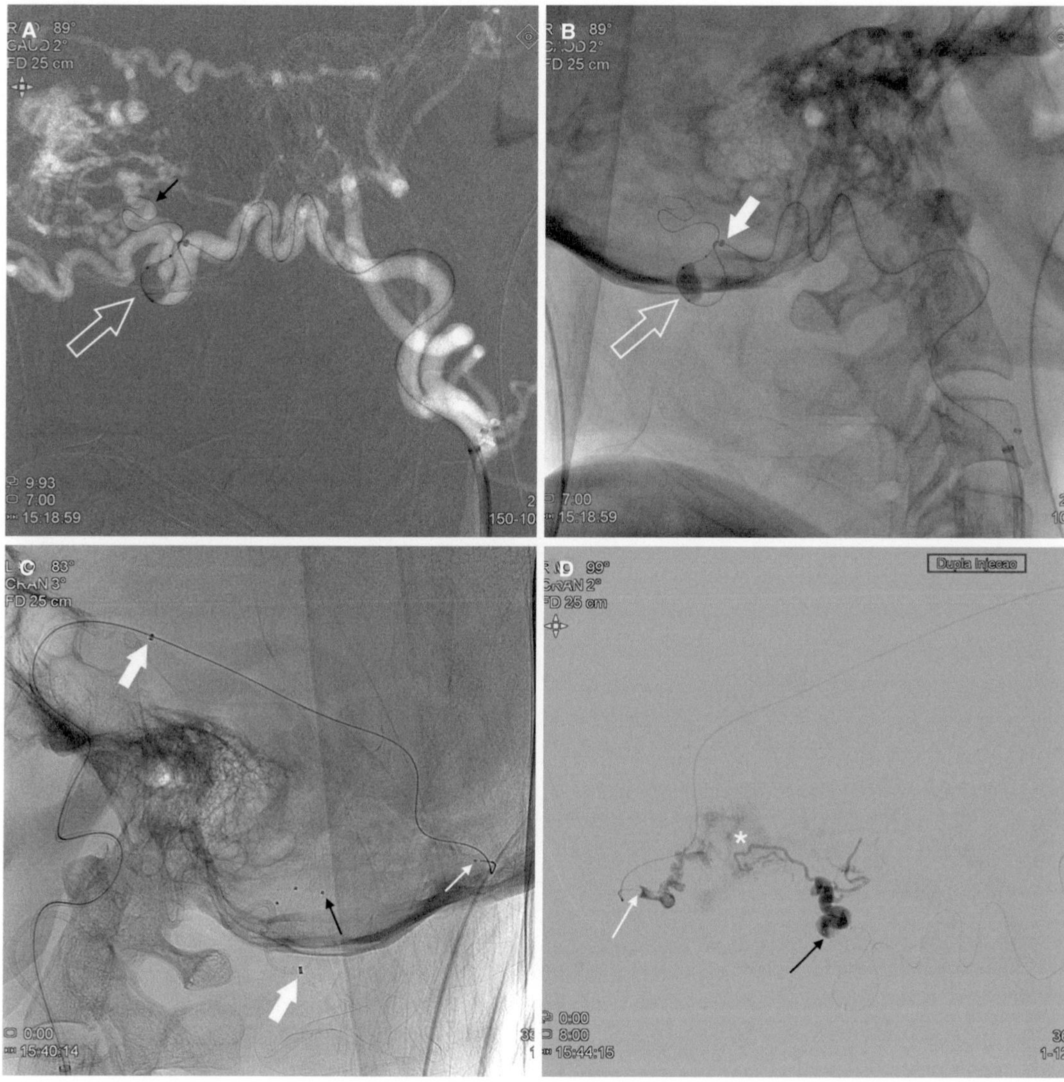

Fig. 11.1 (continued)

c

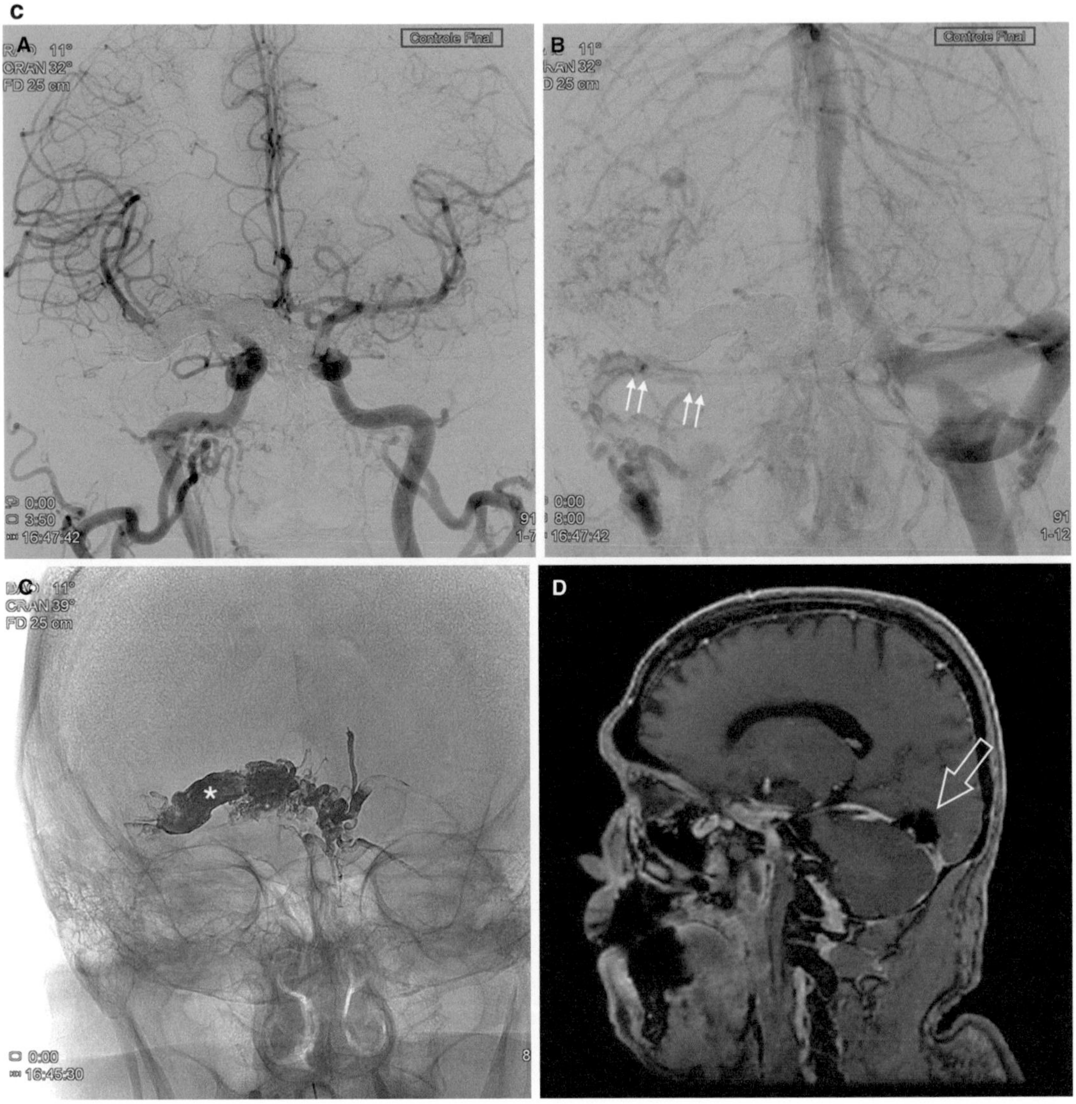

Fig. 11.1 (continued)

occipital artery, which frequently supplies DAVFs, especially at the tentorial region, at the transverse/sigmoid sinuses and torcula, is often very dilated and tortuous, and the control of reflux is difficult due to the great resistance through the transosseous branches [12]. However, with the use of the double-lumen balloon catheter, this artery, which was previously considered a poor access route, can be used with great effectiveness. Ideally, the double-lumen balloon catheter should be positioned inside the mastoid branch; thus, it could prevent both reflux of the embolic agent inside the occipital artery and its distal migration to branches of the scalp [12] (Fig. 11.1c).

The use of two simultaneous arterial accesses, through the middle meningeal artery and occipital artery, should always be considered, since the simple inflation of two balloons promotes a significant reduction in the flow to the fistula, providing better hemodynamic control over the penetration of the embolic agent [12].

Often, during the procedure, spontaneous deflation of the balloon occurs, and depending on the resistance for anterograde migration of the embolic agent, backward movement of the balloon may occur. Thus, the balloon inflation volume must be frequently checked.

The main limiting factor for the use of the double-lumen balloon catheter is anatomical. Very thin and tortuous arteries can prevent navigation to a suitable point for embolization. In these cases, a conventional or detachable tip microcatheter may be preferable [19].

11.6.2 DAVFs Draining to a Dural Sinus

The only balloon on the market dedicated specifically for venous use is the Copernic RC (Balt Extrusion, Montmorency, France). Two sizes are available, 8 × 80 mm and 10 × 80 mm [26–29]. Such balloons are compatible with a 6F guiding catheter. They have only one lumen. Thus, a 0.014 in. guidewire is used for navigation and to occlude the lumen, allowing inflation [19]. Its manufacturer recommends the use of a Transend 14 guidewire (Stryker, Irvine, USA) since other guidewires could allow the leakage of contrast medium from inside the balloon. Contrast medium diluted to 50% should be used. The balloon is DMSO compatible.

The Copernic RC balloon catheter, compared to balloons of the same diameter but dedicated to peripheral angioplasty, has better navigability. It is more flexible and more compliant, conforming better to the sinus wall to seal it.

A careful evaluation should be performed in the preoperative period regarding the patency of the dural sinuses, their diameter and the best access route (ipsilateral jugular or contralateral to the fistula). The direct transjugular route can be an issue if it is necessary to change the side on which the balloon will be navigated.

The balloon is temporarily inflated during the transarterial injection of the embolic agent for a few minutes. A precise maximum time limit for sinus occlusion is not known. However, very prolonged inflations are not recommended [19].

When greater flow of the embolic agent into the dural sinus is desired, the balloon can be deflated intermittently. Attention should be given to the maximum inflation volume to avoid dural venous sinus injury [19]. This type of balloon is not suitable for use inside leptomeningeal veins.

The best scenario occurs when hemodynamic control over the main arterial feeders of the fistula is achieved, as well as over its venous drainage [17]. Therefore, in the case of DAVFs in the wall of a sinus, it would be desirable to position a balloon inside the dural sinus and balloons simultaneously inside the middle meningeal and occipital arteries [15, 19]. In this triple-balloon technique, the progression of the liquid embolic agent is rapid, with a low risk of dural sinus occlusion.

11.7 Results of the Balloon-Assisted Treatment of DAVFs

11.7.1 Transarterial Double-Lumen Balloon Catheter

Before the advent of double-lumen balloon catheters, strategies to control reflux had already been used. Deng et al. reported the treatment of 8 patients with DAVFs using, instead of a double-lumen balloon catheter, single-lumen remodeling balloons in parallel with a microcatheter [13]. Complete occlusion of the fistula was achieved in all cases.

The results of transarterial embolization using the double-lumen balloon catheter are very encouraging. Series with an increasing number of cases have been described [7–10, 14, 15, 18–25].

In a review of the literature, including fistulas with direct leptomeningeal venous drainage and fistulas that drain into the wall of a dural sinus, we gathered a total of 125 DAVFs treated through an arterial approach assisted by a double-lumen balloon catheter (Table 11.1). The most commonly used balloon was Scepter C, followed by Scepter XC. The Ascent balloon was only used in two series.

The most frequent location of DAVFs was in the wall of the transverse/sigmoid sinuses in 57 cases, followed by the superior sagittal sinus [13], tentorial region [12] and other locations. The artery most accessed with the double-lumen

Table 11.1 Summary of major studies reporting the use of transarterial DLBC to treat DAVFs

Author	*n*	Balloon	Location	Access with DLBC	Sessions/patient	Cure rate (%)	Complication
Paramasivam (2012)	7	Scepter XC Ascent	TS (7) Parasagittal (1)	MMA (5) OCC (5)	1.42	71	0%
Jagadeesan (2013)	1	Scepter XC	TS	IMA (2)	1	100	0%
Kim (2013)	1	Scepter C	SSS	MMA (venous[a])	1	100	0%
Spiotta (2014)	1	Scepter C	Convexity	MMA	1	100	0%
Chiu (2014)	6	Scepter C	Convexity (1) SSS (2) TS (2)	MMA (6) (venous balloon[b]—2)	1	100	17% (MMA rupture)
Dabus (2014)	5	Scepter C Ascent	TS (1) Parasagittal (2) Tentorial (2)	OCC (2) (venous[a]—1) MMA (3)	1	100	0%
Clarençon (2016)	2	Scepter XC	TS (2)	OCC (3) MMA (1) STA (1) (Venous balloon[b]—2)	1.5	100	0%
Tao (2016)	1	Scepter C	SSS	MMA	1	100	0%
Kim (2016)	15	Scepter C	TS (6) Cortical (2) Tentorial (3) Sigmoid (3) SSS (1)	MMA (7) OCC (6) STA (1) MHA (3) APA (1)	1	87	7% (Facial palsy)
Piechowiak (2017)	9	Scepter C	TS (6)	MMA (9) (Venous balloon[b]—9)	1	67	0%
Chen (2020)	1	Scepter C	LSW	MMA	1	100	0%
Jang (2021)	35	Scepter	TS (13) Juxta-sinus (13) SPS (5) Torcula (3) LSW (1)	MMA (18) OCC (15) STA (1) APA (1)	1	97	5.7%(Facial palsy) (Cerebral ischemia)
Zamponi (2021)	41	Scepter XC	TS (19) Torcula (8) Tentorial (7) SSS (5) LSW (1) Convexity (1)	OCC (22) MMA (14) MMA + OCC (7) STA (3) APA (1) (Venous balloon[b]—21)	1.14	97.6	12% (Facial palsy—2) (Cerebellar ischemia—1) (Alopecia—1) (Scalp necrosis—1)

APA ascending pharyngeal artery, *DLBC* double lumen balloon catheter, *IMA* internal maxillary artery, *LSW* lesser sphenoid wing, *MHA* meningohypophyseal artery, *MMA* middle meningeal artery, *OCC* occipital artery, *SPS* superior petrosal sinus, *SSS* superior sagittal sinus, *STA* superficial temporal artery, *TS* transverse/sigmoid sinus

[a] Embolization via venous approach

[b] Protective venous balloon associated

balloon catheter was the middle meningeal artery in 74 procedures, followed by the occipital artery in 60 procedures. In 7 cases, simultaneous access was used through the occipital and middle meningeal arteries with two double-lumen balloon catheters.

The number of sessions per patient ranged from 1 to 1.5 (in 76% of the series, a single session per patient was sufficient). Cure rates ranged from 67% to 100%. Of the 125 patients treated, total occlusion was achieved in 116 patients (92.8%).

Complications ranged from 0% to 12%. The series that reported the highest number of complications included minor, transient events [18, 19]. Of the 9 complications reported, the most frequent was facial palsy in 4 cases, followed by cerebral ischemia in 2 cases. Other complications described were alopecia and scalp necrosis. Arterial rupture related to balloon inflation is a rare event, occurring in only 1 case [8].

The only series comparing the use of double-lumen balloon catheters and conventional microcatheters for the treatment of DAVFs via the arterial route, but not randomized, was published by Kim et al. [10]. The balloon group showed complete occlusion of the DAVF in 13 patients and almost complete occlusion in 2 patients. In the microcatheter group, complete occlusion occurred in 5 patients, almost complete occlusion in 5 patients and incomplete occlusion in 4 patients. The balloon group had a shorter mean procedure time, shorter Onyx (Medtronic, Irvine, USA) injection time, and fewer arterial pedicles embolized than the microcatheter group. The complication rate was the same for both groups.

11.7.2 Transvenous "Protection" Balloon Catheter

The use of a transvenous balloon catheter to protect the lumen of the dural sinus in the treatment of DAVFs is relatively recent. In 2014, Jittapiromsak et al. reported 2 cases for the first time, and Ponomarjova et al. reported 4 cases [11, 26]. In these 6 cases, the Copernic RC balloon catheter was used, with complete occlusion of all DAVFs, without complications.

In 11 series reported in the literature, totaling 78 patients, the Copernic RC balloon catheter was used in all, except in one, in which the Hyperglide balloon (Medtronic, Irvine, USA) was used (Table 11.2). The reduced diameter of conventional remodeling balloons is an important limiting factor for their use [3, 7, 8, 11, 15, 18, 19, 26–29].

The balloon catheter was most frequently used to treat DAVFs of the transverse/sigmoid sinuses in 50 cases, followed by the superior sagittal sinus in 9 cases, torcula in 7 cases and marginal sinus in 1 case. The number of sessions per patient ranged from 1 to 2.

Complete occlusion rates ranged from 67% to 100%. In 8 (72.7%) of 11 series, total occlusion was achieved in all cases. In the two largest series in the literature, each including 22 patients treated with transvenous balloons, total occlusion of the fistulous zone was observed in 86% and 100% of cases [19].

The chance of inadvertently occluding the venous sinus is extremely low when a protection balloon is used inside the dural sinus. In 11 series in the literature, only one patient experienced unintentional occlusion of the dural sinus [18]. Volherbst et al. reported 5 (22%) complications, none of which caused a permanent deficit [18]. Two of these complications had venous etiology, including a venous infarction resulting from inadvertent embolization of the vein of Labbé and a hemorrhage secondary to the temporary occlusion of a temporal vein [18]. The intravenous balloon can protect the lumen of the dural sinus; however, it is unable to protect the tributary veins of this sinus. None of the complications reported by Zamponi et al. were related to the presence of a venous balloon [19]. No dural sinus rupture has been reported in the literature.

An arterial double-lumen balloon catheter was associated with a transvenous balloon in 7 of the 11 series. Zamponi et al. used an arterial double-lumen balloon catheter associated with a transvenous balloon catheter in 21 cases [19]. In all cases, complete DAVF occlusion was

Table 11.2 Summary of major studies reporting the use of transvenous "protection" balloon to treat DAVFs

Author	*n*	Balloon	Location	Arterial balloon[a]	Sessions/patient	Sinus occlusion (%)	Cure rate	Complication
Jittapiromsak (2014)	2	Copernic RC	TS (2)	No	1	0	100%	0%
Ponomarjova (2014)	4	Copernic RC	TS (4)	No	1	0	100%	0%
Chiu (2014)	2	Copernic RC	SSS (1) TS (1)	Yes	1	0	100%	50% (MMA rupture)
Zhang (2015)	1	Hyperglide	SSS	No	2	0	100%	100% (Cortical blindness)
Clarençon (2016)	2	Copernic RC	TS (2)	Yes	1.5	0	100%	0%
Ertl (2016)	11	Copernic RC	NM	Yes	1.5	0	71% (General)	0%
Piechowiak (2017)	9	Copernic RC	TS (9)	Yes	1	0	67%	0%
Alturki (2017)	1	Copernic RC	TS	Yes	2	0	100%	0%
Volherbst (2018)	22	Copernic RC	TS (19) SSS (2) Marginal (1)	No	1.1	5	86%	22% (Infarction—2) (Subdural hemorrhage—2) (Intracerebral hemorrhage—1)
Lu (2019)	2	Copernic RC	Torcula (1) TS (1)	Yes	1	0	100%	0%
Zamponi (2021)	22	Copernic RC	TS (11) Torcula (6) SSS (5)	Yes	1.4	0	100%	9% (Alopecia—1) (Scalp necrosis—1)

MMA middle meningeal artery, *NM* not mentioned, *SSS* superior sagittal sinus, *TS* transverse/sigmoid sinus
[a] Embolization through a double lumen balloon associated

observed on control angiography after 6 months. In this same series, 6 of the 18 nonfunctioning dural sinuses that were preserved with the aid of the balloon were shown to be functional on late control angiography (Fig. 11.2a–c). Thus, we believe that the reestablishment of circulation within the nonfunctioning sinus should be a treatment goal.

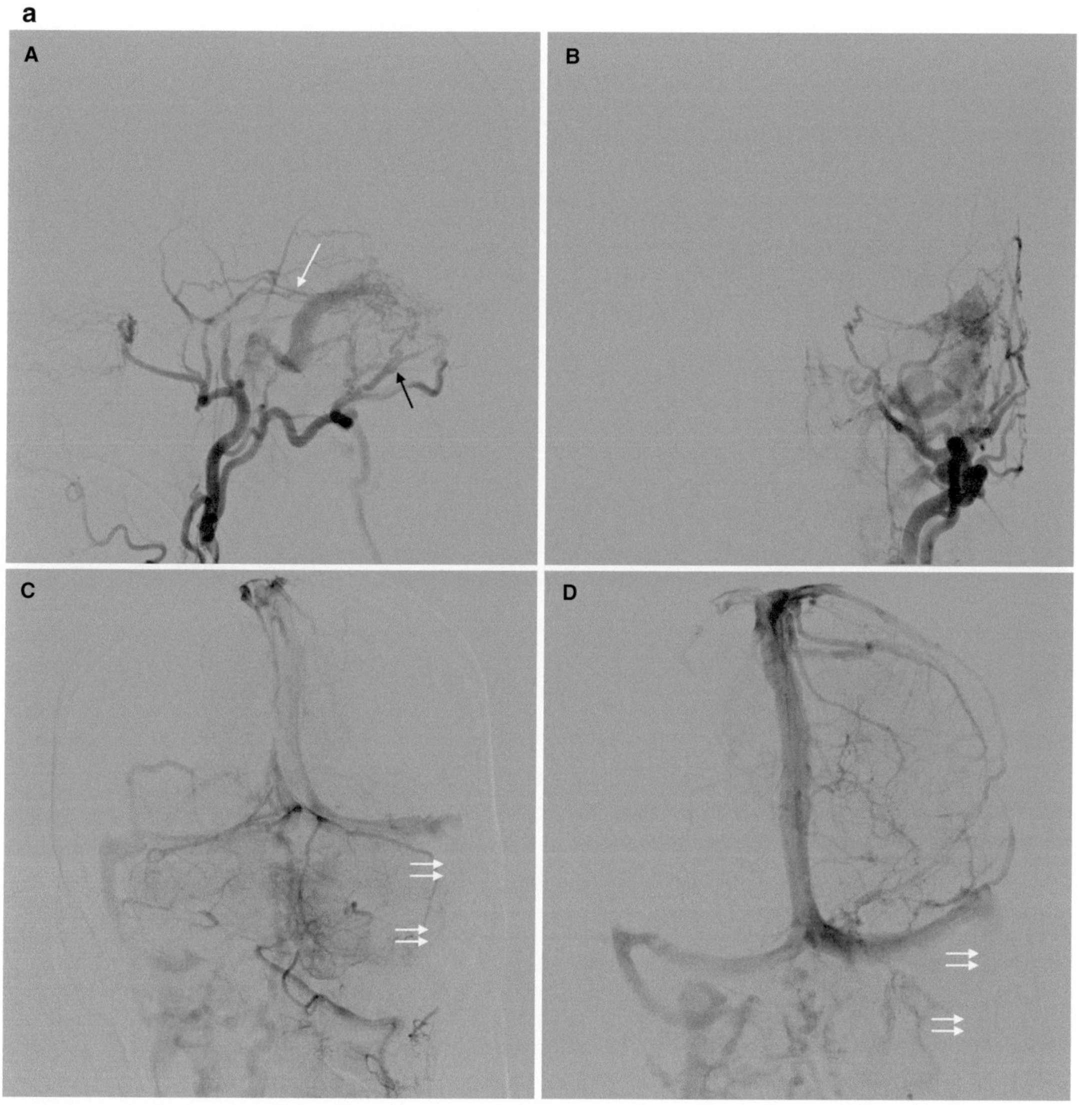

Fig. 11.2 (**a**) (A, B) Angiography (lateral and AP views) shows a transverse/sigmoid sinus DAVF supplied by the occipital artery (black arrow) and the MMA (white arrow). (C, D) Venous phase of the vertebral artery and ICA angiograms demonstrate that the left transverse and sigmoid sinuses are nonfunctioning (double-arrows). (**b**) (A) Fluoroscopy shows the position of the microcatheter (white arrow) inside the petrous branch of the MMA, and the double-lumen balloon catheter (black arrow) inside the mastoid branch of the occipital artery. (B) Note the transvenous balloon catheter is inflated inside the transverse/sigmoid sinuses. (C) Double-injection through the microcatheter and double-lumen balloon catheter demonstrates the fistulous zone. (D) The migration of the embolic agent occurs along the entire sinus wall circumferentially, occluding the fistulous zone. (**c**) (A, B) Control angiography (AP and lateral views) after embolization reveals total occlusion of the DAVF. (C) Note the cast of EVOH along the sinus wall. (D) Venous phase of the ICA control angiogram demonstrates filling of the left transverse and sigmoid sinuses (double-arrows)

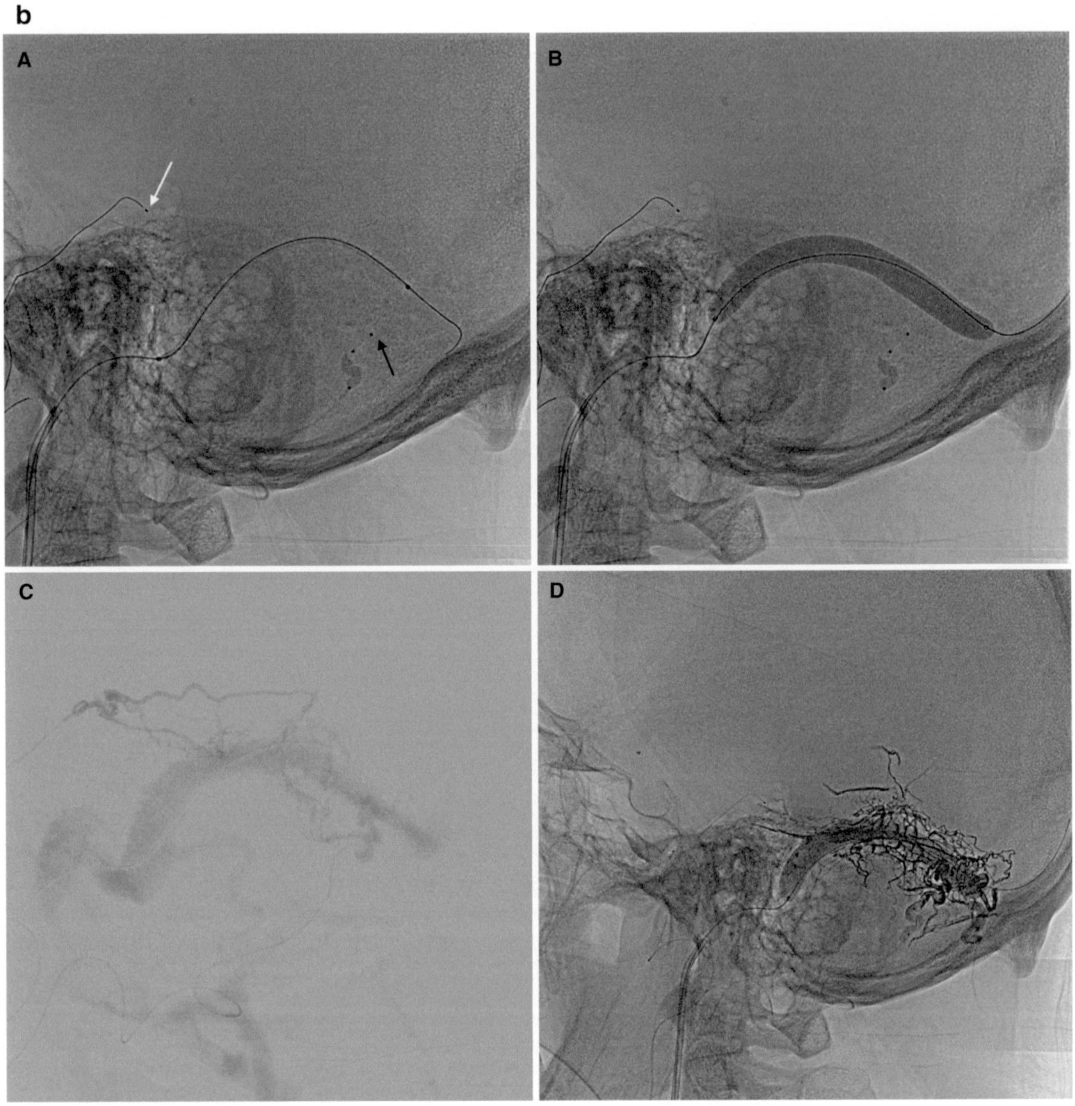

Fig. 11.2 (continued)

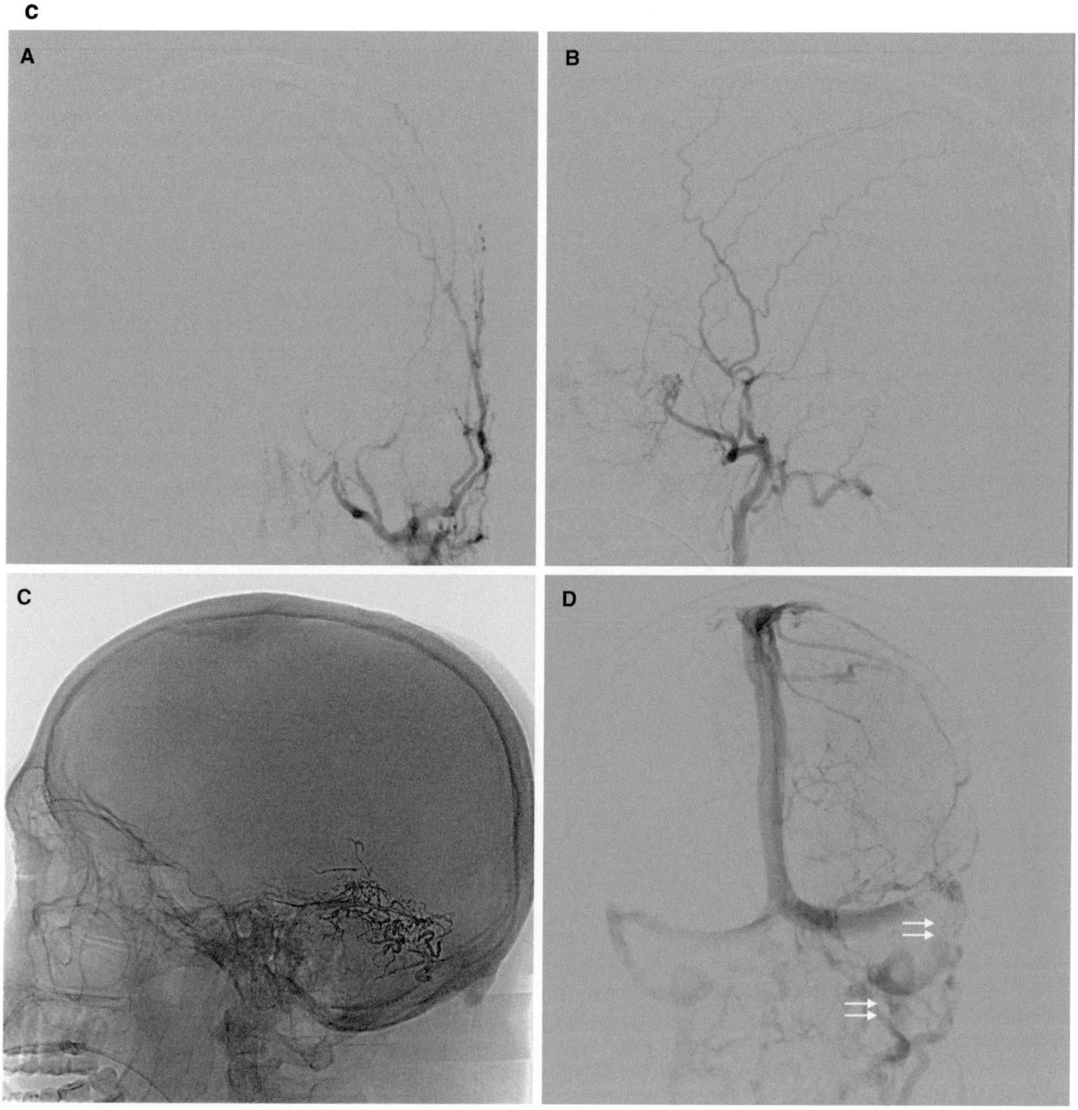

Fig. 11.2 (continued)

11.8 Perspectives

There is no doubt that balloons for flow/pressure control in the treatment of DAVFs will be increasingly used, as well as balloons to protect the venous lumen. The benefit is unquestionable.

Improved flexibility of these balloon catheters and smaller profiles will be imperative, since navigability is still a limiting factor for their use. Attempts already exist, such as the Scepter Mini (Microvention, Tustin, USA).

The use of transvenous balloon catheters is still limited. A wider range of measurements is needed. Improvements in balloon technology will allow selective treatments, preserving the dural sinus lumen.

11.9 Conclusion

Balloon catheters represent an important advance in the management of DAVFs. Transarterial treatment of DAVFs assisted by double-lumen balloon catheters is safe and quite effective. The use of the balloon makes the occipital artery an excellent access route, since the problem of excessive reflux and greater resistance of the transosseous branches is overcome. This route presents results as good as when the middle meningeal artery is used.

The transvenous balloon catheter is also safe and can prevent inadvertent occlusion of the dural venous sinus. Complications related to temporary sinus occlusion are rare.

The association of transvenous and transarterial balloon catheters is very effective, determining high rates of total occlusion of DAVFs. The introduction of two balloons simultaneously, through the middle meningeal artery and the occipital artery, seems to be a very promising approach, since it provides greater control over the flow toward the fistula.

References

1. Cognard C, Gobin YP, Pierot L, et al. Cerebral dural arteriovenous fistulas: clinical and angiographic correlation with a revised classification of venous drainage. Radiology. 1995;164:671–80.
2. Abud TG, Nguyen A, Saint-Maurice JP, et al. The use of Onyx in different types of intracranial dural arteriovenous fistula. AJNR Am J Neuroradiol. 2011;32:2185–91.
3. Ertl L, Brückmann H, Kunz M, et al. Endovascular therapy of low- and intermediate-grade intracranial lateral dural arteriovenous fistulas: a detailed analysis of primary success rates, complication rates, and long-term follow-up of different technical approaches. J Neurosurg. 2017;126:360–7.
4. Rezende MT, Piotin M, Mounayer C, et al. Dural arteriovenous fistulas of the lesser sphenoid wing region treated with Onyx: technical note. Neuroradiology. 2006;48:130–4.
5. Cognard C, Januel AC, Silva NA Jr, et al. Endovascular treatment of intracranial dural arteriovenous fistulas with cortical venous drainage: new management using Onyx. AJNR Am J Neuroradiol. 2008;29:235–41.
6. Lv X, Jiang C, Li Y, et al. The limitations and risks of transarterial Onyx injections in the treatment of grade I and II DAVFs. Eur J Radiol. 2011;80:e385–8.
7. Clarençon F, Di Maria F, Gabrieli J, et al. Double-lumen balloon for Onyx embolization via extracranial arteries in transverse sigmoid dural arteriovenous fistulas: initial experience. Acta Neurochir. 2016;158:1917–23.
8. Chiu AHY, Grace A, Wenderoth JD. Double-lumen arterial balloon technique for Onyx embolization of dural arteriovenous fistulas: initial experience. J Neurointerv Surg. 2014;6:400–3.
9. Dabus G, Linfante I, Galdámez MM. Endovascular treatment of dural arteriovenous fistulas using dual lumen balloon microcatheter: technical aspects and results. Clin Neurol Neurosurg. 2014;117:22–7.
10. Kim JW, Kim BM, Park KY, et al. Onyx embolization for isolated type dural arteriovenous fistulas using a dual-lumen balloon catheter. Neurosurgery. 2016;78:627–36.
11. Jittapiromsak P, Ikka L, Benachour N, et al. Transvenous balloon-assisted transarterial Onyx embolization of transverse-sigmoid dural arteriovenous malformation. Neuroradiology. 2013;55:345–50.
12. Rezende MTS, Trivelato FP, Castro-Afonso LH, et al. Endovascular treatment of tentorial dural arteriovenous fistulas using transarterial approach as a first-line strategy. Oper Neurosurg. 2021;20:484–92.
13. Deng JP, Zhang T, Li J, et al. Treatment of dural arteriovenous fistulas by balloon-assisted transarterial embolization with Onyx. Clin Neurol Neurosurg. 2013;115:1992–7.
14. Paramasivam S, Nimi Y, Fifi J, et al. Onyx embolization using dual-lumen balloon catheter: initial experience and technical note. J Neuroradiol. 2013;40:292–302.
15. Piechowiak E, Zibold F, Dobrocky T, et al. Endovascular treatment of dural arteriovenous fistulas of the transverse and sigmoid sinuses using transarterial balloon-assisted embolization combined with transvenous balloon protection of the venous sinus. AJNR Am J Neuroradiol. 2017;38:1984–9.
16. Chapot R, Stracke P, Velasco A, et al. The pressure cooker technique for the treatment of brain AVMs. J Neuroradiol. 2014;41:87–91.
17. Abud DG, Riva R, Nakiri GS, et al. Treatment of brain arteriovenous malformations by double arterial catheterization with simultaneous injection of Onyx: retrospective series of 117 patients. AJNR Am J Neuroradiol. 2011;32:152–8.
18. Vollherbst DF, Ulfert C, Neuberger U, et al. Endovascular treatment of dural arteriovenous fistulas using transarterial liquid embolization in combination with transvenous balloon-assisted protection of the venous sinus. AJNR Am J Neuroradiol. 2018;39:1296–302.
19. Zamponi JO Jr, Trivelato FP, Rezende MTS, et al. Transarterial treatment of cranial dural arteriovenous fistulas: the role of transarterial and transvenous balloon-assisted embolization. AJNR Am J Neuroradiol. 2020;41:2100–6.
20. Jagadeesan BD, Grigoryan M, Hassan AE, et al. Endovascular balloon-assisted embolization of intracranial and cervical arteriovenous malformations using dual-lumen coaxial balloon microcatheters and Onyx: initial experience. Neurosurgery. 2013;73(ONS Suppl):ons238–43.
21. Kim ST, Jeong HW, Seo J, et al. Onyx embolization of dural arteriovenous fistula, using Scepter C balloon catheter: a case report. Neurointervention. 2013;8:110–4.

22. Spiotta AM, James RF, Lowe SR, et al. Balloon-augmented Onyx embolization of cerebral arteriovenous malformations using a dual-lumen balloon: a multicenter experience. J Neurointerv Surg. 2015;7:721–7.
23. Tao Y, Niu Y, Chen Z, et al. Endovascular treatment of a traumatic dural arteriovenous fistula of the superior sagittal sinus using dual lumen balloon microcatheter. Neuroscience. 2016;21:158–60.
24. Chen S, Ocak PE, Xia Y, et al. Intra-arterial Onyx-18 embolization of a dural arteriovenous fistula of the sphenoparietal sinus using Scepter C balloon microcatheter: case report. Niger J Clin Pract. 2020;23:879–82.
25. Jang CK, Kim BM, Park KY, et al. Scepter dual-lumen balloon catheter for Onyx embolization for dural arteriovenous fistula. BMC Neurol. 2021;21:31.
26. Ponomarjova S, Iosif C, Mendes GAC, et al. Endovascular treatment of transverse-sigmoid sinus type I dural arteriovenous shunts with sinus preservation for patients with intolerable symptoms: four case reports. Clin Neuroradiol. 2015;25:313–6.
27. Zhang Y, Li Q, Huang Q, et al. Embolization of a superior sinus dural arteriovenous fistula under intrasinus balloon protection: a case report. Interv Neuroradiol. 2015;21:94–100.
28. Alturki A, Marulanda AE, Schmalz P, et al. Transarterial Onyx embolization of bilateral transverse-sigmoid dural arteriovenous malformation with transvenous balloon assist—initial US experience with the Copernic RC venous remodeling balloon. World Neurosurg. 2018;109:398–402.
29. Dan L, Chen L, Kang X, et al. The application of Copernic RC balloon in Endovascular treatment of complex intracranial dural arteriovenous fistula of the transverse sigmoid sinus. World Neurosurg. 2019;131:21–6.

Tentorial Dural Arteriovenous Fistulas: Anatomy, Clinical Presentation and Endovascular Treatment

12

Marco Túlio Salles Rezende, Felipe Padovani Trivelato, Alexandre Cordeiro Ulhôa, and Daniel Giansante Abud

Abstract

Tentorial dural arteriovenous fistulas (TDAVFs) located and occur in the (reflected) double dural layer of the tentorium and its attachments. The vast majority have leptomeningeal venous drainage and tend to cause intracranial hemorrhage or progressive neurological deficits. These lesions are often more challenging to treat than DAVFs at other locations and may require multiple treatment sessions and/or combined approaches. Because of their rarity, the number of reports describing TDAVFs and their endovascular management is limited. The introduction of the nonadhesive liquid agent ethylene-vinyl alcohol represents a paradigm shift regarding the endovascular treatment for TDAVFs. Endovascular treatment is a safe and effective therapy for TDAVFs. Transarterial embolization could be used as a primary therapeutic option for most TDAVFs. When a transarterial approach is not possible or does not result in total lesion occlusion, transvenous or combined approaches can be performed, leading to high angiographic occlusion rates.

Keywords

Cerebral angiography · Dural arteriovenous fistula · Embolization · Arteriovenous fistula Tentorium cerebelli

12.1 Introduction

Tentorial dural arteriovenous fistulas (TDAVFs) constitute 4.0–8.4% of all intracranial dural arteriovenous fistulas (DAVFs) [1, 2]. They are deeply located and occur in the (reflected) double dural layer of the tentorium and its attachments [2, 3]. Additionally, most of them are supplied by multiple, small and tortuous arteries [4]. The vast majority have leptomeningeal venous drainage and tend to cause intracranial hemorrhage or progressive neurological deficits [3, 5, 6]. These lesions are often more challenging to treat than DAVFs at other locations and may require multiple treatment sessions and/or combined approaches [3, 6–9]. Because of their rarity, the

M. T. S. Rezende (✉) · F. P. Trivelato · A. C. Ulhôa
Division of Interventional Neuroradiology, Felício Rocho Hospital, Belo Horizonte, Minas Gerais, Brazil

Division of Interventional Neuroradiology, Rede Mater Dei de Saúde, Belo Horizonte, Minas Gerais, Brazil

D. G. Abud
Division of Interventional Neuroradiology, Department of Radiology, Hematology and Oncology, Medical School of Ribeirão Preto, University of São Paulo, Ribeirão Preto, SP, Brazil

X. Lv (ed.), *Intracranial and Spinal Dural Arteriovenous Fistulas*,
https://doi.org/10.1007/978-981-19-5767-3_12

number of reports describing TDAVFs and their endovascular management is limited [3].

The introduction of the nonadhesive liquid agent ethylene-vinyl alcohol represents a paradigm shift regarding the endovascular treatment (EVT) for TDAVFs [9]. In addition to superior clinical results, occlusion rates have also improved, making EVT the current preferred therapeutic option in most cases [9].

In the following chapter, we review anatomical aspects, clinical manifestations and endovascular management of the TDAVFs.

12.2 Epidemiology

A meta-analysis involving 377 patients with DAVFs showed that tentorial fistulas occur less frequently than lesions located in the transverse-sigmoid sinus and cavernous sinus regions (8.4% versus 62.6% and 11.9%, respectively) [1]. Huang et al. [4] treated 122 DAVFs between 2005 and 2008, with 13.1% harboring DAVFs at the tentorial region [4]. Thus, tentorial lesions represent a small portion of all intracranial DAVFs.

Regarding distribution, most TDAVFs are diagnosed in middle-aged men [2, 3]. Men comprise between 61.5% and 91.9% of cases [3, 4].

12.3 Anatomical Considerations

TDAVFs are complex lesions surrounded by critical neurovascular structures located deep in the cranial cavity [7]. According to Zhou et al. [2], they represent a unique subtype of lesion because their fistulous connections are located in the tentorial dura mater and not in the sinus wall. The dura mater of the tentorium and its insertions have two layers [3], and dural arteriovenous fistulas from other topographies involve regions where the dura comprises a single layer.

Despite their proximity to the lateral and sigmoid sinuses, TDAVFs are usually considered separately from fistulas involving these sinuses. This distinction appears to be historical and is based on anatomical, clinical and therapeutic differences [3].

An arteriovenous shunt can occur in any region of the tentorium. In the anteroposterior direction, the tentorial fistulas are distributed from the region of the clinoid processes and petrous apex to the torcula [2, 10]. In the mediolateral direction, they may involve medial locations, such as the free edge of the tentorium, edges of the straight sinus and torcula, or may reach the most lateral portion of the tentorium, adjacent to the lateral sinus [2, 10].

12.4 Vascular Supply

Most TDAVFs are vascularized by several arteries that may come from different vascular axes. Several dural branches emerging from the external carotid artery (e.g., middle meningeal artery), the internal carotid artery (e.g., medial tentorial artery), and the vertebrobasilar system (e.g., posterior meningeal artery) can supply these lesions. Some TDAVFs receive recruitment from pial branches [4, 11].

Lawton et al. found that the arterial supply of TDAVFs can originate from six different sources: (a) tentorial artery; (b) middle meningeal artery; (c) posterior meningeal artery; (d) meningeal branches from the pial arteries; (e) scalp arteries; and (f) miscellaneous branches of the external carotid artery. These results demonstrate that branches of the internal carotid artery, external carotid artery, and vertebrobasilar system may be responsible for irrigating the TDAVFs [7].

Liu et al. (2014) published a series of 26 patients with TDAVFs; all lesions were supplied by multiple vessels [12]. According to Tomak et al., 90.9% of TDAVFs were supplied by more than one artery [6]. Of the 14 TDAVFs treated by Huang et al., only one (7.1%) received a contribution from a single arterial pedicle [4]. Wu et al. found that 35.3% of TDAVFs receive a pial supply [11].

12.5 Venous Drainage

TDAVFs are universally associated with leptomeningeal venous drainage. Most series reporting the results of different treatment modalities for TDAVFs highlighted that 100% of the lesions had direct leptomeningeal venous drainage [2, 6, 8, 13, 14]. However, as described by Iwamuro et al., some TDAVFs do not have direct leptomeningeal venous drainage. This review involved 86 cases and showed that only 5.8% of the lesions drained directly into the venous sinuses, including the superior petrous sinus, straight sinus and transverse sinus. The venous drainage of most (94.2%) of the TDAVFs occurred directly to the leptomeningeal veins from the thrombosed venous sinus. In these cases, the obstruction to the sinusal venous flow precipitated the redirection of venous drainage to the leptomeningeal veins, causing the phenomenon of "arterialization" and development of aneurysms in the involved veins [15].

The TDAVFS that drained into a venous sinus represented 7.1% of the cases in the study of Huang et al. [4], 16.1% in the experience of Picard et al. [10], and 23% in the investigation by Byrne and Garcia [3]. In these studies, even when the TDAVFs presented direct venous drainage into a venous sinus, there was a secondary reflux occurred toward the leptomeningeal veins. In our series, all TDAVFs had direct leptomeningeal venous drainage (Fig. 12.1) [16].

The main drainage pathways for TDAVFs are directly related to the location of the arteriovenous shunt, as described by Picard et al. [10]. Lesions located in the medial part of the tentorium drain primarily into cerebellar cortical veins, and their flow can be directed to the galenic system anteriorly or the torcula and lateral sinuses posteriorly. Some lesions can drain into the spinal venous system. The TDAVFs located in the tentorium notch region drain primarily toward the lateral mesencephalic vein and basal vein of Rosenthal, and their flow can be directed to the supratentorial or infratentorial compartment, even reaching the perimedullary veins. The lateral mesencephalic vein is critical in the drainage of lesions located adjacent to the tentorium notch. It communicates the venous system of the supra- and infratentorial compartments connect-

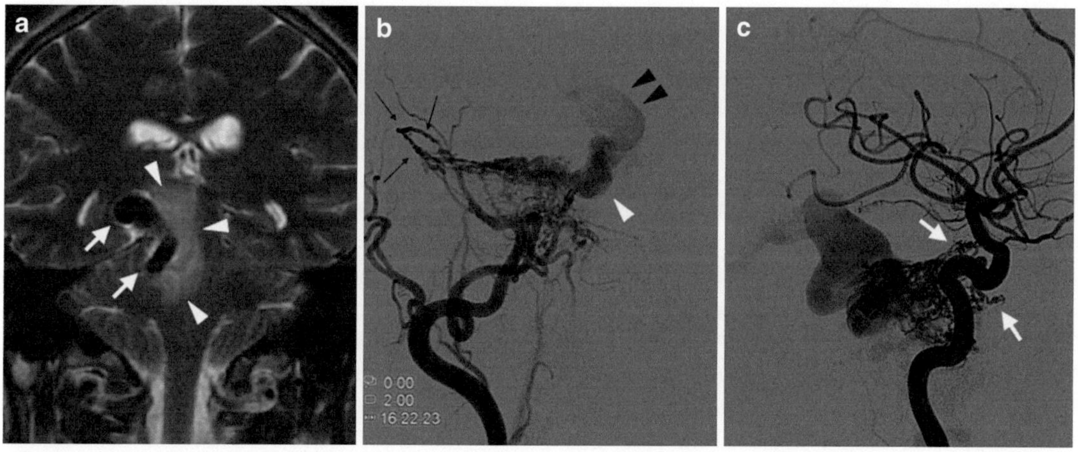

Fig. 12.1 A 32-year-old man with a tentorial dural arteriovenous fistula (TDAVF). (**a**) Coronal magnetic ressonance T2-weighted image of the brain showing a dilated and tortuous flow void signal in the tentorial incisura (white arrows) and brainstem congestion (white arrowheads). (**b**) An anteroposterior view of the right external carotid artery arteriogram showing a marginal TDAVF supplied by the right middle meningeal artery (MMA) (black arrows) draining to the right lateral mesencephalic vein (white arrowhead) presenting venous ectasia (double black arrowheads). (**c**) Lateral view of the right internal carotid arteriogram. Additional supply provided by branches from the right medial tentorial artery (white thick arrows). (**d**) A nondetachable tip microcatheter is navigated in the right MMA. Superselective angiography showing the microcatheter tip in the wedge position (white arrowhead), tortuous and thin distal MMA branches (black arrows) and the level of the spinosum foramen (black arrowhead). (**e**) Lateral unsubtracted image showing the Onyx cast, reflux along the MMA (double white arrows), anterograde progression just to the fistulous connection (black arrowheads) and filling of the proximal portion of the draining vein (white arrowheads). (**f**) Postembolization right external carotid artery arteriogram, anteroposterior view, demonstrating the TDAVF total occlusion

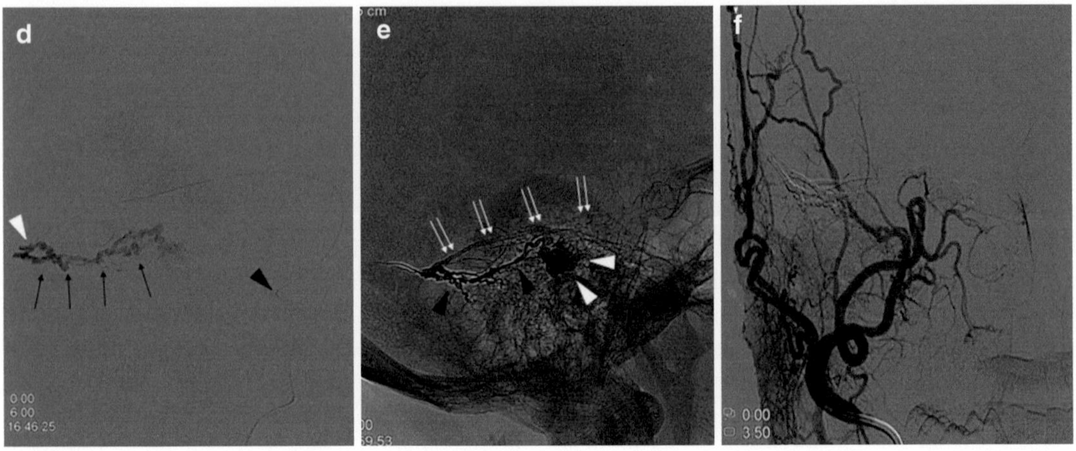

Fig. 12.1 (continued)

ing Rosenthal's basal vein to the petrosal system. According to Cannizzaro et al., the lateral mesencephalic vein is involved in the venous drainage of 31% of TDAVFs [9]. Lesions located in the most lateral portion of the tentorium drain into the cortical veins from the inferolateral surface of the temporal and occipital lobes.

12.6 Clinical Presentation

Several angioarchitectural features of TDAFVs have been linked to the development of aggressive clinical behavior. Among them, are leptomeningeal venous drainage, the formation of venous varices and deep drainage toward the galenic system [1–10].

Because of the effects of venous hypertension, a strong tendency exists for patients to present with intracranial hemorrhage or progressive neurological deficits. Awad et al. reported that TDAVFs have more aggressive neurological behavior than DAVFs in other locations, causing hemorrhage or progressive neurological deficits in 97% of cases [1]. The results of other studies revealed that between 79% and 92% of patients have TDAVFs that determine aggressive neurological behavior and that 38–74% of cases have hemorrhagic presentation [2].

An increasing number of TDAVFs have been diagnosed and treated before their rupture. Several factors can justify this phenomenon, such as the high availability of noninvasive imaging tests and the recognition of venous hypertension as a prominent cause of neurological morbidity. In recent decades, the proportion of patients with TDAVFs with hemorrhagic presentation has dropped from 64.4% (1980–1995) to 43.6% (2006–2014) [9]. In our series, 17 (37.8%) patients reported intracranial hemorrhage [16]. All the patients had received treatment between 2005 and 2019, a period practically similar to the second part of the meta-analysis published by Cannizzaro et al. [9]. A diagnosis before the hemorrhagic manifestation and the subsequent treatment of fistulas are certainly factors that have contributed to the better clinical results obtained in recent decades.

However, the diagnosis of asymptomatic lesions remains infrequent. None of the 19 patients reported by Jiang et al. were asymptomatic, and most (78.9%) exhibited hemorrhage [17]. In the experience of Huang et al., all 14 patients were symptomatic, and 85.7% had intracranial hemorrhage [4]. Even in studies whose hemorrhagic presentation rates were lower, the percentage of asymptomatic patients remained very low. Lawton et al. published the largest series in the literature on the microsurgical treatment of TDAVFs, with 31 patients. Although the bleeding rate found was relatively lower (55%) than that in previous reports, only two (6%) patients were asymptomatic [7].

Our experience encompasses contemporary results. Only three patients were asymptomatic (6.7%), indicating that most TDAVFs continue to be diagnosed when symptomatic [16]. These data confirm that the universal presence of leptomeningeal venous drainage, emphasized by many authors and found in 100% of our patients, determines symptomatic venous hypertension in most patients.

Neurological manifestations resulting from venous hypertension without associated hemorrhage were found in 55.5% (25) of our patients (Fig. 12.2) [16].

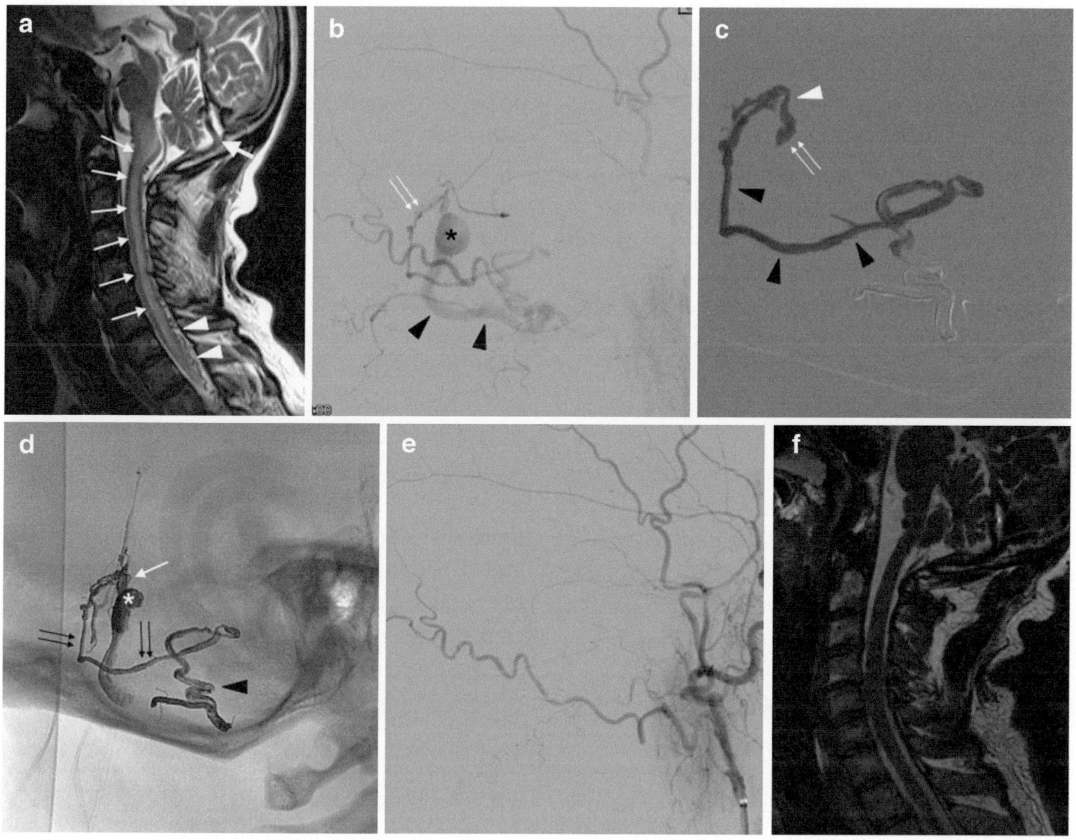

Fig. 12.2 A 64-year-old man presenting cervical pain, dysphagia and tetraparesis. (**a**) Sagittal MRI T2-weighted image of the cranio-cervical junction showing a midline retro cerebellar dilated flow void signal (white thick arrow), medullary and cervical spinal cord patchy edema (white arrowheads) and vessel flow voids dorsally to the spinal cord (double white arrowheads). (**b**) Lateral view of the right external carotid artery angiogram, late arterial phase, demonstrating a medial type TDAVF supplied solely by the dural branch of the mastoid artery (double white arrows) draining to the ectasia (black asterisk) right inferior vermian vein (black arrowheads). (**c**) TAA using the DTM in the OCC mastoid branch. Onyx anterograde progression along the mastoid branch (black arrowheads), penetration into proximal portion of the drainage vein (white arrowhead) and at the venous ectasia (double white arrows). (**d**) Lateral unsubtracted image showing the Onyx cast filling the OCC mastoid branch (black arrowhead), the distal mastoid dural branch (double black arrows), the proximal aspect of the drainage vein (white arrows), and the venous ectasia (white asterisk). (**e**) Postembolization right external carotid artery arteriogram, lateral view demonstrating the TDAVF total occlusion. (**f**) Postoperative sagittal MRI T2-weighted image of the cranio-cervical junction showing resolution of the spinal cord congestion and flow voids disappearance

12.7 Classification

Picard et al. proposed a classification system for DAVFs located exclusively in the tentorium [10]. The tributary veins of the tentorial surface were divided into three regions and the TDAVFs were categorized as follows:

(a) Marginal type: fistulas located along the free edge of the tentorium. They have venous drainage through the basilar and lateral mesencephalic veins. Consequently, they may present drainage into infra- or supratentorial leptomeningeal veins or medullary veins. In rare cases, these fistulas can drain into the cavernous sinus and superior ophthalmic vein.
(b) Lateral type: the lesions are located adjacent to the lateral sinus and receive supratentorial venous drainage through veins on the lateral and inferior surface of the temporal and occipital lobes.
(c) Medial type: fistulas are located adjacent to the torcula and straight sinus. Its venous drainage is infratentorial, coming from veins on the surface of the vermis or cerebellar hemispheres. They drain secondarily into the torcula, lateral sinus or straight sinus.

Anatomical grouping facilitated the radiological identification of the TDAVFs by predicting the venous drainage patterns they might develop. Picard's classification has been the most used by most authors.

To create an algorithm for choosing the best neurosurgical access, Lawton et al. developed a classification system for TDAVFs. Lesions were categorized into six types according to their anatomical location, dural implantation base, involved venous sinus, and direction of venous drainage [7].

Galenic DAVFs (type 1) are located in the midline, on the posterior margin of the tentorial incisura, associated with the vein of Galen as it enters the anterior falcotentorial junction, and their venous drainage can be supratentorial, infratentorial or in both directions. Straight sinus DAVFs (type 2) are located in the midline, along the falcotentorial junction, associated with the straight sinus, with drainage into veins on the inferior surface of the tentorium. Torcular DAVFs (type 3) are located in the midline at the posterior margin of the falcotentorial junction, associated with the torcula and supratentorial venous drainage. Tentorial DAVFs (type 4) are located in the tentorium body, are associated with the tentorial sinus and drain into the occipital (supratentorial) veins. Superior petrosal sinus DAVFs (type 5) are located laterally where the tentorium connects to the middle fossa dura mater and are related to the superior petrosal sinus, draining infratentorially to the petrous vein and its tributaries. Type 6 lesions are called incisural DAVFs. They are located along the free edge of the tentorium, without clear association with a venous sinus, draining into supratentorial veins within and around the cisterna ambiens.

In 2013, Byrne and Garcia proposed a classification system for TDAVFs based on the location of arteriovenous communication [3]. The lesions were divided into two types: (a) dural arteriovenous fistulas in the midline region that could be located in the torcula or falx of the cerebellum and (b) lateral petrotentorial arteriovenous fistulas arranged along the implantation of the tentorium in the petrous bone. The venous drainage patterns found by the authors were similar to the system proposed by Picard et al. [10].

12.8 Treatment

Several therapeutic modalities have been proposed for TDAVFs, such as ligation of the feeding arteries, surgical excision of the fistula, interruption of draining veins, arterial and/or venous embolization, and radiosurgery. Available options can be performed in isolation or in various combinations [6]. However, much debate exists concerning the best treatment option.

Endovascular treatment has become the predominant therapeutic option for most DAVFs because the arterial supply from the external carotid artery can be safely embolized. Additionally, its location on the walls of the dural venous sinuses facilitates its venous access and occlusion. The combination of arterial and venous embolization results in high obliteration rates for most types of DAVFs. However, according to Lawton et al., lesions located in the tentorial region represent an exception [7].

Tentorial dural arteriovenous fistulas have a complex arterial supply. In addition to branches of the external carotid artery, multiple vessels participate in its supply, such as meningeal branches from the internal carotid artery and vertebrobasilar system [7]. These arteries, in addition to being challenging to microcatheterize, are at greater risk when embolized compared with branches originating from the external carotid artery. Because most tentorial dural arteriovenous fistulas drain exclusively into the leptomeningeal veins, venous access has limitations. Microcatheterization of the venous system located deep around the tentorium is challenging [2, 4, 7]. Thus, treatment of TDAVFs may require microsurgery, unlike most other types of DAVFs.

12.8.1 Microsurgical Treatment

Based on the existing concepts that EVT can rarely cure TDAVFs, several authors have defended microsurgery over the last decades as the treatment of choice for these lesions [2, 7, 18, 19].

In 2003, Tomak et al. reported a series of 22 patients with TDAVFs, all Borden type III lesions undergoing endovascular and/or surgical treatment, over a 12-year period. In the early part of the study (1988–1995), the surgical technique used involved disconnecting the arterial supply and draining vein associated with nidal resection. The microsurgical strategy was modified in the most recent period (1995–2000), with only the disconnection of the drainage vein performed without nidal resection. The authors consider that disconnection of the arterial supply and excision of the nidus may be associated with high rates of morbidity and mortality, deeming the procedure unnecessary [6].

More recent publications have shown different types of complications related to microsurgery. Gross and Du described the results of the microsurgical treatment of 14 TDAVFs whose technique used was the simple interruption of the drainage vein. The overall rate of neurological complications was 35.7%. In three cases, transient neurological deficits (cranial nerve palsy or hemiparesis) occurred and one patient developed permanent hemiparesis. One death due to massive intraoperative cerebral edema occurred [20].

Sugiyama et al. published a series of 39 patients with DAVFs who had undergone microsurgical treatment. Ten cases had tentorial lesions. Compared with lesions from other topographies, TDAVFs had higher rates of complications (17.2%; 95% CI 9.7–24.6%) and subtotal angiographic occlusion (8.1%; 95% CI 2.7–13.4%). Cerebral edema after surgery or excessive intraoperative blood loss were the most frequent complications [21].

Although many authors advocate microsurgery as a first-line treatment for TDAVFs, neurological complication rates are considerable [9]. Endovascular treatment, which is less invasive, could become the preferred method if its angiographic occlusion rates are satisfactory [16].

12.8.2 Endovascular Treatment

12.8.2.1 Transvenous Approach

The endovascular treatment of DAVFs using a venous approach has been an efficient option to manage lesions that present direct venous drainage into a dural sinus. In these cases, when the venous sinus is considered excluded from the venous drainage of the supra and infratentorial compartments, it can be occluded.

Most TDAVFs drain exclusively into the leptomeningeal veins. This angioarchitectural characteristic determines that venous access to the fistulous connection point is performed along very dilated, tortuous and thin veins. Venous embolization must be performed to occlude only the portion of the vein immediately adjacent to the fistula, preserving functional venous drainage. The most proximal portion of the drainage vein should be the target of the endovascular occlusion.

Few reports have investigated ETV of TDAVFs using the transvenous approach. The first case was described in 1997 by Kallmes et al. The lesion was occluded with platinum microcoils [22]. In 1999, Deasey et al. described the results of EVT of two TDAVFs using venous access. Lesions drained directly into a venous sinus, an uncommon fact, and were accessed through the internal jugular vein and straight sinus [23]. Tomak et al. reported the results of the transvenous EVT of five TDAVFs. One patient died from ischemia in the posterior fossa after the injection of *n*-BCA into the petrous vein [6]. Jiang et al. used venous access as a complement to arterial access to treat two TDAVFs. One patient died because of venous rupture during EVOH injection [17]. Wanjberg et al. treated eight patients with TDAVFs. In three of them (37.5%), transvenous access was performed. Two patients were treated exclusively using the venous approach, and one was subjected to combined treatment [14].

Huang et al. advised against transvenous embolization of TDAVFs because of the complex anatomy of the involved veins. Because venous varices often have thin walls, a risk of vascular perforation exists. Additionally, partial or distal occlusion of the draining veins can result in redirection of blood flow to the cortical veins, with a risk of venous hypertension or secondary hemorrhage [4].

Therefore, several authors, including Kallmes et al., do not propose transvenous embolization alone as the primary therapy for most TDAVFs. Instead, this approach should be used in combination with or as an alternative to arterial embolization, microsurgery, or radiosurgery [22].

12.8.2.2 Transarterial Approach

Since the first description of DAVF therapeutic embolization, at the beginning of the 1970s [24], several embolizing agents, such as particles [25], liquid silicone [26], cyanoacrylates [27], and EVOH [28] have been used.

Polyvinyl alcohol (PVA) particles were used for preoperative embolization in several microsurgical series of TDAVFs, decreasing their vascularization [2, 7]. However, the occlusion of a TDAVF after isolated PVA injection is uncommon [6].

Tomak et al. treated 11 patients harboring TDAVFs using the transarterial approach (TAA) with glue injection and reported 45% total angiographic occlusion. The TAA with *n*-BCA injection led to an increase in the rates of angiographic occlusion in the EVT of TDAVFs. However, less than half of the patients were cured alone using this strategy. Many cases still required complementary microsurgical treatment during the cyanoacrylate era [6].

The shift from polyvinyl alcohol particles to adhesive liquid agents has slightly improved the occlusion rates [6], but the introduction of ethylene-vinyl alcohol has offered a new perspective.

The first cases of TDAVFs treated using EVOH were described from 2006 onward, and the angiographic occlusion rates proved to be encouraging [29]. Huang et al., using only EVOH injection, obtained 85.7% angiographic occlusion in 14 TDAVFs [4]. Onyx injection through the posterior branch of the MMA has become the first therapeutic option for most TDAVFs [3, 4, 8, 9, 11–14, 17].

12.8.3 Endovascular Treatment Results

The use of EVOH has resulted in a substantial increase in angiographic occlusion rates and has caused changes in treatment strategies for TDAVFs. The proportion of patients treated with microsurgery alone decreased from 38.7% (period 1980–1995) to 20.4% (period 2006–2014). During the same period, the proportion of patients treated using the endovascular route alone has increased from 16.1% to 48.0%. Cannizzaro et al. observed a sustained deviation from the therapeutic option that occurred in the last two decades [9].

The endovascular approach has become the preferred technique to treat TADVFs. In most series, even during the Onyx era, occlusion rates with exclusive EVT rarely exceed 80% [3, 4, 8, 9, 11–13, 17]. In a review of 72 TDAVFs subjected to EVT, 86.1% were occluded at the end of the procedure, but patients who required combined surgery were excluded from the analysis [30].

In 2021, we published the largest series reporting the results for patients with TDAVFs who were treated using an endovascular approach and the TAA as a first-line strategy. An isolated TAA was sufficient to occlude 39 (86.7%) TDAVFs (Fig. 12.3). Some factors contributed to the high rate of total occlusion obtained using the TAA.

12.8.4 Importance of the Preferential Use of the Middle Meningeal Artery

The choice of the middle meningeal artery as the preferred access was a determining factor for the high rate of occlusion obtained in several series [3, 4, 8, 9, 11–14, 17]. This artery has unique characteristics, and even when it does not represent the major vascular supply to the TDAVF, it is recognized as a favorable conduit for EVOH injection.

The MMA is the largest meningeal branch and, consequently, participates in the vascular supply of most DAVFs. Because of the hemody-

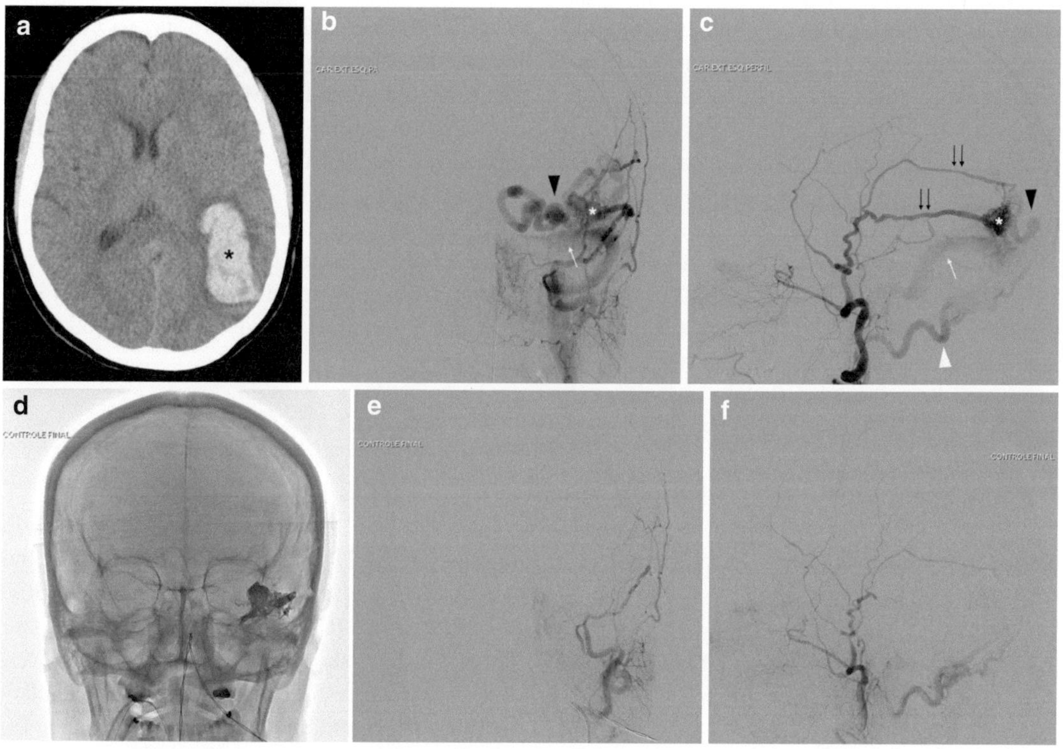

Fig. 12.3 Hemorrhagic presentation. (**a**) Axial cranial computed tomography revealing intraparenchymal hemorrhage (black asterisk). (**b**) An anteroposterior (AP) and (**c**) lateral view of the left external carotid artery arteriogram showing a lateral TDAVF (white asterisk) supplied by the left middle meningeal artery (MMA) (double black arrows) and the left occipital artery (white arrowhead) draining to the left occiptobasal vein (white arrowhead) presenting venous ectasia (black arrowhead) and the ipsilateral lateral sinus (white arrow). (**d**) AP unsubtracted image showing the Onyx cast after isolated left MMA embolization. (**e**) Postembolization left external carotid artery arteriogram, AP view and (**f**) lateral view demonstrating the TDAVF total occlusion

namic stress caused by the arteriovenous shunt, the MMA often becomes larger than normal [31]. The posterior branch of the middle meningeal artery supplies most TDAVFs and provides direct access to its collecting venous system [9]. Puffer et al. reported that the posterior branch of the MMA has a relatively straight course and is dilated in most TDAVFs [13]. These features allow for selective distal catheterization adjacent to the point of fistulous connection. The distal positioning of the microcatheter, almost always in a wedged position, allows the progression of the EVOH, limiting the amount of reflux.

Even when the MMA has a smaller caliber than other pedicles, it should be chosen as the first option for EVOH injection. The main justification for this option is based on anatomical grounds. The MMA and its branches have a relatively straight course along their dural implantation, making their microcatheterization easier relative to the other branches. The extent of reflux does not determine high risks, such as those existing for arteries located in the subdural space. Even in the presence of extensive reflux, the microcatheter can be safely removed because the MMA has a dural anchor. When difficulty exists in removing the microcatheter, the chances of arterial rupture are still much lower when this meningeal branch is chosen. The risks of occlusion of the normal vessels due to reflux are also much lower. The preference to access the TDAVFs by the MMA (66.7%) was one factor that contributed to the high rate of total occlusion obtained in our series [16].

12.8.5 Middle Meningeal Artery Limitations

The middle meningeal artery has unique characteristics, even when it is not the major supplier for the fistula, it is recognized as a favorable conduit [3, 9, 13, 17]. In most series, the MMA was the preferred and most accessed artery [3, 13, 17, 32].

However, there are some limitations in the use of the MMA. First, there is a risk of complications such as microcatheter retention or cranial nerve palsy due to excessive reflux of Onyx [4, 13, 17, 32]. Additionally, in some cases, the injection must be stopped even if occlusion of the fistula has not occurred. In recent years, new tools, such as detachable tip microcatheters (DTMs) and double-lumen balloons (DLBs), have been used for the EVT of TDAVFs [8, 32, 33]. DTMs can be retrieved, even after prolonged injections in distal branch pedicles, often with significant reflux [32, 33]. The use of DTMs can reduce the risks of microcatheter retention, allowing longer and controlled Onyx injections. The rationale for using DLBs is to block reflux and to favor the anterograde migration of Onyx [8, 34], but the size of the MMA should allow a DLB to be insufflated beyond the level of the spinosum foramen.

Second, many TDAVFs are not vascularized by the MMA. In our experience, most fistulas were supplied by the MMA (39/86.7%) [16]. However, according to some authors, its contribution to the TDAVF supply may vary from 33.3% to 88.8% [3, 4, 7, 8, 13].

Third, some anatomical factors, such as the absence of a “sizable” MMA [13] or an exclusive supply from an excessively tortuous artery [4, 8, 13, 17], sometimes make MMA embolization challenging.

12.8.6 Use of an Alternative Arterial Access

Because some TDAVFs are not nourished by the MMA [3, 7, 8], other arterial feeders, such as the occipital artery (OCC) and posterior meningeal artery (PMA), should be considered. However, due to their excessive tortuosity, distal catheterization can be complicated or even impossible [8, 13]. The OCC is surrounded by loose connective tissue and may be very tortuous and dilated, particularly when it accommodates high flow [8]. Although the intracranial segment of the PMA demonstrates a relatively straight configuration, its extracranial portion is tortuous, likely to accommodate the motility of the neck [35].

In our series, all TDAVFs were supplied by at least one of these arteries: the MMA, OCC or

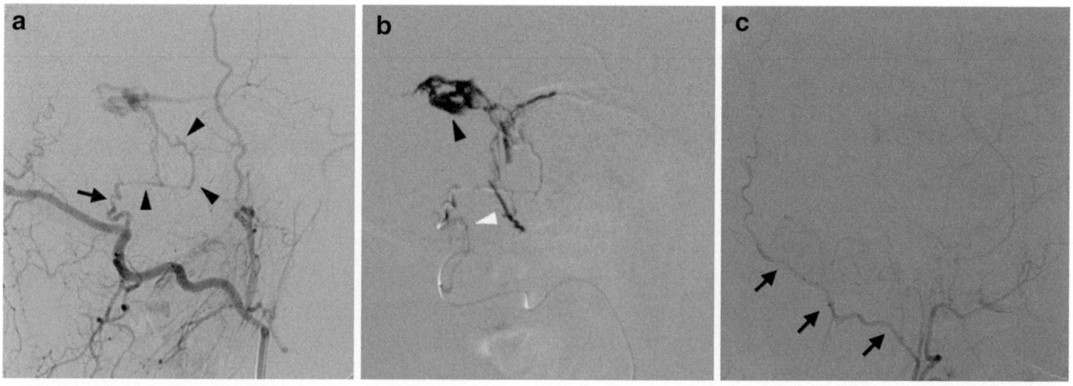

Fig. 12.4 TAA Onyx injection using DLB. (**a**) Lateral right occipital artery selective angiogram demonstrating a tentorial TDAVF supplied solely by dural feeders (black arrowheads) from the OCC mastoid branch (black arrow). (**b**) Tip of the DLB into the mastoid branch (white arrowhead) and anterograde Onyx progression just to the fistulous point and to the "foot" of the drainage vein (black arrowhead). (**c**) Postoperative lateral right OCC angiogram showing total obliteration of the TDAVF and the OCC patency (black arrows)

PMA [16]. Consequently, in all patients, one of them could be catheterized. Nine (20%) TDAVFs were treated by exclusive OCC embolization (Fig. 12.4), and the PMA was accessed in four patients (Fig. 12.5). In our experience, when necessary, with the aid of a distal flexible intracranial catheter, positioning the microcatheter or DLB tip inside the OCC mastoid branch or catheterizing the PMA is possible [16, 34]. The introduction of DTMs and DLBs is another factor that has further facilitated TAA execution in arteries other than the MMA [8, 32–34].

12.8.7 Transvenous and Combined Approaches

A reduced arterial size or excessive tortuosity sometimes make the TAA challenging [4, 8, 13]. These limitations explain why in most EVT series, even in the Onyx era, some TDAVFs are not occluded or treated using the arterial route. The rate of using the TAA in the EVT series varies from 75% to 100% [4, 8, 13, 17, 30]. Puffer et al. obtained 67% of total angiographic occlusion using an isolated TAA with Onyx [13]. Huang et al. described a series of 14 patients harboring TDAVFs treated by transarterial Onyx injection with a 85.7% total angiographic occlusion. They considered the TVA too risky and did not use it for their patients [4]. Until 2020, no series of exclusive TAAs could achieve more than 90% angiographic occlusion [3, 4, 8, 12–14, 17].

Despite some successful outcomes [6, 13, 17, 22, 23], the TVA has been avoided because microcatheter navigation along tortuous, dilated, and potentially fragile leptomeningeal veins is considered challenging and risky [4, 6, 17]. However, to achieve higher occlusion rates solely with EVT, in our opinion, the domain of venous access is fundamental. Wanjberg et al. reported that eight TDAVFs were completely occluded after exclusive EVT. Five patients were treated using the TAA with Onyx injection. Two patients were treated using the TVA, and another was treated with combined endovascular access [14].

Isolated transvenous or combined approaches were performed in four (8.8%) patients in our experience, and all controlled TDAVFs presented with occlusion at the 6-month follow-up. Two TDAVFs were treated by TVA as the primary intention because their arterial supply was judged as inaccessible. Incomplete angiographic occlusion after the TAA occurred in two patients, and both required the TVA. Depending on the leptomeningeal vein involved, the positioning of a hyperflexible distal intracranial catheter into the straight or lateral sinus was crucial to provide support for microcatheter navigation just to the

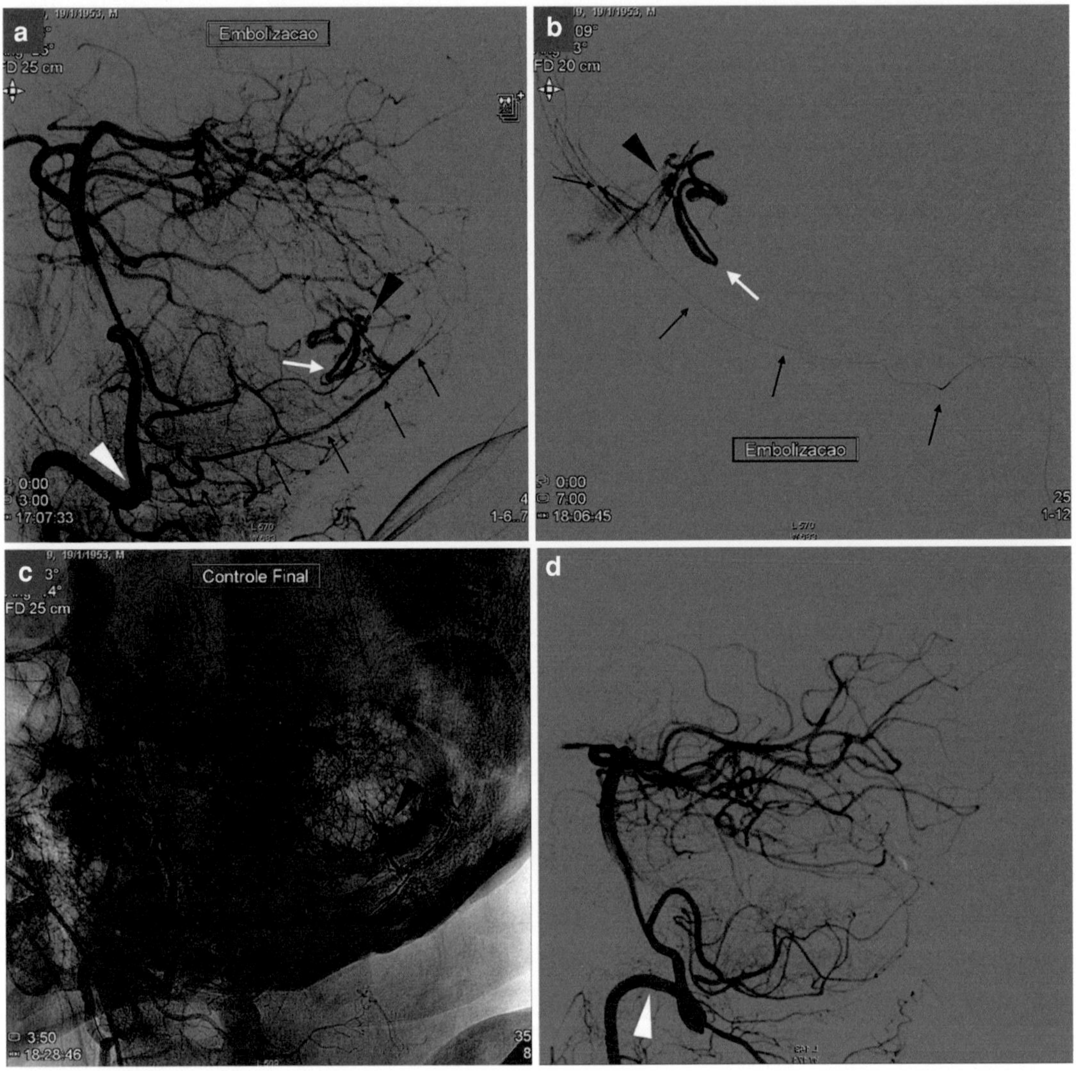

Fig. 12.5 TDAVF supplied by the posterior meningeal artery. (**a**) Oblique left vertebral artery (white arrowhead) selective angiogram demonstrating a medial type tentorial TDAVF (black arrowhead) supplied solely by the posterior meningeal artery (black arrows) draining to the declival vein (white arrow). (**b**) A nondetachable tip microcatheter is navigated in the left PMA (black arrows). Superselective angiography showing the microcatheter tip in the wedge position, the fistulous point (black arrowhead) and the tortuous drainage vein (white arrow). (**c**) Oblique unsubtracted image showing the Onyx cast filling the PMA (black arrows), the fistulous connection (black arrowhead) and the proximal aspect of the drainage vein. (**d**) Postoperative oblique left vertebral angiogram showing total obliteration of the TDAVF and the PMA patency (white arrowhead)

"foot of the vein." We consider that the TVA is a feasible alternative access to treat TDAVFs and should be reserved for situations when arterial access is not possible or insufficient to completely occlude the TDAVF [16].

Only one patient was not treated by an exclusive endovascular approach in our experience. In this patient, a very tortuous MMA originated from the ophthalmic artery (Fig. 12.6). There was no other supply to the TDAVF, and the drainage vein was very dilated and tortuous. Temporal craniectomy followed by direct MMA puncture and Onyx embolization was performed [16]. According to some authors, combined surgical-

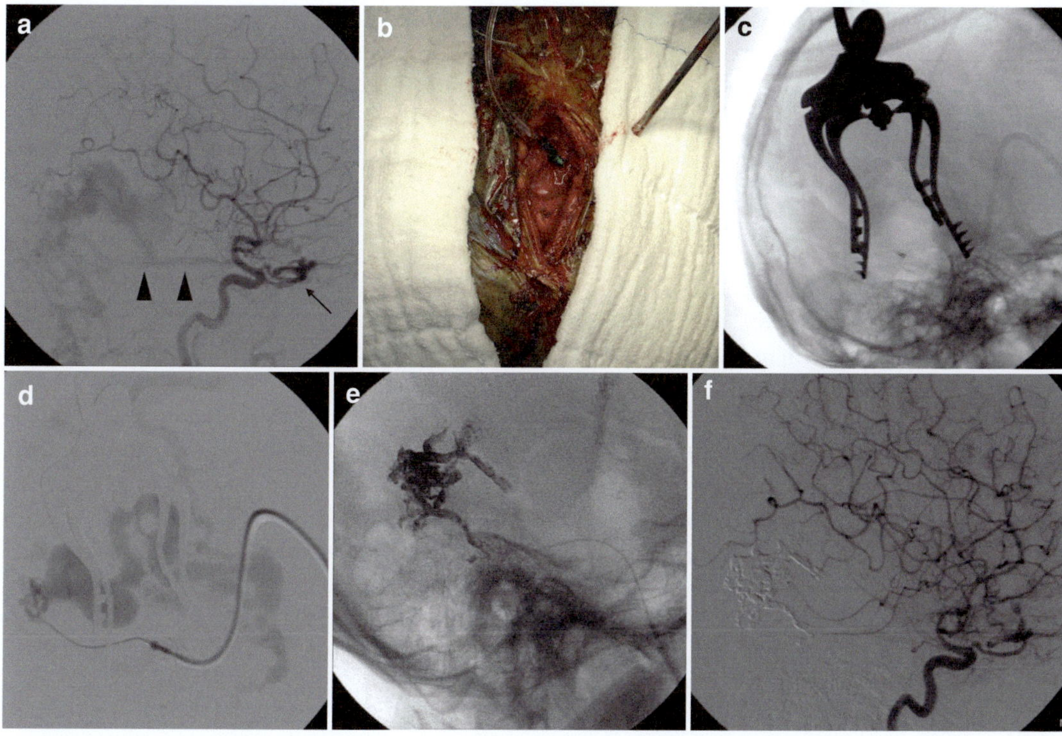

Fig. 12.6 Combined surgical-endovascular approach. (**a**) Oblique right internal carotid artery selective angiogram demonstrating a lateral type tentorial TDAVF supplied solely by the middle meningeal artery (black arrowheads) originating from the ophthalmic artery (black arrows). (**b**) MMA direct puncture. (**c**) Oblique unsubtracted image showing the craniectomy and percutaneous MMA access. (**d**) Superselective angiography showing the microcatheter tip in the wedge position, the fistulous point and the tortuous and dilated drainage vein. (**e**) Unsubtracted image showing the Onyx cast. (**f**) Postembolization right internal carotid artery arteriogram, lateral view demonstrating the TDAVF total occlusion

endovascular techniques can be an alternative for DAVFs that are complicated by a lack of accessibility to an MMA approach [36, 37]. When the TAA is not possible and the TVA is considered high risk, direct MMA puncture should be considered as an alternative approach [16, 36, 37].

12.8.8 Nonadhesive Liquids as the Preferred Embolic Agent

Tomak et al. treated eleven patients harboring TDAVFs using the TAA with glue injection and reported 45% total angiographic occlusion [6]. However, since the first reports on EVT of TDAVFs with Onyx, angiographic occlusion rates have increased [3, 4, 8, 12–14, 16, 17]. Nonadhesive liquids have been the most common material (78.4%) used to treat TDAVFs in the last decade [30], and their advantages over adhesive liquid agents are well established [4, 13, 30, 38]. Recently, other nonadhesive liquid agents, such as Squid (Emboflu, Gland, Switzerland) and Phil (Microvention, Tustin, CA, USA), have been used successfully [8, 30].

We systematically used Onyx as the preferred embolic agent [16]. It was used alone or combined with other agents in all patients except one, who was treated by two sessions with transvenous access. In this patient, the TDAVF was embolized with coils leading to incomplete angiographic occlusion. In the second session, a microcatheter not compatible with dimethyl sulfoxide was used, after subtotal occlusion with coils, glue was injected.

12.8.9 Influence of the Number of Arterial Feeders

TDAVFs are often nourished by multiple vascular groups [4, 7, 8], and only 6.7% of our cases were supplied by a single artery [16]. Liu et al. reported the influence of the number of feeding arteries on the occlusion rates of TDAVFs. According to them, the total occlusion rates using the TAA with Onyx were 85.7%, 53.8%, and 66.7% in the tentorial marginal, lateral, and medial subtypes, respectively. Marginal TDAVFs had fewer feeding arteries and presented higher occlusion rates after the TAA [12]. In our series, all TDAVFs, except one, were completely occluded. The presence of more than four arterial feeders was a predictor of failure for total occlusion after the first treatment session. Other factors, such as bilateral supply and Picard type, were not predictors for occlusion after the first procedure. The high flow secondary to the multiple arterial supply likely causes an increased pressure in the leptomeningeal drainage vein, making it challenging for Onyx to penetrate the shunt during injection into a single arterial pedicle.

To increase the complete occlusion rates using a single procedure, inspired by the concept of double catheterization to treat pial arteriovenous malformations [39], we have adopted a new strategy in recent years. If a TDAVF was supplied by the MMA and OCC, we performed double catheterization [16, 34]. Depending on the caliber and tortuosity of the MMA, a DTM or a DLB was chosen. Inside the mastoid branch of the OCC, another DLB was positioned. Both arteries were blocked, reducing the flow to the shunt and the pressure inside the vein. Simultaneous Onyx injection occluded these lesions in a single session (Fig. 12.7) [16].

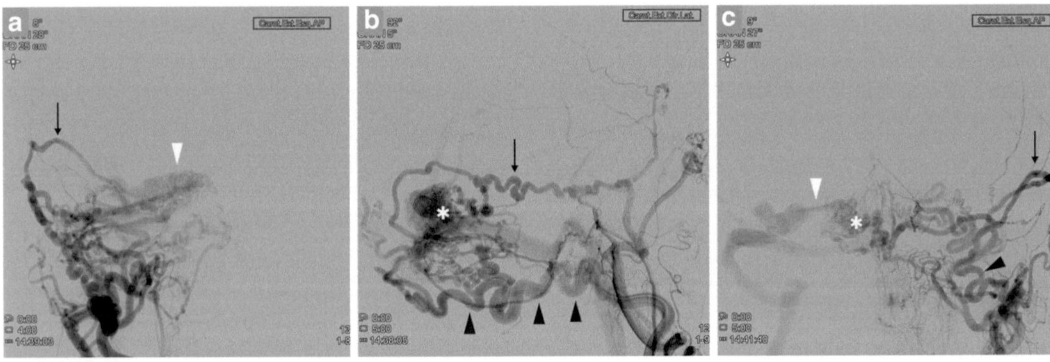

Fig. 12.7 TDAVF supplied by multiple arterial feeders and double catheterization technique. (**a**, **b**) An anteroposterior (AP) and lateral view of the right external carotid artery and (**c**, **d**) left external carotid artery angiogram. TDAVF (white asterisk) supplied by the middle meningeal (black arrows) and the occipital arteries (black arrowheads) from both sides draining directly to a dilated leptomeningeal vein (white arrowhead). (**e**) Lateral right external carotid roadmapping image demonstrating the position of the double lumen balloon (DLB) tip into the mastoid branch of the occipital artery. To obtain support for the DLB navigation, the proximal guiding catheter is positioned in the external carotid artery (white arrowhead), the flexible distal access catheter is navigated along a very tortuous and dilated occipital artery as close as possible to the origin of the mastoid branch (white arrow) and the DLB is inflated (double black arrows). (**f**) Lateral unsubtracted image revealing the position of the flexible distal access catheters in the left middle meningeal artery (black arrowhead) and in the right occipital artery (white arrow). A compatible DSMO microcatheter is positioned distally in the middle meningeal artery (double white arrowheads) and a double lumen balloon is placed inside the mastoid branch (double black arrows). (**g**) Simultaneous superselective angiography showing the microcatheter position in the middle meningeal artery (white arrowheads) and the DLB in the occipital artery (double black arrows). (**h**) Unsubtracted image showing the Onyx cast. (**i**, **j**) Postoperative bilateral common carotid artery angiogram, AP view, arterial and venous phase demonstrating the TDAVF total occlusion

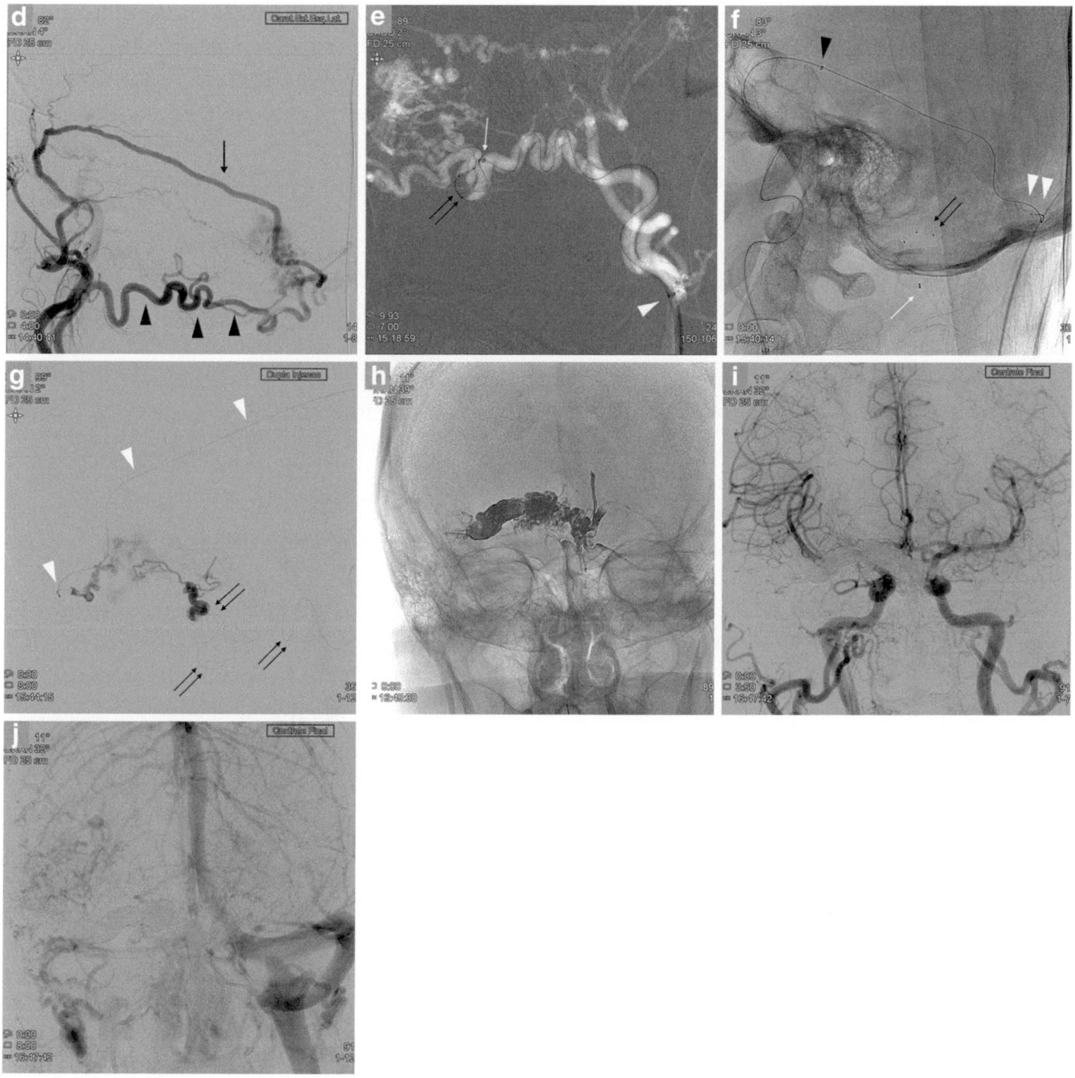

Fig. 12.7 (continued)

12.8.10 Clinical Outcomes

Compared with other therapeutic modalities, EVT resulted in lower perioperative morbidity (6%) and greater resolution of symptoms (82%). In addition, the good long-term neurological outcomes were significantly superior (89%). Due to these clinical results, in recent decades, the endovascular approach has become the standard treatment for most TDAVFs [9].

Despite our aggressive endovascular strategy, where no patient needed complementary direct microsurgical treatment, 41 patients (91.1%) presented good neurological outcomes at 6 months. Most patients with symptomatic unruptured TDAVFs improved [16].

12.8.11 Complications

The reported complication rates of EVT varied from 0% to 13.5% [3, 4, 8, 9, 13, 17, 30, 32]. One of the major challenges related to the intra-arterial injection of liquid agents during the embolization of TDAVFs is the possibility of excessive reflux. Several complications have been described resulting from this phenomenon, such as microcatheter retention and/or rupture, cranial nerve palsy and cerebral ischemia. The force required for microcatheter extraction after the injection of liquid agents is variable and depends on factors such as vascular tortuosity, extent of reflux and proximal access support [33].

Anatomical factors influence microcatheter navigation along dural and pial arteries [4, 6, 8, 13]. Tortuosity and reduced caliber can limit distal catheterization [13]. Depending on the microcatheter tip position, forward Onyx progression is limited, increasing the risk of complications related to excessive reflux [4]. Total occlusion of the TDAVF may not occur after injection in a single artery, requiring additional arterial access and increased risks [16].

In our series, seven (15.6%) patients showed clinical complications after EVT. Five of them experienced transient complications. In most of these cases, multiple arteries were catheterized. In multivariable analysis, clinical complications were related to the number of accessed arteries [16].

12.8.12 Cranial Nerve Deficits After Arterial Embolization

Some arteries that supply the tentorial region also participate in the vascular supply of some cranial nerves [35]. Cranial nerve palsy during the arterial injection of EVOH occurs when the embolic agent migrates toward the vascular supply of the nerve called the vasa nervorum [32]. According to Gioppo et al., the rate of cranial neuropathy associated with endovascular treatment of TDAVFs is 1.2% [30].

12.8.13 Middle Meningeal Artery

Immediately adjacent to the spinous foramen, the middle meningeal artery gives rise to a short arterial trunk that divides into a lateral branch (petrosal artery) and a medial branch (cavernous branch to the trigeminal ganglion). The cavernous branch contributes to the supply of the second and third portions of the trigeminal nerve. The petrous branch penetrates the temporal bone and supplies the tympanic segment and geniculate ganglion of the facial nerve [32, 35]. The occlusion of these branches, resulting from the reflux of EVOH during the injection, can cause deficits of the trigeminal and facial nerves (Fig. 12.8) [32, 40, 41].

To prevent this complication, avoiding Onyx reflux into the petrosal branch is critical [13]. An alternative, is the positioning of a DLB beyond the spinosum foramen level, but the size of the MMA sometimes limits this approach [16].

12.8.14 Medial Tentorial Artery

Despite contributing to the vascular supply in many TDAVFs (50–72%) [4, 7, 8, 42], the medial tentorial artery (MTA) has not been used as a frequent access for the injection of liquid agents. A risk of reflux exists toward the internal carotid artery. Additionally, because the oculomotor and trochlear nerves may derive their blood supply from the MTA, complications such as diplopia may occur [32, 35]. In our series, the MTA supplied 42.2% of the TDAFVs. In only one patient, the MTA was used for Onyx injection, since all fistulas had additional feeding arteries. Transitory diplopia occurred after MMA and MTA Onyx embolization. The MTA was embolized after subtotal occlusion using MMA access. No reflux to the spinosum foramen occurred, and no ischemia was identified on MRI [16]. We recommend that the MTA should be embolized only for TDAVFs for which it is the only feeding artery or if residual filling after embolization occurs by other arterial pedicles. A balloon should be positioned in the internal carotid artery in front of the origin of the MTA. Rooij et al. treated six patients with TDAVFs that were mainly supplied by the tentorial artery. In four patients, the MTA was the only arterial feeder to the fistulas. Three TDAVFs were embolized by glue injection into the MTA with balloon occlusion of the internal carotid artery without complications [42].

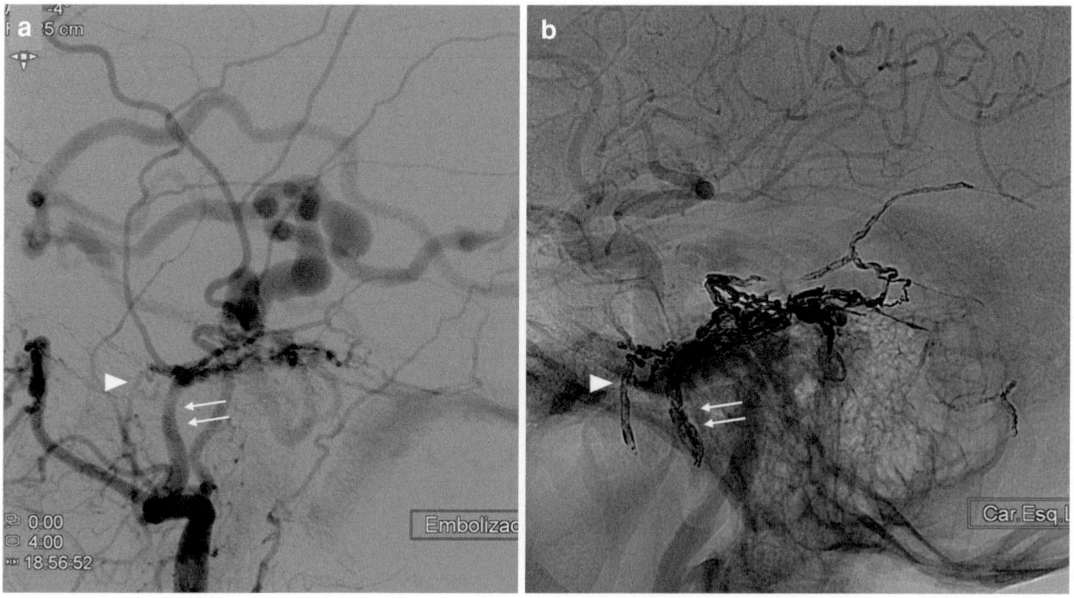

Fig. 12.8 Marginal TDAVF. Facial palsy due to Onyx reflux. (**a**) Lateral view of the right external carotid artery angiography showing a marginal TDAVF supplied by the middle meningeal artery (double white arrows) and accessory meningeal artery (white arrowhead). (**b**) Lateral unsubtracted image demonstrating the Onyx reflux filling retrogradely the middle meningeal artery trunk below the spinosum foramen level (double white arrows) and the accessory meningeal artery trunk (white arrowhead)

12.8.15 Distal Onyx Migration

Onyx migration has been reported during transarterial and transvenous high-flow DAVF embolization [43]. In our experience, this complication occurred in one patient with a lateral TDAVF supplied by six different arterial branches that was embolized by the MMA. During Onyx injection, distal migration occurred. We attribute this complication to the high-flow condition and washout effect related to the multiple arterial feeders. An alternative to avoid this complication is to use Onyx-34 during the initial phases of the injection [44]. During the embolization of pial arteriovenous malformations, double catheterization of the main afferents may decrease flow to the arteriovenous shunt and the risk of Onyx migration [39]. In recent years, when possible, we started to perform double catheterization, and distal venous Onyx migration did not occur [16].

12.8.16 Hemorrhage

Hemorrhagic complications are related to vessel perforation [3, 4], the presence of a pial supply [11], extensive thrombosis of the drainage vein [40], and distal venous occlusion with a residual fistula [17].

Vascular perforation can occur during arterial or venous access. Huang et al. [4] described a series of 14 TDAVFs treated with transarterial injection of EVOH. In one case, arterial perforation occurred during microcatheterization, causing subarachnoid hemorrhage. After embolization through the same artery, subtotal devascularization of the lesion was obtained. The patient evolved uneventfully.

Jiang et al. warned that the migration of liquid embolic agents toward the distal segment of the draining vein can cause venous rupture if there is residual flow in the fistulous connection. These authors reported a fatal complication related to rupture of the draining vein during transvenous injection of EVOH [17].

DAVFs with a pial arterial supply are also called acquired or mixed duropial fistulas. There are rare reports of these lesions [45]. Wu et al. described the results of transarterial injection of EVOH in 17 patients with TDAVFs [11]. Six TDAVFs (35.3%) received an arterial supply from the pial branches. In this series, no DAVF from other topographies received pial vascularization, only tentorial lesions. During embolization, two patients with TDAVFs with a pial supply had hemorrhage. The authors believed that high-flow TDAVF induces the development of pial arteriovenous fistulas. During EVOH injection through a meningeal branch, occlusion of the draining vein and dural arterial supply of the TDAV without involvement of the pial fistula can be observed. Restriction of venous drainage from the pial fistula may lead to hemorrhage. It is postulated that the pial arterial supply may be a risk factor for intraoperative hemorrhage during the embolization of meningeal branches with EVOH. To avoid this complication, endovascular occlusion of the pial supply is suggested before embolization of the dural branches.

After total or subtotal occlusion of a TDAVF with direct leptomeningeal venous drainage, a severe complication may arise. Extensive thrombosis of the arterialized draining vein can cause venous infarction or hemorrhage [40, 46]. Borha et al. reported a bleeding complication attributed to massive thrombosis of the draining vein that occurred 4 days after embolization of a lateral type TDAVF using EVOH and *n*-BCA [46]. To prevent this type of complication, Cognard et al. recommended the postoperative use of intravenous heparin for 48 h and then low molecular weight heparin at a preventive dose for 15–30 days to prevent venous drainage thrombosis. However, in their series, one TDAVF had postembolization hemorrhage secondary to extensive venous thrombosis [40]. This issue remains controversial, and we do not use routine anticoagulation after treatment [16].

12.9 Conclusions

Endovascular treatment is a safe and effective therapy for TDAVFs. A TAA could be used as a primary therapeutic option for most TDAVFs. When a TAA is not possible or does not result in total lesion occlusion, transvenous or combined approaches can be performed, leading to high angiographic occlusion rates.

References

1. Awad IA, Little JR, Akarawi WP, Ahl J. Intracranial dural arteriovenous malformations: factors predisposing to an aggressive neurological course. J Neurosurg. 1990;72:839–50.
2. Zhou LF, Chen L, Song DL, et al. Tentorial dural arteriovenous fistulas. Surg Neurol. 2007;67:472–82.
3. Byrne JV, Garcia M. Tentorial dural fistulas: endovascular management and description of the medial dural-tentorial branch of the superior cerebellar artery. AJNR Am J Neuroradiol. 2013;34:1798–804.
4. Huang Q, Xu Y, Hong B, et al. Use of Onyx in the management of tentorial dural arteriovenous fistulae. Neurosurgery. 2009;65:287–92.
5. Davies MA, ter Brugge K, Willinsky R, Wallace MC. The natural history and management of intracranial dural arteriovenous fistulae. Part 2: aggressive lesions. Interv Neuroradiol. 1997;3:303–11.
6. Tomak PR, Cloft HJ, Kaga A, et al. Evolution of the management of tentorial dural arteriovenous malformations. Neurosurgery. 2003;52:750–60.
7. Lawton MT, Sanchez-Mejia RO, Pham D, et al. Tentorial dural arteriovenous fistulae: operative strategies and microsurgical results for six types. Neurosurgery. 2008;62(3 Suppl 1):110–24.
8. Kortman HG, Boukrab I, Bloemsma G, et al. Tentorial dural arteriovenous fistulas: a single-center cohort of 12 patients. J Cerebrovasc Endovasc Neurosurg. 2017;19:284–90.
9. Cannizzaro D, Brinjikji W, Rammos S, et al. Changing clinical and therapeutic trends in tentorial dural arteriovenous fistulas: a systematic review. AJNR Am J Neuroradiol. 2015;36:1905–11.
10. Picard L, Bracard S, Islak C, et al. Dural fistulae of the tentorium cerebelli. Radioanatomical, clinical and therapeutic considerations. J Neuroradiol. 1990;17(3):161–81.
11. Wu Q, Zhang XS, Wang HD, et al. Onyx embolization for tentorial dural arteriovenous fistula with pial arterial supply: case series and analysis of complications. World Neurosurg. 2016;92:58–64.
12. Liu C, Xu B, Song D, et al. Clinical approach of using Onyx via transarterial access in treating ten-

torial dural arteriovenous fistula. Neurol Res. 2014;36(11):983–91.
13. Puffer RC, Daniels DJ, Kallmes DF, et al. Curative Onyx embolization of tentorial dural arteriovenous fistulas. Neurosurg Focus. 2012;32(5):E4.
14. Wajnberg E, Spilberg G, Rezende MT, et al. Endovascular treatment of tentorial dural arteriovenous fistulae. Interv Neuroradiol. 2012;18:60–8.
15. Iwamuro Y, et al. Tentorial dural arteriovenous fistula presenting symptoms due to mass effect on the dilated draining vein: case report. Surg Neurol. 2006;65:511–5.
16. Rezende MTS, Trivelato FP, de Castro-Afonso LH, et al. Endovascular treatment of tentorial dural arteriovenous fistulas using the transarterial approach as a first-line strategy. Oper Neurosurg. 2021;20(5):484–92.
17. Jiang C, Lv X, Li Y, et al. Endovascular treatment of high-risk tentorial dural arteriovenous fistulas: clinical outcomes. Neuroradiology. 2009;51(2):103–11.
18. Collice M, et al. Surgical treatment of intracranial dural arteriovenous fistulae: role of venous drainage. Neurosurgery. 2000;47:56–67.
19. Grisoli F, et al. Surgical treatment of tentorial arteriovenous malformations draining into the subarachnoid space. Report of four cases. J Neurosurg. 1984;60:1059–66.
20. Gross BA, Du R. Surgical treatment of high grade dural arteriovenous fistulae. J Clin Neurosci. 2013;20:1527–32.
21. Sugiyama T, et al. Complication rate, cure rate, and long-term outcomes of microsurgery for intracranial dural arteriovenous fistulae: a multicenter series and systematic review. Neurosurg Rev. 2021;44(1):435–50.
22. Kallmes DF, Jensen ME, Cloft HJ, et al. Percutaneous transvenous coil embolization of a Djindjian type 4 tentorial dural arteriovenous malformation. AJNR Am J Neuroradiol. 1997;18(4):673–6.
23. Deasey NP, Gholkar AR, Cox TCS, Jeffree MA. Tentorial dural arteriovenous fistulae: Endovascular treatment with transvenous coil embolization. Neuroradiology. 1999;41:308–12.
24. Djindjian R, Cophignon J, Theron J. Embolization by superselective arteriography from the femoral route; review of 60 cases: technique, indications, complications. Neuroradiology. 1973;6:20–6.
25. Grossman RI, et al. Dural malformations with ophthalmic manifestations: results of particulate embolization in seven patients. AJNR Am J Neuroradiol. 1985;6:809–13.
26. Berestein A. Flow controlled silicone fluid embolization. AJR Am J Roentgenol. 1980;134:1213–8.
27. Nelson PK, Russell SM, Woo HH, et al. Use of a wedged microcatheter for curative transarterial embolization of complex intracranial dural arteriovenous fistulas: indications, endovascular technique, and outcome in 21 patients. J Neurosurg. 2003;98(3):498–506.
28. Rezende MT, Piotin M, Mounayer C, et al. Dural arteriovenous fistula of the lesser sphenoid wing region treated with Onyx: technical note. Neuroradiology. 2006;48(2):130–4.
29. Toulgoat F, Mounayer C, Túlio Salles Rezende M, et al. Transarterial embolisation of intracranial dural arteriovenous malformations with ethylene vinyl alcohol copolymer (Onyx18). J Neuroradiol. 2006;33(2):105–14.
30. Gioppo A, Faragò G, Caldiera V, et al. Medial tentorial dural arteriovenous fistula embolization: single experience with embolic liquid polymer SQUID and review of the literature. World Neurosurg. 2017;107:1050.e1–7.
31. Yu J, et al. Clinical importance of the middle meningeal artery: a review of the literature. Int J Med Sci. 2016;13(10):790–9.
32. Tong D, Chen X, Lv X, et al. Current status of endovascular treatment for dural arteriovenous fistulae in the tentorial middle region: a literature review. Act Neurol Belg. 2019;119(1):5–14.
33. Flores BC, See AP, Weiner GM, et al. Use of the Apollo detachable-tip microcatheter for endovascular embolization of arteriovenous malformations and arteriovenous fistulas. J Neurosurg. 2018;130(3):963–71.
34. Zamponi JO Jr, Trivelato FP, Rezende MTS, et al. Transarterial treatment of cranial dural arteriovenous fistulas: the role of transarterial and transvenous balloon-assisted embolization. AJNR Am J Neuroradiol. 2020;41(11):2100–6.
35. Martins C, Yasuda A, Campero A, et al. Microsurgical anatomy of the dural arteries. Neurosurgery. 2005;56(ONS 2):211–51.
36. Lin N, Brouillard AM, Mokin M, et al. Direct access to the middle meningeal artery for embolization of complex dural arteriovenous fistula: a hybrid treatment approach. J Neurointerv Surg. 2015;7(7):e24.
37. Oh JS, Yoon SM, Shim JJ, Bae HG. Transcranial direct middle meningeal artery puncture for the onyx embolization of dural arteriovenous fistula involving the superior sagittal sinus. J Korean Neurosurg Soc. 2015;57:54–7.
38. Rabinov JD, Yoo AJ, Ogilvy CS, et al. ONYX versus n-BCA for embolization of cranial dural arteriovenous fistulas. J Neurointerv Surg. 2013;5:306–10.
39. Abud DG, Riva R, Nakiri GS, et al. Treatment of brain arteriovenous malformations by double arterial catheterization with simultaneous Onyx injection: retrospective series of 17 patients. AJNR Am J Neuroradiol. 2011;32(1):152–8.
40. Cognard C, Januel AC, Silva NA Jr, Tall P. Endovascular treatment of intracranial dural arteriovenous fistulas with cortical venous drainage: new management using Onyx. AJNR Am J Neuroradiol. 2008;29:235–41.
41. Lv X, Jiang C, Li Y, Wu Z. Results and complications of transarterial embolization of intracranial dural arteriovenous fistulas using Onyx-18. J Neurosurg. 2008;109(6):1083–90.

42. van Rooij WJ, Sluzewski M, Beute GN. Tentorial artery embolization in tentorial dural arteriovenous fistulas. Neuroradiology. 2006;48:737–43.
43. Wang H, Lv X, Jiang C, et al. Onyx migration in the endovascular management of intracranial dural arteriovenous fistulas. Interv Neuroradiol. 2009;15(3):301–8.
44. Nogueira RG, Dabus G, Rabinov JD, et al. Preliminary experience with onyx embolization for the treatment of intracranial dural arteriovenous fistulas. AJNR Am J Neuroradiol. 2008;29(1):91–7.
45. Lai CW, et al. Cerebral arteriovenous fistulas induced by dural arteriovenous shunts. AJNR Am J Neuroradiol. 2005;26:1259–62.
46. Borha A, et al. Tentorial dural fistula with giant venous ampulae treated with embolisation and surgery. A case report. Acta Neurochir (Wien). 2010;152(10):1745–53.

Structural Analysis of Tentorial Dural Arteriovenous Fistulae with Special Considerations of Venous Ectasia: Proposing a Simpler Classification

13

Fumitaka Yamane, Yuhei Michiwaki, Tatsuya Tanaka, Akira Matsuno, Shinya Kohyama, Takeshi Uno, Yuta Oyama, and Akihiro Ito

Abstract

Tentorial dural arteriovenous fistulae (TdAVFs) are uncommon lesions in intracranial dural arteriovenous shunts. Dural arteriovenous fistulae (dAVF) with venous ectasia (VE) are known to be related to the aggressive type of dAVF. Most TdAVFs have retrograde cortical VE. In this chapter, we will review the anatomical classification of TdAVF. First, we provide an overview of the classification proposed thus far in literature. Here, we propose a simpler classification. There are four basic categories based on the angioarchitecture of the fistulae: (1) presence of VE, (2) sinus obstruction, (3) involvement of pial feeders, and (4) locations of shunts. The shunt portions were divided into falx cerebelli, torcular, petrotentorial, and marginal. The natural course of TdAVF seems to be determined by the pattern of venous drainage, and many different drainage directions can be distinguished.

Keywords

Tentorial dural AVF · Venous ectasia Classification · Embolization

13.1 Introduction

Tentorial dural arteriovenous fistulae (TdAVFs) are relatively rare, and most patients present with venous dilatation and reflux with symptoms that are often aggressive. Reflux in the venous system often progresses rapidly and can cause direct damage to the central nervous system. There are few reports in literature describing the prevalence of dAVF. Kuwayama [1] reported that the incidence of dAVF in the Japanese population is approximately 0.29 per 100,000 individuals. Subsequently, 1075 cases of dAVF were registered in JR-NET2 [2], with the most common sites being the cavernous sinus (43.6%), trans-

F. Yamane (✉) · Y. Michiwaki · T. Tanaka
A. Matsuno
Department of Neurosurgery, International University of Health and Welfare Narita Hospital, Narita, Chiba, Japan
e-mail: fyamane@iuhw.ac.jp

S. Kohyama
Department of Endovascular Neurosurgery, Saitama Medical University International Medical Center, Hidaka, Saitama, Japan

T. Uno · Y. Oyama
Department of Neurosurgery, Teikyo University School of Medicine, Tokyo, Japan

A. Ito
Department of Neurosurgery, JR Tokyo General Hospital, Tokyo, Japan

X. Lv (ed.), *Intracranial and Spinal Dural Arteriovenous Fistulas*,
https://doi.org/10.1007/978-981-19-5767-3_13

verse sinus, and sigmoid sinus (33.4%). According to JR-NET2, 2.9% of the 1075 cases were slightly more male (68%), and the mean age of the subjects was 59 years. Most cases without venous sinus involvement were classified as Cognard III or IV. In JR-NET2, 42% of patients had cerebral hemorrhage or stroke. Asymptomatic onset is rare. In recent years, the number of cases with minor symptoms such as dizziness and tinnitus that are detected incidentally by magnetic resonance imaging or other methods.

The classification of dAVF has always focused on the venous sinus or venous reflux. Clinical useful classifications are the structure of the venous system. The basic approach to treating dAVF is to understand the relationship between the inflow system and the shunt, to carefully examine the outflow system related to the symptoms, and to obliterate the outflow using endovascular treatment or direct surgery. First, this article outlines the clinical presentation and outcomes of TdAVF. We will review the previously proposed classifications of dAVFs as described by many authors. We will attempt to summarize not only TdAVF but also the various parts of the shunts. It is also important to note that the presence of dAVF with venous ectasia (VE) is known to be related to the so-called aggressive type of dAVF. The presence or absence of symptoms due to venous stasis is related to the structure of the shunt site because most TdAVFs have retrograde cortical VEs (RCVEs). The clinical features of dAVF with RCVE are related to hemorrhage. We also discuss VE and the pathogenesis of stasis in VE [3].

13.2 Clinical Presentations

The symptoms of TdAVF are greatly variable and depend on the degree of venous reflux. The following is a general outline.

Benign presentation: Asymptomatic and incidentally found. Tinnitus, headache, dizziness, conjunctival chemosis, exophthalmos, and decreased visual acuity (not associated with glaucoma).

Aggressive presentation: Progressive neurologic deficit, transitory ischemic attack, epilepsy, intracranial hypertension syndrome, cranial nerve deficits (trigeminal neuralgia [TN], facial nerve paralysis), and glaucoma with an irreversible decrease in visual acuity.

Hemorrhage: Hemorrhage affects many small connections between the branches of intracranial arteries, veins and/or dural venous sinuses [4]. There are two patterns of bleeding: relatively small amounts of bleeding and/or large amounts of bleeding. In the former, the presence of such a network of vessels can easily lead to venous stasis and bleeding. In the latter case, aneurysmal or bleeding of the varix may result in major hemorrhage. The following is a discussion of these issues.

In asymptomatic cases, TdAVFs constitute only 4% of dAVFs but pose a high risk of hemorrhage, especially Borden type III dAVF, which justifies the aggressive treatment after the diagnosis is made [5]. TdAVFs are characterized by a high risk of hemorrhage. Thus, these lesions are treated aggressively on diagnosis. Patients with TdAVF increasingly present with asymptomatic lesions and are treated endovascularly. In addition, they experience higher rates of good neurologic outcomes as endovascular treatment is associated with superior neurologic outcomes but lower occlusion rates, combination of surgical resection and endovascular procedures is best [5].

Although the main symptoms are headache and cranial nerve palsy, TN due to sensory disturbance is also well known and has been reported in many cases. Cranial nerve involvement, headache, ataxia, TN, and quadriparesis have been reported at presentation [6–10]. Even the complete obliteration of the fistula can cause neuralgia recurrence, and the resection of the embolized dilated veins might be effective for treating TN in such cases of recurrence. Many reports disagree as to whether the loss of the shunt improves TN [8, 11–14].

Deep venous congestion due to TdAVF can induce unusual bithalamic lesions and bilateral basal ganglia hemorrhage [15, 16]. There are both clinical and radiographic differences between dAVF-induced thalamic and cortical dementia syndromes. For patients presenting with a rapidly progressive thalamic dementia syndrome, differential diagnosis and radiographic workup are necessary. TdAVF is an aggressive vascular disease, and prompt diagnosis and treatment are required. After dAVF treatment, symptoms resolve rapidly and completely. The most critical anatomical feature is the identification of RCVE. Much data have indicated that within these high risk groups, most of the risk of future injury is within the subgroup presenting with intracerebral hemorrhage (ICH) or nonhemorrhagic neurologic deficits. It is difficult to accurately describe the prognosis simply by the presence of cortical venous drainage (CVD). On the basis of recent data, the annual rate of ICH ranges from 7.4% to 7.6% for patients with symptomatic CVD compared with 1.4% to 1.5% for those with asymptomatic CVD. One study proposed that new categories (symptomatic vs asymptomatic) should be added to the traditional classification [17]. To predict clinical outcomes, recently, an interesting study was reported that the relative signal intensity (rSI) of the draining vessels on time-of-flight magnetic resonance angiography was studied related to clinical behavior [18]. In the study, the authors found that a significant positive correlation was observed between the aggressive and nonaggressive behavior groups in the rSI of the veins with RCVE. There is a growing need to develop methods that can estimate prognosis as simply and accurately as in that article.

As discussed above, the investigators tried to evaluate the risk factors for bleeding of dAVFs [19–26]. The two patterns of bleeding described above were examined as well as in which pathologic conditions rebleeding was more frequent. The hemorrhage type was classified as pure intraparenchymal hemorrhage (pIPH) and subarachnoid hemorrhage (SAH) or subdural hematoma (SDH) with IPH (non-pIPH) [26]. Rebleeding occurred significantly more frequently in the non-pIPH group than in the pIPH group [26]. Thus, early treatment is needed in all dAVFs with ICH. In addition, dAVFs that present with non-pIPH and contain VE on initial angiography may have a higher risk of early rebleeding. The most common presenting symptom was headache without focal neurologic deficits, followed by aphasia [25]. According to Duvernoy et al., there are three patterns of venous runs [27, 28]:

1. The main leptomeningeal veins, which are located on the surface of the cortex.
2. The pial veins that form a highly dense venous network and can merge into a single trunk at the gyrus center.
3. The intracortical veins, which penetrate into the cortical cellular layer.

If the rupture occurs in the main leptomeningeal veins, it can present with SAH or SDH with or without IPH. By contrast, the rupture of the intracortical or pial veins might lead to IPH rather than SAH or SDH as a main hemorrhage type [25, 29]. Duffau et al. [21] found that dAVFs with CVD were associated with a high risk for early rebleeding (35% within 2 weeks after the first hemorrhage). According to Bulters et al. [20], among dAVF patients with CVD, those with RCVE presented with a sevenfold increase in the incidence of hemorrhage (3.5% without and 27% with VE). In the following chapters, we summarize previous reports on the classification and discuss the important factors that should be considered in the classification.

13.3 Summary of Previously Reported Classifications: Anatomy of a Tentorium Cerebelli and TdAVF

The most commonly used classification systems of dAVFs were proposed by Borden et al. and Cognard et al. [30, 31]. RCVE is highly associated with aggressive clinical manifestations such as ICH and can be used in the evaluation of risk factors for dAVF bleeding [19, 20, 22, 23]. The degree of venous reflux is clearly related to prognosis [32].

The venous anatomy of the tentorium cerebelli is described. Depending on the anatomy of the drainer, shunts located at the tentorium can present with a variety of symptoms. The incisura tentorium is surrounded by the basal vein, superior petrosal vein, peduncular veins, lateral mesencephalic veins, and other basal veins that flow into the vein of Galen to straight sinus (SS), as well as inferior temporal veins and basal temporal veins. The venous group of the posterior cranial fossa ultimately includes the torcula system and the transverse sigmoid system, with the Labbe joining the latter. CVD and pial venous reflux are easily caused by the reflux of the dural vessels into the venous sinus or the obstruction of the venous sinus. This results in hemorrhage and ischemia in the brain parenchyma, from which neurologic dropout symptoms arise. Furthermore, CVD into the cerebellopontine vein often results in hemorrhagic events.

Nevertheless, several classification systems have been proposed according to the location and venous drainage patterns of TdAVF [33, 34]. The arterial supply is not an important feature in these descriptions, but with the increased use of endovascular treatment, it is clearly important and may be helpful in classifying and distinguishing TdAVFs from dAVFs located at the tentorial margins. TdAVFs are classified into three groups as proposed by Picard et al. [33]:

1. The tentorial *marginal type* with fistulae located along the free edge of the tentorial hiatus and draining both supra- and infratentorially.
2. The tentorial *lateral type* adjacent to the lateral sinus and draining to supratentorial veins.
3. The tentorial *medial type* with fistulae sited adjacent to the torcular and straight sinuses draining to the infratentorial draining system.

In feeders of TdAVF, the tentorial branches of the ICA, dural branches of the vertebral artery, and external carotid artery are involved. Special attention is drawn to an underrecognized medial dural–tentorial branch of the superior cerebellar artery (SCA) [35] and the tentorial branch of the posterior cerebral artery (PCA), also known as the artery of Davidoff and Schechter (aDS) [36]. In addition, the medial dural–tentorial branch of the SCA supplied only fistulae located at the midline. An additional pial supply, such as the cortical branches of the posterior inferior cerebellar artery and contributions to the subarcuate plexus at the internal acoustic meatus from the anterior inferior cerebellar artery, is also noted. Involvement of pial feeders (PFs) have been discussed extensively in recent years. Osada and Krings [37] reported three predictors of pial feeders: younger age, TdAVF, and VE. That study seems to be important when considering the classification of TdAVF. Therefore, the involvement of pial feeders in addition to impaired venous return should be considered carefully.

The choice of surgical disconnection of the outflow is reasonable. Lawton et al. [34] proposed a classification with six anatomic locations and venous drainage patterns, which, in turn, determined the surgical approach. This classification was based on a larger series of 31 patients and separates midline lesions according to their classification, TdAVFs are divided into the Galenic, SS, torcular, tentorial sinus (TS), superior petrosal sinus, and fistulas around incisura.

Matsushima et al. [38] proposed the following classification of the tentorium from a surgical point of view. They examined variations in the tentorial sinus of cadaver cerebellar tentoria under a surgical microscope. This classification must be considered when classifying TdAVF. Briding veins (BVs) to the tentorium should be considered together with the TS. The authors concluded that the location of BVs can be anticipated when the course of the TS is identified on preoperative venograms.

Group I (69.2%) TS draining the cerebral hemisphere, in which the sinuses receive venous blood from the cerebral hemisphere through BVs. They were frequently present in the posterolateral portion of the tentorium or near the transverse sinus. The TS receive venous blood from the cerebral hemisphere. According to the study by Matsushima et al. [38], the BVs present at this site were as follows: the total number of BVs from the cerebral hemispheres to the tentoria was 155, with an average of six on one side and the greatest number of nine

BVs. These veins drained the basal surface of the temporal and occipital lobes, including the vein of Labbe from the lateral surface of the temporal lobe.

Group II (88.5%) TS draining the cerebellum, in which the sinuses are drained and formed by the terminal portions of the cerebellar hemispheric or vermian veins. The BVs draining into the tentorial sinus of group II were of two kinds: the vermian BV on the vermis in the midline and the hemispheric BV located on the lateral cerebellar surface. In the study, the authors described that because the tentorial sinuses of group II were frequently present as a large sinus, they were separated into five subtypes based on the draining veins and direction of termination.

Group III (42.3%) TS arising in the tentorium. Group III sinuses originate from many tiny tentorial veins. The TS originating in the tentorium were present near the tentorial free edge or the SS.

Group IV (7.6%) TS formed by a BV to the tentorial free edge. A special type of group I or II in which the sinus is formed by a BV. A rarer type of TS was found in two cases. The sinus ran posteriorly from the tentorial edge to the torcular, almost parallel to the straight sinus. In the other case, the peduncular vein running on the midbrain became a BV to the tentorial edge.

The issue of venous reflux is put aside for the moment. There is another classification from a different point of view. This is a classification of the dura mater, which is the shunt origin, from an embryological point of view. On the basis of the association of the epidural venous spaces with the afferent veins from the surrounding calvarium and the central nervous system, Geibprasert et al. [39] classified dAVFs into three categories according to their embryological development. These were the ventral, dorsal, and lateral epidural shunts. TdAVF would fall into the category of lateral epidural shunts, which were found to be more aggressive and were associated with a higher risk of neurologic complications. Tanaka's classification is also based on this concept [40].

13.4 Our Data

In this section, we present our data on TdAVF. The clinical features of dAVF with RCVE, a part of CVR, are related to hemorrhage. To investigate the clinical characteristics of TdAVF in the presence of RCVE, we retrospectively investigated clinical presentations, shunt structures, their anatomical classifications with special attention paid to venous structures, and the results of interventional procedures. In the process, the classification of TdAVF and the occurrence of complications will also be discussed.

13.4.1 Materials and Methods

From April 2007 to September 2021, 21 patients with TdAVF underwent 29 endovascular treatments at Saitama Medical University, International Medical Center, and related hospitals. Initial presentations were hemorrhage in eight cases (38%), dementia and neurologic deficits in seven cases (33%), incidental in three cases (14%), and "other" in three cases (14%). The structures of the shunt pouch and outlet flow to the cortical vein were investigated using three-dimensional digital subtraction angiography (3D-DSA), cone-beam computed tomography with maximum intensity projection, axial 3D digital angiography images, and computed tomography (CT) angiography fusion images.

13.4.2 Results

Transarterial embolization (TAE) was performed in 14 cases. Transvenous embolization (TVE) was performed in three cases, and four cases underwent both TAE and TVE combined. Seven cases had more than two sessions. Finally, 13 patients (68%) had no shunt. Three patients were treated with cyber knife and no shunt. There were no deaths. Complications occurred in six patients: four hemorrhagic and two ischemic complications. Morbidity remained in two patients (10.5%) with hemorrhagic complications. All ischemic complications were transient, with no morbidity. In particular, the following four points were important: (1) presence of VE, (2) sinus obstruction, (3) involvement of pial feeders, and (4) locations of shunts. The shunt portions were divided into four categories: falx cerebelli, torcular, petrotentorial, and marginal.

13.4.3 Case Presentations

Case 1 (Fig. 13.1)
A 69-year-old man with vertigo was referred to our hospital with suspicion of dAVF after undergoing magnetic resonance imaging at another hospital. The diagnosis of TdAVF was made by cerebral angiography. The feeders were the occipital artery, middle meningeal artery (MMA), inferolateral trunk, and posterior meningeal artery (PMA). A shunt was observed posterior to the falx cerebelli, with reflux to the vermian vein and draining into Galen's vein. In terms of the four basic categories, (1) presence of VE = yes, (2) sinus obstruction = no, (3) involvement of pial feeders = no, and (4) locations of shunts = falx cerebelli. The patient was treated with a combination of both TVE and TAE, and the result was no shunt, without morbidity.

Case 2 (Fig. 13.2)
A 64-year-old man experienced a sudden severe headache, vomiting, and loss of consciousness. CT scan revealed a hyperdense area in the cerebellar vermis and perforation of the fourth ventricle, resulting in acute hydrocephalus. For the four basic categories, (1) presence of VE = yes, (2) sinus obstruction = no, (3) involvement of pial feeders = no, and (4) locations of shunts = falx cerebelli. Preoperative cerebral angiography was performed, and a feeder occlusion using 17% NBCA was performed from the PMA. After the procedures, hematoma removal

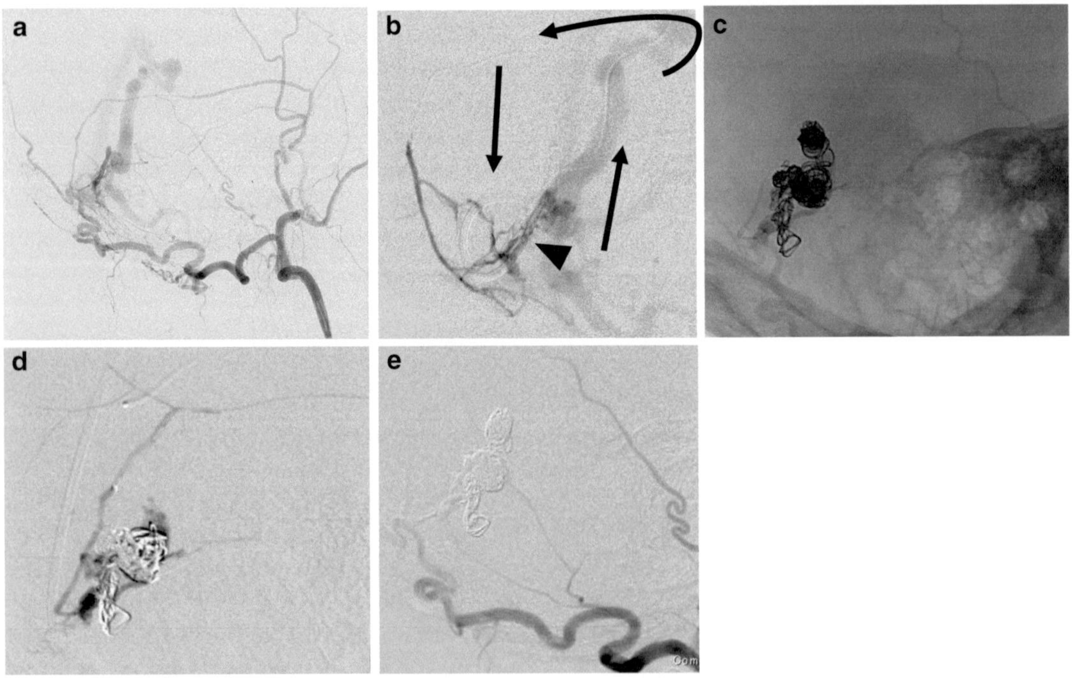

Fig. 13.1 Case 1 detail in text. (**a**) Right external carotid angiogram (ECAG) demonstrated that the shunt was noted in the falx cerebelli, and the feeders were the occipital artery and the MMA. (**b**) The arrowhead shows the position of the shunt, and the arrows are in the direction of the dilated vermian vein flow. (**c**) The shunt and venous outflow are embolized with coils by TVE. (**d**) Embolization using glue from the MMA. (**e**) Final external angiogram. No shunt was observed

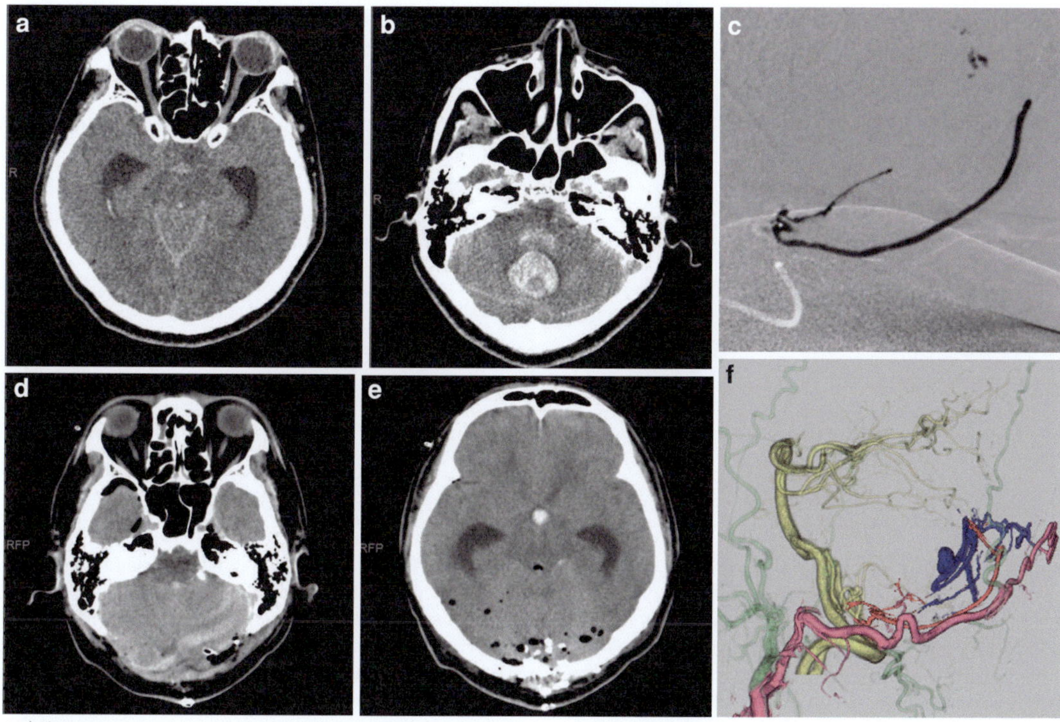

Fig. 13.2 Case 2 detail in text. (**a**, **b**) CT scan of the head showed a massive hemorrhage in the cerebellar vermis, perforating to the fourth ventricles, with associated acute hydrocephalus. (**c**) Following angiography, the microcatheter tip was immediately introduced to the PMA and TAE with glue. (**d**, **e**) Postoperative CT scan showing the removal of the hematoma and external decompression. (**f**) 3D-DSA fusion images with the ECAG and vertebral angiogram (VAG)

and external decompression were performed, and the remaining shunt was removed. The patient was transferred to a rehabilitation hospital with mRS 4.

Case 3 (Figs. 13.3 **and** 13.4)

A 35-year-old woman presented with vertigo and was diagnosed as TdAVF with cerebral angiography and referred to our hospital. The feeding arteries were the MMA, falcian artery (FA), inferolateral trunk, and PMA. The patient also received dural branch inflow from the PCA, and blood flow then drained to the vein of Galen and transverse sinus. For the four basic categories, (1) presence of VE = yes, (2) sinus obstruction = no, (3) involvement of pial feeders = yes, and (4) locations of shunts = marginal. Embolization was performed by TAE and TVE. First, the outflow pouch was occluded using a coil via the sigmoid sinus (TVE), followed by embolization from the MMA and obliteration of the shunt. Simultaneously, mild postoperative hemorrhage was observed. The remaining feeder from the aDS was immediately occluded using glue. The patient developed mild SAH postoperatively but was discharged with mRS 2. Six months after surgery, the patient recovered to mRS 0.

Case 4 (Figs. 13.5 **and** 13.6)

A 68-year-old man presented with progressive cognitive impairment. The feeders were FA from bilateral MMAs, bilateral PMAs, and pial arteries from bilateral PCAs. First, the FA was occluded by coil embolization from the bilateral MMA. The second embolization procedure was performed to obliterate the proximal PMA from the left VA using coils. The third embolization was performed using Onyx (Covidien, Irvine,

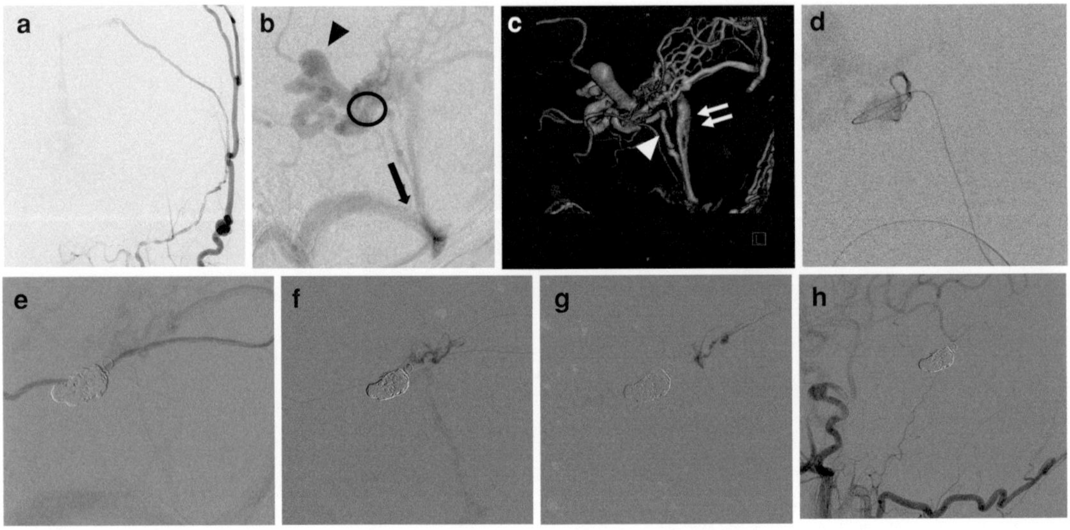

Fig. 13.3 Galenic AVF. Case 3 detail in text. (**a**) In the left ECAG, the feeder FA is shown as a branch of the MMA. (**b**) Left ECAG. Shunt portion (○), vein of Galen (arrowhead), and direction of flow (arrow). (**c**) 3D-DSA of the left ECAG. TVE approach route (arrow head) and straight sinus (double arrows). (**d**) TVE, starting from a feeder over the shunt. (**e**) ECAG showed that the inferior medial shunt disappeared, but a shunt from the upper part remained. (**f**) The remaining shunt was embolized with NBCA from MMA. (**g**) However, the shunt was occluded just before the NBCA injection, and the MMA flowed backward and did not reach the shunt, suggesting that the pial arteries appeared at this point. (**h**) ECAG and VAG were performed, and the disappearance of the shunt was confirmed

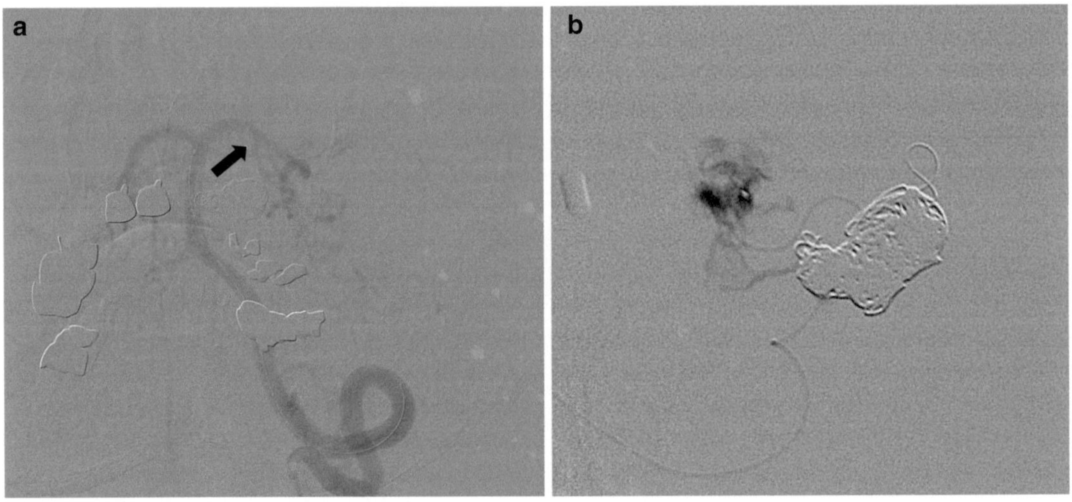

Fig. 13.4 Galenic AVF. Case 3 detail in text. (**a**) On the next day, the patient complained of headache, and CT revealed SAH. The artery of Davidoff and Schechter branching from the PCA (arrow) was observed in the left VAG, and the shunt remained anterior to the coils. (**b**) The microcatheter reached the target position from the PCA and carefully injected NBCA, but extravasation of glue was observed. (**c**) The shunt disappeared in the VAG after injection. (**d**) Postprocedure CT showed mild SAH

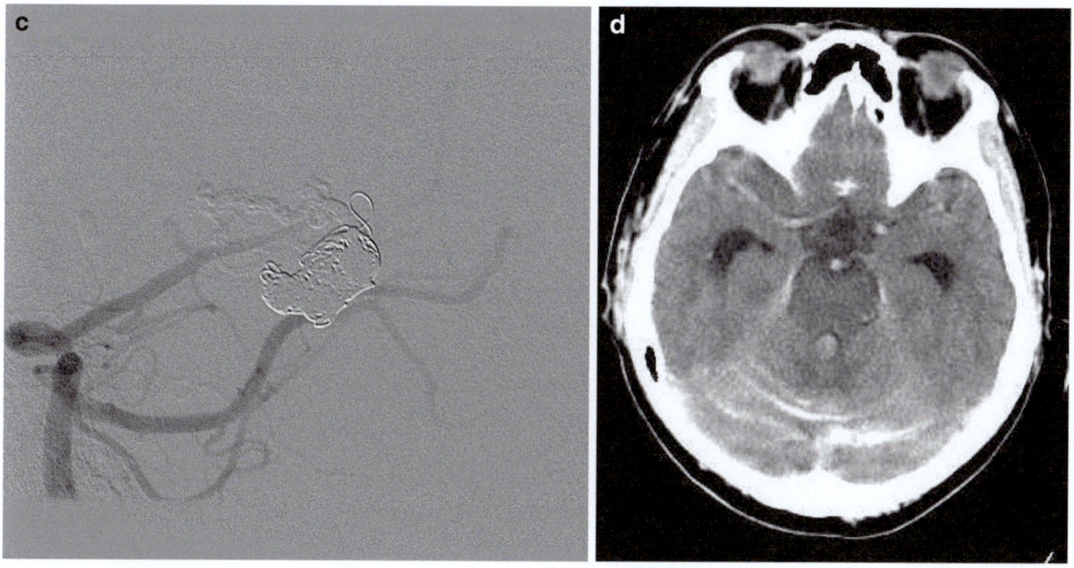

Fig. 13.4 (continued)

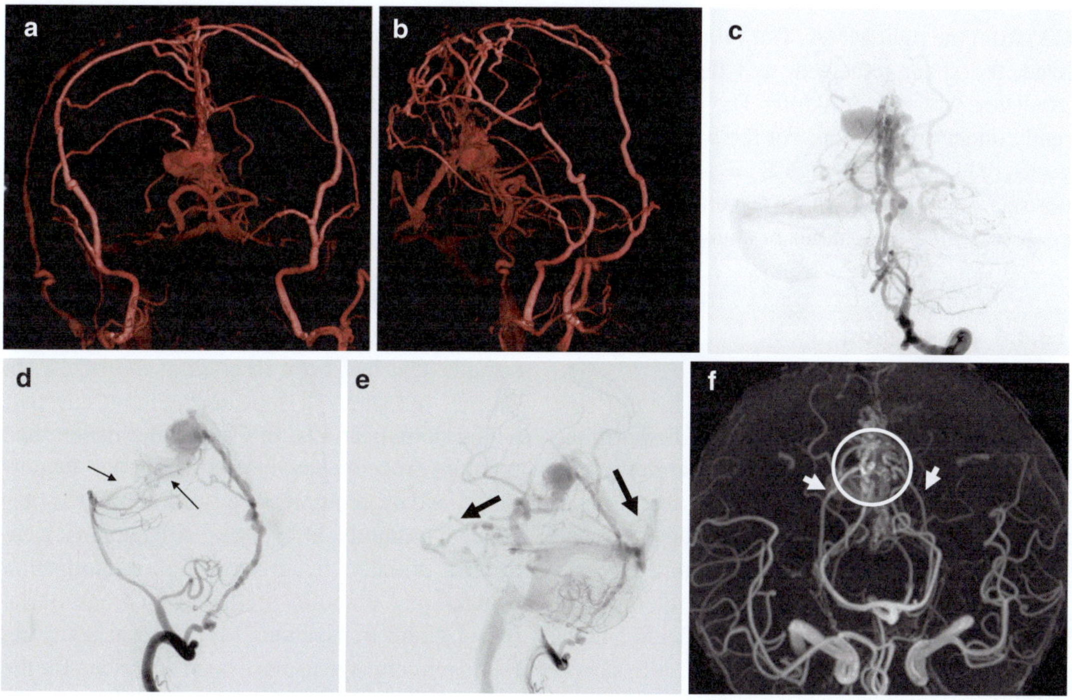

Fig. 13.5 Galenic AVF. Case 4 detail in text. (**a**, **b**) The left and right ECAGs were combined to create a 3D-DSA image. The feeders were multiple FAs, but they branched from the left and right MMAs. (**c**) Left VAG, anterior–posterior (AP) view. Note the aneurysmal dilatation of the vein of Galen. (**d**) Left VAG lateral position. Branches from the PCA and aDSs were observed (arrow). (**e**) Late venous phase of the left VAG. The arrows indicate the direction of venous regurgitation. (**f**) Magnetic resonance angiography showing the shunt structures around the vein of Galen, and the arrows clearly indicate the aDS

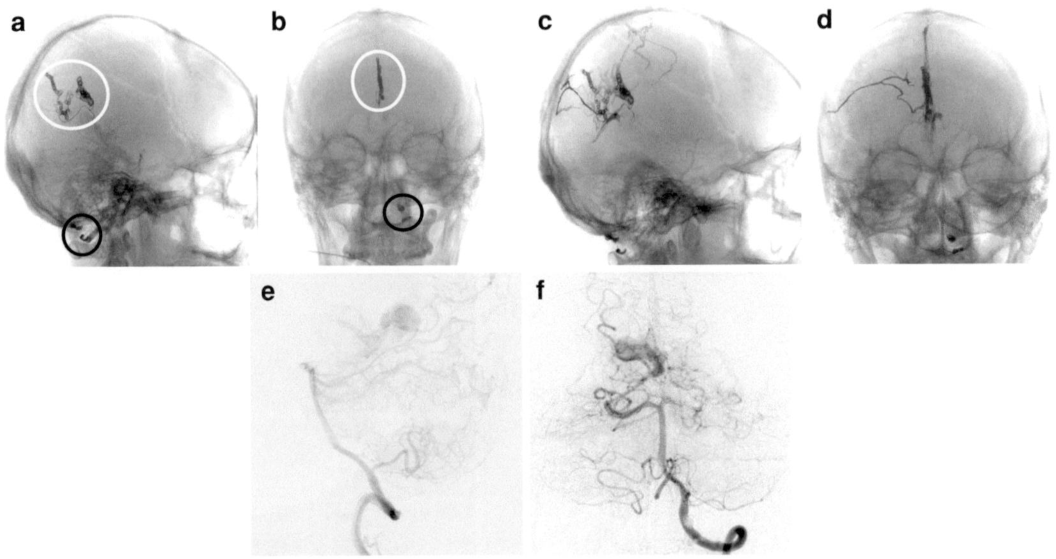

Fig. 13.6 Galenic AVF. Case 4 detail in text. (**a**, **b**) Plain X-ray films. White circles indicate the first treatment and black circles the second treatment. (**c**, **d**) Plain X-ray films. Third TAE treatment with onyx. Final lateral (**e**) and AP (**f**) VAG view after the third embolization. The volume of the shunt was reduced but remained

CA) from the right MMA. The PF was not embolized, the shunt remained, and the patient was irradiated with a cyber knife. The patient is currently under observation. For the four basic categories, (1) presence of VE = yes, (2) sinus obstruction = no, (3) = involvement of pial feeders = yes, and (4) locations of shunts = marginal.

13.4.4 Discussion

dAVF with VE was associated with hemorrhage or edema. In our case series, 38% of hemorrhage onsets and 33% of neurologic disorders (i.e., most cases) were symptomatic and were of the aggressive type. In addition, 14% of cases had minor symptoms such as dizziness, and all cases underwent vigorous endovascular therapy. In particular, because it might be considered a high-flow shunt with long-term duration, VE slowly developed and brain edema and hemorrhage appeared. The natural course of dAVF with VE is determined by many different drainage patterns.

The endovascular results indicated that 13 patients (68%) had no shunts. There were no deaths. Complications occurred in six patients: four hemorrhagic and two ischemic complications. Morbidity remained in two patients (10.5%) with hemorrhagic complications. PFs of TdAVFs can sometimes extend to the subdural space to the shunts and may be involved in severe hemorrhagic complications of curative endovascular treatment using Onyx. Cases 1 and 3 were performed using both TAE and TVE [41]. In Case 1, TVE was performed toward the shunt from the draining vein, which was embolized with coils, and glue was injected through a microcatheter that had been inserted at the MMA. In Case 1, the shunt disappeared without any particular complications. In Case 2, the patient had acute hydrocephalus due to cerebellar hemorrhage, and a decompressive craniotomy was performed promptly after TAE. All patients were treated initially by transarterial embolization using liquid embolic agents. Both transarterial [42, 43] and transvenous [41] approaches using liquid embolic agents have been described for the successful treatment of TdAVFs [44]. Hemorrhagic complications during TAE occur often in patients with aDS [45]. In Case 3, extravascular leakage occurred during the infusion of the embolizing material from the aDS. In addition, if reflux during glue embolization occurs from the aDS, it may flow into P1 and results in serious ischemic complications. On the other hand, in their study, Bhatia et al. [46] reported that using a modified pressure-cooker technique, a highly distal position was achieved with the microcatheter, allowing deposition of small coils to minimize reflux, followed by the administration of Onyx directly to the fistulous point. Injection of a liquid embolic agent from aDS might increase the risk of reflux into the PCA and basilar artery. In this condition, the patient would be subsequently cured by TVA [47]. When conflict flow and a high likelihood of pial supply from the SCA or PCA to a Galenic-type tentorial AVF occur, there seems to be potential difficulties in identifying the aDS supply.

Microneurosurgery is also an important treatment option. Most TdAVFs carry a high risk of hemorrhage, and endovascular approaches can be challenging. Thus, some cases may require microsurgical disconnection [34, 48]. In principle, the operative strategy is based on an optimal surgical approach with an ideally adapted patient position that allows for gravity to retract the brain and interrupt the draining vein. It is reasonable to assume that most fistulas in this location have a potential aDS supply. Therefore, care should be taken to assess the aDS supply using 3D rotational angiography (Fig. 13.2b).

Again, we discuss the venous system in the next chapter. It is regarding the BV and the emissary vein (EV). It should be mentioned that the strict usage of the terms that describe the veins avoids mixing the two structures (BVs and EVs). The way to understand the difference between BVs and EVs is to consider them from the viewpoint of embryology, anatomy, and their functions. For example, in the spinal cord, the venous sinus is not present, therefore it is described anatomically correctly in the term of *bridging–emissary vein*.

13.5 The BVs and the EVs

13.5.1 BV

The BV is derived from the intracranial primitive pial-arachnoid vein and connects the pial veins to the dural sinus or venous plexus. The EV, on the other hands, represents the remaining connections between the superficial venous system and the dural venous system. The venous system of the head is subdivided into the superficial system, which corresponds to the outer skin and soft tissue, the dural system, which lies between the dura mater and bone, and the brain system. [49]. More recent publications indicated some major BVs in unique locations with regard to their relations with the sinuses from an anatomic perspectives [50–53]. All BVs and EVs, regardless of location and group, represent a common anatomic and functional characteristic; that is, both of BVs and EVS can be basically involved in dAVF with direct cortical venous drainage [27]. The sinus occlusion by thrombosis and consequences of BVs and EVs blockade (either as a part of the pathogenesis or as a consequence of the disease) apparently may change this original pathologic tendency of the normal anatomic disposition.

13.5.2 BV Related to TdAVF

Before discussing the details of the pathogenesis of venous reflux, we describe the BV and EV involved in the pathogenesis of TdAVF. Venous reflux determines everything. Here is a brief description of the anatomy of BV and EV structures.

13.5.2.1 Superior Tentorial BVs

This group, in particular, is conventionally referred to as the "lateral type" and belongs to the cerebral BVs, which drain the lateral aspect of the temporal lobe and the basal posterior surface of the temporal and occipital lobes directly either to the upper aspect to the lateral side, to the TS [54], or to the superior petrosal sinuses. A mean numbers of eight BVs per side drain into the transverse sinus [55]. Sakata et al. [56] reported the presence of the temporal BVs, and on the basis of their definitions, they found a transverse sinus exit in 52% of cases, a tentorial exit in 23%, and a petrosal exit in 25%. The tentorial sinuses can drain into the straight, torcular, transverse, or superior petrosal sinus [38] or if more than one sinus present, functioning also as an anastomotic channel.

13.5.2.2 Petrosal BVs or Anterior Metencephalic Group

The tributaries of the superior petrosal vein, namely, the vein of the great horizontal fissure, the brachial vein, the vein of the lateral recess of the fourth ventricle, the lateral pontine vein, and the transverse pontine vein, all of which drain the anterior brain stem and cerebellum, empty into the superior petrosal sinus. In some cases, these tributaries may form separated bridging stems, which drain independently into the superior petrosal sinus [57]. Kiyosue et al. [58] identified a BV connecting the transverse pontine vein to the posterior aspect of the cavernous sinus in 94% of their cases and bilaterally in half of them.

13.5.2.3 Falcine BVs

The veins from the cingulate gyrus and corpus callosum drain into the inferior sagittal sinus through the anterior pericallosal veins as well as the parahippocampal, paraolfactory, and paraterminal gyri; uncus; and anterior part of the calcarine fissure. Also related is the deep venous system (striatal, diencephalic, and choroidal veins) to the straight sinus through the internal cerebral, basal, and great veins. The basal vein is the result of secondary longitudinal and creating horizontal anastomoses from the deep telencephalic vein, ventral diencephalic vein, mesencephalic vein, and superior mesencephalic tributary of the vein of Galen [59] after the elongation and attenuation of the TS due to the posterior expansion of the cerebral hemispheres (as well as from the dorsal diencephalic tributary of the internal cerebral vein), for instance, opening the basal vein into the anterior, middle, or posterior portion of the SS or into the transverse sinus [59, 60] either directly or indirectly via a TS. BVs from the basal vein or the peduncular vein to a sinus coursing in the tentorial edge or to the CS have also been described.

13.5.2.4 Galenic or Superior Group of the Posterior Fossa

This group of veins constitutes the group conventionally referred to as the “marginal type.” These veins exist in close proximity to the surrounding tentorium and falx cerebri and cerebelli. This group belongs to the mesencephalic tributaries, which may join the basal vein, petrosal vein, transverse pontine vein, and precentral vein. However, they do not typically open directly into a specific mesencephalic BV. Rather than reflux directly into a vein, reflux occurs through a shunt such as a tent or falx.

13.5.2.5 Inferior Tentorial BVs or Dorsal Metencephalic Group

This group belongs to the inferior vermian veins and the superior and inferior lateral hemispheric cerebellar veins. The inferior vermian BVs with their tributaries run posterosuperiorly in the paravermian fissure and empty into the SS, torcular sinus, or transverse sinus either directly or indirectly through a TS. Choroidal veins can drain the plexus of the fourth ventricle into the occipital dural plexus [61].

13.5.3 EVs

The cranial nerves that cross the cranial skull apertures (except for the VIII nerve) are accompanied by at least one small EV. The exception is the facial and olfactory nerves, whose accompanying veins do not fulfill the criteria of typical EVs according to the above definition because of the lack of connection with a sinus. The following EVs may be involved in TdAVF.

1. The occipital and mastoid EV can be connected to either the torcular, transverse, or occipital sinus [62, 63].
2. A temporal EV may connect the remnant of the petrosquamosal sinus with the deep temporal vein. The EV of the middle fossa passes through the foramen ovale, rotundum, lacerum, Arnold, and vesalius foramen. **Arnold’s**

nerve is the eponymous name of the **auricular branch**, also known as the **mastoid branch**, of the vagus nerve (CN X). Vesalius foramen is observed in approximately 20% of cases, with the emissary sphenoidal foramen anterior to the medial aspect of the foramen ovale [64].

13.6 Concept of "Directness, Exclusiveness, and Strain" [65]

13.6.1 General Considerations

Although a shunt located on a BV is related to be directly involved in the cortical veins for drainage, on the other hands, a shunt involving primarily an EV is expected to drain mostly to the sinus and not directly to the cortical venous system. The most common of these is the fistula involving a BV that has lost its connection to the parent sinus into which it previously drained. This is characterized by an feeders networks accumulating onto the wall of a BV with CVR. The onset of CVD has often been associated with venous outflow restrictions (VOR). Because of partial or complete thrombosis or stenosis of the involved venous sinus, high-flow shunt, and the location of the lesion in relation to the cranial epidural spaces can be occurred.

The Borden and Cognard classification systems for predicting the clinical behavior of cranial dural arteriovenous shunts focus on venous drainage, particularly the presence of CVD, and on the direction of flow, particularly the presence of retrograde flow. The concept of "directness, exclusiveness, and strain" was proposed by Baltsavias et al. [65]. These authors stated that the terms *direct* and *exclusive* CVD are often used without discrimination to describe the concept of exclusivity [30, 32] or not used at all [17]. A direct CVD was defined by venous drainage that used the BVs without intervening of any sinus. In these cases, the exact location of the shunt was the BV. A nondirect CVD was defined by venous drainage that used the BVs but with the interposition of a sinus, implying that the shunt was primarily or solely located in the wall of the sinus. An exclusive CVD was defined as venous drainage by only the BVs, with its exit to the sinus occluded or because the only exit of the sinus was through the BVs to the leptomeningeal venous system. A nonexclusive CVD was defined by drainage that occurred both by cortical veins and by the venous sinuses, dural veins, or EV. The term *strain* indicates that the CVD shows clear signs of ectasia, congestion, or both, with clear signs of strain. The presence of VE or a congestive pseudophlebitic appearance was recorded as cortical venous strain. All BV shunts had a direct CVD.

Almost all BV shunts and all "isolated" sinus shunts had an exclusive CVD. Venous strain, manifested as ectasia and/or congestion, denotes the decompensation of the cerebral venous system due to the shunt reflux.

13.7 Conclusions

13.7.1 Locations of the Shunt of TdAVF

We considered the angioarchitecture of the shunt locations, including the pattern of arterial feeders, relation with the BVs, primary venous drainage, and VOR. The development of CVD has often been associated with VOR because of partial or complete thrombosis or stenosis of the involved venous sinus, high-flow shunt, and the location of the lesion in relation to the cranial epidural spaces. The great majority of these shunts present thrombotic phenomena. The exact location of the shunt with regard to the BVs is a key factor in the development of CVD [66]. The main angioarchitectural feature of the [30] Borden type 2 shunts with mixed sinusal–CVD was the presence of a diffuse arterial network of vessels converging onto a site in the wall of the dural sinus, with CVR following the opacification of the sinus. In particular, we differentiated the dAVF primarily located in the wall of a sinus from that located primarily in the wall of a BV, which normally drains into the sinus [67]. The most common was the fistula engaging a BV that had lost its connection to the parent sinus into which it previously drained. The other patterns were those of an "isolated" sinus segment characterized by arterial feeders converging onto the wall of the dural sinus with CVD following the opacification of the sinus. As a rule, the draining BVs varied in distance from the shunt site, and the sinus was opacified prior to the BVs.

On the basis of the above considerations, the following four points are important when considering the classification of TdAVF:

1. Presence of VE
2. Sinus obstruction
3. Involvement of pial feeders
4. Locations of the shunts (falx cerebelli, torcular, petrotentorial, and marginal)

The presence of VE cannot be ignored in relation to clinical symptoms. Furthermore, it is important to carefully consider both BV and EV reflux. The presence or absence of venous sinus obstruction is important in the determination of lesion progression. Although the presence of PFs has been considered rare, it can occur by a variety of routes and requires careful management. These four points should be kept in mind in the endovascular treatment for TdAVF, and each category should be analyzed carefully.

Disclosure None of the authors declared any conflict of interest.

References

1. Kuwayama N. Epidemiologic survey of dural arteriovenous fistulas in Japan: clinical frequency and present status of treatment. Acta Neurochir. 2016;123:188. https://doi.org/10.1007/978-3-319-29887-0_26.
2. Hiramatsu M, Sugiu K, Hishikawa T, et al. Epidemiology of dural arteriovenous fistula in Japan: analysis of Japanese Registry of Neuroendovascular therapy (JR-NET2). Neurol Med Chir (Tokyo). 2014;54:63–71.
3. Hacein-Bey L, Konstas AA, Pile-Spellman J. Natural history, current concepts, classification, factors impacting endovascular therapy, and pathophysiology of cerebral and spinal dural arteriovenous fistulas. Clin Neurol Neurosurg. 2014;121:64–75.
4. Awad IA, Little JR, Akarawi WP, et al. Intracranial dural arteriovenous malformations: factors predisposing to an aggressive neurological course. J Neurosurg. 1990;72:839–50.
5. Cannizzaro D, Brinjikji W, Rammos S, et al. Changing clinical and therapeutic trends in tentorial dural arteriovenous fistulas: a systematic review. AJNR Am J Neuroradiol. 2015;36:1905–11.
6. Zhou LF, Chen L, Song DL, et al. Tentorial dural arteriovenous fistulas. Surg Neurol. 2007;67:472–82.
7. Benndorf G, Schmidt S, Sollmann WP, et al. Tentorial dural arteriovenous fistula presenting with various visual symptoms related to anterior and posterior visual pathway dysfunction: case report. Neurosurgery. 2003;53:222–7.
8. Rahme R, Ali Y, Slaba S, et al. Dural arteriovenous malformation: an unusual cause of trigeminal neuralgia. Acta Neurochir (Wien). 2007;149:937–41.
9. Khan S, Polston DW, Shield W Jr, et al. Tentorial dural arteriovenous fistula presenting with quadriparesis: case report and review of the literature. J Stroke CVD. 2009;18:428–34.
10. Ito M, Sonokawa T, Mishina H, et al. Dural arteriovenous malformation manifesting as tic douloureux. Surg Neurol. 1996;45:370–5.
11. Jiang L, Qi M, Ye M, et al. Recurrent secondary trigeminal neuralgia caused by obliterated tentorial dural arteriovenous fistula cured with surgical resection: case report and literature review. World Neurosurg. 2019;121:243–8.
12. Lu X, Qin X, Ni L, et al. Tentorial dural arteriovenous fistula manifesting as contralateral trigeminal neuralgia: resolution after transarterial onyx embolization. BMJ Case Rep. 2013;2013:1–4.
13. Akhaddar A, Gazzaz M, Elmostarchid B, et al. Trigeminal neuralgia and dural arteriovenous fistula in an edentulous man. Headache. 2010;50:861–2.
14. Ge H, Lv X, Jin H, et al. Role of endovascular embolization for trigeminal neuralgia related to cerebral vascular malformation. Interv Neuroradiol. 2016;22:600–5.
15. Holekamp TF, Mollman ME, Murphy RKJ, et al. Dural arteriovenous fistula-induced thalamic dementia: report of 4 cases. J Neurosurg. 2016;124:1752–65.
16. Kashiwagi H, Matsubara N, Ikeda N, et al. Tentorial dural arteriovenous fistula with bithalamic lesions and bilateral basal ganglia hemorrhage: a case report (JPN). No Shinkei Geka. 2019;47:1247–54. https://doi.org/10.11477/mf.1436204111.
17. Zipfel GJ, Shah MN, Refai D, et al. Cranial dural arteriovenous fistulas: modification of angiographic classification scales based on new natural history data. Neurosurg Focus. 2009;26:E14.
18. Ryu B, Sato S, Mochizuki T, et al. Relative signal intensity on time-of-flight magnetic resonance angiography as a novel indicator of aggressive presentation of intracranial dural arteriovenous fistulas. J Cerebral Blood Flow Metab. 2021;41:1428–36.
19. Brown RD Jr, Wiebers DO, Nichols DA. Intracranial dural arteriovenous fistulae: angiographic predictors of intracranial hemorrhage and clinical outcome in nonsurgical patients. J Neurosurg. 1994;81:531–8.

20. Bulters DO, Mathad N, Culliford D, et al. The natural history of cranial dural arteriovenous fistulae with cortical venous reflux—the significance of venous ectasia. Neurosurgery. 2012;70:312–8; discussion 318–9.
21. Duffau H, Lopes M, Janosevic V, et al. Early rebleeding from intracranial dural arteriovenous fistulas: report of 20 cases and review of the literature. J Neurosurg. 1999;90:78–84.
22. Jolink WM, van Dijk JM, van Asch CJ, et al. Outcome after intracranial haemorrhage from dural arteriovenous fistulae; a systematic review and case-series. J Neurol. 2015;262:2678–83.
23. Satomi J, Ghaibeh AA, Moriguchi H, et al. Predictability of the future development of aggressive behavior of cranial dural arteriovenous fistulas based on decision tree analysis. J Neurosurg. 2015;123:86–90.
24. Singh V, Smith WS, Lawton MT, et al. Risk factors for hemorrhagic presentation in patients with dural arteriovenous fistulae. Neurosurgery. 2008;62:628–35; discussion 628.
25. Zhao LB, Suh DC, Lee DG, et al. Association of pial venous reflux with hemorrhage or edema in dural arteriovenous fistula. Neurology. 2014;82:1897–904.
26. Choi JH, Jo KI, Kim KH, et al. Early rebleeding of intracranial dural arteriovenous fistulas after an intracranial hemorrhage. Acta Neurochir. 2017;159:1479–87.
27. Duvernoy HM. Vascularization of the cerebral cortex. Rev Neurol (Paris). 1999;155:684–7.
28. Duvernoy HM, Delon S, Vannson JL. Cortical blood vessels of the human brain. Brain Res Bull. 1981;7:519–79.
29. Daniels DJ, Vellimana AK, Zipfel GJ, et al. Intracranial hemorrhage from dural arteriovenous fistulas: clinical features and outcome. Neurosurg Focus. 2013;34:E15.
30. Borden JA, Wu JK, Shucart WA. A proposed classification for spinal and cranial dural arteriovenous fistulous malformations and implications for treatment. J Neurosurg. 1995;82:166–79.
31. Cognard C, Gobin YP, Pierot L, et al. Cerebral dural arteriovenous fistulas: clinical and angiographic correlation with a revised classification of venous drainage. Radiology. 1995;194:671–80.
32. Davies MA, TerBrugge K, Willinsky R, et al. The validity of classification for the clinical presentation of intracranial dural arteriovenous fistulas. J Neurosurg. 1996;85:830–7. https://doi.org/10.3171/jns.1996.85.5.0830.
33. Picard L, Bracard S, Islak C, et al. Dural fistulae of the tentorium cerebelli: radioanatomical, clinical and therapeutic considerations. J Neuroradiol. 1990;17:161–81.
34. Lawton MT, Sanchez-Mejia RO, Pham D, et al. Tentorial dural arteriovenous fistulae: operative strategies and microsurgical results for six types. Neurosurgery. 2008;62:110–24.
35. Byrne JV, Garcia M. Tentorial dural fistulas: endovascular management and description of the medial dural-tentorial branch of the superior cerebellar artery. AJNR Am J Neuroradiol. 2013;34:1798–804.
36. Wollschlaeger PB, Wollschlaeger G. An infrantentorial meningeal artery [in German]. Radiologe. 1965;5:451–2.
37. Osada T, Krings T. Intracranial dural arteriovenous fistulas with pial arterial supply. Neurosurgery. 2019;84:104–15.
38. Matsushima T, Suzuki SO, Fukui M, et al. Microsurgery anatomy of the tentorial sinuses. J Neurosurg. 1989;71:923–8.
39. Geibprasert S, Pereira V, Krings T, et al. Dural arteriovenous shunts: a new classification of craniospinal epidural venous anatomical bases and clinical correlations. Stroke. 2008;39:2783–94.
40. Tanaka M. Embryological consideration of dural arteriovenous fistulas. Neurol Med Chir (Tokyo). 2016;56:544–51.
41. Beer-Furlan A, Dasenbrock HH, Joshi KC, et al. Transarterial and transvenous approaches for embolization of tentorial dural arteriovenous fistula. Neurosurg Focus. 2019;46:V10.
42. Puri AS. Dural arteriovenous fistula supplied by the artery of Davidoff and Schechter. Radiol Case Rep. 2010;5:375.
43. Choudhri O, Marks MP. Endovascular treatment of a tentorial dural arteriovenous fistula. Neurosurg Focus. 2014;37:1.
44. Gioppo A, Farago G, Caldiera V, et al. Medial tentorial dural arteriovenous fistula embolization: single experience with embolic liquid polymer SQUID and review of the literature. World Neurosurg. 2017;107:1050.e1–57.
45. Sato K, Matsumoto Y, Endo H, Tominaga T. A hemorrhagic complication after Onyx embolization of a tentorial dural arteriovenous fistula: a caution about subdural extension with pial artery supply. Interv Neuroradiol. 2017;23:307–12.
46. Bhatia KD, Kortman H, Wälchli T, et al. Artery of Davidoff and Schechter supply in dural arteriovenous fistulas. AJNR Am J Neuroradiol. 2020;41:300–4. https://doi.org/10.3174/ajnr.A6380.
47. Chu CL, Chu YC, Lam CT, et al. Endovascular treatment of medial tentorial dural arteriovenous fistula through the dural branch of the pial artery. Front Neurol. 2021;12:736919. https://doi.org/10.3389/fneur.2021.736919.
48. Radovanovic I, Wallace M. Cranial dural arteriovenous fistula disconnection. In: Jandial R, McCormick P, Black P, editors. Core techniques in operative neurosurgery. Philadelphia: Elsevier; 2019.
49. Baltsavias G, Parthasarathi V, Aydin E, et al. Cranial dural arteriovenous shunts. Part 1. Anatomy and embryology of the bridging and emissary veins. Neurosurg Rev. 2015;38:253–63; discussion 263.
50. Dagain A, Vignes JR, Dulou R, et al. Junction between the great cerebral vein and the straight sinus: an ana-

tomical, immunohistochemical and ultrastructural study on 25 human brain cadaveric dissections. Clin Anat. 2008;21:389–97.
51. Dagain A, Vignes R, Dulou R, et al. Study of the junction between the cortical bridging veins and basal cranial venous sinus. Neurochirurgie. 2009;55:19–24. https://doi.org/10.1016/j.neuchi.2008.10.011.
52. Han H, Tao W, Zhang M. The dural entrance of cerebral bridging veins into the superior sagittal sinus: an anatomical comparison between cadavers and digital subtraction angiography. Neuroradiology. 2007;49:169–75. https://doi.org/10.1007/s00234-006-0175-z.
53. Vignes JR, Dagain A, Guérin J, et al. A hypothesis of cerebral venous system regulation based on a study of the junction between the cortical bridging veins and the superior sagittal sinus. laboratory investigation. J Neurosurg. 2007;107:1205–10. https://doi.org/10.3171/JNS-07/12/1205.
54. Gibbs E, Gibbs FA. The cross section areas of the vessels that form the torcular and the manner in which flow is distributed to the right and to the left lateral sinus. Anat Rec. 1934;59:419–26.
55. Han H, Yao Z, Wang H, et al. Dural entrance of the bridging vein into the transverse sinus provides a reliable measure for preoperative planning: an anatomic comparison between cadavers and neuroimages. Neurosurgery. 2008;62(Suppl 2):ONS289–95. https://doi.org/10.1227/01.neu.0000326009.46197.ab.
56. Sakata K, Al-Mefty O, Yamamoto I. Venous consideration in petrosal approach: microsurgical anatomy of the temporal bridging vein. Neurosurgery. 2000;47:153–60; discussion 160–1.
57. Tanriover N, Abe H, Rhoton AL Jr, et al. Microsurgical anatomy of the superior petrosal venous complex: new classifications and implications for subtemporal transtentorial and retrosigmoid suprameatal approaches. J Neurosurg. 2007;106:1041–50.
58. Kiyosue H, Tanoue S, Sagara Y, et al. The anterior medullary-anterior pontomesencephalic venous system and its bridging veins communicating to the dural sinuses: normal anatomy and drainage routes from dural arteriovenous fistulas. Neuroradiology. 2008;50:1013–23. https://doi.org/10.1007/s00234-008-0433-3.
59. Salamon G, Huang YP. Radiologic anatomy of the brain. New York: Springer; 1976.
60. Padget D. The cranial venous system in man in reference to development, adult configuration, and relation to the arteries. Am J Anat. 1956;98:307–55.
61. De Miquel MA, Mateu JMD, Cusi V, et al. Embryogenesis of the veins of the posterior fossa: an overview. In: As H, editor. Surgery of the intracranial venous system: embryology, anatomy, pathophysiology, neuroradiology, diagnosis, treatment. London: Springer; 1996. p. 14–25.
62. San Millan Ruiz D, Gailloud P, Rufenacht DA, et al. The craniocervical venous system in relation to cerebral venous drainage. AJNR Am J Neuroradiol. 2002;23:1500–8.
63. Matsushima K, Kawashima M, Matsushima T, et al. Posterior condylar canals and posterior condylar emissary veins-a microsurgical and CT anatomical study. Neurosurg Rev. 2014;37:115–26. https://doi.org/10.1007/s10143-013-0493-7.
64. Lasjaunias P, Berenstein A, ter Brugge K. Surgical neuroangiography: clinical vascular anatomy and variations, vol. 1. 2nd ed. Berlin: Springer; 2001, P649, Table 7.3.
65. Baltsavias G, Peter R, Valavanis A. Cranial dural arteriovenous shunts. Part 3. Classification based on the leptomeningeal venous drainage. Neurosurg Rev. 2015;38:273–81.
66. Baltsavias G, Kumar R, Aydin E, et al. Cranial dural arteriovenous shunts. Part 2. The shunts of the bridging veins and leptomenindeal venous drainage. Neurosurg Rev. 2015;38:265–72.
67. Gaston A, Chiras J, Bourbotte G, et al. Meningeal arteriovenous fistulae draining into cortical veins. 31 cases. J Neuroradiol. 1984;11:161–77.

Dural Arteriovenous Fistula in Moyamoya Angiopathy

14

Shambaditya Das, Souvik Dubey, and Biman Kanti Ray

Abstract

Moyamoya angiopathy (MMA) is an idiopathic, progressive intracranial occlusive vasculopathy leading to formation of abnormal vascular network of collaterals. Dural arteriovenous fistula (DAVF) has been rarely reported to co-exist with MMA. A paucity of literature has limited the elucidation of the pathophysiological association between the two conditions. It may be hypothesized that a chronic cerebral ischemic state in MMA and subsequent angiogenesis leading to the formation of collaterals might lead to the formation of DAVF. At present, there are no definite guidelines for treatment of DAVF in MMA. However, it may be reasonable to practice conservative management with close follow-up in case of asymptomatic DAVF or those without cerebral venous drainage, while high grade DAVF may be subjected to endovascular or open surgery to prevent future intracranial hemorrhage.

Keywords

Moyamoya angiopathy · Dural arteriovenous fistula · DAVF · Moyamoya disease Angiogenesis

S. Das (✉) · S. Dubey · B. K. Ray
Department of Neurology, Institute of Post Graduate Medical Education and Research, Bangur Institute of Neurosciences, Kolkata, India

14.1 Introduction

Moyamoya angiopathy (MMA) is a chronic progressive occlusive intracranial vasculopathy characterized by angiographic findings of stenosis or occlusion at the terminal portion of the internal carotid artery (ICA) or proximal anterior cerebral artery (ACA) and/or middle cerebral artery (MCA) together with the abnormal vascular network (classically appears to be like "puff of smoke") at the base of the brain [1, 2]. It can present with wide array of transient and fixed neurological manifestations and is a frequently overlooked cause of stroke [3–5]. MMA has been reported with various vascular malformations like intracranial aneurysms, arterio-venous malformations and primitive carotid-basilar anastomosis. Dural arteriovenous fistula (DAVF) is intra-cranial condition characterized by abnormal connections between meningeal arteries and dural venous sinuses, meningeal veins or cortical veins [6]. Both MMA and DAVF have extremely rare occurrence and their co-existence have only been uncommonly reported [6–12].

14.2 Pathophysiology

The pathogenesis of MMA is yet to be fully elucidated. Both genetic and inflammatory factors have been implicated. Adult DAVF is generally an acquired lesion [13–16]. Dural sinus thrombo-

X. Lv (ed.), *Intracranial and Spinal Dural Arteriovenous Fistulas*,
https://doi.org/10.1007/978-981-19-5767-3_14

sis or stenosis has been known play a pivotal role in the pathogenesis of DAVF. Besides, trauma, craniotomy or treatment of another DAVF has also been reported to be associated with formation of DAVF [6, 9].

Because the co-occurrence of MMA and DAVF is quite rare, a robust research related to the exact etio-pathogenetic connection between the two conditions is lacking. The proposed hypothesis is open-ended, wherein MMA can lead to the formation of DAVF and vice-versa [6, 12].

MMA is a chronic vaso-occlusive condition where a persistent cerebral ischemia is inevitable [1]. This contributes to release of pro-angiogenic factors like basic fibroblast growth factor (bFGF), vascular endothelial growth factor, transforming growth factor β-1, hepatocyte growth factor, intracellular adhesion molecules, matrix metalloproteinases and hypoxia-inducing factor 1α. It has been seen that this pro-angiogenic factors especially bFGF and vascular endothelial growth factor are elevated in the dura of both MMA and DAVF. It can be contemplated that this increased pro-angiogenic factors contribute to the angiogenesis, leading to formation of Moyamoya collaterals as well as formation of DAVF [6, 9–12].

Furthermore, cases of DAVF formation following revascularization surgery (especially extracranial-intracranial bypass) in MMA has been seen. It is not unusual that the cortical veins near the bypass graft may have intra-operative traumatic affection, thus, entertaining the possibility of an iatrogenic basis of DAVF in MMA [6, 9, 11]. Liu et al. [9] and Feroze et al. [11] described a similar situation wherein DAVF developed following the revascularization surgery for MMA.

As an extrapolation, it may also be postulated that MMA initiation and progression secondary to DAVF may occur as a consequence to increased turbulence proximal to DAVF, often in the distal ICA causing accentuated intimal hyperplasia and progressive occlusive changes of MMA [10, 12, 17]. While in three of the previously reported seven cases, MMA and DAVF were detected simultaneously, in rest four cases, DAVF was detected later to the diagnosis of MMA. Thus, the plausibility of the mechanism of chronic ischemia of MMA precluding the DAVF formation seems more [6–12].

Another theory suggests that head trauma, known to herald both DAVF and MMA, may lead to altered angiogenesis within the dura and subsequent sinus venous thrombosis and DAVF. This is supported by the case described by Zaletel et al., wherein DAVF and MMA were detected simultaneously following a history of head injury several years ago [12].

14.3 Management

MMA is a progressive disease with recurrent cerebrovascular events and progressive cognitive decline and merits revascularization surgery aimed at improving cerebral blood supply [1, 18]. There are no clear guidelines on the management of concomitant MMA and DAVF, and must be individualized depending on the clinical presentation and invasiveness [6]. While an asymptomatic DAVF and those without cortical venous drainage may be managed conservatively with a close follow-up, a high-grade DAVF should be managed aggressively through endovascular route or open surgery. DAVF with cortical venous drainage is a risk factor for future hemorrhagic events and deserves to be intervened (Fig. 14.1) [6]. Another consideration that the treating neurologist needs to be mindful of while intervening DAVF in the background of MMA with revascularization surgery is that the integrity of the bypass graft might get compromised during fistula disconnection by transarterial glue embolization or microsurgery [11]. While four of the seven reported cases underwent conservative management for DAVF [6, 8, 11, 12], three were intervened due to severe clinical symptomatology or higher Cognard classification, two of them underwent transvenous embolization and one underwent both transarterial and subsequent transvenous embolization [7, 9, 10].

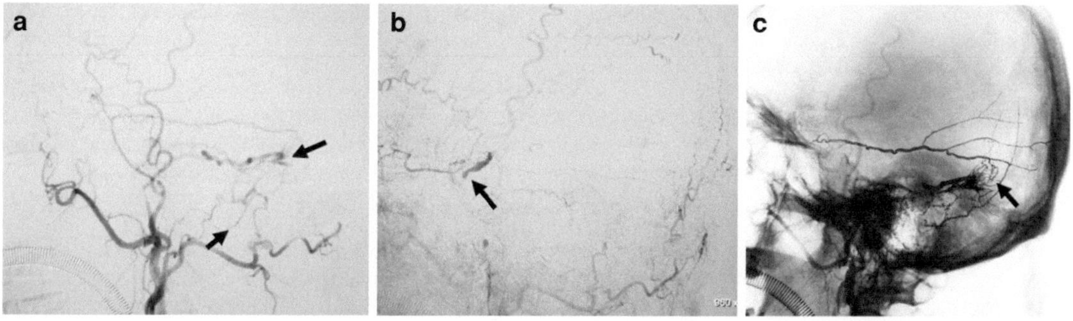

Fig. 14.1 A case of a Borden type-III and Cognard type-III DAVFs involving the transverse sinus co-existed with MMA (arrow in panel **a**). The shunt was obliterated with Onyx injection (arrows in panel **c**). (**a**) Preoperative the left external carotid angiogram. (**b**) Postoperative carotid angiogram showing the obliteration of the distal internal carotid artery and the proximal internal carotid artery was retrogradely filled from the ophthalmic artery (arrow). The DAVF was completely obliterated. (**c**) Postoperative craniogram showing the Onyx casts (arrow)

14.4 Conclusion

MMA can rarely be associated with DAVF during various stages of its disease course. Chronic cerebral ischemia and subsequent angiogenesis might be the missing link between the two conditions. Management of DAVF in the background greatly depends on the symptomatology and invasiveness.

Funding The authors did not receive any funding or sponsorship.

The manuscript has not been published in any preprint server.

Disclosure Dr. Shambaditya Das, (Prof.) Dr. Souvik Dubey, and (Prof.) Dr. Biman Kanti Ray have no disclosures to make.

Authorship Agreement Dr. Shambaditya Das take full responsibility for the data, the analyses and interpretation, and the conduct of the research. I have full access to all the data and have the right to publish any and all data, separate and apart from the guidance of any sponsor.

Conflict of Interest The authors have stated explicitly that there are no conflicts of interest in connection with this article.

References

1. Das DS, Dubey DS, Acharya DM, Ghosh DR, Chatterjee DS, Hazra PA, et al. The disease presentation of Moyamoya angiopathy in Eastern India. J Stroke Cerebrovasc Dis. 2020;29(8):104957.
2. Das S, Dubey S, Acharya M, Chatterjee S, Lahiri D, Das G, et al. Thalassemia and Moyamoya syndrome: unfurling an intriguing association. J Neurol. 2019;266(11):2838–47 [cited 2020 Aug 30]. Available from: https://pubmed.ncbi.nlm.nih.gov/31422456/.
3. Das S, Ray BK, Dubey S. Temporal lobe epilepsy with nocturnal wandering leading to discovery of Moyamoya angiopathy. Acta Neurol Belgica. 2021:1–3 [cited 2021 Dec 2]. Available from: https://link.springer.com/article/10.1007/s13760-021-01830-y.
4. Das S, Ghosh R, Dubey S, Pandit A, Ray BK, Kraemer M. Limb-shaking TIA in Moyamoya angiopathy. Clin Neurol Neurosurg. 2021;207:106783 [cited 2021 Jul 5]. Available from: https://linkinghub.elsevier.com/retrieve/pii/S0303846721003127.
5. Dubey S, Ghosh R, Chatterjee S, Dubey MJ, Ray BK, Das S, et al. Spicy foods triggering clinical symptoms in Moyamoya angiopathy. J Neurosurg Sci. 2021;65(1):85–88 [cited 2021 Mar 18]. Available from: https://pubmed.ncbi.nlm.nih.gov/32550609/.
6. Hou K, Zhao Y, Chen X, Xu K, Yu J. Moyamoya disease concurrent with dural arteriovenous fistula: a case report and literature review. Exp Ther Med. 2020;20(6):161 [cited 2022 Jan 17]. Available from: https://www.ncbi.nlm.nih.gov/pmc/articles/PMC7571339/.
7. Killory BD, Gonzalez LF, Wait SD, Ponce FA, Albuquerque FC, Spetzler RF. Simultaneous unilateral moyamoya disease and ipsilateral dural arteriovenous fistula: case report. Neurosurgery. 2008;62(6):E1375–6 [cited 2022 Jan 17]. Available from: https://pubmed.ncbi.nlm.nih.gov/18824958/.
8. Koduri S, Andrew Wilkinson D, Griauzde JM, Gemmete JJ, Maher CO. Development of bilateral dural arteriovenous fistulae following pial synangiosis for moyamoya syndrome: case report. J Neurosurg Pediatr. 2019;24(1):9–13.
9. Liu AF, Li C, Yu W, Lin LM, Qiu HC, Zhang YQ, Lv XL, Wang K, Liu C, Jiang WJ. Dissection-related

carotid-cavernous fistula (CCF) following surgical revascularization of chronic internal carotid artery occlusion: a new subtype of CCF and proposed management. Chin Neurosurg J. 2020;6:2.
10. Liu P, Xu Y, Lv X, Ge H, Lv M, Li Y. Progression of unilateral moyamoya disease resulted in spontaneous occlusion of ipsilateral cavernous dural arteriovenous fistula: case report. Interv Neuroradiol. 2016;22(3):362–4.
11. Feroze AH, Kushkuley J, Choudhri O, Heit JJ, Steinberg GK, Do HM. Development of arteriovenous fistula after revascularization bypass for moyamoya disease: case report. Oper Neurosurg. 2015;11(1):E202–6.
12. Zaletel M, Surlan-Popović K, Pretnar-Oblak J, Žvan B. Moyamoya syndrome with arteriovenous dural fistula after head trauma. Acta Clin Croatica. 2011;50:115–20 [cited 2022 Jan 17]. Available from: https://pubmed.ncbi.nlm.nih.gov/22034792/.
13. Das S, Ray BK, Ghosh R, Sengupta S, Pandit A, Dubey S. Impact of COVID-19 pandemic in natural course of Moyamoya angiopathy: an experience from tertiary-care-center in India. Egypt J Neurol Psychiatry Neurosurg. 2021;57(1):1–6. Available from: https://ejnpn.springeropen.com/articles/10.1186/s41983-021-00412-2.
14. Das S, Dubey S, Pandit A, Ray BK. Moyamoya angiopathy unmasking systemic lupus erythematosus. BMJ Case Rep. 2021;14(1):e239307 [cited 2021 Jul 5]. Available from: https://casereports.bmj.com/content/14/1/e239307.
15. Mikami T, Suzuki H, Komatsu K, Mikuni N. Influence of inflammatory disease on the pathophysiology of moyamoya disease and quasi-moyamoya disease. Neurol Med Chir (Tokyo). 2019;59(10):361 [cited 2021 Jul 30]. Available from: https://www.ncbi.nlm.nih.gov/pmc/articles/PMC6796064/.
16. Kim JS. Moyamoya disease: epidemiology, clinical features, and diagnosis. J Stroke. 2016;18(1):2–11 [cited 2021 Dec 16]. Available from: https://pubmed.ncbi.nlm.nih.gov/26846755/.
17. Mawad ME, Hilal SK, Michelsen WJ, Stein B, Ganti SR. Occlusive vascular disease associated with cerebral arteriovenous malformations. Radiology. 1984;153(2):401–8 [cited 2022 Jan 17]. https://doi.org/10.1148/radiology15326484172. Available from: https://pubs.rsna.org/doi/abs/10.1148/radiology.153.2.6484172.
18. Mikami T, Suzuki H, Komatsu K, Mikuni N. Influence of inflammatory disease on the pathophysiology of moyamoya disease and quasi-moyamoya disease. Neurol Med Chir (Tokyo). 2019;59(10):1–10 [cited 2020 Aug 30]. Available from: https://www.ncbi.nlm.nih.gov/pmc/articles/PMC6796064/.

Spinal Dural Arteriovenous Shunts 15

Sirintara (Pongpech) Singhara Na Ayudhaya

Abstract

Spinal dural arteriovenous shunt (SDAVS) is the most common vascular shunt of the spine. SDAVS occurs predominantly in men (more than 80% patients), commonly involves the thoracolumbar spine, and usually causes progressive myelopathy because of venous hypertension of the spinal cord. Recent advances in imaging technology can visualize the detailed angioarchitecture of the SDAVS, and provide more information of the regional microanatomy related with the SDAVS. Based on these data, classifications for SDAVSs was reviewed. Endovascular embolization is an increasingly effective therapy in the treatment of SDAVSs, and can be used as a definitive intervention in the majority of patients. As surgery is required for refractory cases or those not amenable to embolization, a multidisciplinary approach to the treatment of these lesions is required.

Keywords

Spinal dural arteriovenous shunt
Classification · Presentation · Treatment

S. (P). S. Na. Ayudhaya (✉)
Radiology (INR), Mahidol University,
Bangkok, Thailand

Abbreviations

AK	Artery of Adamkiewicz
ASA	Anterior SPINAL Artery
NBCA	*N*-butyl cyanoacrylate
PSA	Posterior spinal artery
RM	Radioculomedullary artery
RP	Radiculopial artery
SAVS	Spinal arteriovenous shunt(s)
SDAVF/SDAVM	Spinal dural arterio-venous fistula/malformation
SDAVS	Spinal dural arterio-venous shunt(s)
Th	Thoracic

15.1 Introduction

Spinal dural arteriovenous shunt (SDAVS) is acquired arteriovenous shunt located within or adjacent to dura along the spinal canal. It is an abnormal arteriovenous shunt in the dura, most commonly at the thoracolumbar level [1–3].

They are the most frequent spinal arteriovenous shunt (AVS) and frequently occur in older adults. They usually present with an 85% (male:female = 5:1) male predominance after the fourth or fifth decade of life. The locations of the SDAVS have been reported throughout the spinal canal, from the foramen magnum to the level of the sacrum. The venous drainage can be very extensive and reach the intracranial veins even if the SDAVS

X. Lv (ed.), *Intracranial and Spinal Dural Arteriovenous Fistulas*,
https://doi.org/10.1007/978-981-19-5767-3_15

is at the sacral level or conversely reach the thoracic perimedullary venous plexus level from an intracranial dural arteriovenous shunt.

The arterial supply of SDAVSs mostly arises from a dural (radicular) branch of the dorsospinal artery in the region of the intervertebral foramen. The spinal cord veins pierce the dura at the nerve roots. In this venous disposition, a potential radicular arterial supply to the SDAVS can be demonstrated. There is a single extradural arterial pedicle that gives rise to a small SDAVS that is within the dura itself in the great majority of patients. A single highly tortuous draining vein emerges from this SDAVS. This vein pierces the dura several millimeters from the accompanying nerve root (either above or below it) to reach the perimedullary venous system and then produces venous congestion of the medullary veins [1, 2, 4, 5].

Advances in noninvasive imaging contribute greatly to establish the timely diagnosis of SDAVSs. The plain films, myelography, and computed tomography have been taken over by MR imaging (MRI), which can reliably demonstrate the presence of signal changes within the cord, signifying the imaging equivalent of the clinical symptomatology. The non-specific slight enhancement following intravenous contrast administration and the absence of significant mass effect favor the non-neoplastic or non-demyelinating cause of these MRI findings [6–8]. Abnormal flow voids can be demonstrated additionally, representing the prominent perimedullary venous plexus associated with the retrograde venous flow from the SDAVS. These findings on MR imagings are non-specific for the actual location of the SDAVS, but are highly specific for their impact. Epidural, dural, and perimedullary AVSs may all have similar MRI findings. Therefore, their clinical symptoms may be similar and angiography is necessary to separate out these different etiologies and confirm the exact location of the AVS. Improvements in MRI and MRA techniques have resulted in the high sensitivity and specificity to demonstrate the actual location of the AVS along the dura noninvasively, which will help to focus the spinal angiogram on a specific segmental level, decreasing time for diagnostic spinal angiogram and helping treatment planning more accurately [6, 9, 10].

15.2 Classification of the SDAVSs (Fig. 15.1, Tables 15.1 and 15.2) [1, 2]

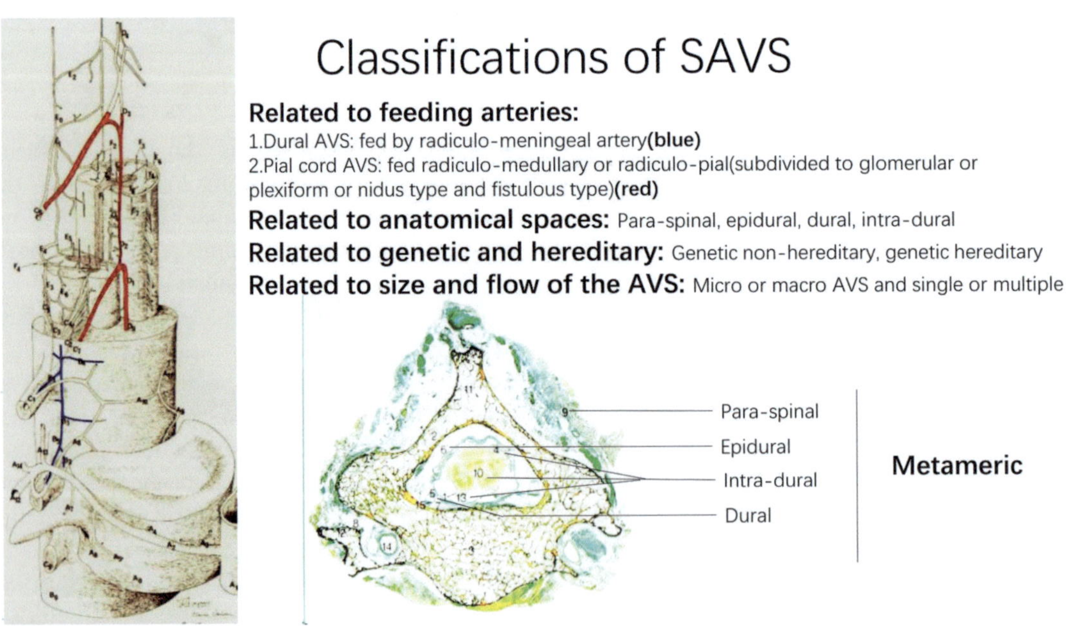

Fig. 15.1 Drawing and picture from Surgical Neuroangiography vol. 1 (Lasjaunias et al) [1] with permission

Table 15.1 Classification of spinal vascular lesions following anatomical spaces [1, 11]

Types	Descriptions	Associated diseases
Parachordal arteriovenous shunts	Spinal extradural and paraspinal arteriovenous shunts Isolated (VVF and other locations)	Systematized dysplasia, von Recklinghausen's
Spinal dural arteriovenous shunts	Isolated or multiple	None
Spinal cord vascular malformation	Perimedullary/superficial/deep location; isolated or multiple arteriovenous malformation, arteriovenous shunt	None
Spinal Arteriovenous Metameric Syndrome (SAMS)	Cobb and other syndromes-SAMS	Rendu-Osler-Weber and Klippel-Trenaunay syndromes and others (spinal cord telangiectasias)
Cavernous vascular malformations	Cavernomas	None

Table 15.2 Incidence of SDAVSs, SCAVMs, and metameric AVMs in 296 patients (Surg. Neuroangiogr. Vol. 3, Lasjaunias P. et al. with permission)

Series	SDAVSs	SCAVMs	Metameric/other	Total
Djindjian	46	74	10	130
Rosenblum	27	51	3	81
Berenstein	31	50	4	85
Total	104 (35%)	175 (59%)	17 (6%)	296 (100%)

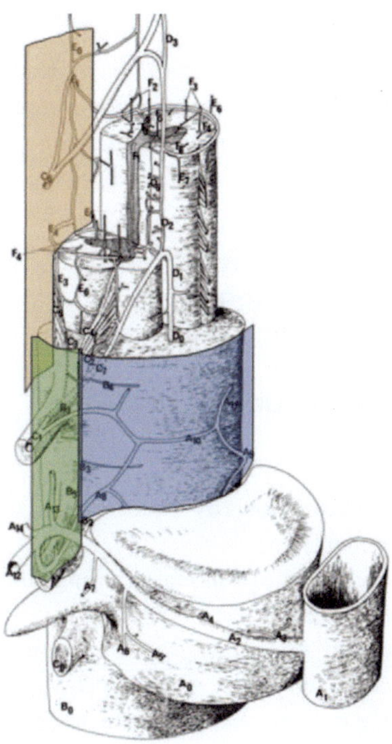

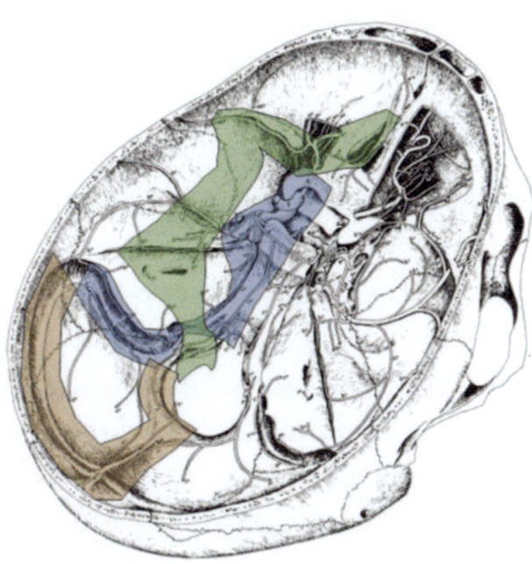

Types of AV shunts	Academic name
Ventral epidural group	Ventral epidural shunts
Dorsal epidural group	Dorsal epidural shunts
Lateral epidural group	Lateral epidural shunts

Fig. 15.2 Classification of cranio-spinal DAVS reported by Geibprasert(2008) [2]

15.3 Natural History and Age Onset, Clinical Presentation Corresponding to Each Type of Classification [2, 6, 12]

Three centers (Bicetre Hospital/France, Ramathibodi Hospital/Thailand and Brazillian gr./South America) had analyzed Epidural spaces of spine and base skull correlated with DAVS cases, the results can predict angiographic findings and clinical presentation (Fig. 15.2).

(a) Lateral epidural space: always have pial venous reflux causing aggressive clinical course and always clinically worsen if not treated.
(b) Dorsal and ventral group lesion: pial venous reflux will occur only if there is thrombosis of the venous outlet of a high flow shunt.

15.3.1 Spinal SDAVS

This confined to the micro-AVS at the dural entrance of the artery; usually at the nerve root level; drain immediately into intradural veins and also medullary veins; either cephalad or caudad direction [1–3, 6, 8].

Differential diagnosis is the epidural AVS which same arterial feeder opens into thrombosed epidural venous segment and drains back into radicular vein and finally perimedullary veins. The radicular AVM which was grouping within the SCAVS and sometimes with the SCAVM when the intradural single draining vein was wrongly interpreted as continuing artery. Another two differential diagnosis are filum terminale AVS and micro perimedullary AVS which can be presented with same clinical symptoms as well as mimic each other in imaging findings.

SDAVS locates within or adjacent to dura mainly at intervertebral foramen level along the spinal canal.

- Presented after fourth to fifth decade of life.
- 85% male predominant or M:F = 5:1 opposite to dural at skull base which F ≫ M.
- Can be located from sacral level to Foramen Magnum level.
- Mainly located at T-L regions.
- Venous drainage can be extensive: reach dural sinus even shunt located at sacral level.

15.3.2 Pathology: Clinical Presentation

- Arterial supply mostly arises from a radicular artery (a dural ranch of the dorsospinal artery) at intervertebral foramen level.
- Mostly small AVS.
- Venous drainage: single tortuous draining vein pierces dura (adjacent to accompanying nerve root) to reach perimedullary venous plexus.
- Produces venous hypertension of the medullary veins within the spinal cord.

15.3.3 SDAVS: Pathophysiology

- Patients with more symptoms are: anterior and posterior drainage > posterior alone; downward/caudal drainage > upward/cephalad.
- Typical spinal cord changes in long standing lesion are "neocapillaries" within the spinal cord.
- Primarily congested intrinsic venous network of the spinal cord causes secondarily chronic extensive hypoxia from long standing venous congestion.

15.4 Treatment Options: Need Full Information from Imaging Findings

15.4.1 SDAVS: Treatment Indications [6, 8, 11]

- Indications: all patients (by endovascular or surgical treatment).
- Aim cure (occlude the proximal draining vein and the micro AVS).
- Contraindication for endovascular treatment (the anterior spinal artery (ASA) originates from the same radicular supplier, which superselective catheterization cannot be safely done or the extra spinal longitudinal anastomosis cannot be clarified to prevent accidentally embolization of the ASA).

15.4.2 SDAVS: Endovascular Treatment [1, 3, 6, 8, 13]

- Afferent arteries size 40–60 μm.
- Liquid embolic material reaches the shunt and the proximal vein, but particles will not be effective.
- Results: up to 80% of the patients showed clinical improvement from endovascular treatment.
- Depends on a shorter history between onset of symptoms and treatment.
- Anti-coagulation: clinical improvement is stopped; SDAVS with descending venous drainage; absence of radicular veins opacified at T level for AVS at L-S level.

15.4.3 SDAVS: Treatment Surgery

- Interruption of drainage vein by coagulation and excision of the dura at the site using bipolar coagulation.
- Cluster of abnormal vessels at inner aspect of the dura are usually seen at surgery.
- Duroplasty at the level of the lesion.
- Average same result as endovascular treatment if exact site of the AVS was found.

15.5 Imaging of Spinal DAVS

15.5.1 MRI Imaging of Spinal DAVS (Fig. 15.3) [1, 6–8]

(a) T2 hyperintense signal within edematous cord accompany with perimedullary dilated vessels.
(b) Various types of cord enhancement from chronic venous congestion (chronic ischemic change).
(c) Later-cord atrophy.
(d) Location of dilated vessel or cord abnormality does not relate with AVS location.

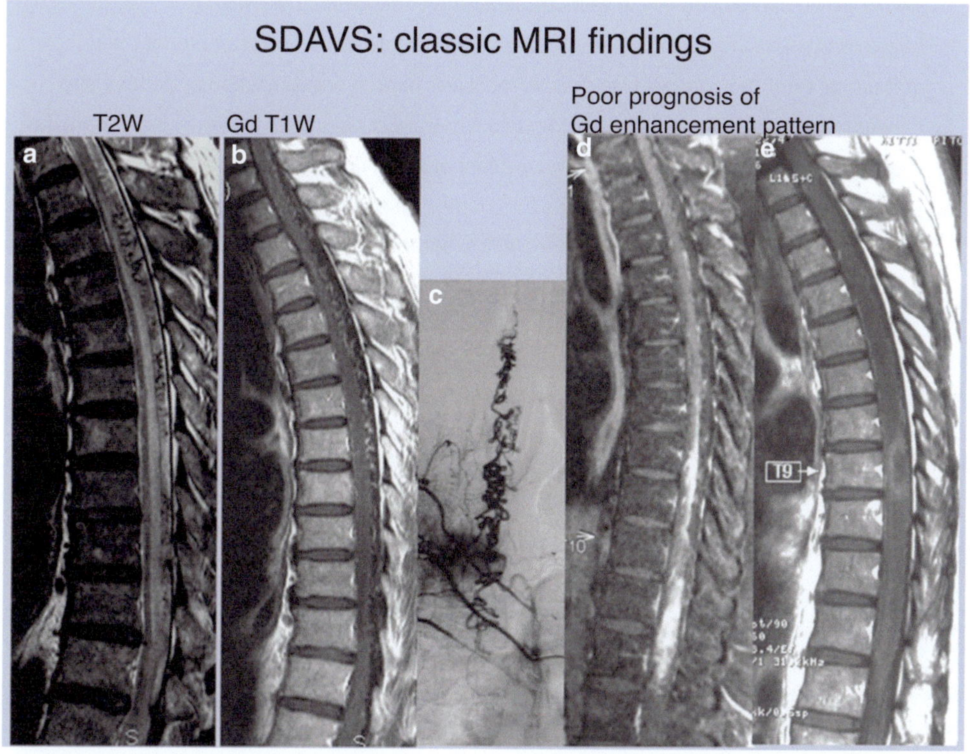

Fig. 15.3 (**a**, **b**) Sag T2W and Gd T1W MRI Th spine showed classic signal changes of cord congestion as well as dilated perimedullary veins. (**c**) Selective segmental artery injection showed classic arterial feeder (Rt Th) to the AVS at transdural portion of the nerve root, then drained into radicular vein and perimedullary veins (in this case upward direction). (**d**, **e**) Two pattern of cord enhancement in poor prognosis (usually chronic cord congestion) are patchy enhancement (**d**) and ring enhancement (**e**)

15.5.2 Current Imaging Protocol [1, 4, 6, 7, 9, 14, 15]

1. MRI of the symptomatic spinal levels: routine sequences with Gd study (Fig. 15.4 and Table 15.3), usually screening whole spine is valued (T2W) (Figs. 15.5 and 15.6).
2. CE spinal MRA (dynamic study: if SAVS are suspected from 1).
3. Spinal angiography: is still the goal standard of imaging in all SAVS patients due to highest temporal and spatial resolutions (Figs. 15.7, 15.8, 15.9 and 15.10).

15.5.3 Special Consideration in Pediatric Spinal Arteriovenous Shunts

Types of the Spinal Arterio-Venous Shunts: in Analysis of pediatric spinal AVS [3, 16–18] cases [19, 20] (Lekhong et al. total 40 cases), there was no DAVSs in children population [12]. But SDAVS can occur after surgical removal the malformation in children.

SAVS: accuracy of shunt detection, localization and subtype of discrimination by manual syringe contrast injection spinal MRA

MR technique:

- 1.5T MR image system-eight channel cervical-thoracic-lumber spine array coil.
- 3-phase 3D fast-spoiled gradient echo pulse sequence with centric k-space filling, 400mm FOV in craniocaudal direction, 512× 256 matrix, 0.5mm thick sagittal sections acquired, TR of 4.9 ms, TE of 1.4 ms, FA 30 degree and 40-46 seconds acquisition time of each phase.
- IV access was obtained using no smaller than a 20-gauge intravenous catheter at the right antecubital vein. The contrast injection protocol was hand syringe injection of gadobenate dimeglumine (MultiHance) 0.15 mmol/kg and a maximum volume of 20 ml, with an approximate injection flow rate of 3 ml/sec, followed by 25 ml of saline flush at the same rate.
- MR fluoroscopy was used to determine the optimal scan delay time, which was the time required to visualize the maximal enhancement of the entire aorta down to the aortic bifurcation.

Fig. 15.4 MR technique for accurate diagnosis of SDAVS [9]

Table 15.3 Sensitivity, specificity, accuracy, PPV and NPV of spinal MRA for detecting and elevating SDAVS

Variable	Sensitivity (95% CI)	Specificity (95% CI)	Accuracy (95% CI)	PPV (95% CI)	NPV (95% CI)
Detection of AVS	100 (100.0–100.0)	100 (100.0–100.0)	100 (100.0–100.0)	100 (100.0–100.0)	100 (100.0–100.0)
Subtype discrimination	94.12 (83.81–104.43)	100 (100.0–100.0)	97.06 (91.29–100.0)	100 (100.0–100.0)	75 (56.02–93.98)
Shunt localization	88.24 (74.11–102.36)	100 (100.0–100.0)	94.12 (86.22–100.0)	100 (100.0–100.0)	60 (38.53–81.47)
Dominant feeder detection	52.94 (31.07–74.82)	100 (100.0–100.0)	76.47 (64.24–88.7)	100 (100.0–100.0)	27.27 (7.75–46.79)

NPV negative predictive value, *PPV* positive predictive value

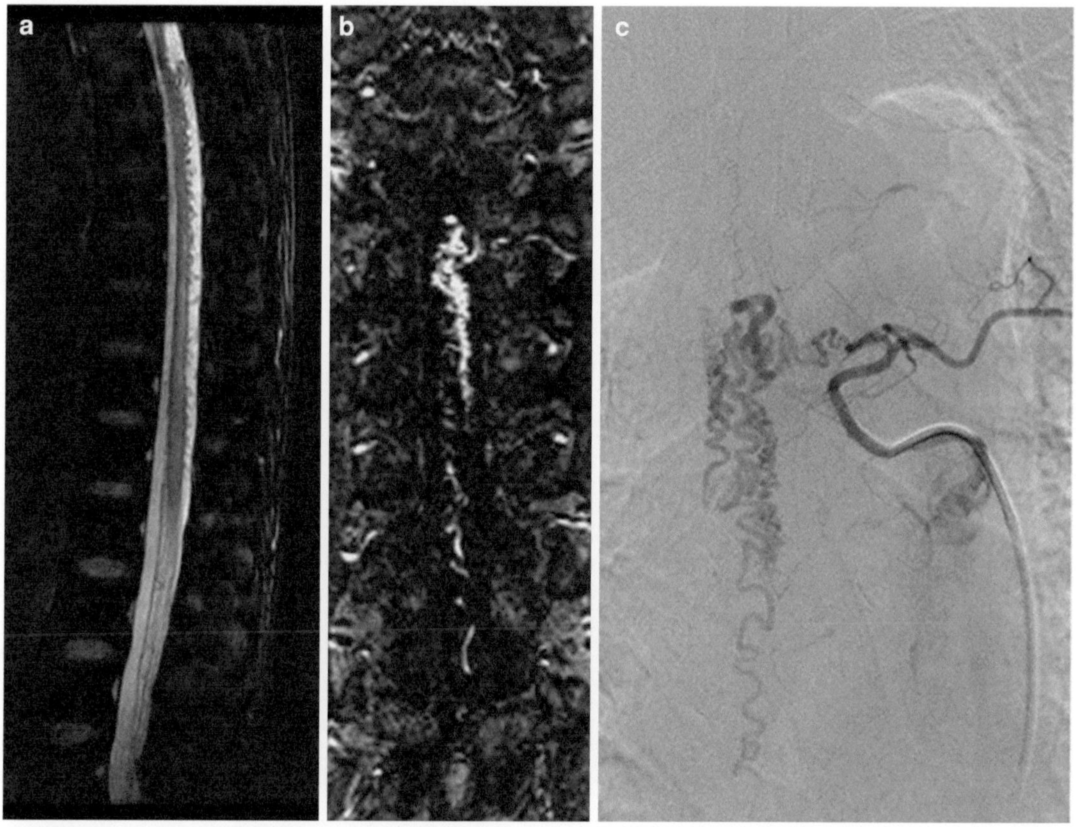

Fig. 15.5 (**a**) Classic T2W sagittal MRI Th spine showed venous congestion and signal voids of dilated perimedullary veins around the cord. (**b**) Coronal arterial phase of spinal MRA showed arterialized dilated perimedullary veins as well as Lt Th arterial feeder. (**c**) Correlated selective spinal angiogram of same Th level showed similar findings of the arterial feeder, AVS and draining veins

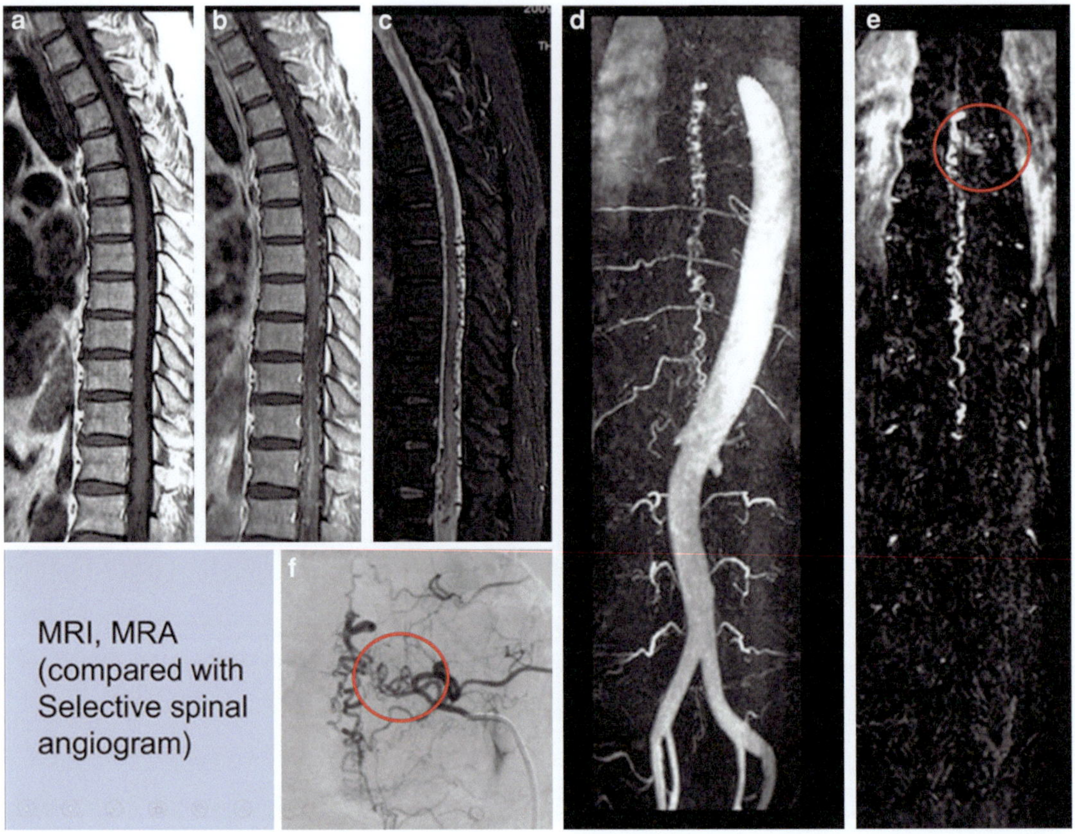

Fig. 15.6 (**a–c**) Sag T1W, Gd T1W and T2W MRI Th spine showed venous congestion, pattern of shaggy enhancement of Conus Medullaris and signal voids of dilated perimedullary veins around the cord. (**d**, **e**) Global MRA of the spine including aorta showed arterial veins coming off the lower Th segmental artery on Lt side, while coronal early arterial phase MRA study showed exact level of the arterial feeder to the AVS. (**f**) Superselective segmental spinal angiogram showed similar findings (circle) as MRA (which provide faster time of spinal angiogram and good information prepared for the treatment)

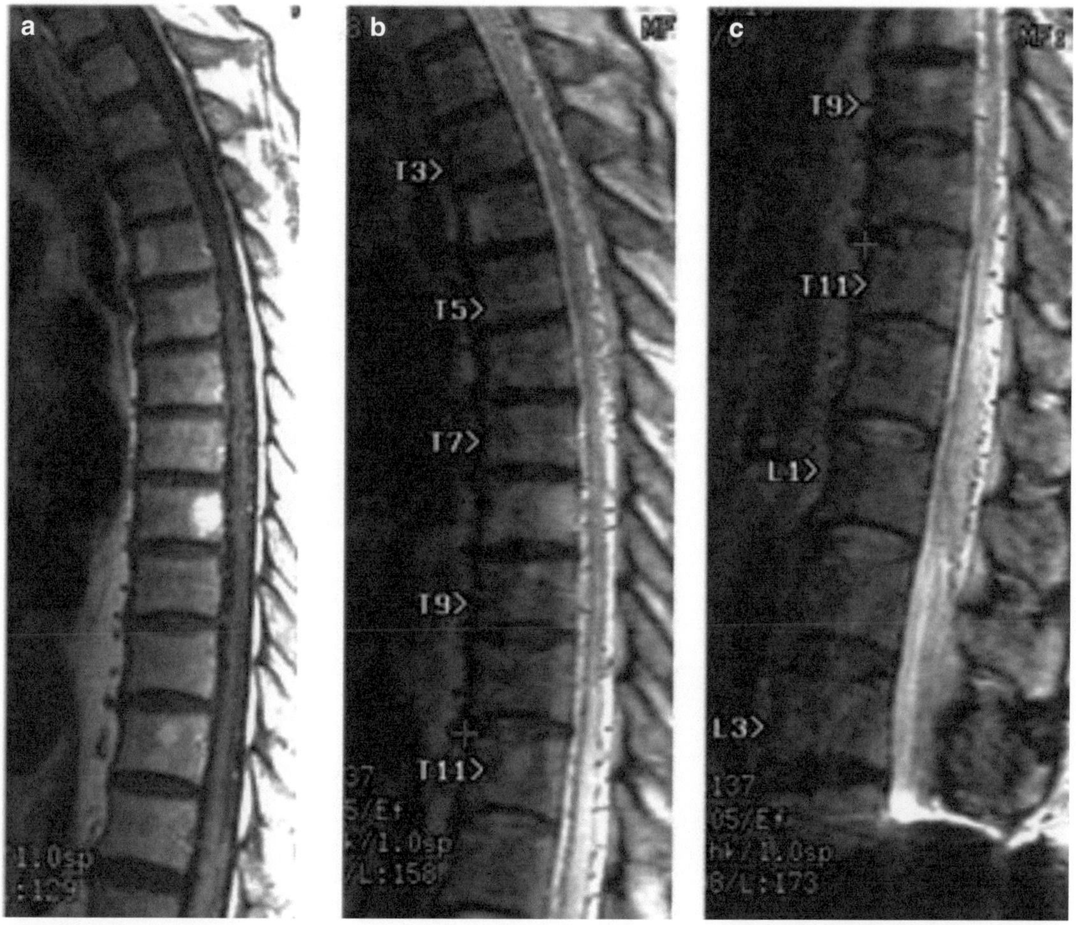

Fig. 15.7 Classic presentation post laminectomy of L5–S1 level. A 60-year-old man; s/p back surgery 5 years with internal fixator for the spondylolisthesis; 4-month PTA: hypoesthesia and weakness both legs, atrophy gluteus/hip muscle, sphincter problems. (**a–c**) Sag T1W, T2W MRI Th and lumbar spine showed classic Conus Medullaris and lower Th spinal cord congestion as well as diffuse dilated perimedullary veins ventral and dorsal to the cord. Figure showing DAVS from bilateral L4 feeders; oblique projections are needed to get working position for good analysis and treatment planning (arrow point to the AVS). (**d**, **e**) Selective segmental spinal angiogram in this case were limited due to large metallic surgical instrument, some oblique or lateral projection as well as Town or Caldwell projection may be needed to see clearly the angioarchitecture of the SDAVS. (**f–h**) Images with bony structures may add more information of the previous disease and treatment

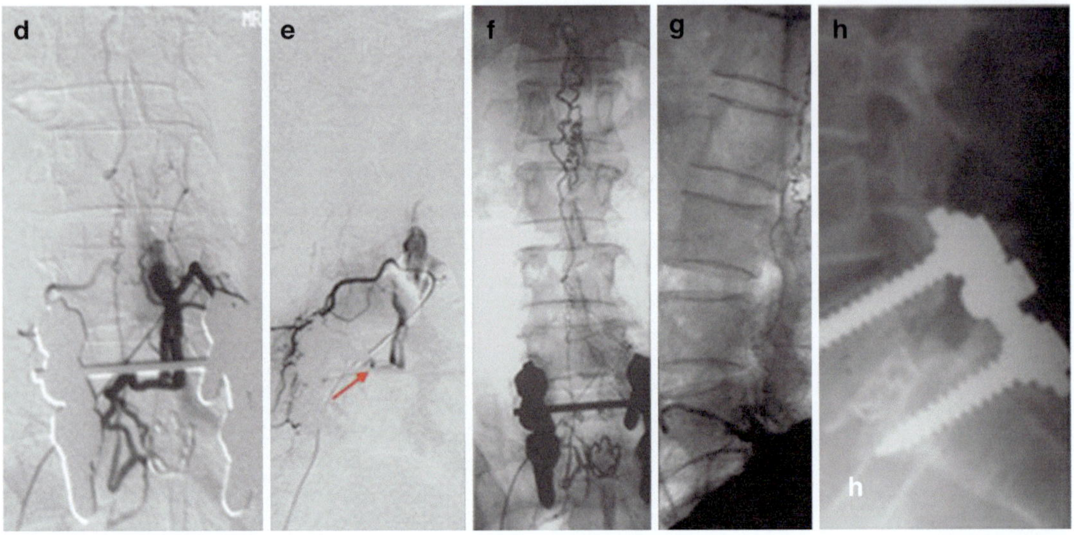

Fig. 15.7 (continued)

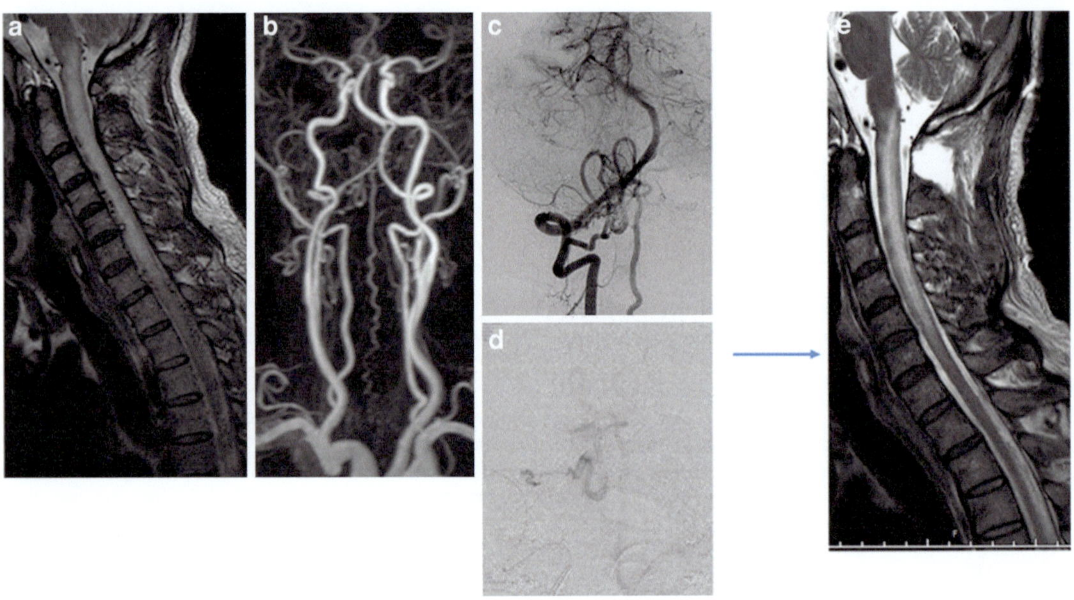

Fig. 15.8 SDAVS can occur at the most cephalad level at foramen magnum. (**a**, **b**) MRI C spine Sag hyper T2W upper C cord congestion and dilated perimedullary veins are seen and MRA demonstrated AVS located from Rt upper C segmental artery. (**c**, **d**) RVA angiogram and superselective catheterization into Rt C1 segmental arterial feeder showed DAVS at this level. (**e**) Seven days post embolization showed no further seen dilatation of the perimedullary veins and some improvement of the C cord congestion

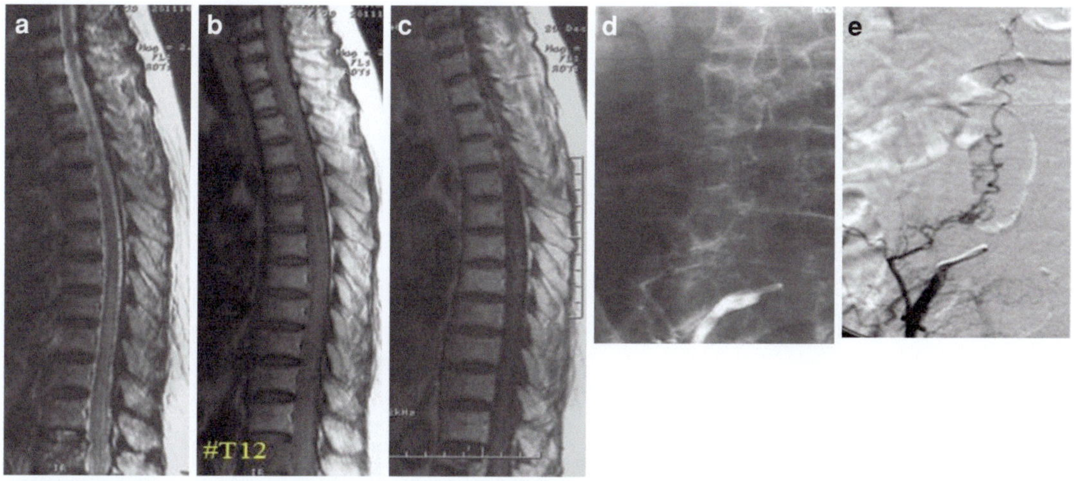

Fig. 15.9 SDAVS can occur at the most caudad level: lateral sacral arterial feeder level. A 71-year-old woman presented with paraparesis without sphincter problems. (**a–c**) Sagittal T2W, T1W, Gd T1W MRI Th spine showed conus medullaris and lower Th spinal cord congestion as well as diffuse dilated perimedullary veins ventral and dorsal to the cord. (**d**, **e**) Special oblique position for stabilize catheterization of the guiding system from ipsilateral Rt Iliac artery which clearly showed the DAVS fed from Rt lateral sacral artery

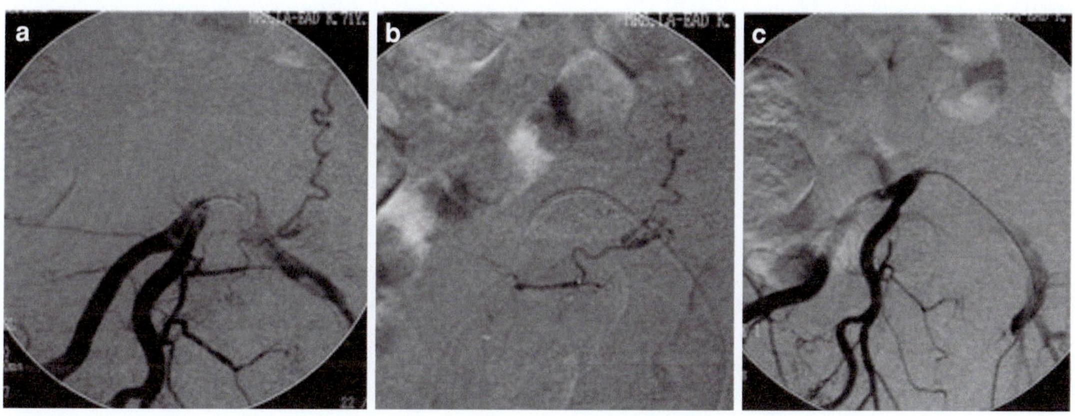

Fig. 15.10 Superselective catheterization into the arterial feeder and DAVS. NBCA cast within the AVS and proximal vein. Post embolization control angiogram showed complete obliteration of the shunt. (**a**, **b**) After failure to microcatheterization into the feeder from same side; contralateral approach was done with better view for superselective microcatheterization. (**c**) Control angiogram post NBCA proper embolization showed complete cure result

15.5.4 Differential Diagnosis

15.5.4.1 Spinal Dural Arteriovenous Shunts

As this condition can be mis-diagnosed from the MRI study as the spinal cord congestion or edema can be seen in other diseases, and if the dilated perimedullary veins are not large enough to be clearly seen in routine MRI study. Also contrast study MRI may mimic diagnosis of myelitis (transverse or ascending myelitis) (Fig. 15.11a, b)

1. *Epidural SDAVS*. One differential diagnosis of SDAVS is the epidural SDAVS. The AV

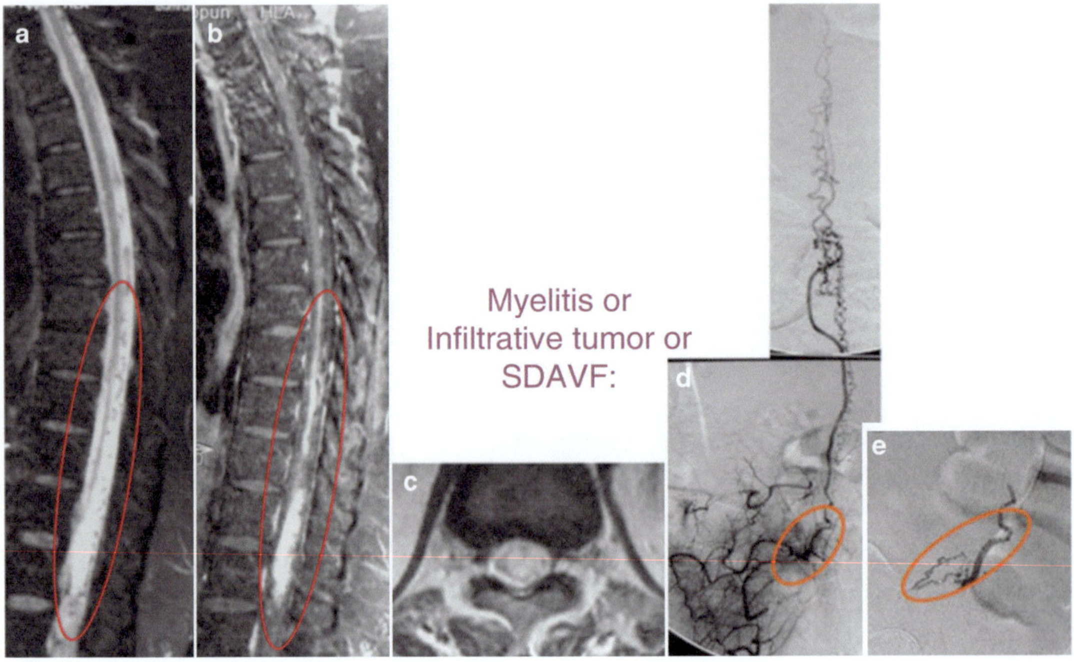

Fig. 15.11 (**a**–**c**) Sagittal T2W and CE T1W MRI of the whole spine and axial study showing diffuse cord congestion seen as diffuse hyper T2W signal more at level of the conus medullaris up to mid Th level and diffuse abnormal contrast enhancement, while the abnormal signal void structures were seen along the dorsal aspect of the subarachnoid space of the lower cord level. (**d**, **e**) Superselective Rt lateral sacral angiogram demonstrated the SDAVS which were the cause of cord congestion (perimedullary venous congestion). Transarterial liquid embolic material embolization which cover the AVS and foot of venous drainage (circle) will provide curative result

shunt may occur at the transdural portion of nerve root or at the epidural venous segment, then drain back via dura into perimedullary venous refluxes creating venous congestion of the spinal cord [21] (Figs. 15.11c–e, 15.12 and 15.13).

2. *Radicular AVM*. Another differential diagnosis of SDAVS is the radicular AVM [22], which is located along the intradural portion of the nerve root (Fig. 15.14), drains into short radicular vein into perimedullary vein and can congest the spinal cord. Clinical presentation could include radiculopathy as well as myelopathy and treatment options could be considered same as SDAVS.
3. *Micro perimedullary AVF and filum terminale AVF*. Another two differential diagnoses of SDAVS are micro perimedullary AVF, filum terminale AVF and intracranial DAVS (Figs. 15.15, 15.16, 15.17, 15.18 and 15.19) [5, 21]. The first one belongs to intradural spinal cord superficial AVF, occurs more

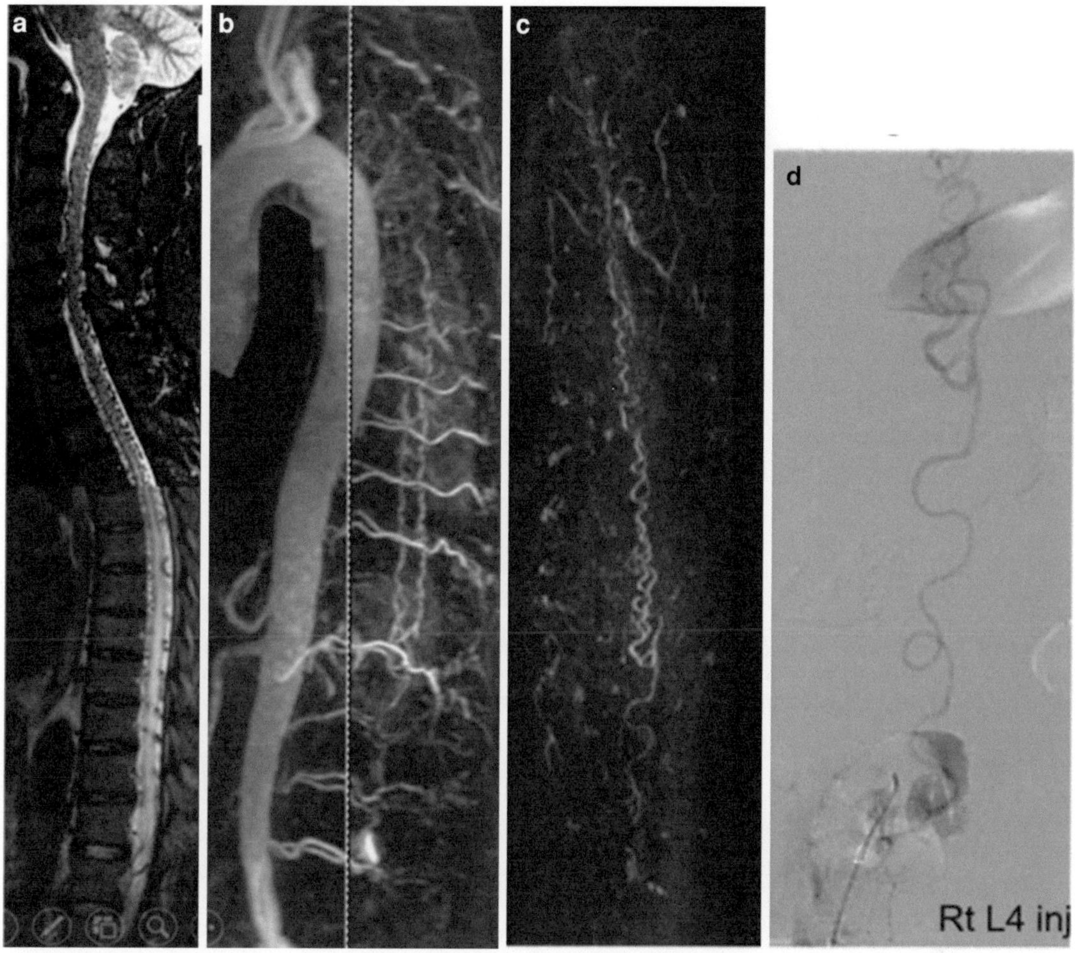

Fig. 15.12 A case of epidural SDAVS draining into intradural veins. (**a**) Sagittal T2W MRI of the whole spine showed diffuse cord congestion as diffuse hyper T2W signal more intense at the conus medullaris extended up to upper Th level. Visualization of the multiple signal void structures along the entire dorsal and ventral aspect of the subarachnoid space around the cord. (**b**, **c**) Proper techniques of spinal MRA were performed to include lower Lumbar level that we found the focal epidural AVS draining into filum terminale vein into perimedullary vein which was the cause of venous congestion. (**d**) The lesions were confirmed by superselective Rt L4 spinal angiogram for proper endovascular treatment

common in pediatric group and can presented with hemorrhagic symptoms as well as cord congestion. The latter is the micro AVF at the level of filum terminale below the basket (anastomosis between anterior and posterior spinal arterial systems) drains up into the filum terminale vein and finally perimedullary veins. Both can present with same signs and symptoms as well as imaging findings.

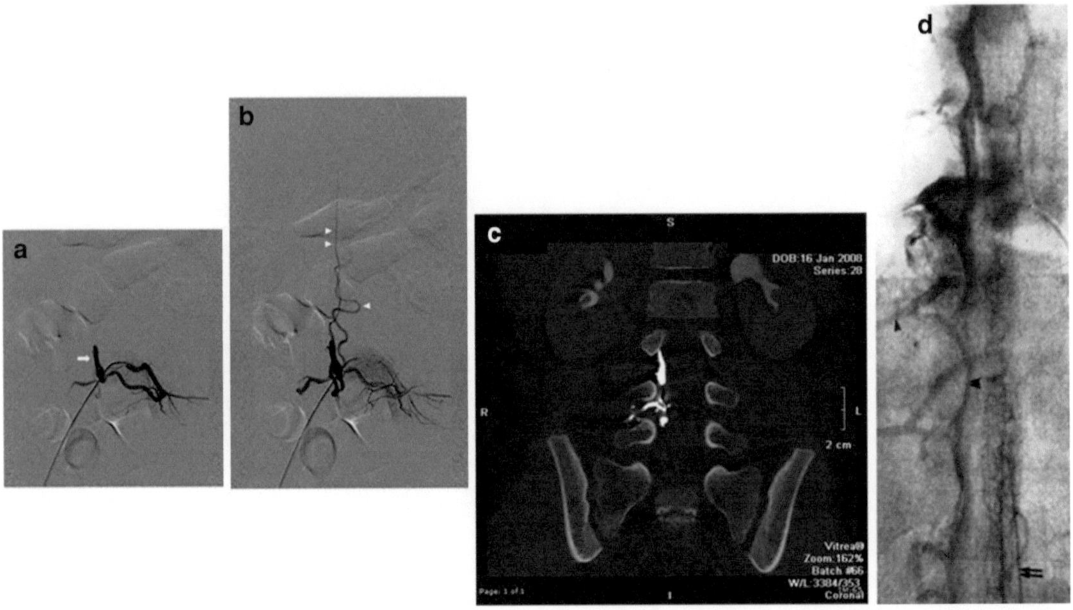

Fig. 15.13 Spinal epidual AVS. (**a**) Arrow point to epidural segment. (**b**) Arrows point to perimedullary intradural vein. (**c**, **d**) The CT in coronal study after proper NBCA cast deposition in endovascular treatment was confirmed to be located within the short epidural segment (arrow in panel **d**)

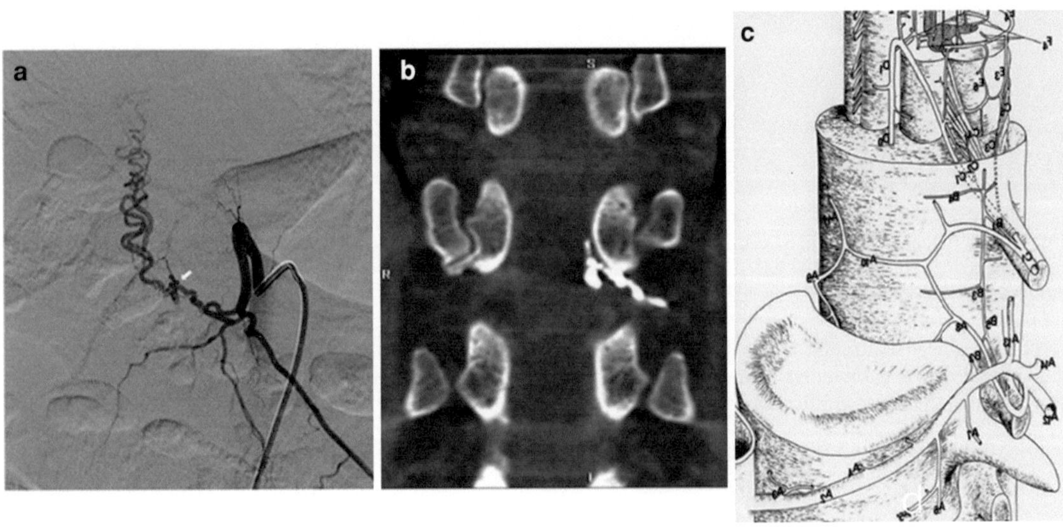

Fig. 15.14 (**a**) A case of radicular AVM located along the intradural portion of the nerve root, drains into short radicular vein into perimedullary vein and can congest the spinal cord (arrow). (**b**) The CT in coronal study showed NBCA cast along the nidus of the nerve root in post-operation. (**c**) Drawing of the radicular artery

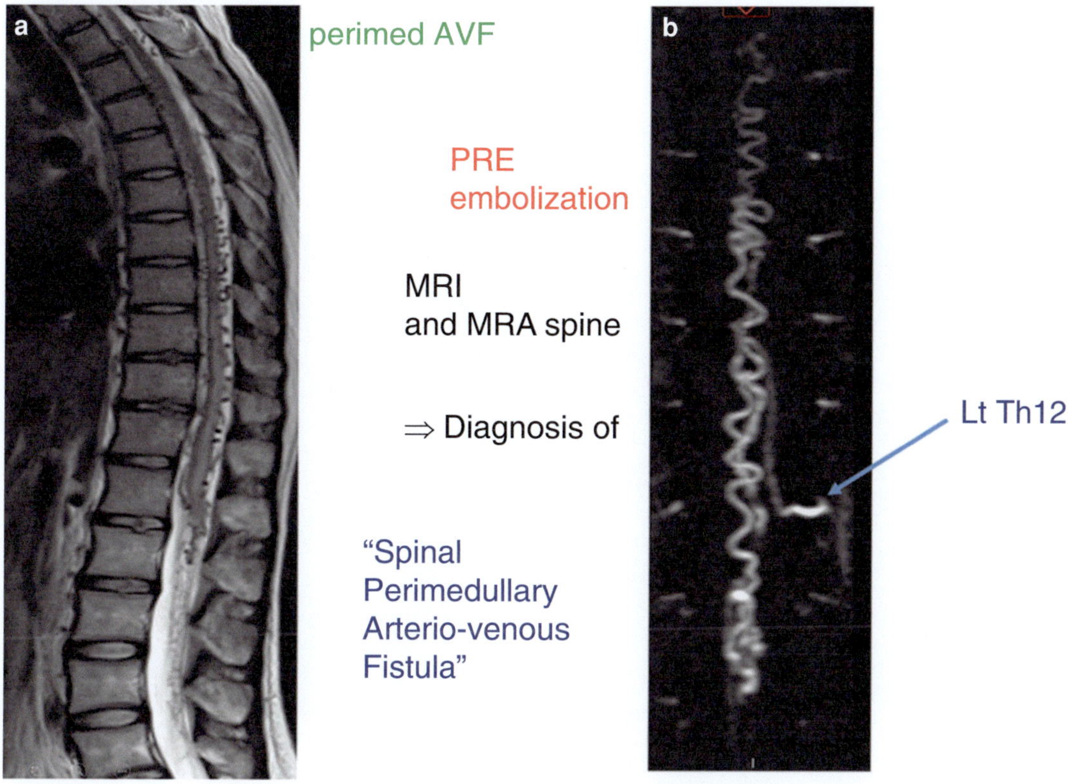

Fig. 15.15 Example of micro AVF at Lt Th12 level, same MRI findings as SDAVS (**a**) but good quality spinal MRA could provide proper diagnosis of radicular artery open via micro AVF into perimedullary vein at Lt Th12 (**b**, arrow)

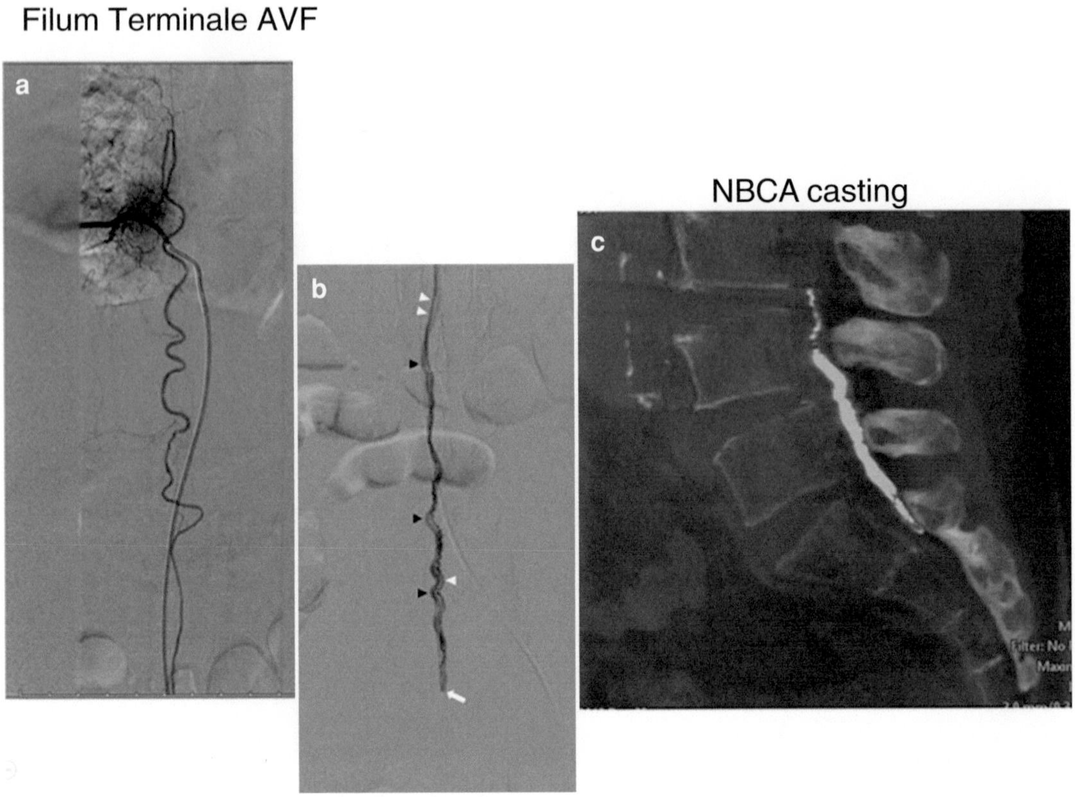

Fig. 15.16 Example of the filum terminale AVF which the arterial feeder is the Adamkiewicz (dominant RM artery) reaching ASA which at the level of filum terminale level (**a**), open into Filum Terminale vein running up into perimedullary vein (**b**) creating cord congestion. Sagittal reconstruction CT study post op showed NBCA cast properly located within the AV shunt (**c**)

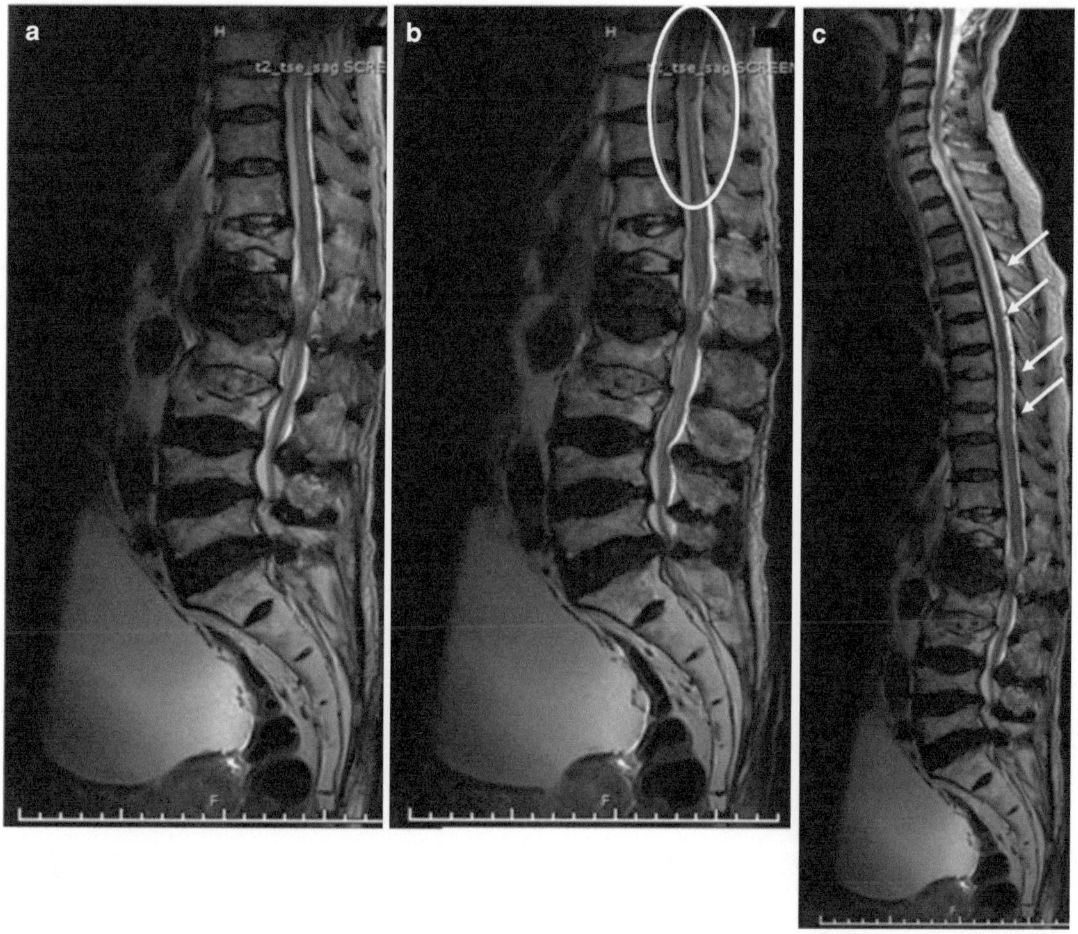

Fig. 15.17 An 85-year-old man presented with progressive paraparesis for 2 months. (**a**, **b**) T2W sagittal MRI L-S spine showed multiple spinal body collapsed from degenerative changes/spondylosis which may distract radiologist NOT to notice the signal void structures dorsal aspect of lower Th cord as well as mild hyper T2W at lower Th cord (circle). (**c**) Radiologist must extend the study to cover whole spinal screening which will clearly demonstrate the signal void structures dorsal aspect of lower Th cord and mild hyper T2W at lower Th cord which explained the myelopathy (arrows). *Notes*: Due to sphincter dysfunction from the congested conus medullaris, radiologists should notice the full bladder and constipation condition too

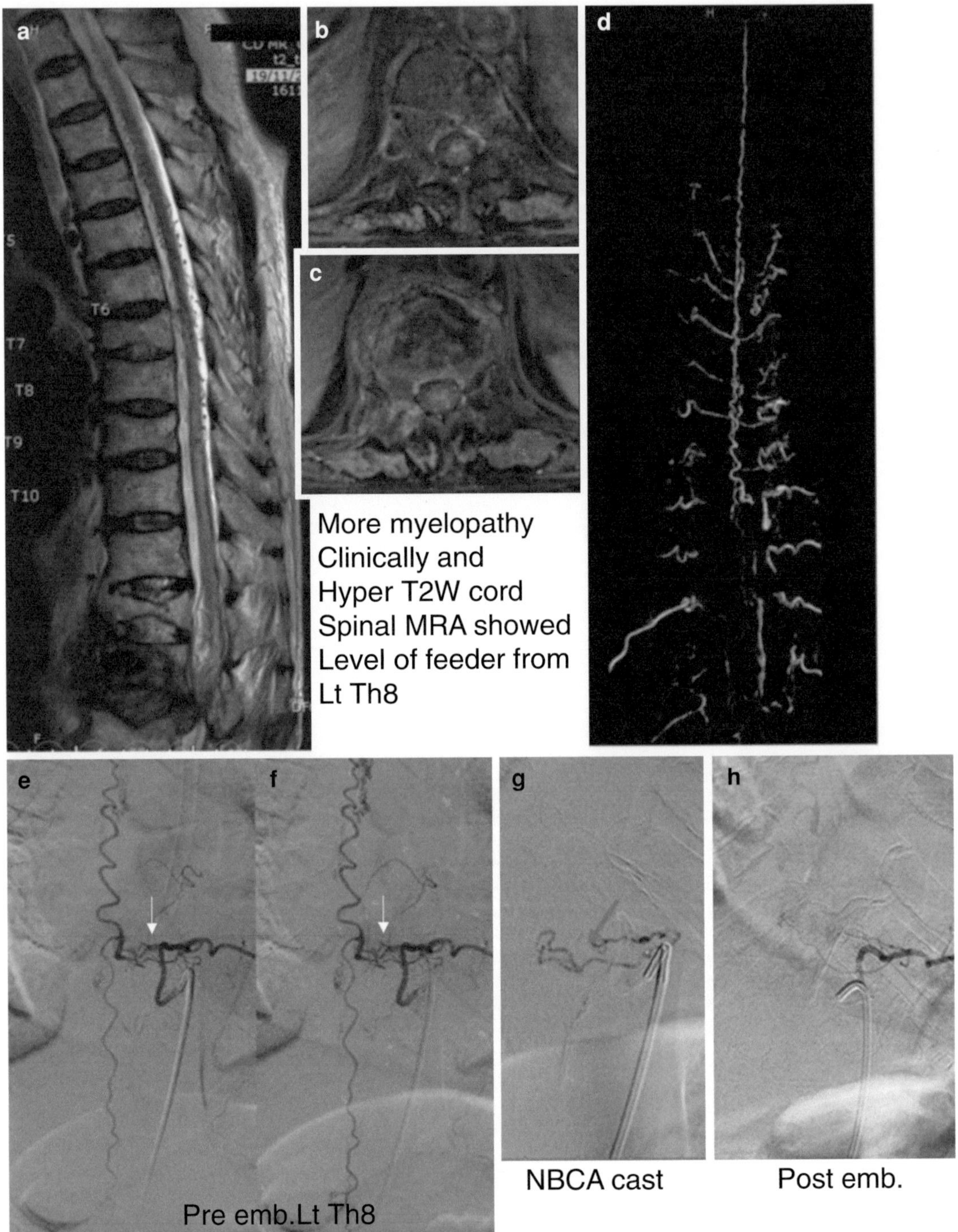

Fig. 15.18 (**a**–**c**) Sagittal T2W and axial T2W MRI Th-L spine showed cord venous congestion from mid Th level to Conus Medullaris and diffuse dilated perimedullary veins around the mid to upper Th level. (**d**) Radiologists must perform proper technique of spinal MRA which demonstrate the arterialized perimedullary veins draining the SDAVS and prominent Lt Th8 Radicular artery as the feeder. (**e**, **f**) Lt Th8 superselective injection showed radiculomeningeal artery fed SDAVS (arrow) drained into perimedullary veins. (**g**) The NBCA cast was seen covering from the AVS, foot of veins and arterial feeder. (**h**) Lt Th8 superselective injection showed curative result of the proper treatment

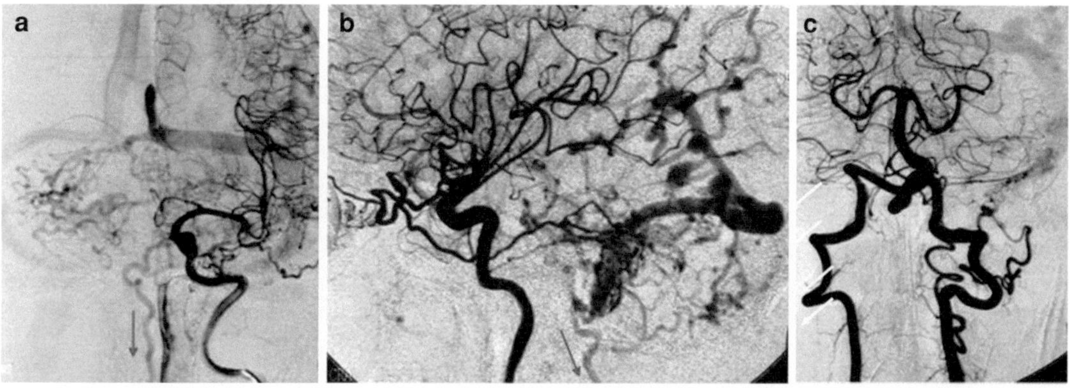

Fig. 15.19 An 80-year-old woman presented with progressive myelopathy upto C level; dementia; MRI C spine showed abnormal vessels at C cord level. Angiogram showed DAVS at left sigmoid sinus; partial occlusion at jugular bulb with retrograde venous reflux into posterior fossa veins and spinal vein. (**a**–**c**) Intracranial DAVS at Lt TS-SS with spinal venous drainage; (red arrows) which clinical could mimic SDAVS

15.6 Spinal Vascular Anatomy and Imaging (Figs. 15.20, 15.21 and 15.22) [1, 4, 7, 9, 15]

15.6.1 Routine Protocol in the Work-Up of the Spinal AV Shunt in the Spinal Angiogram (Figs. 15.23, 15.24, 15.25, 15.26 and 15.27)

1. Identify the AV shunts
2. Rule out the possible collateral supply from another adjacent segmental a
3. Identify the level of artery of Adamkiewicz
4. Identify the angioarchitecture that have higher chance of complication during treatment

15.6.2 Technique: ±Under GA

Controlled respiration: Apnea technique 5–20 s each time
Route: usually femoral (rarely axillary)
Material/methods: low osmolarity contrast and special catheters (double right angle distal end/tip very tapering/5Fr size
Recommended protocol: usually AP view only (rarely lateral or oblique)
Contrast injection: each segmented arteries: 2 cc/s for 2 s; for AK: 1 cc/s for 10 s
3D rotational spinal angiography was not performed routinely

Diagnostic spinal angiography can have the same risks as the cerebral angiography which are spi-

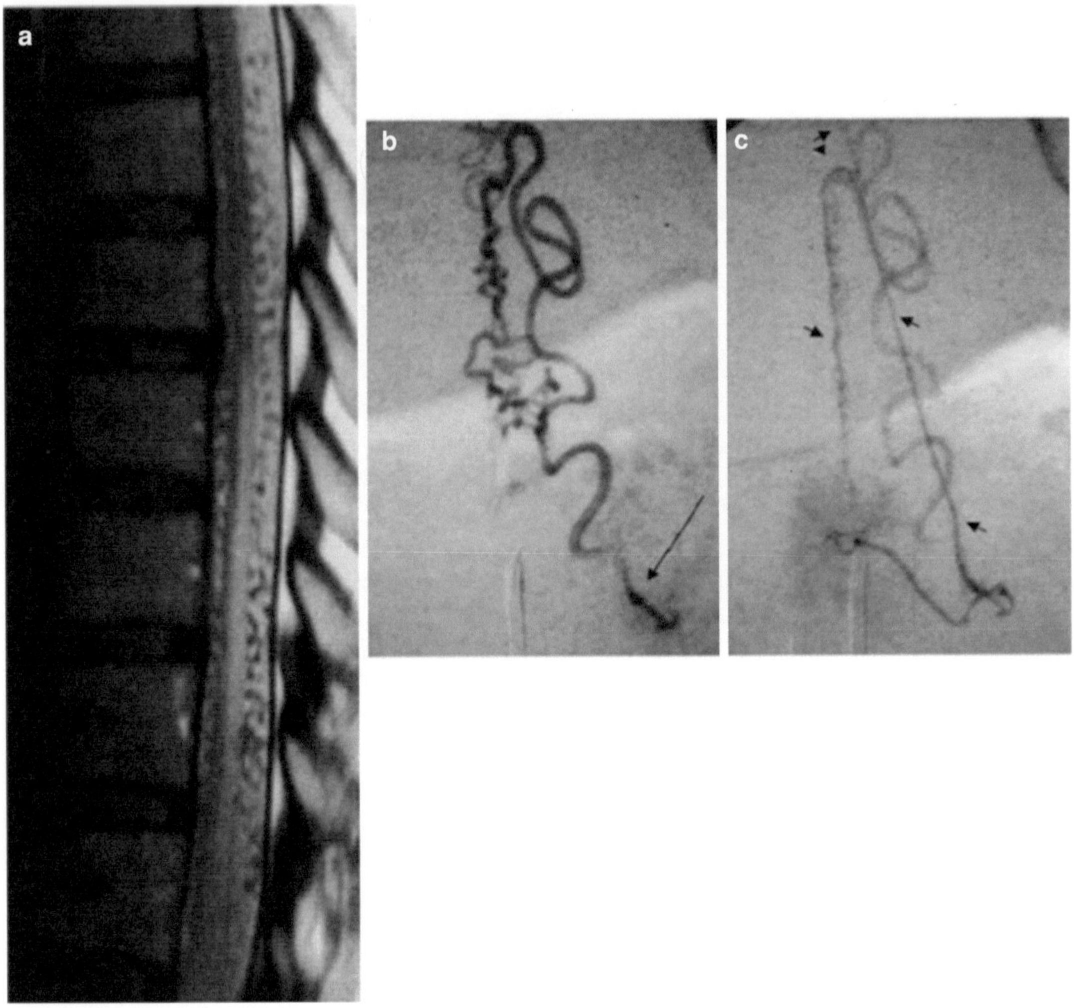

Fig. 15.20 Showing the common trunk of the radicular artery supplying the cord (RM to ASA) and the DAVS (Surg. Neuroangiogr. Vols. 1 and 3, Lasjaunias et al. with permission). (**a**) MRI T2W Sagittal Thoracic spine showed hyper T2W signal in cord (lower cord congestion) and abnormal dilated tortuous signal void structures dorsal and ventral aspect of the cord which are perimedullary veins dilatation. (**b**) Superselective Lt lower Th segmental arteriogram demonstrated a Radiculomeningeal artery feeder to SDAVS (long arrow) which drained into those perimedullary veins. (**c**) Minimal movement the tip of microcatheter 1–2 mm. may demonstrate the common trunk of dominant radiculomedullary artery (Adamkiewicz.) which contribute to ASA (short arrow)

nal cord ischemic events from thromboembolism or air embolism, patients could manifest symptoms of myelopathy as well as causing vessel dissection or ruptured atherosclerotic plaques. There are reports of transient myelopathy 0–2.2% of all spinal angiography procedures but the irreversible myelopathy is extremely rare [12, 14, 21].

The anatomical differentiation of the spinal vessels which have the oblique direction, hair-pin shape vessel with ascending and descending branches may be the artery (ASA or PSA) or the vein (Radicular vein and perimedullary vein). The segmental artery which gives radiculomedullary artery, if we follow the descending branch at the conus, we will see the anastomosis with PSA as we call "basket." While the Radicular veins, even have the same shape but are usually larger size and more tortuous, if drain AVS may congest

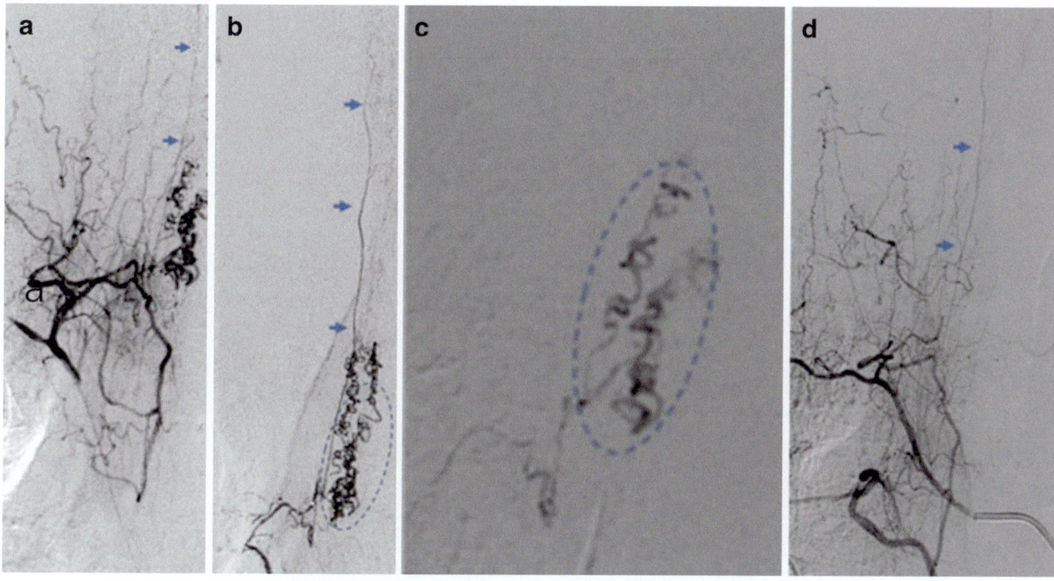

Fig. 15.21 RP to PSA is the common trunk with arterial supply to SDAVS. (**a**, **b**) Superselective Rt upper Th segmental arteriogram demonstrated the radiculomeningeal artery feeder to SDAVS which drained into dilated tortuous perimedullary veins. Interventional neuroradiologist notice a paramedian upward artery ascended up (posterior spinal artery PSA) as well as noticed also the intrinsic arterial network filling the contralateral PSA (arrows). (**c**) Superselective microcatheterization beyond the common trunk to PSA (safe enough) to inject the NBCA liquid embolic material with NO reflux. (**d**) Curative result with good preservation of the PSA (arrow)

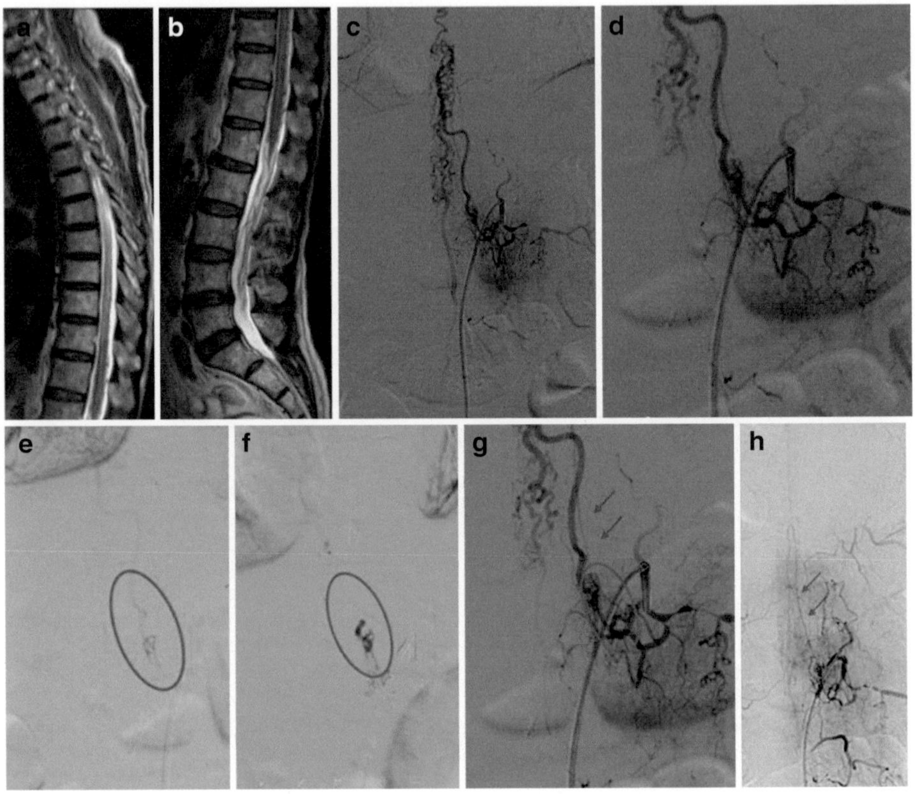

Fig. 15.22 A 65-year-old male presented with progressive myelopathy. Superselective spinal angiogram demonstrated arterial feeder to the DAVS. Small radiculomedullary artery was originated from the same segmental artery as the radiculomeningeal feeder to the AVS, as the risk of liquid embolic material reflux into RM is high (creating major deficits) if we did not recognize this anatomy. (**a**, **b**) Sagittal T2W MRI Th-L spine showed subtle lower Th cord hyper T2W changes as well as some dilated perimedullary veins. (**c**, **d**) Superselective segmental artery injection showed the Radiculomeningeal arterial feeder to the AVS then dilated draining veins which small oblique vessel is noted originated from same trunk as the feeder artery. (**e**, **f**) Superselective microcatheterization into distal arterial feeder followed by diluted NBCA proper embolization (cover distal arterial feeder, AVS and foot of draining vein). (**g**, **h**) Compare pre and post embolization segmental spinal angiogram showed that the small vessels (red arrows) are actually the radiculomedullary artery to the ASA axis with classic hairpin shape and descending/ascending branches. (**i**, **j**) Sag T2W and Gd FS T1W MRI. Th spine at 2 months follow up showed less cord congestion and no further seen dilated perimedullary veins, small areas of shaggy enhancement at the residual congested cord were noted

Fig. 15.23 (**a**) Proper selective segmental spinal angiogram study showed the diagnostic catheter (usually Cobra shape 5Fr) tip was put into the junction of the branches to avoid the contrast refluxes. The dominant radiculomedullary (Adamkiewicz) artery was seen contributing the ASA axis down with visualization of the two (Rt and Lt) PSA anastomosis filling up at basket level. Also, the anastomosis to segmental artery one level up and down as well as contralateral one is seen. (**b**, **c**) Late phase (body spine staining) showed filling of the oblique vessel which in normal situation, drained out from the spinal cord to the epidural venous plexuses, classic for radicular vein. (**d**) Another example of proper selective segmental spinal angiogram study showed the diagnostic catheter (usually Cobra shape 5Fr) tip was put into the junction of the branches to avoid the contrast refluxes. The dominant radiculomedullary (Adamkiewicz) artery (double arrows) was seen contributing the ASA axis down with visualization of the two (Rt and Lt) PSA anastomosis filling up at basket level. Another smaller oblique artery originated from same segmental trunk is also seen running up in more narrow Hairpin shape reach "paramedian" vertical axis of PSA was seen, as example of the radiculopial artery contribute to Lt PSA. (**e**) Later phase showed multiple oblique vessels draining out into Rt and Lt epidural venous plexuses (arrows), these are the radicular veins (diagram **g**). (**f**) Later phase of the spinal angiogram study showed the epidural venous plexuses system as well as the specimen injection example (**h**). (Surg. Neuroangiogr. Vols. 1, 3. Lasjaunias et al. with permission)

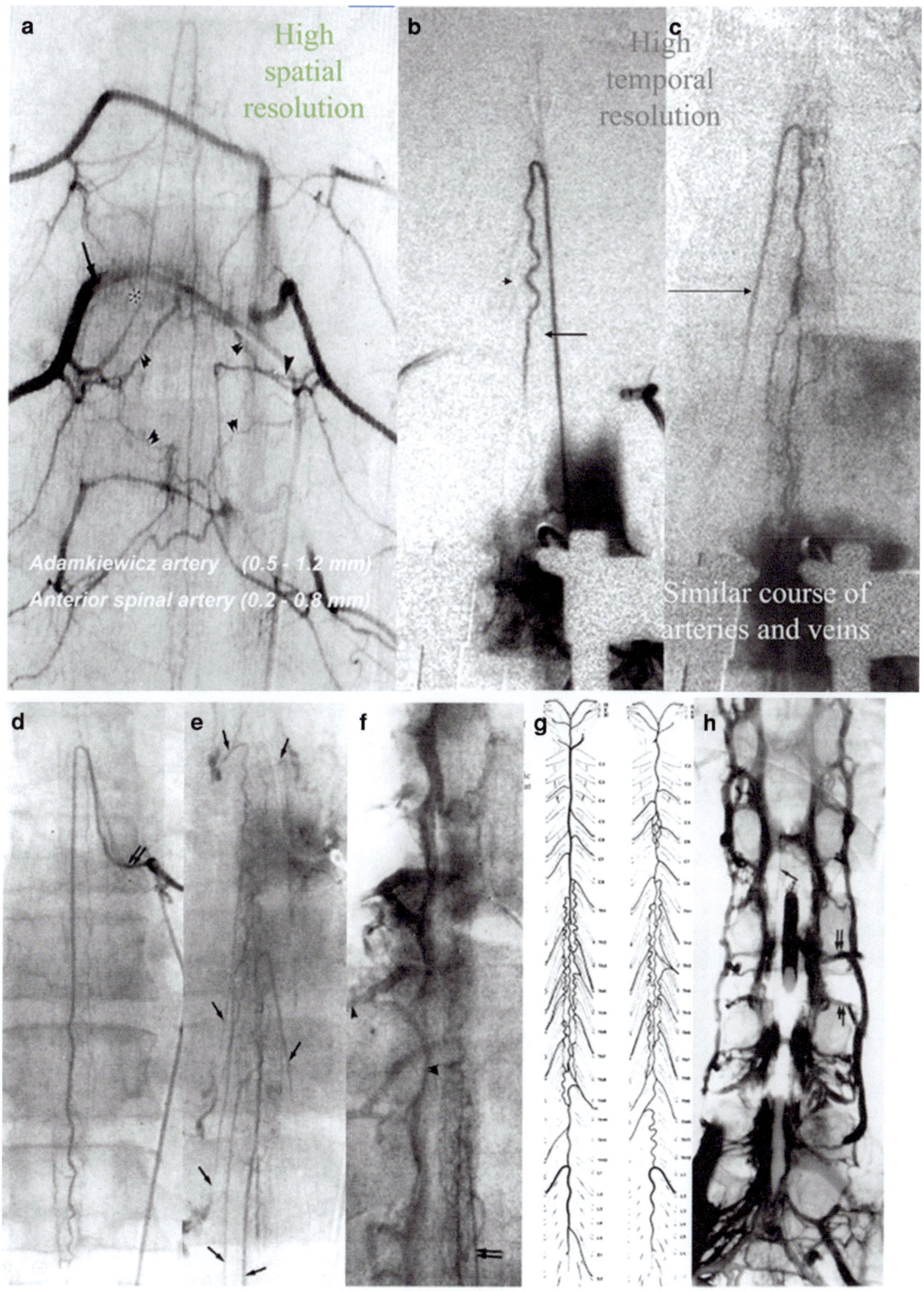
a
High
spatial
resolution
Adamkiewicz artery (0.5 - 1.2 mm)
Anterior spinal artery (0.2 - 0.8 mm)
b
High
temporal
resolution
c
Similar course of
arteries and veins
d
e
f
g
h

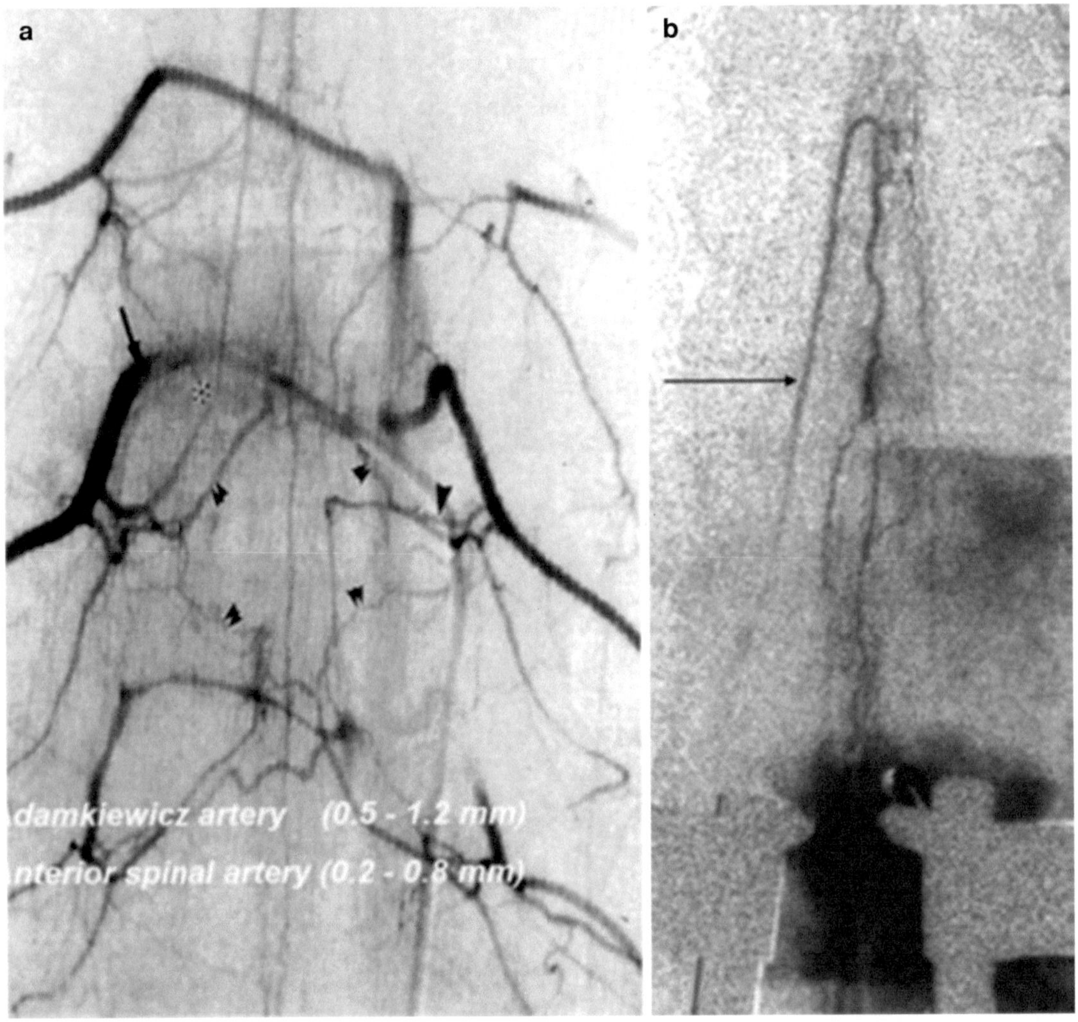

Fig. 15.24 (**a**) Lumbar artery injection (arrow) showed radiculomedullary artery, ASA, basket and PSA as well as the extradural anastomosis (double arrows). (**b**) Late phase angiogram showed radicular veins (arrow). (Surg. Neuroangiogr. Vols. 1, 3. Lasjaunias et al. with permission)

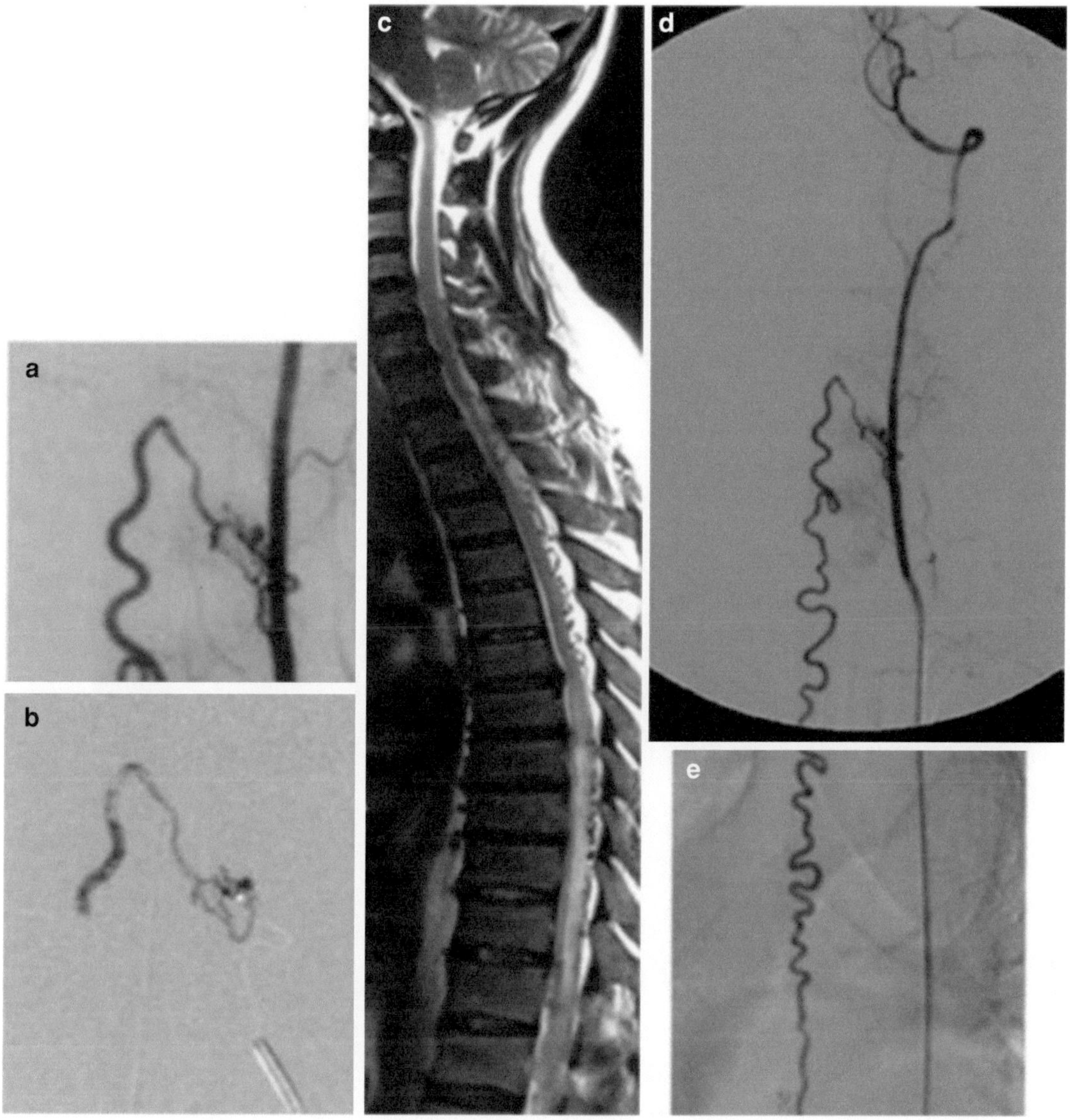

Fig. 15.25 (**c**) MRI whole spine T2W sagittal showed venous congestion mid Th to conus level dilated tortuous perimedullary veins suggesting SDAVS, epidural AVF or radicular AVF. (**a**, **d**, **e**) LVA angiograms. Showed a SDAVS Lt C5 root or radicular AVM around Lt C5 root. (**b**) NBCA cast superselective embolization AVS foot of draining vein

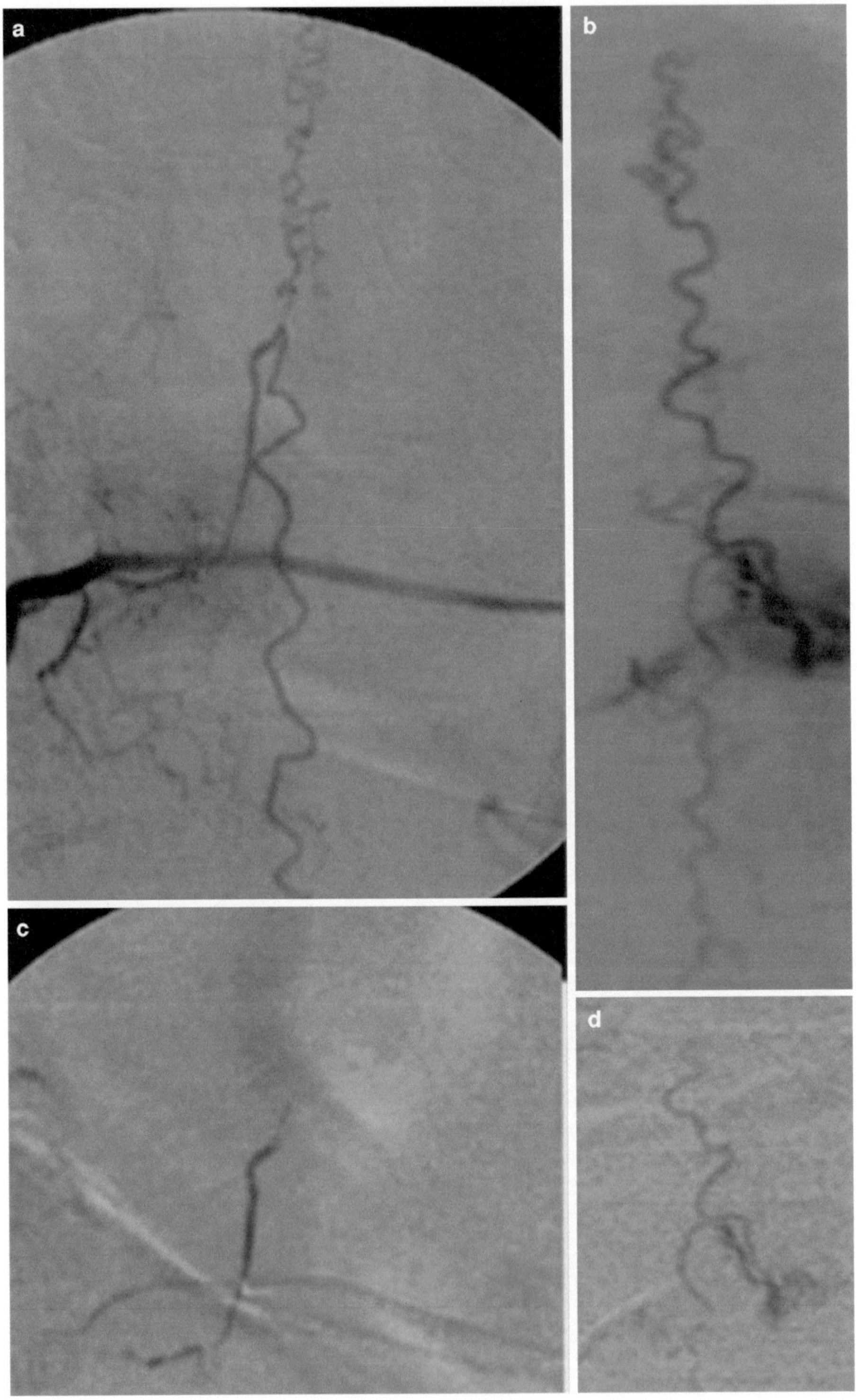

Fig. 15.26 (**a**, **b**) Spinal angiogram injected from Rt Th segmental artery showed oblique hair-pin shape vessel with ascending and descending branches. Diagnosis was SDAVS and the vessels are draining veins (**b** was the NBCA cast). (**c**, **d**) Another spinal angiogram and microcatheter injected from Lt Th segmental artery also showed oblique hair-pin shape vessel with ascending and descending branches. Diagnosis was SDAVS and most of the vessels seen were draining veins

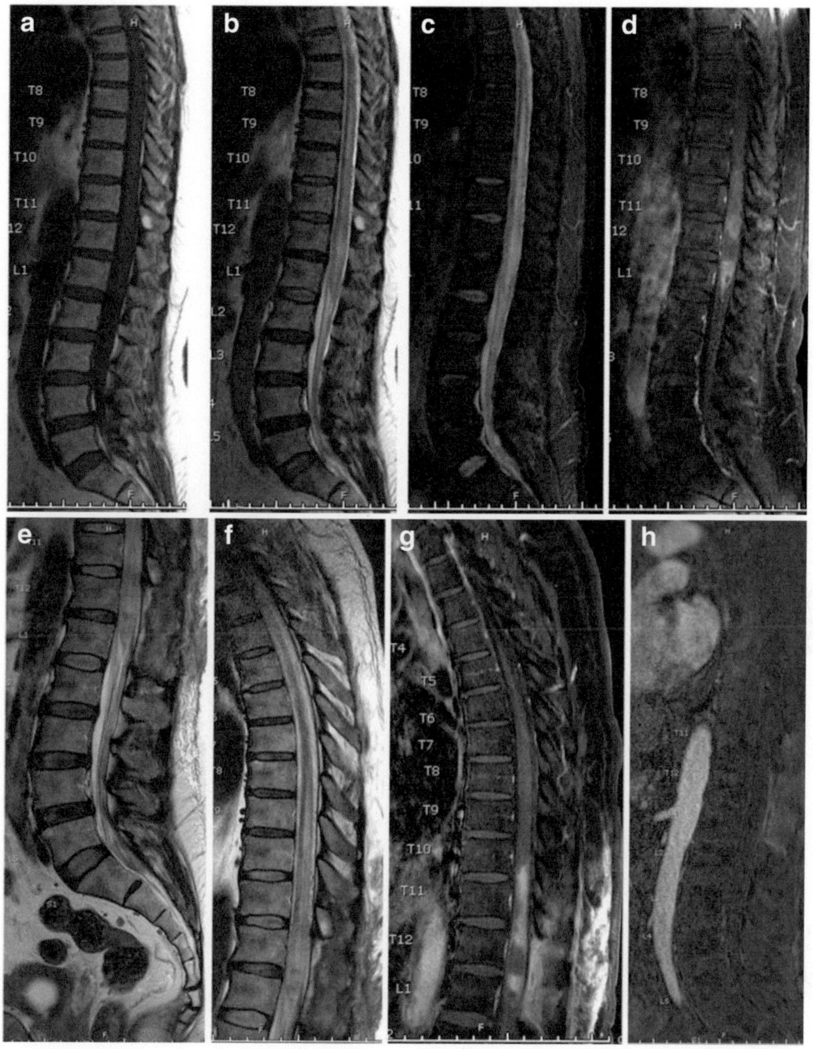

Fig. 15.27 A 71-year-old man on consultation from "Known case of spinal cord tumor, was sent for evaluation of primary cancer." (**a–d**) Sag T1W, T2W, FS T2W and Gd T1W MRI of Th-L spine showed the diffuse hyper T2W signal along the Th cord and conus medullaris; with shaggy enhancement at the lower Th and conus congested level; suggestive of long-standing process of cord congestion and imaging can mimic infiltrative cord lesions, i.e., tumors. Even tiny signal void structures at dorsal aspect of the mid Th level can be seen already. (**e–h**) The lesion at T10-L1 level S/P T12 laminectomy and partial L1 laminectomy has been developed persistent back pain1 month later. The patient had been operated but the clinical was worsening. MRI still showed more intense cord congestion and larger area of enhancement. The screening MRA confirmed abnormal vessels around the conus. (**i–k**) Adamkiewicz artery and ASA study: delayed emptying of the ASA and no venous drainage (radicular veins and epidural veins at 20 s, which represent delayed spinal cord circulation time). Proper superselective injection of the dominant RM artery (Adamkiewicz) up to 20 s should demonstrated the venous phase of the spinal cord circulation. In this case due to cord congestion (from AVS drained into perimedullary veins), the spinal cord cannot drain in proper circulating time, finding of prolong filling of the contrast in ASA axis and no demonstrable radicular/epidural veins at 20 s are demonstrated. (**l–n**) Selective spinal angiogram was performed all levels until an AVS was found at right lateral sacral artery injection. Special curve of guiding catheter into the Rt lateral sacral artery angiogram showed dilated early filling of the Filum Terminale vein draining from the AVS and drained upward direction to congest all the perimedullary veins along the entire Th cord. (**o–r**) Special guiding catheter was deeply placed in the arterial feeder for microcatheter wedging and contrast testing. Superselective microcatheterization into the distal arterial feeder followed by diluted NBCA proper embolization (cover distal arterial feeder, AVS and foot of draining vein). The curative result was proved in control post embolization Rt lateral sacral artery contrast injection (**r**). (**s, t**) Sagittal follow-up T1W and FS T2W MRI Th spine at 4 months showed no further hyper T2W signal of cord congestion anymore, as well as no further seen abnormal dilated perimedullary vessels

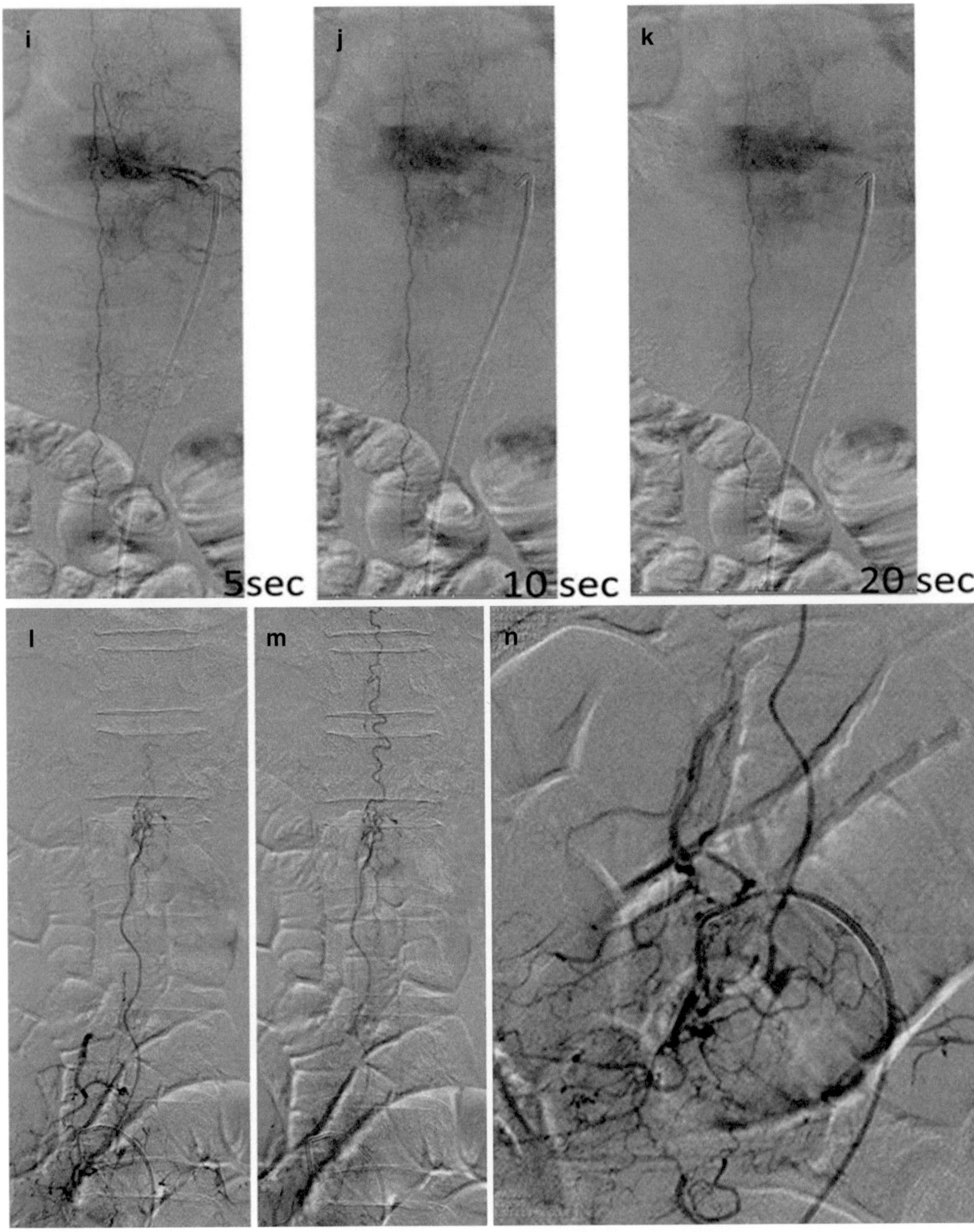

Fig. 15.27 (continued)

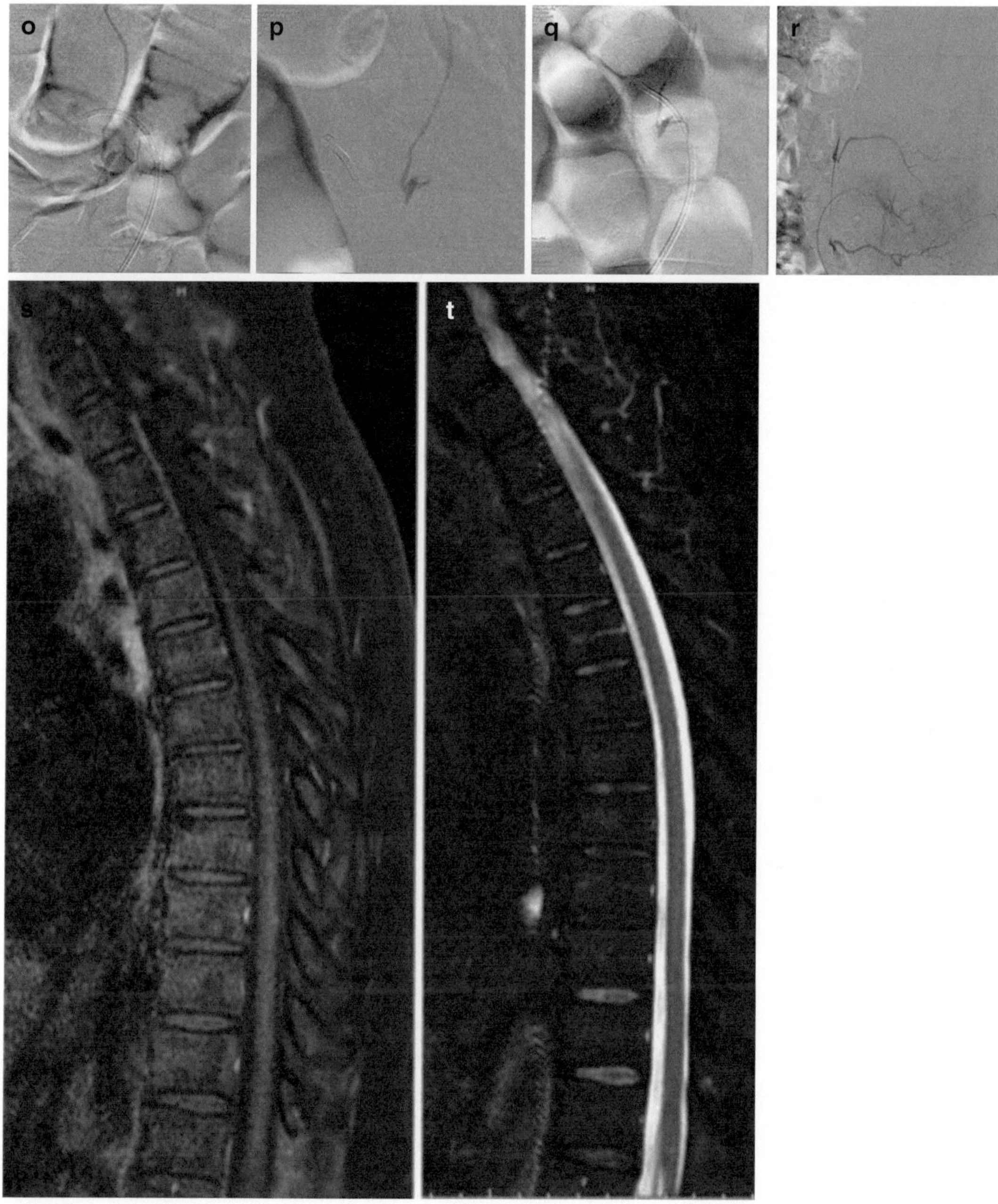

Fig. 15.27 (continued)

spinal cord, but in normal situation will drain out into epidural venous plexus. Radiologists must be caution in case AVS, the veins in early arterial phase and mimic arteries.

15.7 Follow Up Imaging of Spinal Vascular Lesions

- Clinical follow up: The last symptoms will recover first up to the duration of the presenting symptoms.
- MRI: Gold standard for F/U improvement of the dural shunt by mean of congestion of the medullary veins and degree of myelopathy; grossly follow up size of abnormal vessels; intravascular thrombosis; perilesional edema and changes of cord condition.
- Spinal angiogram: In case of suspicious remaining shunt to determine angioarchitecture or anastomosis of other arterial feeders to the shunting for further treatment planning (Fig. 15.28).

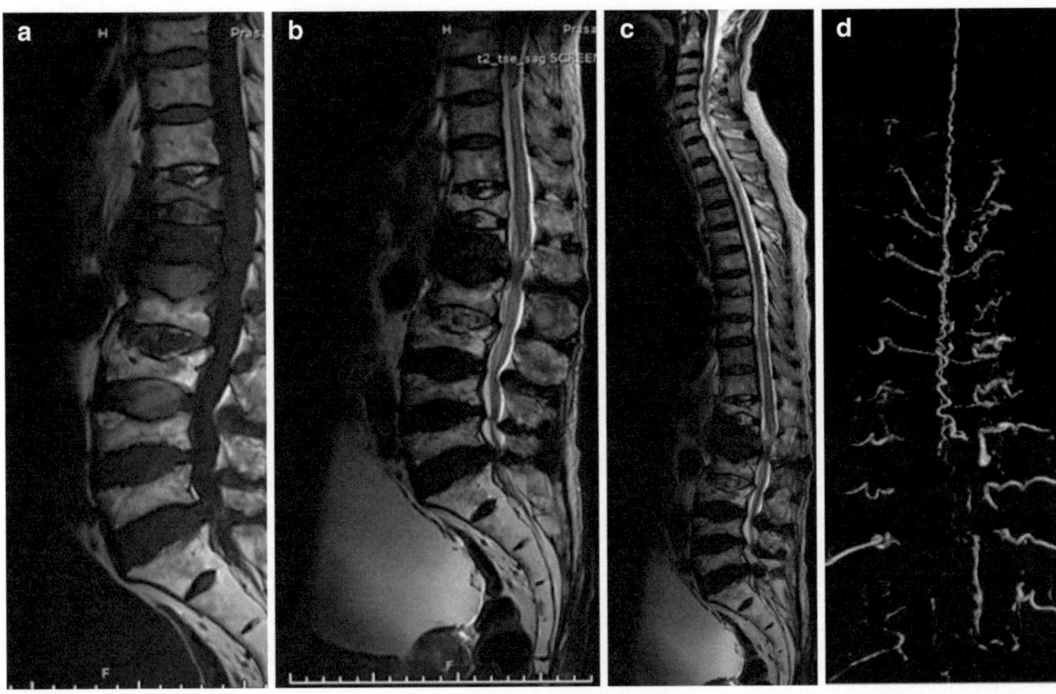

Fig. 15.28 An 85-year-old man presented with progressive paraparesis for 2 months. (**a–d**) Sagittal T1W, T2W, screening sag T2W whole spine and MRA (**d**) confirmed diagnosis of SDAVS and arterial feeder from Lt mid Th segmental artery and draining perimedullary veins upward. (**e–g**) Arterial feeder to the SDAVS is at left Th8, well correlated with the MRA, making treatment possible and more effective. (**h–j**) Superselective segmental artery injection followed by NBCA injection, the NBCA cast was seen too proximal mainly in arterial and partially in the AVS zone but not into the foot of draining vein (confirmed the cast in NCCT coronal study in panel **j**). This patient recover partially and need another session of treatment for curative result

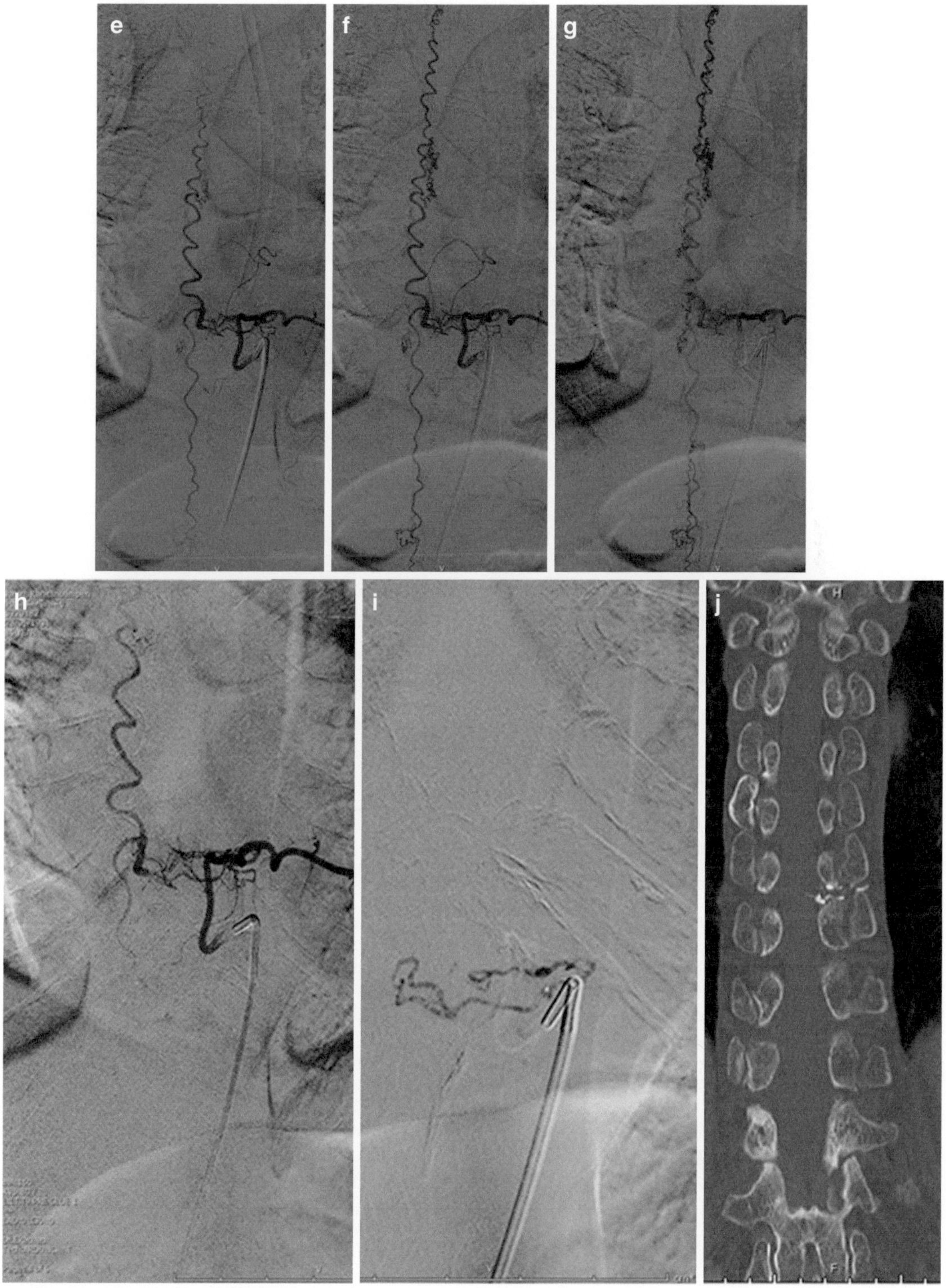

Fig. 15.28 (continued)

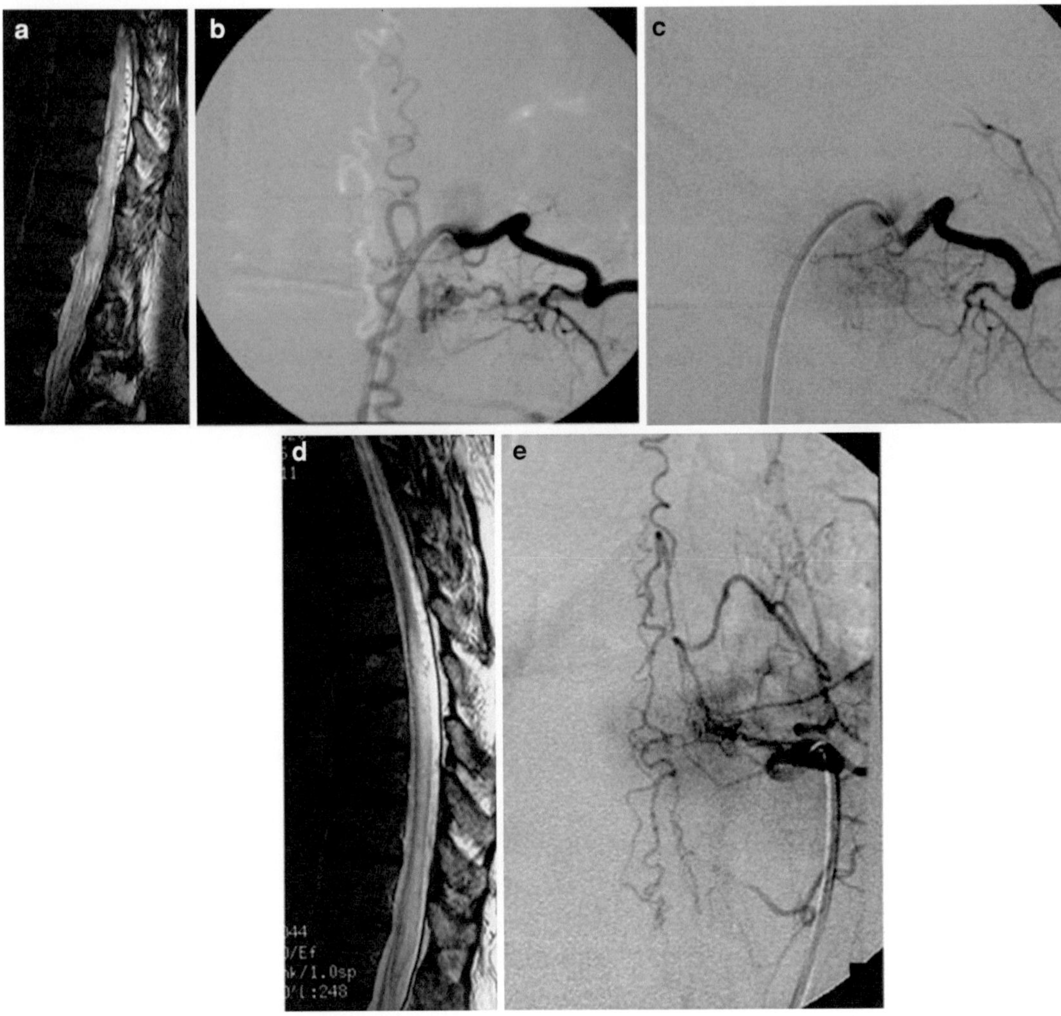

Fig. 15.29 A 61-year-old man presented with 11 months history of progressive myelopathy SDAVS fed from the left Th9. (**a**) Sagittal T2W MRI showed diffuse cord congestion and dilated perimedullary veins. (**b**, **c**) Selective segmental spinal angiogram showed SDAVS fed from this level (Lt Th9); pre and post treatment angiogram showed complete curative result. (**d**, **e**) Partial improvement of the symptoms then worsening of the symptoms at 16 months suggested the possibility of multiple lesions that was not diagnosed at the beginning. In this case the patient was having another location SDAVS fed from Lt Th6 feeder (**e**)

15.7.1 Recurrence Symptoms After Endovascular Treatment

1. Residual AVS caused by proximal supplier embolization without occlusion of the proximal compartment of the draining vein.
2. Multiple SDAVS, not recognized at the first treatment time (Fig. 15.29) [6, 20, 23].

References

1. Lasjaunias P, Ter Brugge KG, Berenstein A. Surgical neuroangiography. Clinical and interventional aspect in children, vol. 15. 2nd ed. Heidelberg: Springer; 2006. p. 721–66.
2. Giebprasert S, Pereira V, Krings T, Jiarakongmun P, Toulgoat F, Pongpech S, Lasjaunias P. Dural arterio-venous shunts: a new classification of craniospinal

epidural venous anatomical bases and clinical correlations. Stroke. 2008;39(10):2783–94.
3. Rodesch G, Hurth M, Alvarez H, Ducot B, Tadie M, Lasjaunias P. Spinal cord intradural arteriovenous fistulae: anatomic, clinical, and therapeutic consider series of 32 consecutive patients seen between 1981 and 2000 with emphasis on endovascular therapy. Neurosurgery. 2005;57(5):973–83.
4. Taeshineetanakul P, Wirojtananugoon C, Singhara Na Ayudhaya S. Elliptical contrast-enhanced MRA to detect abnormal spinal vasculature in Ramathibodi Hospital. Asean J Radiol. 2009;15(3):68–77.
5. Chanthanaphak E, Pongpech S, Jiarakongmun P, Kobkitsuksakul C, Vhi CT, Terbrugge KG. Filum terminale arteriovenous fistulas: the role of endovascular treatment. J Neurosurg Spine. 2013;19(1):49–56.
6. Krings T, Lasjaunias P, Reinges MHT, Mull M, Hans FJ, Thron AK. Spinal vascular malformations. Diagnostic and therapeutic management. Clin Neuroradiol. 2006;16:217–27.
7. Krings T, Lasjaunias P, Hans FJ, et al. Imaging in spinal vascular disease. Neuroimaging Clin N Am. 2007;17:57–72.
8. Rodesch G, Lasjaunias P. Spinal cord arteriovenous shunts: from imaging to management. Interv Neuroradiol. 2003;46(3):221–32.
9. Unsrisong K, et al. Spinal arteriovenous shunts: accuracy of shunt detection, localization and subtype discrimination using spinal magnetic resonance angiography and manual contrast injection using a syringe. J Neurosurg Spine. 2016;24(4):664–70.
10. Farb R, et al. Spinal dural arteriovenous fistula localization with a technique of first-pass gadolinium-enhanced MR angiography: initial experience. Radiology. 2002;222(3):843–50.
11. Rodesch G, Hurth M, Alvarez H, et al. Classification of spinal cord arteriovenous shunts: proposal for a reappraisal. The Bicetre experience with 155 consecutive patients treated between 1981 and 1999. Neurosurgery. 2002;51:374–9.
12. Matsumaru Y, Pongpech S, Laothamas J, Alvarez H, Rodesch G, Lasjaunias P. Multifocal and metameric spinal cord arteriovenous malformations. Review of 19 cases. Interv Neuroradiol. 1999;5(1):27–34.
13. Jiarakongmun P, Chewit P, Pongpech S. Ruptured anterior spinal artery aneurysm associated with coarctation of aorta. Case report and literature review. Interv Neuroradiol. 2002;8(3):285–92.
14. Lindenholz A, et al. The accuracy and utility of contrast enhanced MR angiography for localization of spinal dural arteriovenous fistilas: the Toronto experience. Eur Radiol. 2014;24(11):2885–94.
15. Rodesch G, Hurth M, Alvarez H, Ducot B, Tadie M, Lasjaunias P. Angio-architecture of spinal cord arteriovenous shunts at presentation. Clinical correlations in adults and children. Acta Neurochir. 2004;46:217–27.
16. Rodesch G, Pongpech S, Alvarez H, Zerah M, Hurth M, Sebire G, Lasjaunias P. Spinal cord arteriovenous malformations in a pediatric population: children below 15 years of age: the place of endovascular management. Interv Neuroradiol. 1995;1:29–42.
17. Cullen S, Alvarez H, Rodesch G, Lasjaunias P. Spinal arteriovenous shunt presenting before 2 years of age: analysis of 13 cases. Childs Nerv Syst. 2006;22(9):1103–10.
18. Chen CC, Wang CM, Chu NK, Wu KPH, Tang SFT, Wong AMK. Spinal cord arteriovenous malformation presenting as chest pain in child. Spinal Cord. 2008;46:456–8.
19. Davagnanam I, Toma AK, Brew S. Spinal arteriovenous shunts in children. Neuroimaging Clin N Am. 2013;23(4):749–56.
20. Lekkhong E, Jiarakongmun P, Lasjaunias P, Singhara Na Ayudya S. Multiple spinal arteriovenous fistulas: two pediatric cases report. Asean J Radiol. 2011;17(2):132–7.
21. Mull M, et al. Spinal epidural arteriovenous fistula with perimedullary venous reflux: clinical and neuroradiological features of and underestimated vascular disorder. AJNR Am J Neuroradiol. 2018;39(11):2095–102.
22. Giebprasert S, Pongpech S, Jiarakongmun P, Krings T. Cervical spine dural arteriovenous fistuls presenting with congestive myelopathy of the conus. J Neurosurg Spine. 2009;11(4):427–31.
23. Rodesch G, Hurth M, Alvarez H, et al. Embolization of spinal cord arteriovenous shunt: morphological and clinical follow up and results-review of 69 consecutive cases. Neurosurgery. 2003;53(1):40–50.

Intraoperative Imaging Techniques in the Surgical Management of Spinal AV Fistulas

16

Morgan Broggi, Francesco Acerbi, Elio Mazzapicchi, Marco Schiariti, Francesco Restelli, Jacopo Falco, Ignazio G. Vetrano, Paolo Ferroli, and Giovanni Broggi

Abstract

Introduction, diagnosis and treatment: Spinal dural arteriovenous fistula (SDAVF) is a rare disease with an estimated annual incidence of 5–10 per million population mostly affecting middle age and elderly men. The etiology of SDAVF is still unknown, as they are identified as part of heterogenous group of spinal vascular malformations.

SDAVF diagnosis can be challenging. The presenting symptoms are often non-specific and consist of sensory and/or motor deficits up to, in a late stage, severe myelopathy with bladder incontinence and sexual dysfunction. This is mostly due to venous congestion and spinal cord edema. The variable disease course and misleading findings can lead to a delayed or missed diagnosis. The definitive diagnostic technique of SDAVF is spinal digital subtraction angiography (DSA); however, magnetic resonance (MR) imaging is the first tool in the diagnostic disease workup. Spontaneous occlusion of a SDAVF is very rare; therefore, treatment is almost always required and consists by disconnecting the draining radicular vein of the fistula at the point of dural attachment (AKA point of fistula, PoF). There are two main options: endovascular treatment and open surgery, alone or in combination.

The aim of this chapter is to present the "state of the art" of the intraoperative imaging techniques in the surgical management of SDAVF.

Intraoperative imaging techniques for surgical management of SDAVF: Surgical occlusion of the SDAVF is simple and safe. It involves hemilaminectomy/laminotomy, followed by dural opening and identification of the arterialized radicular vein under the microscopic view; then, following the vein to its dural attachment, the PoF should be coagulated and cut or clipped. Effective occlusion of the SDAVF is indicated by an immediate change in color of the arterialized intradural vein(s).

However, exact identification of the PoF can be sometimes challenging; moreover, it is crucial to obtain confirmation of the complete fistula occlusion and restoration of normal blood flow to avoid ischemic complications. Intraoperative or postoperative DSA are the

M. Broggi · F. Acerbi · E. Mazzapicchi · M. Schiariti
F. Restelli · J. Falco · I. G. Vetrano · P. Ferroli
Department of Neurosurgery, Fondazione IRCCS
Istituto Neurologico Carlo Besta, Milan, Italy

G. Broggi (✉)
Department of Neurosurgery, Fondazione IRCCS
Istituto Neurologico Carlo Besta, Milan, Italy

Fondazione I.E.N., Milan, Italy

X. Lv (ed.), *Intracranial and Spinal Dural Arteriovenous Fistulas*,
https://doi.org/10.1007/978-981-19-5767-3_16

"gold standard" to achieve these goals, but they are invasive, expensive and time consuming.

For these reasons, in recent times, several intraoperative imaging techniques have been introduced to improve surgical results of SDVAF treatment; these include the following:

- *Intraoperative indocyanine green videoangiography (ICGV)*

  In the last two decades, intraoperative indocyanine green (ICG) videoangiography (ICGVA) has widely spread as a safe and simple adjunctive tool able to provide real-time information about the precise location of spinal and cranial DAVFs and confirmation of their complete occlusion.

  The operative field is illuminated by a light source of a wavelength that covers part of the ICG absorption band (700 ± 850 nm, maximum 805 nm). ICG is then injected into a peripheral/central vein line as a bolus. The fluorescence light (780–950 nm, maximum 835 nm) is then recorded by a non-intensified video camera, with optical filtering. Thus arterial, capillary and venous angiography can be observed on the video screen in real-time; semiquantitative measurement of blood flow is possible too. ICGVA can be used several times throughout the procedure. A dedicated microscope is necessary for this technique.
- *Ultrasound*

  Intraoperative ultrasound (ioUS) associated with contrast enhanced ultrasound (CEUS) have been successfully introduced into oncological and vascular brain and spinal surgery.

  In literature, the experience on the application of ioUS in spinal SDAVF is extremely limited.

  The association of standard B-mode imaging, color-doppler US and CEUS represent an effective intraoperative tool to define vascular features of the SDAVF and their anatomical relationship with the spinal cord, allowing to recognize vessels deeper than the only pial surface or in any case, not directly illuminated by the microscope.
- *Sodium fluorescein*

  More recently, sodium fluorescein video angiography (SFVA) seemed to be a valuable alternative in vascular neurosurgery. SFVA has been explored in aneurysm and cerebral arterio-venous malformation (AVM) surgery, but there are few studies reporting the use of fluorescein in SDAVF. Sodium fluorescein (SF) fluoresces with wavelengths of 520–530 nm in response to excitation with light at 465–490 nm. In practice, this results in yellowish-green fluorescence that can be detected by video angiography. SFVA allows a better visualization of the operative field than ICG, especially concerning very small vessels, and it is a low-cost technique. The main drawback of SFVA is the extravascular leakage of fluorescein, so the best visualization can be obtained with the fist injection and an interval of at least 20 min is necessary between two SF injections. A dedicated microscope is necessary for this technique.

Keywords

Spinal dural arteriovenous fistula
Intraoperative indocyanine green videoangiography · Ultrasound · Sodium fluorescein · Spine neurosurgery

16.1 Introduction, Diagnosis and Treatment

16.1.1 Introduction

Spinal dural arteriovenous fistula (SDAVF) is a rare disease with an annual incidence of 5–10 out of a million people [1]. SDAVF is an acquired disease with greater occurrence in middle age and elderly men (man:female ratio 6:1) [2–4]. It represent about 60% of all cases of spinal vascular malformations and is mostly located in the middle or upper tract of the spine [5]. The etiology of SDAVFs is still unknown, as they are identified as part of a larger group of spinal vascular malformations.

Table 16.1 Spetzler classification and clinical characteristics of spinal AVFs [6]

Characteristic	Extradural	Dorsal intradural	Ventral intradural
Pathophysiology	Spinal cord compression, venous congestion, vascular steal	Venous congestion, rare hemorrhage	Compression (venous aneurysm), hemorrhage, vascular steal
Presentation	Progressive myelopathy	Progressive myelopathy	Progressive myelopathy
Diagnostic modality	MR imaging, angiography	MR imaging, angiography	MR imaging, angiography
Previous nomenclature	Epidural	Dural AVF, long dorsal, type IA, others	Types IVA (small), B (medium), and C (large), perimedullary

The classification proposed by Spetzler et al. [6] divides all types of vascular spinal cord alterations into three groups: neoplastic vascular lesions, aneurysms and arteriovenous lesions. The latter is further divided into arteriovenous malformations (AVMs) and arteriovenous fistulas (AVFs). AVFs are subdivided into extradural, dorsal intradural or ventral intradural fistulas. Ventral AVFs correspond to the peri-medullary fistulas (fistulas that connect pial arterial branches with pial veins in the subarachnoid space), while dorsal AVFs correspond to "classic" SDAVFs. SDAVFs are also dichotomized into two types based on the number of feeders: AVFs with one feeder are categorized as type A, while those with multiple feeders as type B (Table 16.1).

To understand the pathogenesis and treatment of these lesions, it is essential to know the vascular anatomy from which SDAVFs originate. Spine vascularization is supplied by segmental arteries [7]. From its origin, each segmental artery moves dorsally and, after passing the neural foramina, it divides into three major trunks: (1) a radicular artery, which supplies the dura and the nerve roots; (2) a dorsal branch that supplies the posterior spinal musculature and the facet regions; and (3) a lateral branch, a continuation of the segmental artery that circumferentially wraps around the chest or abdominal wall from the dorsal to the ventral side [8]. Both radiculo-pial and radiculo-medullary branches originate from the radicular artery.

As far as the venous drainage is concerned, it can be divided into an intradural portion (an intrinsic venous network draining spinal cord parenchyma), an extrinsic system (which, amongst others, includes surface veins of spinal cord linking the intradural venous system) and the extradural venous plexus (Batson's plexus).

The radicular arteries are the vessels often involved in SDAVFs, connecting one or more radiculo-dural branches with an intradural radicular vein to form the proper arteriovenous fistula. Due to an increased spinal venous pressure, caused by the SDAVF, the normal spinal cord venous drainage is altered, resulting in a subsequent venous congestion and intramedullary edema. The diminished arteriovenous pressure gradient, as well as the reduced outflow of the other radicular veins due to partial thrombosis [1], is the cause of chronic hypoxia, spinal cord damage and progressive myelopathy [9–11].

16.1.2 Diagnosis

Diagnosing SDAVFs could be challenging [12]. In the first phase of the disease, SDAVFs could mimic polyneuropathy or radiculopathy, since symptoms are often nonspecific and include gait difficulties, sensory deficit, motor weakness and radicular pain [13]. Patients often present symptoms and signs of upper and lower motor neuron deficits which may lead to a misdiagnosis [3, 13, 14]. Bladder symptoms, sexual dysfunctions or sensory impairments in the perineal region could strongly support this diagnosis. Additional rare symptoms and signs like headaches could be associated to a hemorrhage into the spinal or intracranial subarachnoid space.

Based on clinical suspicion, a proper imaging study should be carried out to confirm the diagnosis and location of SDAVF. A total axis (or thoracolumbar) spine magnetic resonance (MR) scan is the most common procedure in these cases, which usually demonstrates the combination of intramedullary signal alteration with a perimedullary vessels enlargement [15]. On T2-weighted images, spinal cord edema appears as a central hyperintensity over multiple segments. On T1-weighted images, the swollen cord is slightly hypointense and enlarged. After intravenous (i.v.) contrast administration, the chronic venous congestion could appear as a diffuse intramedullary enhancement due to a blood-spinal cord barrier breakdown. In the late stages of the disease, the spinal cord may appear atrophic. In SDAVFs, the dilated ad tortuous vessels are mainly located on the dorsal part of perimedullary space, and they can be easily observed in T2-weighted images as a flow void signal. However, for small dural AVFs, venous congestion could be seen only after contrast agent administration [4] (Fig. 16.1).

MR can identify the level and location of the nidus in relation to the spinal cord and dura, especially when combined with a spinal contrast-enhanced dynamic magnetic resonance angiogram (MRA). This technique can demonstrate early venous filling, which may indicate the level of the shunt. Computed tomography angiography (CTA) can also provide spinal vessel images showing the surrounding bony structure [16]. Even though MR, MRA, and CTA are less invasive, their findings often do not provide all the hemodynamic information needed to plan surgical therapy. Therefore, conventional spinal digital subtraction angiography (DSA), although being more invasive, more expensive and requiring a higher level of expertise, is still considered the "gold standard" diagnostic technique for SDAVFs.

When imaging exams clearly suggest the presence of a fistula, or when the exact level cannot

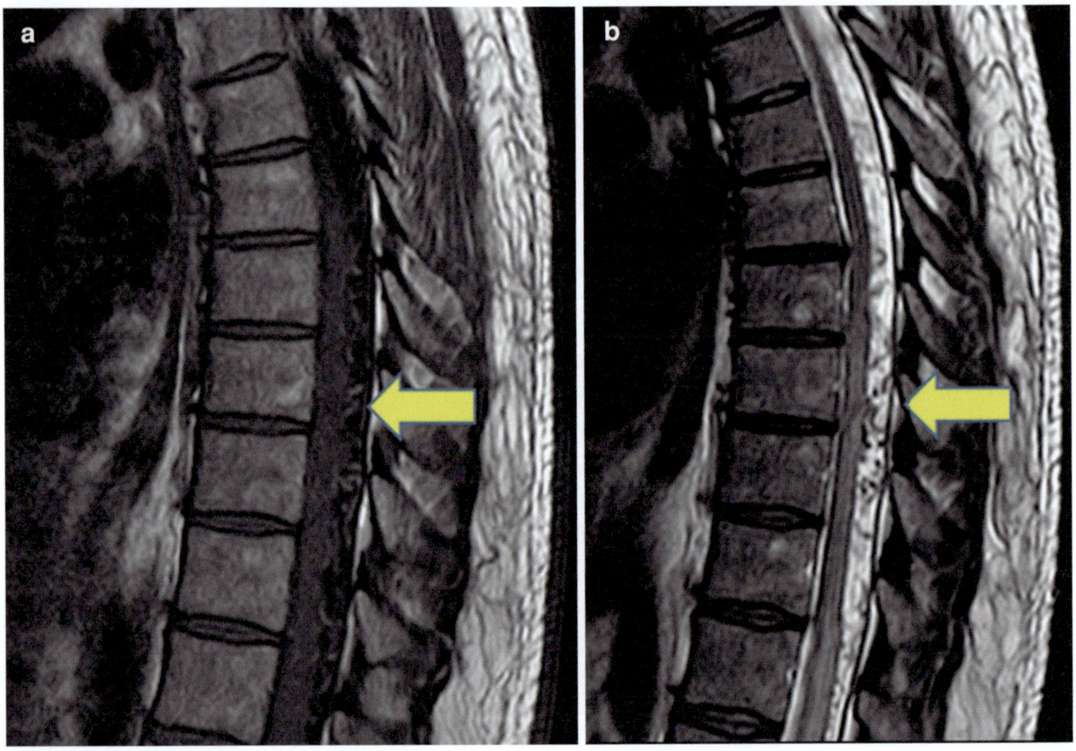

Fig. 16.1 (**a**) Sagittal T1-wieghted with i.v. contrast administration MR showing multilevel dilated and tortuous vessels (*yellow arrow*) on the dorsal part of perimedullary space secondary to a right D7 SDAVF. (**b**) Sagittal T2-wieghted MR showing the same case as (**a**); the pathological vessels can be seen as flow void signals (*yellow arrow*)

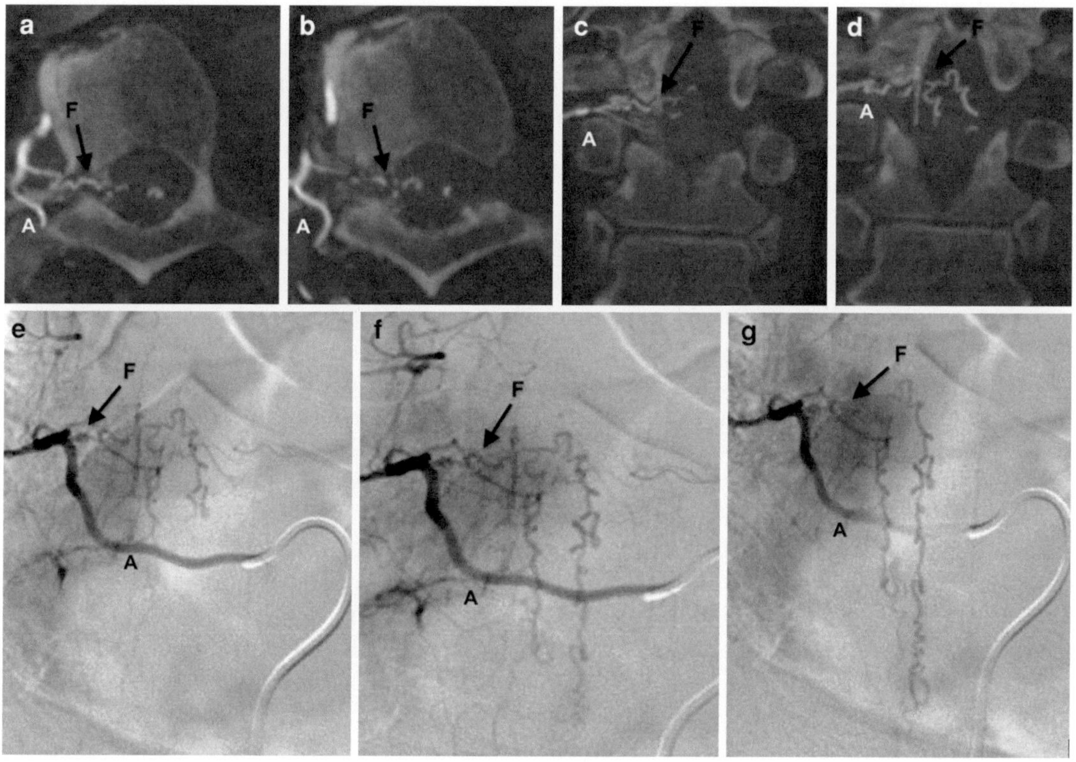

Fig. 16.2 (**a**, **b**) Axial Dyna-CT with i.v. contrast administration showing a right D5 SDVAF; note the artery (*A*) outside the foramina and the fistula (*F*) at the level of the foramina. (**c**, **d**) Coronal Dyna-CT with i.v. contrast administration showing a right D5 SDVAF; note the artery (*A*) outside the foramina and the fistula (*F*) at the level of the foramina. (**e–g**) Early arterial, mid arterial and late arterial spinal DSA images showing the same case as (**a–d**); note the artery marked as *A* and the fistula marked as *F*

be determined, patients should undergo DSA (it is advisable to perform this exam under general anesthesia so that embolization, if feasible, could be executed at the same time). If the fistula level is unknown, all spinal segments should be evaluated. Since 70–80% of SDAVFs are located at the mid-lower thoracic spine, this segment should be searched first. If the fistula is still not identified, the upper thoracic segmental vessels, the subclavian arteries and their branches should be explored. The angiographic hallmark of SDAVF is the early filling of an enlarged radicular vein and then filling of multiple enlarged draining veins in several directions. The anterior spinal artery (ASA), if found, could be identified as a vessel characterized by slow flow and stasis due to spinal cord edema and venous congestion. SDAVF is excluded if no fistula is found on angiography and the radiculo-medullary injection shows good ASA flow with no venous delay [7] (Fig. 16.2).

The differentiation between SDAVFs and peri-medullary fistulas is difficult to detect through an MR exam alone. On conventional spinal angiographies, peri-medullary fistulas drain into the intradural veins, as SDAVFs. However, in contrast to SDAVFs, they are supplied by pial arterial branches and present an increased flow in the pial arteries and veins due to abnormal pial connections.

16.1.3 Treatment

The spontaneous occlusion of SDAVFs very rarely occurs. Treatments are therefore almost always mandatory, aimed at arresting the progression of symptoms or even reversing them, when possible. Endovascular treatment and open surgery, alone or combined [17], are the two main alternatives when it comes to SDAVFs treatment. Both choices require the disconnection of the draining radicular veins involved in the fistula at the point of dural attachment (AKA point of fistula, PoF), in order to solve the venous system congestion causing the spinal cord edema [3, 4, 18]. Indications on treating patients with asymptomatic fistulas remain controversial, as symptoms may appear different years after an incidental finding [19]. Therefore, patients should be followed with serial clinical assessments and MR and be treated as soon as any new relevant clinical sign appears.

In endovascular surgery for SDAVF, embolic material (e.g., glue and Onyx) is injected to occlude the venous drainage of the fistula. Angiography must explore all the segmental arteries to have a complete understanding of vascular architecture around the lesion and choose the feeder to embolize. The vessels must be checked again at the end of the procedure to detect any remnants [14, 20]. The proper concentration of embolic fluid injected is determined by the rate of flow of the fistula, the location of the catheter and the configuration of the radicular vein. When the venous side of the fistula is filled with embolic agents, the SDAVF is considered cured [21, 22]. If a proper closure of fistula does not occur, the patients should immediately undergo surgical treatment; it is therefore recommended, if not mandatory, that SDAVF are treated in big case load centers where both experienced endovascular and neurosurgical teams are available. The two main reasons behind the failure of endovascular treatments are associated with placing the microcatheter in the wedge position or too far from the lesion. Overall, for both glue and Onyx, if radiculo-medullary branches such as the radiculo-medullary magna (also known as artery of Ademkiewicz) arise from the same segmental branch of the fistula, surgical treatment is preferred over endovascular embolization. Furthermore, compared to surgical treatment, endovascular therapy has been associated with a lower rate of fistula closing and consequently a higher rate of recurrence, from 15% to 44% [23, 24]. Among the several authors that have compared surgical versus endovascular treatment, Eskandar et al. and Ruiz-Juretschke et al. reported, respectively, a failure rate of 39% and 44% for endovascular procedures, as well as a failure rate of 0.5% for surgical therapy [25, 26]; in addition, Gokhale et al. demonstrate a recurrence rate of 30% after endovascular procedure [23]. In their meta-analysis, Bakker et al. [27] showed that the initial success rate of surgical treatment was 96.6% compared to 72.2% for endovascular therapy. The possible reason of the different rate of success and recurrence could be explained by the fact that these fistulas are often fed by multiple dural arteries with a single draining vein. The inability to occlude all arterial feeders through an endovascular approach can lead to the recanalization or development of collaterals, resulting in the recurrence of SDAVFs [28]. In addition, due to the rapid technological changes that characterize endovascular techniques, it is difficult to estimate the real complication rate of these procedures, which are surely not harmless (e.g., Song et al. [29] have reported 15% of post-embolization neurologic deterioration). In the case series proposed by Guillevin et al. [30], in 19% of patients the procedure was aborted and repeated several days later due to renal malfunction (12%) or spasm of the SDAVF to be filled (7%).

Surgical treatment for SDAVFs is often definitive and curative. Best results are obtained in patients treated before the onset of severe symptoms, as recovery from previous deficits can be limited. If the procedure is carried out in big caseload centers with experienced neurosurgical teams, there are low post-operative risks, higher fistulas obliteration rates with rapid resolution of the venous congestion. Briefly, to treat typical thoracolumbar SDAVFs, patients are placed in prone position with the interested spine segment centrally located in neutral or slightly kyphotic position. The correct spine level is then confirmed through intraoperative fluoroscopy. A midline vertical skin incision is made down to the muscular fascia, and paraspinal muscles are dissected from the midline until the articular facets on both sides are identified. A two or more-level laminotomy/hemilaminectomy is carried out centered on the feeding radicular artery. The opening must be wider enough to identify the PoF (see next paragraphs). Once the exposure is completed, SDAVFs must be identified. Whilst they are often fed by a singular artery, sometimes feeders from levels above or below the fistula may reach the lesion through transdural connection. Following the identification of the level, the dura is opened longitudinally and retracted with stay sutures to visualize the spinal cord and the nerve root. The draining vein is thickened by the chronic effects of arterialization. A temporary clip is then placed on this vein; after receiving the confirmation that the fistula is interrupted (see next paragraphs), the interested vein is then coagulated intradurally and divided between two titanium hemoclips. Effective occlusion of the SDAVF is indicated by an immediate change in color of the arterialized intradural vein(s). The fistula is then bipolar cauterized to obliterate both intradural and extradural surfaces, to reduce or even eliminate the possibility of recurrences. Arteries that supply the spinal cord must be preserved. In addition, to monitor any spinal cord damages, intraoperative motor and sensory-evoked potential monitoring is often used, and it is strongly recommended, throughout the procedure. Finally, the mean arterial pressure should be kept not below 80 mmHg to prevent severe hypotension and avoid cord hypoperfusion risk.

16.2 Intraoperative Imaging Techniques

As said above, surgical occlusion of SDAVF is simple, safe and, most of the times, effective. However, in some cases, the exact identification of the PoF can be challenging: when the PoF is not correctly identified, the procedure may fail and/or can be aborted in order to avoid spinal cord damages. Moreover, it is crucial to obtain confirmation of the complete fistula occlusion and restoration of normal blood flow to avoid ischemic complications. Intraoperative or postoperative DSA are the "gold standard" to achieve these goals, but they are, once again, invasive, expensive and time consuming.

For these reasons, in recent times, several intraoperative imaging techniques have been introduced to improve surgical results of SDVAF treatment.

16.2.1 Indocyanine Green Videoangiography (ICGVA)

Indocyanine Green (ICG) is a tri-carbo-cyanine firstly used in the diagnostic investigations of cardiac output, liver function and hepatic blood circulation. Its use was approved by the FDA in 1956, in the context of the evaluation of cardiocirculatory and liver functions, as well as in 1975 for ophthalmic angiography. In recent times, ICG video-angiography (ICGVA) spread widely also in vascular neurosurgery as a helpful and simple tool able to provide an intraoperative real-time evaluation of local circulation. The absorption and emission peaks of ICG are respectively of 805 and 835 nm. Typically, ICGVA is performed with i.v. bolus injection (1–2 s, preferred in the central line) of 12.5–25 mg of ICG dissolved in saline solution. Once ICG is injected, it primarily binds a1-lipoproteins and other globulins and carried to the systemic circulation. ICG is then excreted by the liver with a half-life time of 4 min. The maximal daily dose should not exceed 5 mg/kg. Microscope-integrated ICG fluorescence angiography can be utilized to evaluate flow-dynamic information of surgical outcome for intracranial and spinal vascular diseases. Neurosurgical applications of ICG and technical details have been previously described by several authors [31–33].

Indocyanine green videoangiography can provide flow-dynamic information such as flow direction, velocity, and alteration. Using occlusion tests in different vessels and observing the real-time alterations in the filling pattern allow to clearly visualize the difference phases of filling and thus to identify the feeders, the draining vein(s), and the shunts. A small dose in a single bolus and the feasibility of repeating several injections without adverse events are clear advantages of this technique providing precise flow-dynamic information throughout the procedure. Horie et al. [34] firstly described the efficacy of ICGVA for spinal AVFs. To our knowledge, Schuette et al. [35] reported one of the largest series in using ICGVA for the management of SDAVFs. Evidence presented by the authors demonstrates that ICGVA matched with postoperative DSA in all cases, and this technique added only 1–3 min at each injection to the operating time without any ICG-related complications.

During SDAVF surgical occlusion, ICGVA is generally performed at least at two stages throughout the procedure before and after the clipping and disconnection of the PoF. Specifically, initial ICG angiography is done to obtain information about the exact localization of the PoF, the afferent artery, the arterialized vein or veins and to study the venous flow congestion due to the fistula. Secondly, ICG analysis is done at the end of the occlusion to confirm the disconnection of the PoF and to check the patency of adjacent arteries and veins along with the restoration of the normal flow in the spinal parenchyma affected by the fistula.

Furthermore, to provide more information about flow dynamics, the use of the ICGVA has recently been associated with the application of the software FLOW 800. The software employs a color-coded semi-automatically generated map to identify the direction and sequence of blood flow in the observed surgical cavity. This tool makes it easier to distinguish arterial and venous flows and to identify eventual fistulous points and draining veins. Different reports have demonstrated the utility of this technique in vascular neurosurgery [36–38]. Shi et al. [39] firstly evaluate the efficacy of FLOW 800 in the management of SDAVFs. They discovered that paralesional parenchymal perfusions significantly improved after a successful treatment of the SDAVF, and that the transit time was shorter following fistula occlusions. Many factors like ICG injection speed, microscope position, illumination intensity, cardiac output, hepatic excretory function and cerebrospinal fluid or blood accumulation could influence FLOW 800 analyses. Therefore, this technique should be used in specific cases, particularly those in which intraoperative assessments of flow dynamics or rapid monitoring of parenchymal perfusions are needed.

Most authors agree that the major limitation of ICGVA is that it captures only what is exposed in the surface of the surgical field and, as a consequence of this, it requires that the parenchyma and vessels must be clear of any tissue, blood clots, cottonoids, et cetera; furthermore, the position of the microscope influences the quality of ICGVA images and should be carefully evaluated. Finally, the availability of a microscope with the dedicated filter and software can be considered another intrinsic limitation of the technique.

Spiotta et al. in 2011 concluded that the use of intraoperative ICGVA assists in diagnosing angiographic occult DAVFs, evaluating DAVFs flow, and confirming fistula closure by possibly avoiding the need for postoperative angiography [40] (Figs. 16.3 and 16.4).

16.2.2 Intraoperative Ultrasound (ioUS)

Intraoperative ultrasound (ioUS), in combination with contrast enhanced ultrasound (CEUS), has been introduced into oncological and vascular neurosurgery in recent years [41]. However, there are very limited reports on the use of ultrasound in SDAVFs [42, 43]. After the identification of the spinal level and following laminectomy/laminotomy, US doppler scan could be performed to evaluate the perimedullary flow and identify the appropriate point to open the dura. Then, CEUS could be performed extradurally, allowing the visualization of the arterialized vein with inverted flow from radicular dural sleeve to the perimedullary plexus. After dural opening, a new CEUS scan can confirm pre-occlusion blood flow dynamics of the SDAVF. This scan often shows an inverted direction of microbubble from radicular sleeve toward to perimedullary dilatated plexus, which appears characterized by chaotic high flow of microbubbles. Once fistula occlusion and coagulation are completed, CEUS scan

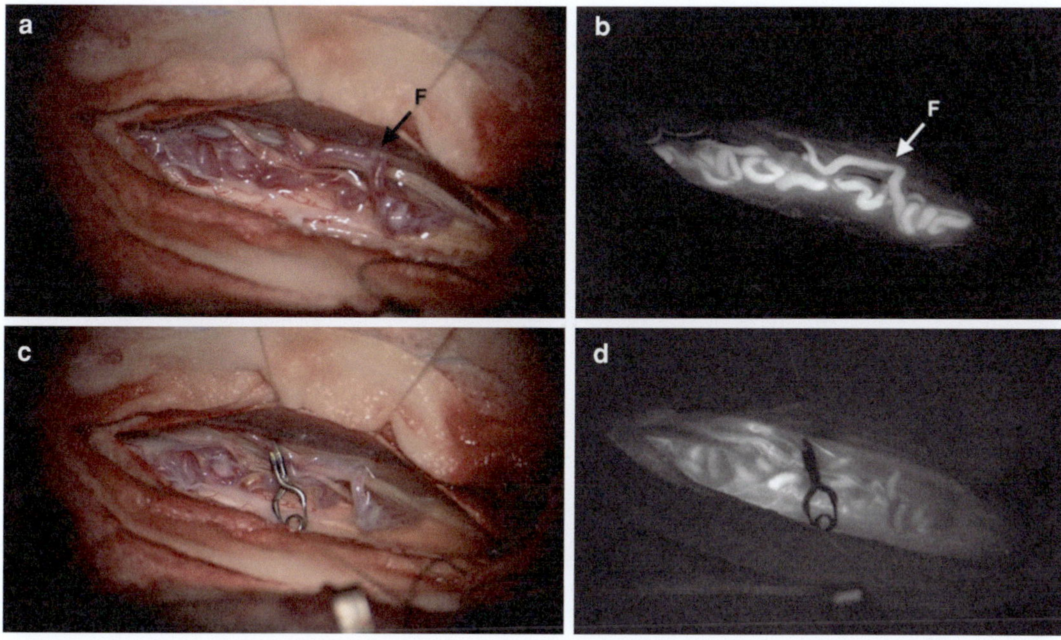

Fig. 16.3 (**a**) Intraoperative microscopic exposure of a left D6 SDAVF; the fistula is marked as *F.* (**b**) ICGVA of the same case as (**a**); the fistula is marked as *F*. (**c**, **d**) A clip has been placed at the PoF (**c**) and ICGVA confirms that the pathological drainage has been stopped by the clip (**d**). The PoF can be now coagulated and cut

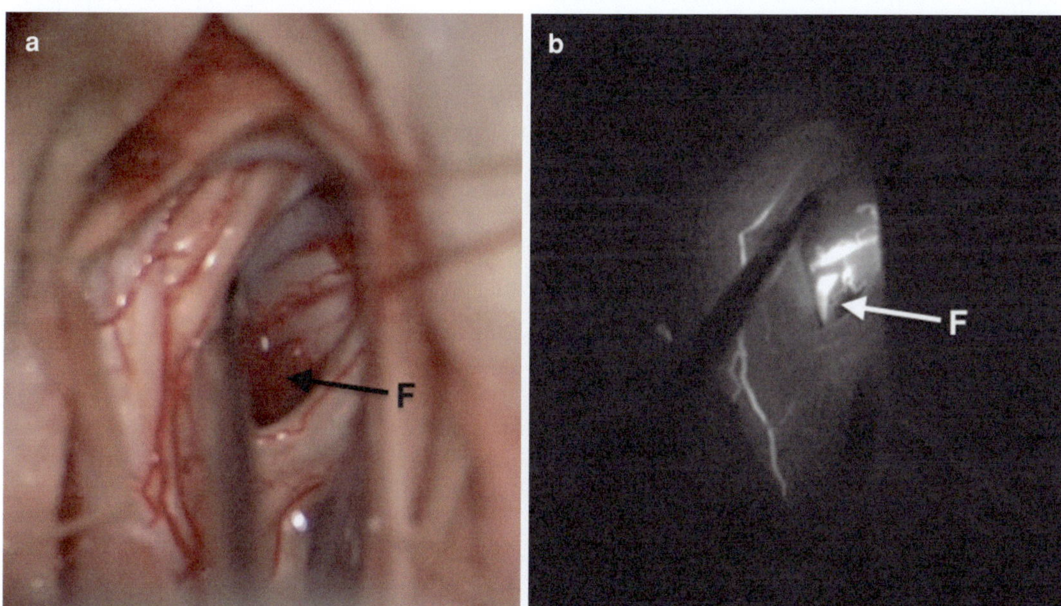

Fig. 16.4 (**a**) Intraoperative microscopic exposure of a left C5 SDAVF; the fistula is marked as *F.* (**b**) ICGVA of the same case as (**a**); the fistula is marked as *F*. (**c**) ICGVA with flow800 analysis shows the high flow at the level of the fistula (*F*)

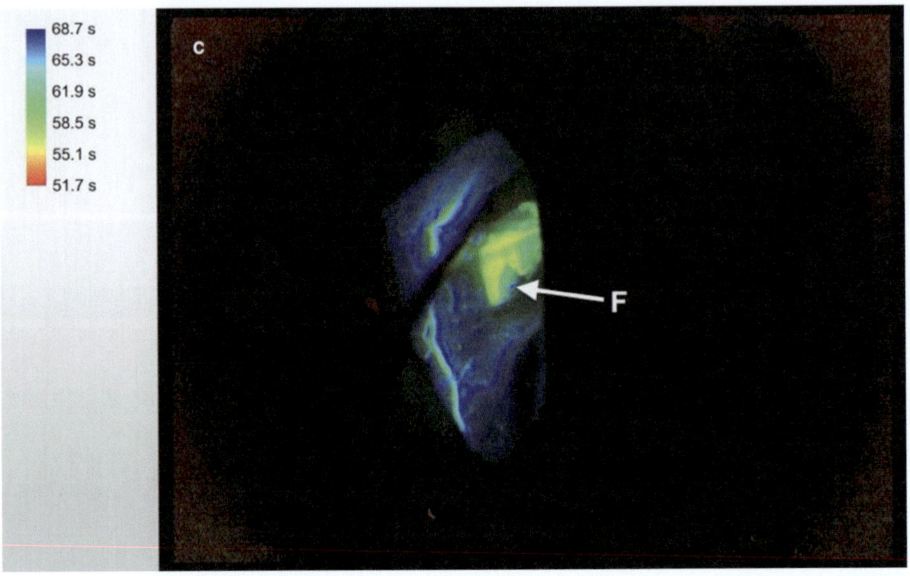

Fig. 16.4 (continued)

could confirm the interruption of arterialized vein(s) and provide information about normal blood flow restoration in perimedullary plexus and in spinal cord.

The association of standard B-mode imaging, color-doppler and CEUS provides important information about SDAVF anatomical relationships, nerve roots position, vessels alteration, and flow dynamics. In addition, ioUS and CEUS allow to visualize hidden anatomical and pathological structures that are not exposed in surgical field, thus minimizing unnecessary surgical exposition, defining anatomical relationships and reducing surgical manipulation. Currently, there is no evidence about the comparison of ioUS/CEUS and ICGVA in literature; however, each technique has different advantages and drawbacks. ICGVA is a simple and feasible technique that provides precise flow dynamic information, but it allows to investigate only vessels at the pial surface or directly illuminated by the microscope. Therefore, proper intraoperative assessments can be limited if draining vessels or fistulous points are in unfavorable anatomical positions, as stated above. CEUS provides rapid and real-time information on the anatomical position of fistula, while color-doppler allows to confirm the arterialization of the flow at the PoF and eventual flow dynamic changes after treatment (Figs. 16.5 and 16.6).

Some of the limitations of ioUS include the fact that the procedure is operator-dependent, with a steeper learning curve than ICGVA since this image modality is much less familiar to neurosurgeons. The recent introduction of US navigated probes, however, allows an easier integration of US and MR to improve the correct identification of structures. In addition, the scanning window can visualize only a limited part of the lesion at time.

Intraoperative US and ICGVA can be both used as complementary tools to provide a better and global flow dynamic information of SDAVFs and improve surgical outcomes.

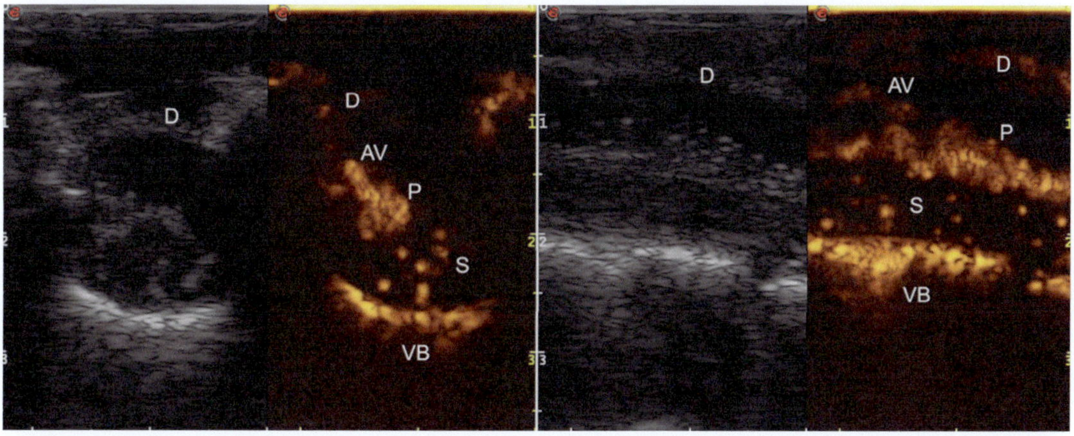

Fig. 16.5 Pre-ligation CEUS scan of D6 dorsal SDAVF acquired before dural opening (left—axial scan; right—sagittal scan). These images show the location of the intact dura mater (*D*) and the arterial veins (AV) ending in the enlarged peri-medullary plexus (P). The spinal cord (*S*) CEUS signal is stronger than the physiological state due to congestion and increased blood flow in the intramedullary capillaries. The medulla oblongata is displaced relative to the vertebral body (*VB*) [42]. (Courtesy of Dr. Francesco Prada, Department of Neurosurgery, Fondazione IRCCS Istituto Neurologico C. Besta, Milan, Italy)

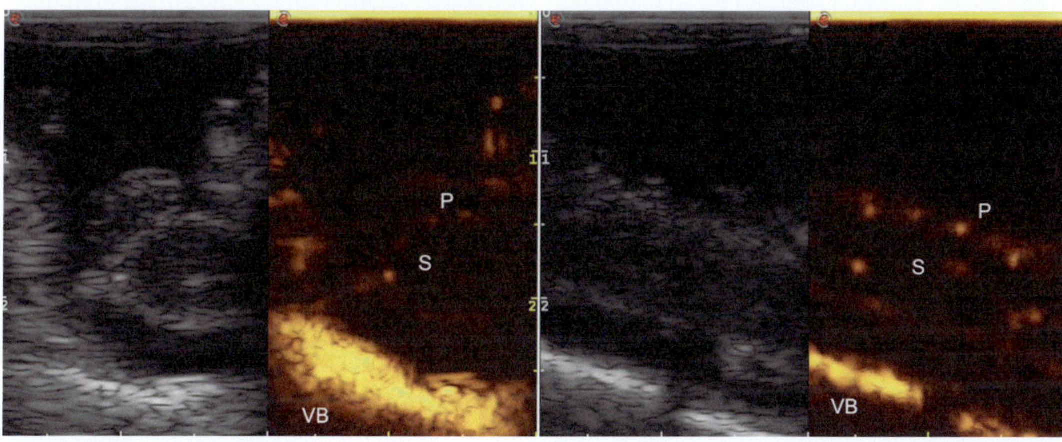

Fig. 16.6 Post-ligation CEUS scan of D6 dorsal SDAVF (left—axial scan; right—sagittal scan). Arterialized veins are no longer visible. The previously dilated peri-medullary plexus (*P*) is now less crowded and less visible at CEUS. The CEUS signal from the spinal cord (*S*) is still visible, but less than the previous signal and more similar to the physiological aspect. The spinal cord is no longer displaced respect to the vertebral body (VB)43. (Courtesy of Dr. Francesco Prada, Department of Neurosurgery, Fondazione IRCCS Istituto Neurologico C. Besta, Milan, Italy)

16.2.3 Sodium Fluorescein

Sodium fluorescein (SF) has been used to evaluate retinal blood flows since 1881 [44]. More recently, it was adopted to better visualize glial tumor during surgical resection and biopsy [45–50]. The application of SF in vascular neurosurgery was firstly reported in 1971 [51]; however, since then, the number of studies that analyze SF videoangiography (SFVA) has been very limited: it has been explored in aneurysm and cerebral AVM surgery, but there are very few studies reporting the use of fluorescein in SDAVF.

After i.v. administration, SF binds to plasma globulins and is then metabolized by the liver. Sodium fluorescein fluoresces with wavelengths of 520–530 nm in response to excitation with light at 465–490 nm. In practice, this results in yellowish-green fluorescence that can be detected under microscopic view, that is visible even under conventional white light illumination. However, the use of specific filter integrated into the microscope (namely, yellow560 filter) greatly improve image quality and allow for high resolution video-angiography. Despite several indications, SF dose should not exceed 20 mg/kg body weight; complications such as cardiac alteration, respiratory reaction or seizure have been rarely reported, with a rate of adverse effects lower than 1 in 1900 [52, 53]. Sodium Fluorescein administration for vascular neurosurgical procedures usually requires lower doses: the medium dosage of a single i.v. injection ranges from 75 to 500 mg or 1 to 1.5 mg/kg per bolus. Doses of intraarterial (i.a.) injection of SF are lower, ranging from 10 to 50 mg per bolus. In their study, Kuroda et al. reported that 10 ml of 0.01% of SF was enough to detect intracranial vessels. While i.v. bolus could be administrated in central or peripheral venous accesses, i.a. administration needs additional vascular access sites with associated perioperative risks. However, i.a. SF injections enable to visualize arterial phase in no more than two seconds and venous phase in less than 1 min. Furthermore, since i.v. injections require higher doses, i.a. SF administrations present less risk of vessel wall staining and provide a better intra-extravascular contrast.

Although the application of ICGVA in vascular neurosurgery came at a later stage than the use of SF [32], it is currently much wider used than SFVA. Nevertheless, ICGVA presents several drawbacks already cited above, making ICGVA and SFVA two complementary tools that, if employed together, can both provide benefits in different neurosurgical scenarios. In fact, differently from ICG, SF presents excitation and emission of wavelengths within the visible spectrum. Therefore, SFVA provides less contrast than ICGV, but allows for a better visualization of the angiogram in the three-dimensional and visible background anatomy, which can enable a direct and real-time manipulation on surgical field under fluorescent visualization, which is not possible with ICG. Furthermore, SFVA is able to show precisely the course and the patency of even very small vessels (perforators and even capillaries), which again is not possible with ICGVA, especially in deep or poorly illuminated surgical fields. Finally, SF is a cheap dye, easy to use and generally well tolerated at the aforementioned dosages; however, as for ICGVA, it requires a dedicated filter in the surgical microscope to provide angiographic images effectively helpful during surgery. Recently, endoscopes equipped with SF dedicated filter are available on the market as well.

The main drawback of SFVA is the extravascular leakage of Fluorescein, requiring an interval of more than 20 min between two injections [54].

To our knowledge, the study proposed by Bretonnier et al. [55] is the only one that analyzes the use of SFVA in the SDVAFs treatment. The authors used SF to assess the occlusion of SDAVFs in six patients, reporting a 100% success rate and demonstrating that SFVA is a safe, feasible and helpful tool also for SDAVFs surgery (Fig. 16.7).

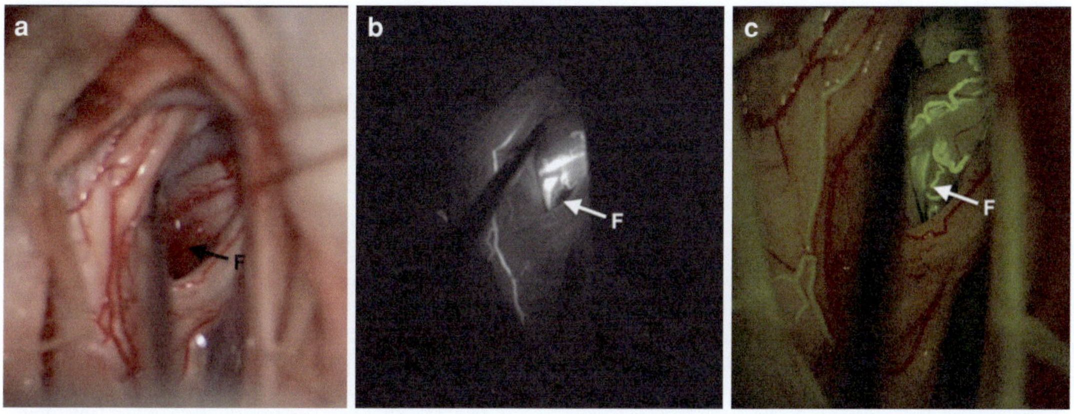

Fig. 16.7 (**a**) Intraoperative microscopic exposure of a left D5 SDAVF; the fistula is marked as *F.* (**b**) ICGVA of the same case as (**a**); the fistula is marked as *F*. (**c**) The same case as (**a**) and (**b**) in which also SF has been i.v. injected: the fistula is marked as *F*. Note how SF is able to show with high resolution very small vessels compared to ICGVA

16.3 Conclusions

Spinal dural AV fistulas are rare, but benign and curable vascular lesions; they can be insidious to diagnose and to treat, when the PoF is not clearly recognizable. Several intraoperative imaging techniques were developed to improve surgical results in treating SDAVF, without the absolute need for intra and postoperative DSA control. Of these, the greater experience has been gained with ICGVA, which is able most of the times to show the PoF before treatment and to confirm complete fistula occlusion with restorage of normal spinal cord flow at the end of the procedure. However, other new imaging tools may reveal helpful as an adjunct to ICGVA. Intraoperative US, along with CEUS and color-doppler US can be utilized several times throughout the procedure to confirm the right target (i.e. the PoF) and to provide a better and global flow dynamic information during SDAVF surgical treatment. Finally, although current results are still preliminary, SF could further improve our management of this disease, providing useful information on microcirculation involvement in SDAVF and on its preservation after treatment in such an eloquent tissue as the spinal cord. All these techniques are complementary one to each other and not in contraposition; these innovations must be welcome and, after adequate training, they should be available and well known by vascular neurosurgical teams that manage SDAVF.

Disclosure All the authors are aware of the content of the paper and do not have any financial or other interests that might be construed as a conflict of interest.

This research did not receive any specific grant from any source.

References

1. Thron A. [Spinal dural arteriovenous fistulas]. Radiologe. 2001;41(11):955–60. https://doi.org/10.1007/S001170170031.
2. Li X, Wang D, Yang N, et al. The diagnosis of spinal dural arteriovenous fistulas. Spine (Phila Pa 1976). 2013;38(9) https://doi.org/10.1097/BRS.0B013E31828A38C4.
3. Jellema K, Tijssen CC, Van Gijn J. Spinal dural arteriovenous fistulas: a congestive myelopathy that initially mimics a peripheral nerve disorder. Brain. 2006;129(Pt 12):3150–64. https://doi.org/10.1093/BRAIN/AWL220.

4. Krings T, Geibprasert S. Spinal dural arteriovenous fistulas. AJNR Am J Neuroradiol. 2009;30(4):639–48. https://doi.org/10.3174/AJNR.A1485.
5. Gilbertson JR, Miller GM, Goldman MS, Marsh WR. Spinal dural arteriovenous fistulas: MR and myelographic findings. Am J Neuroradiol. 1995;16(10):2049–57.
6. Spetzler RF, Detwiler PW, Riina HA, Porter RW. Modified classification of spinal cord vascular lesions. J Neurosurg. 2002;96(2 Suppl):145–56. https://doi.org/10.3171/SPI.2002.96.2.0145.
7. Krings T, Lasjaunias PL, Hans FJ, et al. Imaging in spinal vascular disease. Neuroimaging Clin N Am. 2007;17(1):57–72. https://doi.org/10.1016/J.NIC.2007.01.001.
8. Lasjaunias P, Berenstein A, ter Brugge KG. Clinical vascular anatomy and variations. Clin Vasc Anat Var. 2001; https://doi.org/10.1007/978-3-662-10172-8.
9. Hassler W, Thron A, Grote EH. Hemodynamics of spinal dural arteriovenous fistulas. An intraoperative study. J Neurosurg. 1989;70(3):360–70. https://doi.org/10.3171/JNS.1989.70.3.0360.
10. Van Rooij WJ, Nijenhuis RJ, Peluso JP, Sluzewski M, Beute GN, Van Der Pol B. Spinal dural fistulas without swelling and edema of the cord as incidental findings. AJNR Am J Neuroradiol. 2012;33(10):1888–92. https://doi.org/10.3174/AJNR.A3082.
11. Kataoka H, Miyamoto S, Nagata I, Ueba T, Hashimoto N. Venous congestion is a major cause of neurological deterioration in spinal arteriovenous malformations. Neurosurgery. 2001;48(6):1224–30. https://doi.org/10.1097/00006123-200106000-00004.
12. Grandin C, Duprez T, Stroobandt G, Laterre EC, Mathurin P. Spinal dural arterio-venous fistula: an underdiagnosed disease? Acta Neurol Belgium. 1997;97(1):17–21. https://pubmed.ncbi.nlm.nih.gov/9107340/. Accessed 27 Dec 2021.
13. Jellema K, Canta LR, Tijssen CC, Van Rooij WJ, Koudstaal PJ, Van Gijn J. Spinal dural arteriovenous fistulas: clinical features in 80 patients. J Neurol Neurosurg Psychiatry. 2003;74(10):1438–40. https://doi.org/10.1136/JNNP.74.10.1438.
14. Van Dijk JMC, TerBrugge KG, Willinsky RA, Farb RI, Wallace MC. Multidisciplinary management of spinal dural arteriovenous fistulas: clinical presentation and long-term follow-up in 49 patients. Stroke. 2002;33(6):1578–83. https://doi.org/10.1161/01.STR.0000018009.83713.06.
15. Fugate JE, Lanzino G, Rabinstein AA. Clinical presentation and prognostic factors of spinal dural arteriovenous fistulas: an overview. Neurosurg Focus. 2012;32(5):E17. https://doi.org/10.3171/2012.1.FOCUS11376.
16. Lai PH, Ben PH, Yang CF, et al. Multi-detector row computed tomography angiography in diagnosing spinal dural arteriovenous fistula: Initial experience. Stroke. 2005;36(7):1562–4. https://doi.org/10.1161/01.STR.0000170048.94718.07.
17. Saladino A, Atkinson JLD, Rabinstein AA, et al. Surgical treatment of spinal dural arteriovenous fistulae: a consecutive series of 154 patients. Neurosurgery. 2010;67(5):1350–7. https://doi.org/10.1227/NEU.0B013E3181EF2821.
18. Afshar JKB, Doppman JL, Oldfield EH. Surgical interruption of intradural draining vein as curative treatment of spinal dural arteriovenous fistulas. J Neurosurg. 1995;82(2):196–200. https://doi.org/10.3171/JNS.1995.82.2.0196.
19. Houdart E, Redondo A, Saint-Maurice JP, Merland JJ. Natural history of an incidentally discovered spinal dural arteriovenous fistula. Neurology. 2001;57(4):742–3. https://doi.org/10.1212/WNL.57.4.742.
20. Kaufmann TJ, Morris JM, Saladino A, Mandrekar JN, Lanzino G. Magnetic resonance imaging findings in treated spinal dural arteriovenous fistulas: lack of correlation with clinical outcomes. J Neurosurg Spine. 2011;14(4):548–54. https://doi.org/10.3171/2010.11.SPINE10178.
21. Sherif C, Gruber A, Bavinzski G, et al. Long-term outcome of a multidisciplinary concept of spinal dural arteriovenous fistulae treatment. Neuroradiology. 2008;50(1):67–74. https://doi.org/10.1007/S00234-007-0303-4.
22. Jellema K, Sluzewski M, van Rooij WJ, Tijssen CC, Beute GN. Embolization of spinal dural arteriovenous fistulas: importance of occlusion of the draining vein. J Neurosurg Spine. 2005;2(5):580–3. https://doi.org/10.3171/SPI.2005.2.5.0580.
23. Gokhale S, Khan SA, McDonagh DL, Britz G. Comparison of surgical and endovascular approach in management of spinal dural arteriovenous fistulas: a single center experience of 27 patients. Surg Neurol Int. 2014;5 https://doi.org/10.4103/2152-7806.125628.
24. Hall WA, Oldfield EH, Doppman JL. Recanalization of spinal arteriovenous malformations following embolization. J Neurosurg. 1989;70(5):714–20. https://doi.org/10.3171/JNS.1989.70.5.0714.
25. Eskandar EN, Borges LF, Budzik RF, Putman CM, Ogilvy CS. Spinal dural arteriovenous fistulas: experience with endovascular and surgical therapy. J Neurosurg. 2002;96(2 Suppl):162. https://doi.org/10.3171/JNS.2002.96.1.0162.
26. Ruiz-Juretschke F, Perez-Calvo JM, Castro E, et al. A single-center, long-term study of spinal dural arteriovenous fistulas with multidisciplinary treatment. J Clin Neurosci. 2011;18(12):1662–6. https://doi.org/10.1016/J.JOCN.2011.03.008.
27. Bakker NA, Uyttenboogaart M, Luijckx GJ, et al. Recurrence rates after surgical or endovascular treatment of spinal dural arteriovenous fistulas: a meta-analysis. Neurosurgery. 2015;77(1):137–44. https://doi.org/10.1227/NEU.0000000000000727.
28. Park SB, Han MH, Jahng TA, Kwon BJ, Chung CK. Spinal dural arteriovenous fistulas: clinical experience with endovascular treatment as a primary therapeutic modality. J Korean Neurosurg Soc. 2008;44(6):364–9. https://doi.org/10.3340/JKNS.2008.44.6.364.

29. Song JK, Viñuela F, Gobin YP, et al. Surgical and endovascular treatment of spinal dural arteriovenous fistulas: long-term disability assessment and prognostic factors. J Neurosurg. 2001;94(2 Suppl):199–204. https://doi.org/10.3171/spi.2001.94.2.0199.
30. Guillevin R, Vallee JN, Cormier E, Lo D, Dormont D, Chiras J. n-Butyl 2-cyanoacrylate embolization of spinal dural arteriovenous fistulae: CT evaluation, technical features, and outcome prognosis in 26 cases. Am J Neuroradiol. 2005;26(4):929–35.
31. Imizu S, Kato Y, Sangli A, Oguri D, Sano H. Assessment of incomplete clipping of aneurysms intraoperatively by a near-infrared indocyanine green-video angiography (Niicg-Va) integrated microscope. Minim Invasive Neurosurg. 2008;51(4):199–203. https://doi.org/10.1055/S-2008-1080916/ID/19.
32. Raabe A, Beck J, Gerlach R, et al. Near-infrared indocyanine green video angiography: a new method for intraoperative assessment of vascular flow. Neurosurgery. 2003;52(1):132–9. https://doi.org/10.1097/00006123-200301000-00017.
33. Raabe A, Nakaji P, Beck J, et al. Prospective evaluation of surgical microscope-integrated intraoperative near-infrared indocyanine green videoangiography during aneurysm surgery. J Neurosurg. 2005;103(6):982–9. https://doi.org/10.3171/JNS.2005.103.6.0982.
34. Horie N, So G, Debata A, et al. Intra-arterial indocyanine green angiography in the management of spinal arteriovenous fistulae: technical case reports. Spine (Phila Pa 1976). 2012;37(4) https://doi.org/10.1097/BRS.0B013E31822BA834.
35. Schuette AJ, Cawley CM, Barrow DL. Indocyanine green videoangiography in the management of dural arteriovenous fistulae. Neurosurgery. 2010;67(3):658–62. https://doi.org/10.1227/01.NEU.0000374721.84406.7F.
36. Fukuda K, Kataoka H, Nakajima N, Masuoka J, Satow T, Iihara K. Efficacy of FLOW 800 with indocyanine green videoangiography for the quantitative assessment of flow dynamics in cerebral arteriovenous malformation surgery. World Neurosurg. 2015;83(2):203–10. https://doi.org/10.1016/J.WNEU.2014.07.012.
37. Uchino H, Nakamura T, Houkin K, Murata JI, Saito H, Kuroda S. Semiquantitative analysis of indocyanine green videoangiography for cortical perfusion assessment in superficial temporal artery to middle cerebral artery anastomosis. Acta Neurochir (Wien). 2013;155(4):599–605. https://doi.org/10.1007/S00701-012-1575-Y.
38. Horie N, Fukuda Y, Izumo T, Hayashi K, Suyama K, Nagata I. Indocyanine green videoangiography for assessment of postoperative hyperperfusion in moyamoya disease. Acta Neurochir (Wien). 2014;156(5):919–26. https://doi.org/10.1007/S00701-014-2054-4.
39. Shi W, Qiao G, Sun Z, Shang A, Wu C, Xu B. Quantitative assessment of hemodynamic changes during spinal dural arteriovenous fistula surgery. J Clin Neurosci. 2015;22(7):1155–9. https://doi.org/10.1016/J.JOCN.2015.01.024.
40. Spiotta AM, Bain M, Moskowitz S. Intraoperative indocyanine green angiography as a substitute for conventional angiography in the surgical management of spinal dural arteriovenous fistulae. J Neurointerv Surg. 2011;3(2):182–5. https://doi.org/10.1136/JNIS.2010.003210.
41. Vetrano IG, Prada F, Nataloni IF, Del Bene M, DiMeco F, Valentini LG. Discrete or diffuse intramedullary tumor? Contrast-enhanced intraoperative ultrasound in a case of intramedullary cervicothoracic hemangioblastomas mimicking a diffuse infiltrative glioma: technical note and case report. Neurosurg Focus. 2015;39(2):E17. https://doi.org/10.3171/2015.5.FOCUS15162.
42. Prada F, Del Bene M, Faragò G, DiMeco F. Spinal dural arteriovenous fistula: is there a role for intraoperative contrast-enhanced ultrasound? World Neurosurg. 2017;100:712.e15–8. https://doi.org/10.1016/J.WNEU.2017.01.045.
43. Della Pepa GM, Sabatino G, Sturiale CL, et al. Integration of real-time intraoperative contrast-enhanced ultrasound and color doppler ultrasound in the surgical treatment of spinal cord dural arteriovenous fistulas. World Neurosurg. 2018;112:138–42. https://doi.org/10.1016/J.WNEU.2018.01.101.
44. Norton EW, Gutman F. Diabetic retinopathy studied by fluorescein angiography. Ophthalmologica. 1965;150(1):5–17. https://doi.org/10.1159/000304822.
45. Cavallo C, De Laurentis C, Vetrano IG, et al. The utilization of fluorescein in brain tumor surgery: a systematic review. J Neurosurg Sci. 2018;62(6):690–703. https://doi.org/10.23736/S0390-5616.18.04480-6.
46. Vetrano IG, Acerbi F, Falco J, et al. Fluorescein-guided removal of peripheral nerve sheath tumors: a preliminary analysis of 20 cases. J Neurosurg. 2019;134(1):260–9. https://doi.org/10.3171/2019.9.JNS19970.
47. Acerbi F, Broggi M, Schebesch KM, et al. Fluorescein-guided surgery for resection of high-grade gliomas: a multicentric prospective phase II study (FLUOGLIO). Clin Cancer Res. 2018;24(1):52–61. https://doi.org/10.1158/1078-0432.CCR-17-1184.
48. Falco J, Cavallo C, Vetrano IG, et al. Fluorescein application in cranial and spinal tumors enhancing at preoperative MRI and operated with a dedicated filter on the surgical microscope: preliminary results in 279 patients enrolled in the FLUOCERTUM prospective study. Front Surg. 2019;6 https://doi.org/10.3389/FSURG.2019.00049.
49. Acerbi F, Cavallo C, Schebesch KM, et al. Fluorescein-guided resection of intramedullary spinal cord tumors: results from a preliminary, multicentric, retrospective study. World Neurosurg. 2017;108:603–9. https://doi.org/10.1016/J.WNEU.2017.09.061.
50. Moore GE, Peyton WT. The clinical use of fluorescein in neurosurgery; the localization of brain tumors. J

Neurosurg. 1948;5(4):392–8. https://doi.org/10.3171/JNS.1948.5.4.0392.
51. Feindel W, Yamamoto YL, Hodge CP. Red cerebral veins and the cerebral steal syndrome. Evidence from fluorescein angiography and microregional blood flow by radioisotopes during excision of an angioma. J Neurosurg. 1971;35(2):167–79. https://doi.org/10.3171/JNS.1971.35.2.0167.
52. Shinoda J, Yano H, Yoshimura SI, et al. Fluorescence-guided resection of glioblastoma multiforme by using high-dose fluorescein sodium. Technical note. J Neurosurg. 2003;99(3):597–603. https://doi.org/10.3171/JNS.2003.99.3.0597.
53. Yannuzzi LA, Rohrer KT, Tindel LJ, et al. Fluorescein angiography complication survey. Ophthalmology. 1986;93(5):611–7. https://doi.org/10.1016/S0161-6420(86)33697-2.
54. Rey-Dios R, Cohen-Gadol AA. Technical principles and neurosurgical applications of fluorescein fluorescence using a microscope-integrated fluorescence module. Acta Neurochir. 2013;155(4):701–6. https://doi.org/10.1007/S00701-013-1635-Y.
55. Bretonnier M, Morandi X, Le Reste PJ. Fluorescein-guided surgery for spinal dural arteriovenous fistulas: a short series. J Clin Neurosci. 2019;70:226–8. https://doi.org/10.1016/J.JOCN.2019.08.036.

Embolization of Spinal Dural Arteriovenous Fistulae Using a Nonadhesive Liquid Embolic Agent Delivered Via a Dual-Lumen Balloon Catheter

17

Muhammet Arslan, Celal Cinar, and Ismail Oran

Abstract

A spinal dural arteriovenous fistula is the most common type of spinal vascular malformation. The principal aim of endovascular treatment is to occlude the fistula site and the proximal part of the draining vein. However, this is not always possible because selective catheterization can be difficult in patients with tortuous feeding arteries, and there is a risk of liquid embolic agent reflux. Herein, we present a novel technique. We use a dual-lumen balloon catheter to inject a liquid embolic agent into the fistula. The pre-inflated balloon prevents proximal reflux and also engages in forward pushing that augments distal penetration of the embolic agent. An absolute prerequisite is a lack of radiculomedullary branches arising from the same segmental feeding artery; careful angiographic examination is mandatory. Use of the dual-lumen balloon catheter technique when long tortuous feeding arteries supply the spinal dural arteriovenous fistula ensures safe and successful embolization with a low risk for complications.

M. Arslan
Department of Radiology, Pamukkale University Medical School, Denizli, Turkey

C. Cinar · I. Oran (✉)
Department of Radiology, Ege University Medical School, Izmir, Turkey
e-mail: ismail.oran@ege.edu.tr

Keywords

Spinal dural arteriovenous fistulae · Dual lumen balloon catheter · Embolization Nonadhesive liquid embolic agent Endovascular treatment

17.1 Spinal Vascular Anatomy

To safely treat a spinal dural arteriovenous fistula (SDAVF), it is essential to know the vascular anatomy of the spinal cord. The main vessels that supply the cord are the anterior spinal artery (ASA) and the posterior spinal artery (PSA). The ASA runs along the anterior sulcus of the spinal cord and descends to the conus medullaris. Along its long course, the ASA is supplied by medullary branches (the so-called anterior radiculomedullary arteries) from the cervical region to the conus medullaris. Therefore, the ASA should not be considered a single feeding vessel, rather as a series of sequential anastomotic lines. Above T3, the segmental anterior radiculomedullary arteries are formed by branches from the vertebral arteries, posterior inferior cerebellar arteries, ascending cervical arteries, deep cervical arteries, and supreme intercostal artery in the cervical and upper thoracic region. Below the level of T3 and in the upper lumbar spine, they originate from the lumbar and intercostal arteries. The median sacral artery and the lateral sacral arteries

X. Lv (ed.), *Intracranial and Spinal Dural Arteriovenous Fistulas*,
https://doi.org/10.1007/978-981-19-5767-3_17

(branches of the internal iliac artery) also feed the cauda equina fibers [1].

The radiculomedullary arteries are thin vascular branches and are clearly visible only on good-quality catheter angiograms. The radiculomedullaris magna artery, also known as the Adamkiewicz artery (the most prominent anterior radiculomedullary artery), is easily recognized on angiograms. It arises in the thoracolumbar region (between T7 and L2 in 95% of cases); in 77% of cases, it lies on the left [2]. This radiculomedullary artery arises from the spinal branch of the intercostal or lumbar artery. The artery makes a characteristic "hairpin turn" at the point of anastomosis with the ASA. Damage to this vessel can cause spinal cord infarction; the artery is the dominant supplier of the thoracolumbar spinal cord.

The two posterolateral spinal arteries (PSAs) originate from the vertebral artery or the posterior inferior cerebellar artery. The PSAs descend along the right and left posterolateral surfaces of the spinal cord and feature rich communications via the surface arterial network. As the PSAs descend posterolaterally, they receive the posterior radiculomedullary branches of the intercostal or lumbar arteries. All radiculomedullary branches supplying either the ASA or the PSAs exhibit characteristic hairpin turns, although these are less prominent than the turn of the Adamkiewicz artery [3].

In terms of venous cord drainage, the intrinsic sulcal and radial veins drain the substance of the cord to the extrinsic system. The latter consists of anterior and posterolateral veins that mirror their arterial counterparts. They exhibit rich collateral communications (over the surface of the spinal cord) with the longitudinal collector veins termed the "perimedullary veins." These veins first drain into the internal vertebral plexuses (via the radicular veins of each segment), then into the external vertebral plexuses, and finally into the azygos and hemiazygos venous systems [4].

17.2 Pathophysiology

The precise etiology of SDAVF remains unknown but it is assumed that the disease is acquired. An arteriovenous shunt lies in the inner aspect of the dural layer at the level of the posterior wall of the dural sleeve, where the arterial blood emerges from the radiculomeningeal branch. Venous drainage runs via the radicular vein toward the perimedullary veins (thus in a reverse manner), triggering venous congestion within the spinal cord. Prolonged venous congestion induces venous ischemia, followed by cord dysfunction. Although infrequent, other mechanisms that may give rise to clinical symptoms include subarachnoid or intraparenchymal hemorrhage, vascular compression, and vascular steal [5, 6].

17.3 Diagnostic Angiography

Digital subtraction angiography is the gold standard for diagnostic confirmation of any spinal vascular malformation. In general, after a suspicion is raised in magnetic resonance imaging, the most likely feeding arteries should be identified via magnetic resonance angiography. Sometimes, a complete spinal angiogram may be required; all possible arteries should be bilaterally investigated (Table 17.1). In an SDAVF, the fistula is typically located on the posterior surface of the dural sheath surrounding the radix. The precise fistulation point is characterized by a sudden

Table 17.1 Possible feeding arteries evident in a spinal angiogram

Intercostal arteries
Lumbar arteries
Inferior hypogastric artery
Median and lateral sacral arteries
Vertebral arteries
Ascending/deep cervical arteries
Thyrocervical trunk
External carotid artery

change in vessel diameter and/or direction evident angiographically. Venous drainage within the dura runs toward the spinal perimedullary veins. During selective angiography, the perimedullary veins are opacified along the entire spinal cord on the cranial or caudal side of the fistula, but the radicular veins connecting the (dilated and engorged) perimedullary veins outside the dura are typically not opacified. When an arterial feeder of an SDAVF is localized, the adjacent bilateral intercostal or lumbar arteries should be catheterized to exclude the possibility of multiple feeding arteries.

17.4 Management

SDAVF features progressive deterioration; treatment is essential. Untreated SDAVFs can progress to the development of serious symptoms and irreversible neurological damage [7, 8]. The clinical success of treatment is directly related to symptom severity and duration at the time of treatment [9]. If the disease is treated early, the probability of complete recovery without any neurological deficit is high. If treatment is delayed, clinical improvement will be minimal, even after successful treatment. Treatment options include endovascular embolization and surgical occlusion of the fistula.

Surgery remains the first treatment of choice for SDAVF [10–12]; occlusion rates as high as 98% have been reported [12]. A fistula located in the posterior wall of the dural sheath can be seen when the dura is cut longitudinally via an ipsilateral laminectomy. Surgery should be performed immediately in patients with very thin/tortuous feeding arteries and/or low-flow fistulae that are not amenable to microcatheterization, or in patients whose radiculomedullary arteries supplying the spinal cords arise from the same segmental artery. If the liquid embolic agent does not attain the venous site during embolization, fistula persistence/recurrence will be possible in clinical/radiological follow-up [13]. In such a circumstance, surgery should proceed without delay [14]. If surgery is planned, a small coil should be placed in the proximal segmental artery during diagnostic angiography. This allows accurate fluoroscopic localization of the fistula level during surgery [15].

Nonadhesive liquid embolizing agents (NLEAs) are preferred to cyanoacrylate glue when treating SDAVFs. The NLEA penetrate more distally into target vessels and the risk for microcatheter sticking is low. Over the last 20 years, endovascular embolization has increasingly been used to treat SDAVFs because it is not very invasive, and both embolic agents and microcatheter technology have improved over time [16]. Occlusion rates as high as 85% have been reported [17]. The goal of endovascular treatment is to occlude both the fistula and the first 1–2 cm of the proximal draining vein [8, 18].

17.5 NLEAs

The neurointerventional NLEAs include Onyx (Medtronic, Irvine, CA, USA), Squid (Balt, Montmorency, France), and PHIL (MicroVention, Tustin, CA, USA) [19]. All are nonadhesive, nonabsorbable, permanent liquid embolic agents. Onyx, a widely used NLEA, features an elastic polymer with an ethylene-vinyl alcohol (EVOH) co-polymer dissolved in dimethyl sulfoxide (DMSO), with a micronized tantalum powder to ensure radio-opacity. When Onyx contacts water or blood, the material precipitates because of rapid DMSO diffusion, forming an elastic, soft, spongy, radiopaque cohesive cast inside the vessel lumen, which solidifies completely after about 10 min. The viscous nature of the material and the slow polymerization facilitate delivery and penetration of the agent. Squid is also based on an EVOH/DMSO system with micronized tantalum powder. However, there is a low-viscosity variant that guarantees more distant penetration. PHIL includes a copolymer dissolved in DMSO. Unlike Onyx and Squid, PHIL features an iodine component chemically bound to the copolymer, ensuring radio-opacity for fluoroscopic visualization. A potential advantage is that PHIL does not require shaking before delivery, thus avoiding time-consuming preparation. In addition, as PHIL does not contain tantalum, there are fewer CT artifacts.

17.6 Dual-Lumen Balloon Catheters

Dual-lumen (double-lumen) balloon catheters feature a central lumen (for injection) and a separate external lumen for balloon inflation and deflation. They are also termed occlusion balloon catheters. They were employed to improve NLEA penetration during embolization of intracranial arteriovenous malformations and fistulae. The dual-lumen balloon catheters afford temporary vascular occlusion; they selectively stop or control blood flow. After balloon inflation, they also prevent back-flow (reflux) and push the embolizing agent forward. They thus afford controlled delivery of embolizing agent to the target.

Currently, four double-lumen balloon catheters produced by three different manufacturers are available: Ascent (Codman Neurovascular, Raynham, MA, USA); Scepter (MicroVention Terumo); Copernic 2L (Balt Extrusion); and Eclipse (Balt Extrusion). All are DMSO-compatible and accommodate a 0.014 in. guidewire (Table 17.2).

17.7 Embolization Using a Dual-Lumen Balloon

All procedures should be performed with the patient under general anesthesia; NLEA embolization is very painful. A 5 or 6 Fr introducer sheath is inserted into the femoral artery to allow arterial access. The procedure is performed under systemic heparinization, which usually commences with maintenance of the activated clotting time (ACT) at a level two- to three-fold above the baseline (generally, a 100 IU/kg heparin bolus is given followed by constant infusion at 1000 IU/h). Given the awkward position of the intercostal/lumbar segmental arteries, an exchange maneuver over a hydrophilic 0.035-in. guidewire may be necessary to achieve selective insertion of a 5 Fr guiding catheter with a soft tip. In patients with a tortuous elongated aorta and a more cranial target segmental artery (i.e., an artery at a high thoracic level), initial insertion of a 6 Fr long sheath may ensure more stable positioning of the inner 5 Fr guiding catheter.

First, it is necessary to determine whether the segmental artery supplying the SDAVF features any anterior or posterior radiculomedullary artery that supplies the spinal cord. If so, the operation should be cancelled (Fig. 17.1). The operator should prefer the use of a dual-lumen balloon catheter if standard selective microcatheterization of the fistula feeder is impossible or fails. The main branches of the segmental (intercostal or lumbar) artery supplying the distal paraspinal

Table 17.2 Dual lumen balloon catheters

Catheter	Scepter	Eclipse	Ascent	Copernic
Length of the balloon (mm)	10, 11[a], 15, 20	7, 9, 12, 15, 20	7, 9, 10, 15	10, 15, 20, 30
Diameter of the balloon (mm)	2.2–2.7[b], 4	2–6	4, 6	3–5
Length of the tip (mm)	5	3, 7	3	12
Shaft outer diameter (French)	2.8	3.3 × 2.7	2.9	3.7 × 2.7
Inner lumen (in.)	0.0165	0.0161	0.0170	0.0240
Manufacturer	MicroVention Terumo	Balt Extrusion	Codman	Balt Extrusion

[a] Scepter XC X-tra compliant balloon catheter
[b] Scepter mini dual lumen balloon catheter

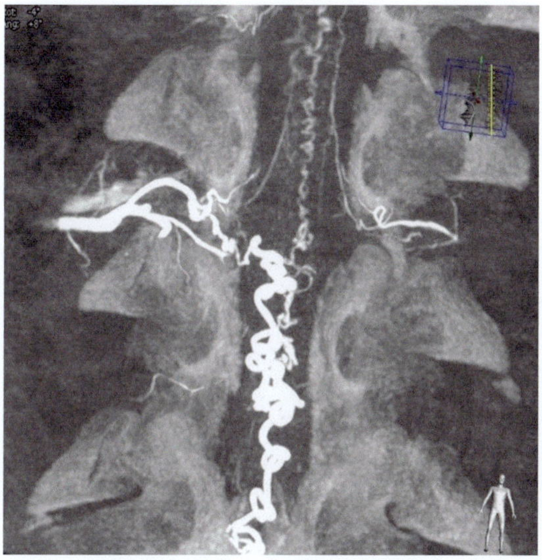

Fig. 17.1 Cone-beam CT angiography during selective injection through the right T8 intercostal artery in a patient with SDAVF. The right radiculomedullary artery arising from the same segmental artery which feeds the posterior spinal artery with typical hairpin appearance makes the patient not suitable for embolization

soft tissues should be initially occluded by coils (pushable or detachable) to avoid possible tissue ischemia associated with NLEA. Then a dual-lumen balloon catheter is prepared, advanced through the guide catheter, and placed in the main trunk of the segmental artery just before the artery feeding the SDAVF (Fig. 17.2). After balloon inflation, an angiogram must be obtained for final validation just before embolization. Then NLEA, prepared as recommended by the manufacturer, is injected slowly through the catheter under road-mapping guidance while the balloon is inflated. After the fistula and the proximal part of the draining vein are filled with NLEA, the balloon is deflated and removed. A control angiogram is performed via the diagnostic catheter (Fig. 17.3).

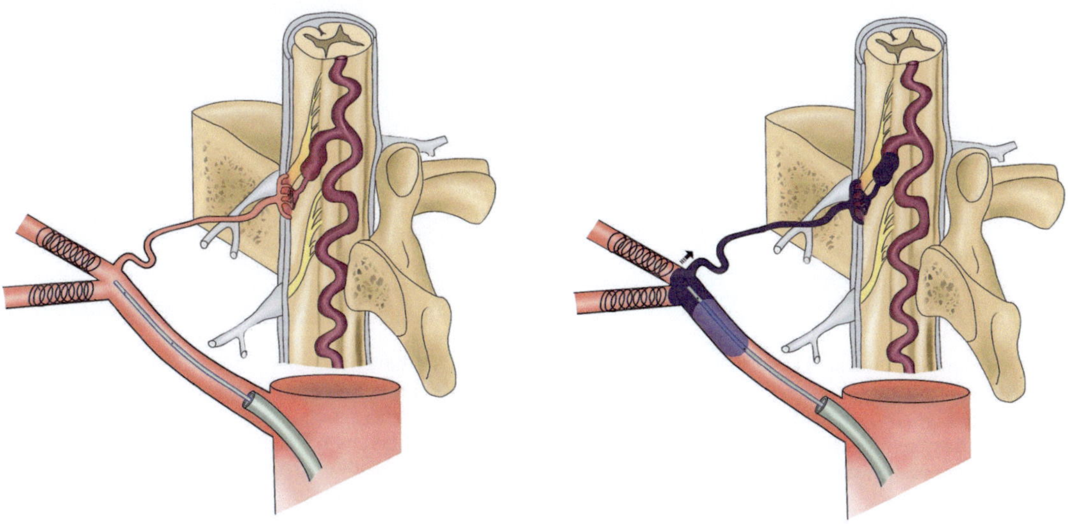

Fig. 17.2 Dual-lumen balloon catheter embolization of an SDAVF. The distal main branches of the segmental artery are first occluded by coils to prevent paraspinal tissue ischemia, and then the dual-lumen balloon catheter is placed in the main trunk of the segmental artery (left image). The liquid embolic agent is carefully injected as the balloon is inflated; this ensures distal penetration to the proximal venous site (right image)

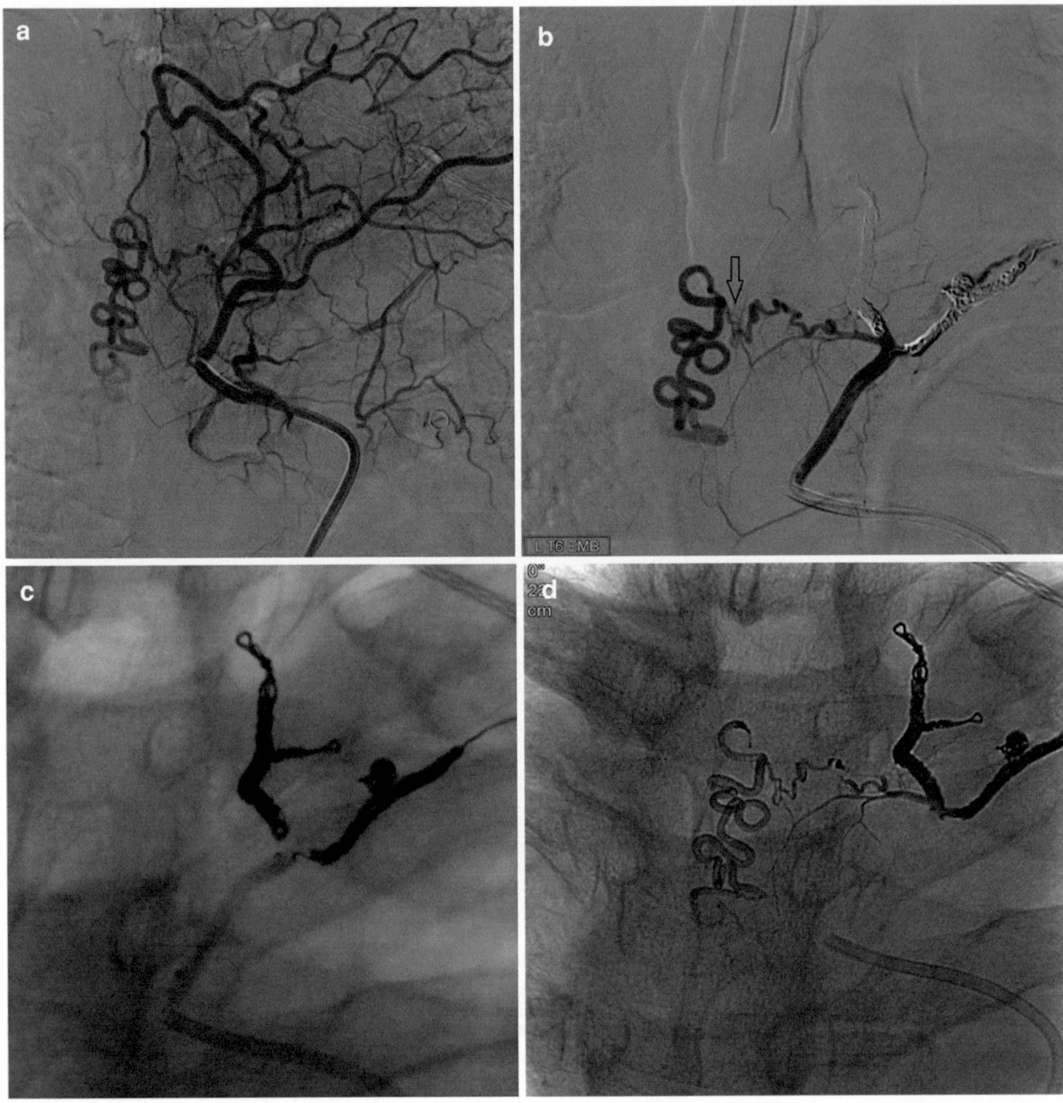

Fig. 17.3 Embolization of SDAV arising from the left T6 intercostal artery. (**a**) Initial angiogram. (**b**) Angiogram after selective coil occlusion of distal paraspinal branches of the left T6 intercostal artery. Arrow indicates the fistula point. (**c**) Fluoroscopy image showing the inflated balloon of the dual-lumen balloon catheter, just before NLEA injection. (**d**) Fluoroscopy image showing the tiny feeding artery, the fistula point, and the proximal perimedullary vein, all are filled with NLEA

17.8 Dual-Lumen Balloon Catheter Use to Treat an SDAVF

Dual-lumen balloon catheters have been successfully used for embolization of intracranial arteriovenous malformations and fistulae; such catheters facilitate the penetration of liquid embolic agents. Initial reports revealed good catheter navigability and enhanced penetrability [20]. In 2017, the dual-lumen balloon catheter was reported for the first time in a patient having SDAVF [21]. Only a few later cases have been reported [22–24]; the catheter has been reported effective and safe in treating SDAVF. The pressure cooker technique, another technique that enhances distal penetration of liquid embolic agents, features double microcatheterization of the main arterial feeder, proximal plugging via the first microcatheter, and distal penetration of the embolic fluid via the second microcatheter. Although this technique seems to be more complicated during procedural preparation, the working principle is the same as that of the dual-lumen balloon catheter. The pressure cooker technique has recently been used to treat 15 patients with SDAVF [25]. Fistula occlusion was observed in all cases (15/15) and angiographic follow-up (of 12 cases) showed that complete occlusion persisted in 11 of them (91.7%). No major complication (and only one minor complication) (6.6%) was reported.

17.9 Follow-Up

After treatment of the fistula, the patient should be clinically and radiologically evaluated in a multidisciplinary clinic [26]. Routine magnetic resonance imaging (including contrast examination) is required 3–6 months after treatment regardless of the clinical status (postoperative imaging features sometimes do not correlate with clinical outcomes). The cord T2 hyperintensity and enhancement should decrease with time, but these features can persist for even more than 6 months. Similarly, the enlarged perimedullary veins should have shrunken at the time of the first magnetic resonance imaging, although normalization can require up to 12 months. If persistent perimedullary vessels are evident in follow-up magnetic resonance imaging and/or the patient evidences clinical deterioration, a spinal angiogram is required not only for definitive evaluation but also to guide subsequent surgery. In patients with favorable follow-up magnetic resonance imaging results who exhibit clinical stabilization or improvement, follow-up imaging is repeated after a further 6–12 months.

17.10 Conclusion

Few patients with SDAVF have been treated using the dual-lumen balloon catheter technique. Employment of such a catheter to perform NLEA embolization is acceptable and feasible, and may increase the complete endovascular cure rate. Careful angiographic examination is essential before use of such a catheter. It is essential to avoid spinal ischemic complications.

Teaching Points

- When treating an SDAVF, the aim is to occlude the fistula site and the proximal part of the draining vein; this affords ideal embolization.
- The use of a dual-lumen balloon catheter to deliver nonadhesive liquid embolic agents affords safe and successful embolization.
- A careful angiographic examination is obligatory prior to such treatment.
- Endovascular treatment is absolutely contraindicated when the radiculomedullary artery arises from the same segmental artery.
- The diameter and length of the feeding artery must be large enough to allow inflation of the balloon.
- The aim is to avoid uncontrolled retrograde reflux of the embolic agent and to increase the distal penetration of that agent.

References

1. Santillan A, Nacarino V, Greenberg E, Riina H, Gobin Y, Patsalides A. Vascular anatomy of the spinal cord. J Neurointerv Surg. 2011;4:67–74.
2. Taterra D, Skinningsrud B, Pękala P, Hsieh W, Cirocchi R, Walocha J, Tubbs R, Tomaszewski K, Henry B. Artery of Adamkiewicz: a meta-analysis of anatomical characteristics. Neuroradiology. 2019;61:869–80.

3. Hong M, Hong M, Pan W, Wallace D, Ashton M, Taylor G. The angiosome territories of the spinal cord: exploring the issue of preoperative spinal angiography. J Neurosurg Spine. 2008;8:352–64.
4. Sethuraman M. Chapter 4: Neurophysiology. In: Essentials of neuroanesthesia. 1st ed. London: Academic Press; 2017.
5. Krings T, Geibprasert S. Spinal dural arteriovenous fistulas. Am J Neuroradiol. 2009;30:639–48.
6. Kataoka H, Miyamoto S, Nagata I, Ueba T, Hashimoto N. Venous congestion is a major cause of neurological deterioration in spinal arteriovenous malformations. Neurosurgery. 2001;48:1224–30.
7. Qi X, Lv L, Han K, Xu Z, Mei Q, Chen H, Huang C, Bai R, Hou L, Lu Y. Analysis of the embolization spinal dural arteriovenous fistula and surgical treatments on 52 cases of the patients. Int J Clin Exp Med. 2014;7:3062–71.
8. Jeng Y, Chen D, Hsu H, Huang Y, Chen C, Tseng Y. Spinal dural arteriovenous fistula: imaging features and its mimics. Korean J Radiol. 2015;16:1119.
9. Kirsch M, Berg-Dammer E, Musahl C, Bäzner H, Kühne D, Henkes H. Endovascular management of spinal dural arteriovenous fistulas in 78 patients. Neuroradiology. 2013;55:337–43.
10. Goyal A, Cesare J, Lu V, Alvi M, Kerezoudis P, Brinjikji W, Nasr D, Lanzino G, Bydon M. Outcomes following surgical versus endovascular treatment of spinal dural arteriovenous fistula: a systematic review and meta-analysis. J Neurol Neurosurg Psychiatry. 2019;90:1139–46.
11. Bakker N, Uyttenboogaart M, Luijckx G, Eshghi O, Mazuri A, Metzemaekers J, Groen R, Van Dijk J. Recurrence rates after surgical or endovascular treatment of spinal dural arteriovenous fistulas. Neurosurgery. 2015;77:137–44.
12. Steinmetz M, Chow M, Krishnaney A, Andrews-Hinders D, Benzel E, Masaryk T, Mayberg M, Rasmussen P. Outcome after the treatment of spinal dural arteriovenous fistulae: a contemporary single-institution series and meta-analysis. Neurosurgery. 2004;55:77–88.
13. Patsalides A, Santillan A, Knopman J, Tsiouris A, Riina H, Gobin Y. Endovascular management of spinal dural arteriovenous fistulas. J Neurointerv Surg. 2010;3:80–4.
14. Koch M, Stapleton C, Agarwalla P, Torok C, Shin J, Coumans J, Borges L, Ogilvy C, Rabinov J, Patel A. Open and endovascular treatment of spinal dural arteriovenous fistulas: a 10-year experience. J Neurosurg Spine. 2017;26:519–23.
15. Fox S, Hnenny L, Ahmed U, Meguro K, Kelly M. Spinal dural arteriovenous fistula: a case series and review of imaging findings. Spinal Cord Ser Cases. 2017; https://doi.org/10.1038/scsandc.2017.24.
16. Westphal M, Koch C. Management of spinal dural arteriovenous fistulae using an interdisciplinary neuroradiological/neurosurgical approach: experience with 47 cases. Neurosurgery. 1999;45:451–8.
17. Morris J. Imaging of dural arteriovenous fistula. Radiol Clin N Am. 2012;50:823–39.
18. Warakaulle D, Aviv R, Niemann D, Molyneux A, Byrne J, Teddy P. Embolisation of spinal dural arteriovenous fistulae with Onyx. Neuroradiology. 2003;45:110–2.
19. Vollherbst D, Chapot R, Bendszus M, Möhlenbruch M. Glue, Onyx, Squid or PHIL? Liquid embolic agents for the embolization of cerebral arteriovenous malformations and dural arteriovenous fistulas. Clin Neuroradiol. 2021; https://doi.org/10.1007/s00062-021-01066-6.
20. Paramasivam S, Niimi Y, Fifi J, Berenstein A. Onyx embolization using dual-lumen balloon catheter: initial experience and technical note. J Neuroradiol. 2013;40:294–302.
21. Nakae R, Nagaishi M, Hyodo A, Suzuki K. Embolization of a spinal dural arteriovenous fistula with ethylene-vinyl alcohol copolymer (Onyx) using a dual-lumen microballoon catheter and buddy wire technique. Surg Neurol Int. 2017;8:166.
22. Trivelato F, Rezende M, Ulhoa A, Nakiri G, Abud D. Dual-lumen balloon to increase onyx venous penetration in the treatment of spinal dural arteriovenous fistulas. J Neuroradiol. 2018;45:142–6.
23. Arslan M, Cınar C, Oran I. Dual-lumen balloon catheter technique for Onyx embolization of spinal dural arteriovenous fistula. J Vasc Interv Neurol. 2019;10:34–7.
24. Clarençon F, Shotar E, Pouvelle A, Premat K, Lenck S, Drir M, Guillaumet G, Maillart E, Sourour N. Spinal epidural arteriovenous fistula embolization with ethylene vinyl alcohol (EVOH) copolymer using the Scepter Mini dual-lumen balloon. J Neurointerv Surg. 2020;13:492.
25. Clarençon F, Stracke C, Shotar E, Wallocha M, Mosimann P, Boch A, Sourour N, Chapot R. Pressure cooker technique for endovascular treatment of spinal arteriovenous fistulas: experience in 15 cases. Am J Neuroradiol. 2021;42:1270–5.
26. van Dijk J, TerBrugge K, Willinsky R, Farb R, Wallace M. Multidisciplinary management of spinal dural arteriovenous fistulas. Stroke. 2002;33:1578–83.

Predicting Outcomes of Stereotactic Radiosurgery for Dural Arteriovenous Fistulas

18

Anirudha S. Chandrabhatla, Panagiotis Mastorakos, Ching-Jen Chen, and Jason Sheehan

Abstract

Stereotaxic radiosurgery (SRS) is an important alternative, additive or salvage intervention for the treatment of dural arteriovenous fistulas (dAVF). Treatment with SRS can offer favorable rates of dAVF obliteration and offers a solution to dAVF not amenable or refractory to surgical or endovascular treatment. It is important to identify the factors associated with favorable outcomes following SRS. Recent studies suggest that anatomic location, angiographic and clinical criteria can affect the outcome of SRS. Established grading scales based on angiographic criteria are primarily focused on hemorrhage risk stratification and provide guidance regarding management but do not adequately predict effectiveness of SRS. The primary goal of this chapter is to outline the factors that predict dAVF obliteration as described in recent studies. We also describe a practical grading system by Nasser et al. that incorporates angiographic, anatomic and clinical parameters to specifically predict dAVF outcomes following SRS. Our goal is to help clinicians predict SRS outcomes on an individual basis and as such aid the decision-making process.

Keywords

Dural arteriovenous fistula · Stereotaxic radiosurgery · Grading scales · Predictors

18.1 Chapter Overview

Stereotactic radiosurgery (SRS) is an important intervention in dural arteriovenous fistulas (dAVF) treatment. Due to immediate obliteration that can be achieved with endovascular and surgical treatments, SRS is often reserved for complex lesions that cannot be adequately treated with endovascular or surgical approaches, and for patients with high surgical risks. Despite this, SRS confers favorable dAVF obliteration rates that range between 41% and 90% in the literature [1].

Optimal therapeutic strategies based on patient and lesion characteristics remain undefined, and there continues to be significant variations among centers. Optimal patient selection for SRS is unclear, and our ability to predict SRS outcomes in dAVF patients leaves room for improvement. As unique adverse events, such as

A. S. Chandrabhatla · P. Mastorakos (✉) · J. Sheehan
School of Medicine, University of Virginia, Charlottesville, VA, USA
e-mail: pm5mt@virginia.edu; PM5MT@hscmail.mcc.virginia.edu

C.-J. Chen
Department of Neurosurgery, University of Virginia Health System, Charlottesville, VA, USA

Department of Neurosurgery, Thomas Jefferson University Hospital, Philadelphia, PA, USA

X. Lv (ed.), *Intracranial and Spinal Dural Arteriovenous Fistulas*,
https://doi.org/10.1007/978-981-19-5767-3_18

radiation-induced changes (RIC) and hemorrhage during the latency period, pertain to SRS treatment, clinically relevant prediction models that adequately capture these can be challenging and is of high clinical importance.

Anatomical location combined with angiographic and clinical characteristics affect SRS outcomes in dAVFs (Table 18.1). Prior grading scales, based on angiographic characteristics, have focused on untreated dAVF hemorrhage risk

Table 18.1 Key takeaways from relevant analyses in the literature

PMID	Author	Year	Study size	Type of predictor	Key takeaways
33582776	Chen et al.	May 2021	345 Patients	Anatomical and physiologic	Intervention (e.g., embolization, SRS) for low-grade dAVFs achieved superior obliteration compared to conservative management, but did not improve functional or neurological outcomes.
34608140	Chen et al.	September 2021	415 Patients	Anatomical and physiologic	Functional outcomes were similar between SRS and observation for unruptured high-grade dAVFs (Borden type II or III) Obliteration was higher for embolization and surgery compared to observation
29777886	Chen et al.	August 2018	41 Patients	Patient history/ demographics	Obliteration without permanent neurological deficit was achieved in 62% of high grade dAVF cases Presentation with non-hemorrhagic neurological deficit was an independent predictor of permanent neurological deficit after SRS
25479123	Chen et al.	February 2015	729 Patients	Anatomical	No significant difference in obliteration rates between cavernous sinus (CS) and non-cavernous sinus (non-CS) dAVFs
31384943	Hung et al.	May 2020	131 Patients	Anatomical	CS dAVFs: (1) higher obliteration rates, (2) higher max dose predicted better outcomes (e.g., post-SRS obliteration without hemorrhage), (3) symptoms improved regardless of obliteration Non-CS dAVFs: (1) symptoms improved with obliteration
30790731	Mohammed et al.	May 2019	96 Patients	Patient history/ demographics	Older patients (>65 years old): transverse sinus predicted obliteration; 47.7% and 78% 3 and 5 year post-SRS obliteration Younger patients: cavernous sinus predicted obliteration; 56% and 70% 3 and 5 year post-SRS obliteration

Table 18.1 (continued)

PMID	Author	Year	Study size	Type of predictor	Key takeaways
31584074	Mohammed et al.	August 2020	120 Patients	Anatomical, physiologic, and patient history/ demographics	Multivariable regression identified: (1) cortical venous flux, (2) prior ICH, and (3) non-cavernous sinus location as factors in a new classification scheme for predicting outcomes after SRS ROC analysis showed superior predictive ability compared to established grading systems
34507278	Samaniego et al.	September 2021	342 Patients	Anatomical and physiologic	Multiple, complimentary interventions achieved increased complete obliteration rate (55.2% after combined radiosurgery and open surgery)
30875690	Starke et al.	March 2019	147 Patients	Anatomical, physiologic, and patient history/ demographics	Presence of cortical venous drainage (CVD), convexity or torcula location increased likelihood of hemorrhage Presence of non-hemorrhagic neural deficits or past endovascular treatments were independent predictors of hemorrhage
30611144	Starke et al.	January 2019	114 Patients	Anatomical and physiologic	Middle fossa and tentorial dAVFs or margin dose greater than 23 Gy predicted less favorable outcome (e.g., post-SRS hemorrhage) Commonly used grading scales (Borden and Cognard) were not predictive of outcomes Female sex, absent venous ectasia, and cavernous carotid are predictors of obliteration
29547086	Tonetti et al.	March 2018	42 Patients	Anatomical and physiologic	Non-aggressive dAVFs with CVD are good candidates for SRS as they have a low risk of subsequent hemorrhage or radiation-related complications

stratification, and provided guidance regarding management [2–4]. But they do not adequately predict dAVF outcomes after SRS treatment. Hence the primary goal of this chapter is to summarize our current understanding of dAVF outcome predictors after SRS treatment. Here, we also highlight a recent grading scales that incorporates angiographic, anatomic, and clinical parameters to specifically predict dAVF outcomes after SRS.

18.2 Current Grading Scales

Intracranial dAVFs are often classified based on the presence of cortical venous drainage (CVD) or lack thereof. There are three main grading scales that have classically been employed to predict dAVF natural history and risk of hemorrhage. The Borden scale considers venous drainage site and presence of cortical venous drainage (CVD) to classify dAVFs as "benign" or low grade and "aggressive" or high grade, with direct cortical venous drainage associated with the highest risk [2]. A subsequent modification to the Borden scale integrates clinical presentation [4]. The more elaborate Cognard scale includes flow pattern in venous sinuses (anterograde versus retrograde) and presence of venous ectasia as additional factors in the classification [3]. Finally, the Barrow classification, specific for cavernous-carotid fistulas, essentially classifies fistulas as direct or indirect fistulization based on whether blood shunts into the cavernous sinus from the internal carotid artery (ICA) or branches of the ICA and/or external carotid arteries, respectively [5]. Although these grading scales can be used to predict SRS outcomes, they were not specifically designed to assess SRS outcomes, and their ability to discriminate SRS outcomes have shown to be poor [6].

18.3 Predictors of Obliteration

There are several factors that have been reported to predict obliteration in patients with dAVFs treated with SRS. Broadly, these factors can be categorized as pertaining to anatomical characteristics, physiologic behavior, and clinical characteristics.

18.3.1 Anatomy

Although some treatment algorithms have indicated that SRS offers good outcomes for dAVFs independent of their anatomy [7], larger and more recent studies have indicated that the anatomy of a patient's dAVF plays a significant role in determining the likelihood of adverse events and favorable outcomes.

SRS can be used for both non-cavernous sinus (non-CS) and indirect cavernous sinus (CS) dAVFs [8]. Compared to non-CS dAVFs, dAVFs in the CS often achieve higher rates of obliteration after SRS [9–11]. The reasons for this higher rate of obliteration are multifaceted and include earlier detection due to visual or facial symptoms and smaller size. Moreover, CS dAVFs are more tolerant of higher radiation dose because of their extradural location. Maximal radiation doses of greater than 45 Gy were associated with favorable outcomes in CS dAVFs (i.e., obliteration without radiation-induced changes or post-SRS hemorrhage and radiological follow-up at 12 months or later). It should be noted that patients with CS dAVFs often report symptomatic improvement with or without obliteration [9]. On the contrary, symptomatic improvement is in fact dependent on obliteration in non-CS dAVFs. CS and non-CS dAVFs should be analyzed in different ways when assessing likelihood of favorable outcomes. When focusing on non-CS dAVFs, overall obliteration rates after SRS are approximately 68%, and actuarial obliteration rates are 82% at the 10-year mark. However, middle fossa or tentorial dAVFs are less likely to be obliterated (OR = 2.4) [12].

18.3.2 Physiology

Cortical venous drainage (CVD) is considered a driving prognostic factor in the natural history of dAVFs, as exemplified by the Borden and Cognard grading systems [2]. The absence of CVD has been shown to positively correlate with dAVF obliteration post-SRS [6, 8]. The underlying physiology of this correlation is not yet well understood. It is hypothesized that CVD may represent a surrogate marker of larger fistulous vessel diameter. The processes of endothelial damage, intimal reaction and thrombosis that have been well characterized in the arteriovenous malformation literature are more likely to occlude dAVFs with smaller diameter fistulous vessels [13].

Grading of dAVFs (e.g., low- or high-grade) can also help determine treatment approach and predict outcomes. Hemorrhage and neurological deficits are rarely associated with low-grade dAVFs, with annual neurological morbidity and mortality incidences of 0–0.6% [14–16]. As such, high level of evidence supporting a clinical benefit of intervention (e.g., embolization, open surgery, SRS) for low-grade dAVFs is lacking. The data show that any intervention for these low-grade dAVFs resulted in greater rates of obliteration compared to conservative management [17]. However, intervention did not improve functional or neurological outcomes as assessed by the modified Rankin Scale or other metrics such as symptomatic improvement and mortality. This indicates that while low-grade dAVFs are more likely to be obliterated by SRS, they do not necessarily require treatment unless symptomatic [17].

In contrast, high-grade dAVFs are associated with a considerably more aggressive natural history, with annual morbidity and mortality incidences of 15% and 10.4%, respectively [18]. Studies of unruptured high-grade dAVFs have assessed outcomes of different interventions versus observation [19]. Functional outcomes were similar between all interventions—including SRS—compared to the observation cohort. SRS, embolization, and surgery had low hemorrhage rates and non-hemorrhagic neurological deficits were similar between all groups. Overall, embolization and surgery were most likely to result in obliteration of unruptured high-grade dAVFs (43% and 86%, respectively), compared to observation (17%). Ultimately, these results suggest SRS is a viable treatment option for appropriately selected unruptured high grade dAVFs.

18.3.3 Clinical Characteristics

Finally, patient age has also been shown to impact response to SRS for dAVFs. In a cohort of 415 patients, those over 65 had post-SRS obliteration rates of roughly 48% and 78% at the 3- and 5-year time points, respectively. In these patients, transverse sinus location predicted obliteration. Patients younger than 65 had higher short-term, but worse long-term post-SRS obliteration rates of roughly 56% and 70% at the 3- and 5-year time points. In this younger cohort, cavernous sinus location predicted obliteration, and margin dose greater than 25 Gy predicted unfavorable outcomes (e.g., non-obliteration). There is heterogeneity in some predictive variables with respect to patient age, which should be accounted for when developing techniques for risk stratification [20].

18.4 Predictors of Adverse Events

The predictors of adverse events can be categorized similarly to factors predicting obliteration. The most studied post-SRS complication is hemorrhage. Multiple studies have found that post-SRS hemorrhage risk is similar to the natural risk of hemorrhage, leading to the conclusion that rupture risk remains not appreciably altered until obliteration is achieved [13].

18.4.1 Anatomy

Several studies have suggested that convexity or torcula location of the dAVF are associated with post-SRS hemorrhage [9, 21, 22]. Moreover, the predictors of adverse events depend on the anatomic location of the dAVF. Namely, non-CS dAVF patients with adverse events are more likely to be male, have multiple arterial feeding fistulas, and be treated with a lower maximum dose (<45 Gy). Patients with longer clinical follow-up also tend to have lower rates of adverse events [9], underscoring the need for consistent post-intervention care. Though the patients with CS dAVFs have higher rates of adverse events, no independent predictive factors could be identified to explain this unlike the three factors identified for non-CS dAVFs. Interestingly, some studies also report that higher margin doses (>23 Gy) are more likely to result in adverse events such as RIC [9]. The anatomy of dAVFs undoubtedly plays a role in determining adverse events with SRS treatment. As such, more consistent clinical guidelines must be established to help clinicians assess potential patient risk.

18.4.2 Physiology

The annual post-SRS dAVF hemorrhage rate is 0.84% [23]. A particularly strong predictor of hemorrhage in a multivariate analysis of SRS-treated dAVFs was presence of CVD [23]. This correlation is limited to dAVFs in the convexity or torcula, indicating that the interplay between anatomy and physiology must be taken into consideration when assessing patient risk.

Interestingly, some have found that CVD is not always as significant a risk factor as previously believed. Non-aggressive dAVFs—those that present without non-hemorrhagic neurological deficit or hemorrhage—are reasonable candidates for SRS even in the presence of CVD [24]. In fact, there were no complications post-SRS in 19 patients with nonaggressive dAVFs with CVD. Compiling an additional 155 cases from the literature also showed zero hemorrhages or radiation-related complications in nonaggressive dAVFs. Long term follow-up revealed that nonaggressive dAVFs with CVD did not bleed after SRS over almost 280 patient years, compared with a 3% hemorrhage rate for aggressive dAVFs over 165 patient years [24].

18.4.3 Clinical Characteristics

Apart from the intrinsic anatomy and physiology of dAVFs, patient history and demographics are undoubtedly important in assessing candidacy for SRS. As described above for non-CS dAVFs, female patients and patients with longer clinical follow-up tend to have lower rates of adverse events [9].

Additionally, the history of hemorrhage drastically alters the effect of SRS. It is well established that untreated dAVFs with CVD have a distinct pretreatment annual risk of hemorrhage depending on whether they are unruptured (1.5%) or previously ruptured (7.4%) [25]. While for unruptured dAVFs this risk remains unchanged post treatment until obliteration is achieved, for ruptured dAVFs SRS decreased the annual risk of hemorrhage to approximately 1% [23]. However, due to the high recurrent hemorrhage risk of ruptured dAVFs, SRS is a suboptimal therapy in many cases of ruptured dAVFs due to the latency period between treatment and obliteration which is typically 3 years after SRS [7].

Patients presenting with non-hemorrhagic neurological deficits (NHND) and those who had prior endovascular treatments are more likely to experience hemorrhage following radiosurgery [23]. Interestingly, a seizure at presentation was linked to a higher annual post-SRS hemorrhage rate compared to other NHND (40% vs 2.3%) [23]. Presentation with a non-hemorrhagic neurological deficit was also an independent predictor of a new and permanent neurologic deficit after SRS [26]. These findings are not contraindications for SRS. However, the increased risk of adverse events in these patient populations should warrant consideration and heightened precautions.

18.5 Next Steps

There are multiple opportunities for clinicians and researchers to build upon the recent, exciting work in this field. One way is to leverage analyses of predictive variables to define new classification criteria that better reflect relative patient risk.

In 2020, Mohammed et al. designed a new grading system that could help clinicians predict outcomes after SRS for dAVFs [6]. Using an international cohort of 120 dAVF patients treated with SRS, the group used logistic regression to identify factors that predicted obliteration without post-SRS hemorrhage. These factors were then combined with variables from other studies that examined a total of 736 patients. Backwards multivariate regression was employed to identify the best predictors of the group.

The three best predictors of favorable post-SRS outcomes (i.e., dAVF obliteration without post-SRS hemorrhage) were: (1) cortical venous reflux, (2) prior intracerebral hemorrhage or neurological deficit due to dAVF, and (3) non-cavernous sinus location. As expected, these factors represent the anatomical/physiological and patient demographic categorization of the predictive variables we present here. Using these variables, the group developed a scoring system where points were assigned based on how many of the three predictive variables applied to a specific patient (Table 18.2). The rate of favorable outcomes was found to be 80% for Grade I (0–1 point), 57% for Grade II (2 points), and 37% for Grade III (3 points). Kaplan-Meier analysis showed statistically significant survival differences between the three subclasses and this SRS specific scoring system better predicted outcomes

Table 18.2 Grading system for dAVFs presented by Mohammed et al. Points are allocated based on dAVF characteristics and patient history. Grade I dAVFs (0–1 points) have a favorable outcome rate of 80%, followed by Grade II (2 points) of 57%, and Grade III (3 points) of 37%

Predictor variable	Presence or absence	Points
Cortical venous reflux	Absent	0
	Present	1
Prior ICH or neurological deficit due to dAVF	Absent	0
	Present	1
Location	Cavernous	0
	Non-cavernous	1

compared to the traditional grading systems. Of note this new grading system has not yet undergone external validation.

More studies are needed with larger patient populations to continue developing new grading systems like the one proposed by Mohammed et al. Databases such as the CONDOR registry, which has data on dAVFs from more than 1000 patients [27], will be useful in the pursuit of this aim. Machine learning models may also have a role in further studies, to delineate complex, nonlinear relationships between anatomic, radiographic, and patient demographic data points. The development of novel strategies for predicting outcomes post-SRS will contribute to improve patient selection for SRS, and thus improve safety and efficacy of SRS as a treatment approach.

References

1. Hasegawa H, Yamamoto M, Shin M, Barfod BE. Gamma knife radiosurgery for brain vascular malformations: current evidence and future tasks. Ther Clin Risk Manag. 2019;15:1351–67. https://doi.org/10.2147/TCRM.S200813.
2. Borden JA, Wu JK, Shucart WA. A proposed classification for spinal and cranial dural arteriovenous fistulous malformations and implications for treatment. J Neurosurg. 1995;82(2):166–79. https://doi.org/10.3171/jns.1995.82.2.0166.
3. Cognard C, Gobin YP, Pierot L, et al. Cerebral dural arteriovenous fistulas: clinical and angiographic correlation with a revised classification of venous drainage. Radiology. 1995;194(3):671–80. https://doi.org/10.1148/radiology.194.3.7862961.
4. Zipfel GJ, Shah MN, Refai D, Dacey RG, Derdeyn CP. Cranial dural arteriovenous fistulas: modification of angiographic classification scales based on new natural history data. Neurosurg Focus. 2009;26(5):E14. https://doi.org/10.3171/2009.2.FOCUS0928.
5. Corbelli I, De Maria F, Eusebi P, et al. Dural arteriovenous fistulas and headache features: an observational study. J Headache Pain. 2020;21(1):1–9. https://doi.org/10.1186/s10194-020-1073-1.
6. Mohammed N, Hung YC, Chen CJ, et al. A proposed grading scale for predicting outcomes after stereotactic radiosurgery for dural arteriovenous fistulas. Neurosurgery. 2020;87(2):247–55. https://doi.org/10.1093/neuros/nyz401.
7. Chen CJ, Lee CC, Ding D, et al. Stereotactic radiosurgery for intracranial dural arteriovenous fistulas: a systematic review. J Neurosurg. 2015;122(2):353–62. https://doi.org/10.3171/2014.10.JNS14871.
8. Cifarelli CP, Kaptain G, Yen CP, Schlesinger D, Sheehan JP. Gamma knife radiosurgery for dural arteriovenous fistulas. Neurosurgery. 2010;67(5):1230–5. https://doi.org/10.1227/NEU.0b013e3181eff6f7.
9. Hung YC, Mohammed N, Kearns KN, et al. Stereotactic radiosurgery for cavernous sinus versus noncavernous sinus dural arteriovenous fistulas: outcomes and outcome predictors. Neurosurgery. 2020;86(5):676–84. https://doi.org/10.1093/neuros/nyz260.
10. Yang H-C, Kano H, Kondziolka D, et al. Stereotactic radiosurgery with or without embolization for intracranial dural arteriovenous fistulas. Neurosurgery. 2010;67(5):1276–85. https://doi.org/10.1227/NEU.0b013e3181ef3f22.
11. Wu HM, Pan DHC, Chung WY, et al. Gamma knife surgery for the management of intracranial dural arteriovenous fistulas. J Neurosurg. 2006;105(Supplement):43–51. https://doi.org/10.3171/sup.2006.105.7.43.
12. Starke RM, McCarthy DJ, Chen CJ, et al. Evaluation of stereotactic radiosurgery for cerebral dural arteriovenous fistulas in a multicenter international consortium. J Neurosurg. 2019;132(1):114–21. https://doi.org/10.3171/2018.8.JNS181467.
13. Söderman M, Edner G, Ericson K, et al. Gamma knife surgery for dural arteriovenous shunts: 25 years of experience. J Neurosurg. 2006;104(6):867–75. https://doi.org/10.3171/jns.2006.104.6.867.
14. Satomi J, van Dijk JMC, Terbrugge KG, Willinsky RA, Wallace MC. Benign cranial dural arteriovenous fistulas: outcome of conservative management based on the natural history of the lesion. J Neurosurg. 2002;97(4):767–70. https://doi.org/10.3171/jns.2002.97.4.0767.
15. Shah MN, Botros JA, Pilgram TK, et al. Borden-Shucart type I dural arteriovenous fistulas: clinical course including risk of conversion to higher-grade fistulas: clinical article. J Neurosurg. 2012;117(3):539–45. https://doi.org/10.3171/2012.5.JNS111257.
16. Gross BA, Du R. The natural history of cerebral dural arteriovenous fistulae. Neurosurgery. 2012;71(3):594–603. https://doi.org/10.1227/NEU.0b013e31825eabdb.
17. Chen CJ, Buell TJ, Ding D, et al. Observation versus intervention for low-grade intracranial dural arterio-

venous fistulas. Neurosurgery. 2021;88(6):1111–20. https://doi.org/10.1093/neuros/nyab024.

18. van Dijk JMC, terBrugge KG, Willinsky RA, Wallace MC. Clinical course of cranial dural arteriovenous fistulas with long-term persistent cortical venous reflux. Stroke. 2002;33(5):1233–6. https://doi.org/10.1161/01.STR.0000014772.02908.44.
19. Chen CJ, Buell TJ, Ding D, et al. Intervention for unruptured high-grade intracranial dural arteriovenous fistulas: a multicenter study. J Neurosurg. 2021;136:1–9. https://doi.org/10.3171/2021.1.JNS202799.
20. Mohammed N, Hung YC, Xu Z, et al. A propensity score-matched cohort analysis of outcomes after stereotactic radiosurgery in older versus younger patients with dural arteriovenous fistula: an international multicenter study. World Neurosurg. 2019;125:e1114–24. https://doi.org/10.1016/j.wneu.2019.01.253.
21. Li C, Wang Y, Li Y, Jiang C, Yang X, Wu Z. Clinical and angioarchitectural risk factors associated with intracranial hemorrhage in dural arteriovenous fistulas: a single-center retrospective study. PLoS One. 2015;10(6):e0131235. https://doi.org/10.1371/journal.pone.0131235.
22. Peng T, Liu A, Jia J, et al. Risk factors for dural arteriovenous fistula intracranial hemorrhage. J Clin Neurosci. 2014;21(5):769–72. https://doi.org/10.1016/j.jocn.2013.07.024.
23. Starke RM, McCarthy DJ, Chen CJ, et al. Hemorrhage risk of cerebral dural arteriovenous fistulas following Gamma Knife radiosurgery in a multicenter international consortium. J Neurosurg. 2019;132(4):1209–17. https://doi.org/10.3171/2018.12.JNS182208.
24. Tonetti DA, Gross BA, Jankowitz BT, et al. Reconsidering an important subclass of high-risk dural arteriovenous fistulas for stereotactic radiosurgery. J Neurosurg. 2018;130(3):972–6. https://doi.org/10.3171/2017.10.JNS171802.
25. Söderman M, Pavic L, Edner G, Holmin S, Andersson T. Natural history of dural arteriovenous shunts. Stroke. 2008;39(6):1735–9. https://doi.org/10.1161/STROKEAHA.107.506485.
26. Chen CJ, Buell TJ, Diamond J, et al. Stereotactic radiosurgery for high-grade intracranial dural arteriovenous fistulas. World Neurosurg. 2018;116:e640–8. https://doi.org/10.1016/j.wneu.2018.05.062.
27. Guniganti R, Giordan E, Chen CJ, et al. Consortium for Dural Arteriovenous Fistula Outcomes Research (CONDOR): rationale, design, and initial characterization of patient cohort. J Neurosurg. 2021;136:1–11. https://doi.org/10.3171/2021.1.JNS202790.

19 Complications During Endovascular Embolization of Dural Arteriovenous Fistulas

Huachen Zhang and Xianli Lv

Abstract

Endovascular Onyx embolization has now been accepted as the primary treatment strategy to manage dural arteriovenous fistulas (DAVFs). Side effects of this procedure include trigeminal cardiac reflex, perforation or rupture of intracranial vessels, cranial nerve palsy, and worsening of venous congestion. Liquid embolics can reflux into arterial feeders and further reflux into normal arterial territories causing ischemia of normal tissue during transvenous embolization. Intracranial abscess has also been reported related to transvenous DAVF embolization. The permanent neurological deficits are rare, but transient neurological complications are noted in up to 10% of patients. After successful transvenous DAVF embolization, delayed development of a second fistula at a different site is also possible. This chapter detailed information concerning the complications related to endovascular embolization of DAVFs.

Keywords

Endovascular · Embolization · Complications Dural arteriovenous fistula

H. Zhang · X. Lv (✉)
Department of Neurosurgery, Beijing Tsinghua Changgung Hospital, School of Clinical Medicine, Tsinghua University, Beijing, China

A little error may lead to a large discrepancy.
—Yi-Jing

19.1 Introduction

The incidence of dural arteriovenous fistulas (DAVFs) is reported to be 0.3 per 100,000 per year [1]. Current endovascular therapy includes transvenous Onyx embolization and transarterial glue or Onyx embolization [2]. Complication rates associated with endovascular embolization range from 5% to 10%, including permanent neurologic deficits [3]. The aim of this chapter is to report complications that resulted from endovascular treatment of DAVFs.

19.2 Trigeminal Cardiac Reflex

Trigeminocardiac reflex (TCR) has been described in the literature as a reflexive response of bradycardia, hypotension during Onyx embolization of DAVF [4–6]. TCR has been observed during transarterial or transvenous Onyx embolization of DAVFs [7]. The TCR rate is 7.7% in patients treated intraarterial Onyx embolization [7]. This phenomenon of TCR was not observed in transvenous GDC (Guglielmi detachable coil) and *n*BCA (*n*-butyl cyanoacrylate) embolization of cavernous DAVF [4–7]. TCR was observed in 33.3% patients treated with transvenous Onyx embolization for cavernous DAVFs [7]. The TCR

X. Lv (ed.), *Intracranial and Spinal Dural Arteriovenous Fistulas*,
https://doi.org/10.1007/978-981-19-5767-3_19

has been described during endovascular treatment DAVFs adjacent to the cavernous sinus, tentorium, transverse sinus and the torcular [4–7] (Fig. 19.1). The dura mater of the posterior fossa is innervated partly by branches of the trigeminal nerve and receives vascular supply from branches

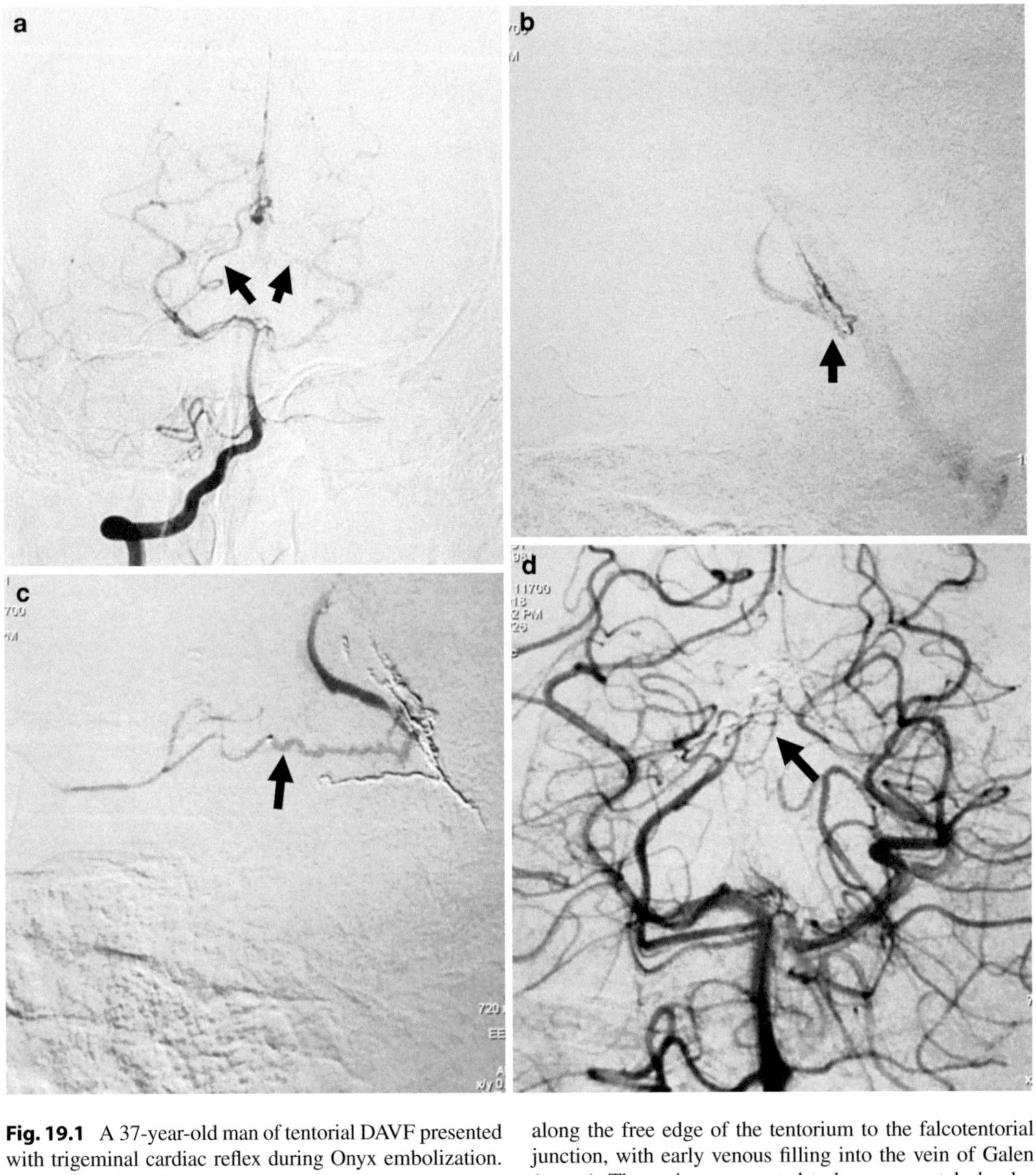

Fig. 19.1 A 37-year-old man of tentorial DAVF presented with trigeminal cardiac reflex during Onyx embolization. (**a**) Anterior-posterior projection of a right vertebral artery injection shows a tentorial DAVF supplied by the bilateral arteries of Davidoff and Schechter (arrows). (**b**) Lateral projection of a microcatheter injection within the right artery of Davidoff and Schechter shows the early venous filling into the vein of Galen (arrow). (**c**) Lateral projection of a microcatheter injection within the left artery of Davidoff and Schechter shows the course of the vessel along the free edge of the tentorium to the falcotentorial junction, with early venous filling into the vein of Galen (arrow). The patient was noted to become acutely bradycardic, and proceeded to asystole during dimethyl sulfoxide injection and there was a return of spontaneous circulation while ceasing injection. After addition to 5 mg Atropine, the procedure was completed without any side effects. (**d**) Anterior-posterior projection of a right vertebral artery injection after Onyx embolization shows no residual early venous filling with cure of the DAVF

of the posterior branch of middle meningeal artery and/or posterior meningeal artery (arising from the vertebral artery) as well as transosseous branches of the occipital artery [4]. Hence, Onyx embolisation of these vessels can irritate the trigeminal nerve and cause a TCR. We think that direct stimulation of the dura matter by dimethyl sulfoxide (DMSO) and injection pressure, which induce neuronal signals via the Gassarian ganglion to the sensory nucleus of the trigeminal nerve, forming the afferent pathway of the reflex arc. This afferent pathway continues along the short internuncial nerve fibers in the reticular formation to connect with the efferent pathway in the motor nucleus of the vagus nerve and causes bradycardia [4].

It is not possible to predict which patients will present with this response. Therefore, our recommendation is that interventionalists need to be aware of the possibility of this response during Onyx embolization procedures for dural fistulas. A brief 'pause' prior to Onyx injection to inform anesthesia colleagues of any potential instability is our standard practice. When the patient's heart beat rate drops, treatment of hemodynamic instability consists of ceasing procedure and administering anticholinergic drugs without permanent sequelae. Atropine is effective to eliminate the TCR in following Onyx injection procedure. Anticholinergic drugs are not for regular use in Onyx embolization because they can cause refractory arrhythmias [4].

19.3 Cranial Nerves Palsy

Liquid embolic materials, such as NBCA and Onyx, penetrates into the vasa nervosum will cause cranial nerve palsy, such as oculomotor nerve palsy (III) (Fig. 19.2), trigeminal nerve

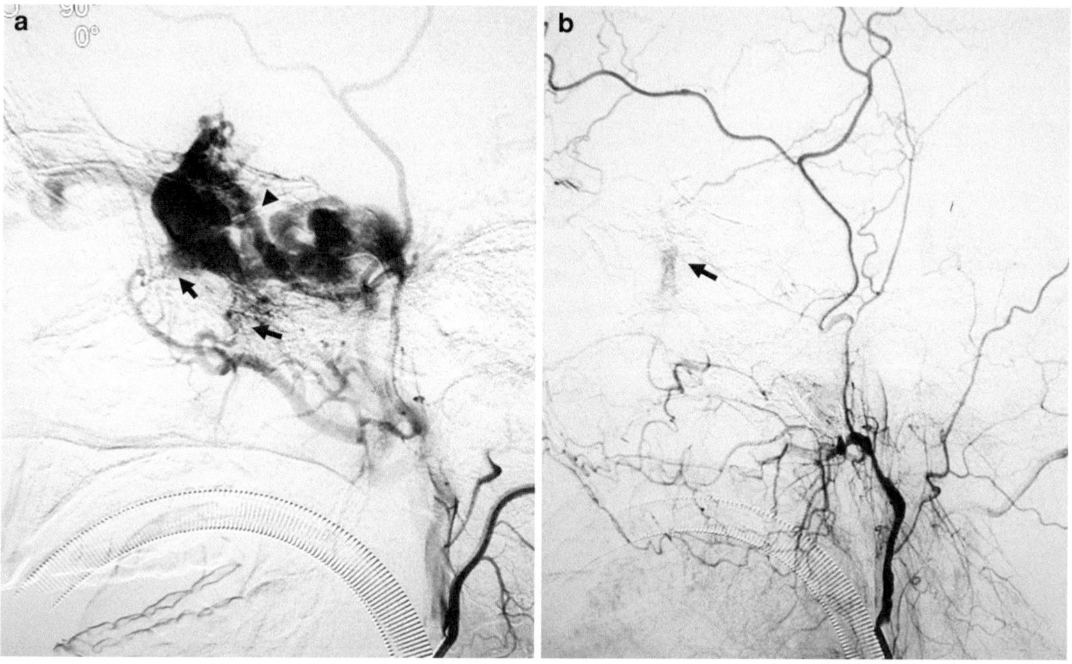

Fig. 19.2 A case of cavernous sinus DAVF treated with transarterial Onyx embolization causing oculomotor nerve palsy. (**a**) Preoperative external carotid angiogram (lateral view) shows the shunt in the cavernous sinus fed by the anterior branch of the middle meningeal artery (arrowhead), the artery of the foramen rotundum (short arrow) and the artery of the foramen ovale (long arrow) arising from the internal maxillary artery. (**b**) The postoperative external carotid artery angiogram (lateral view) shows a small residual of the fistula. The patient suffered the left oculomotor nerve palsy after embolization

palsy (V), facial nerve palsy (VII), and the lower cranial nerves (IX–XII) [8–10]. The most important external carotid artery supplies to the cranial nerves are the supplies to CN III, V, VII and IX–XII. Supply of the geniculate ganglion of the facial nerve consists of the petrous branch of the MMA (Fig. 19.3). Many external carotid branches like the middle meningeal, accessory meningeal, deep temporal artery, and the artery of foramen rotundum give rise to branches feeding the cranial nerves around the middle fossa (CN III, IV, V and VI) (Fig. 19.4). The middle meningeal, ascending pharyngeal, occipital artery, and posterior meningeal branch of the vertebral artery also

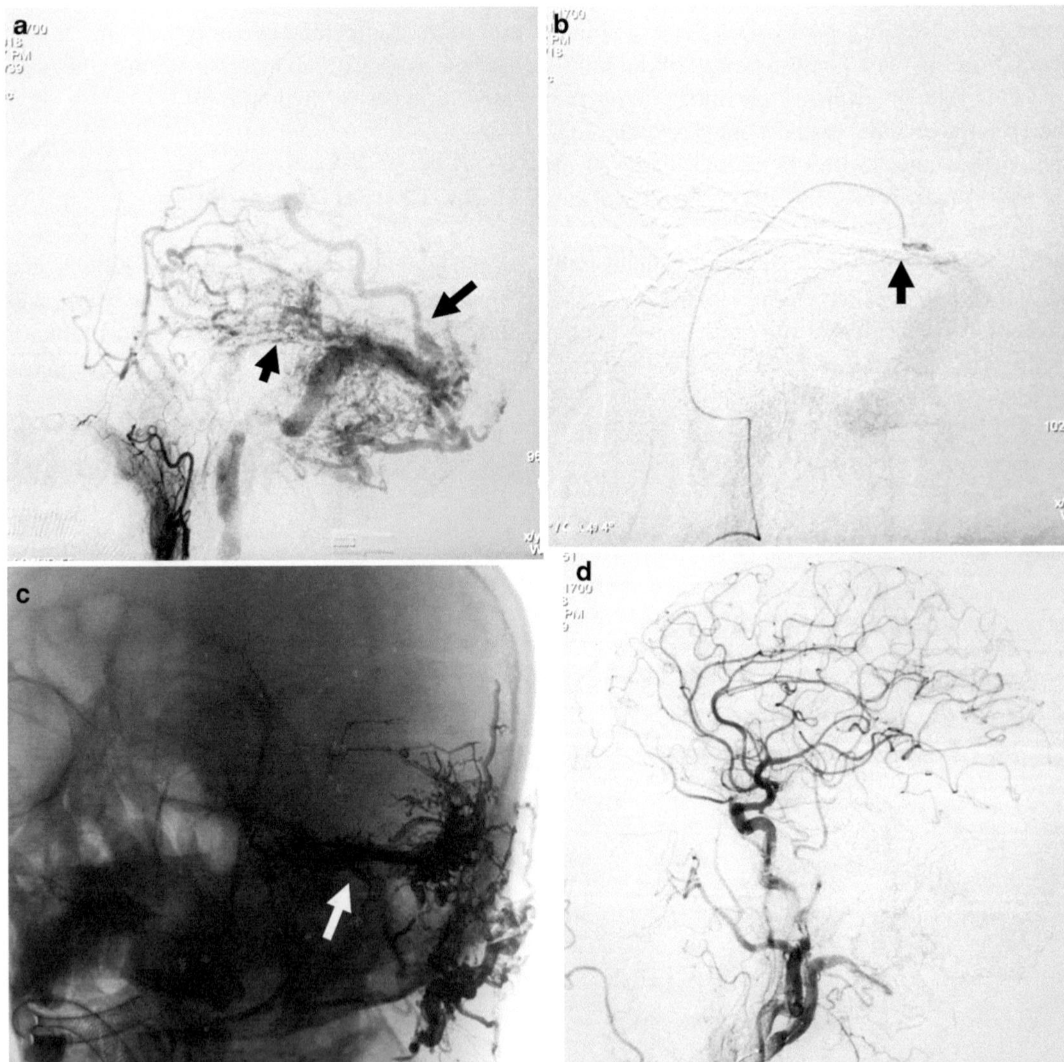

Fig. 19.3 A case of the transverse-sigmoid sinus DAVF treated with transarterial Onyx embolization causing facial nerve palsy. (**a**) Preoperative external carotid angiogram (lateral view) shows the shunt in the transverse-sigmoid sinus fed by the dural branches of the middle meningeal artery (short arrow) and the occipital artery with reflux to the Labbé vein (long arrow). (**b**) Lateral projection of a microcatheter injection within the posterior branch of the middle meningeal artery shows the early venous filling into the transverse-sigmoid sinus. (**c**) Postoperative craniogram showing the Onyx cast. Note the Onyx within the petrosal branches of the middle meningeal artery (arrow). (**d**) The postoperative common carotid artery angiogram (lateral view) shows complete occlusion of the fistula. The patient suffered the left facial nerve palsy after embolization

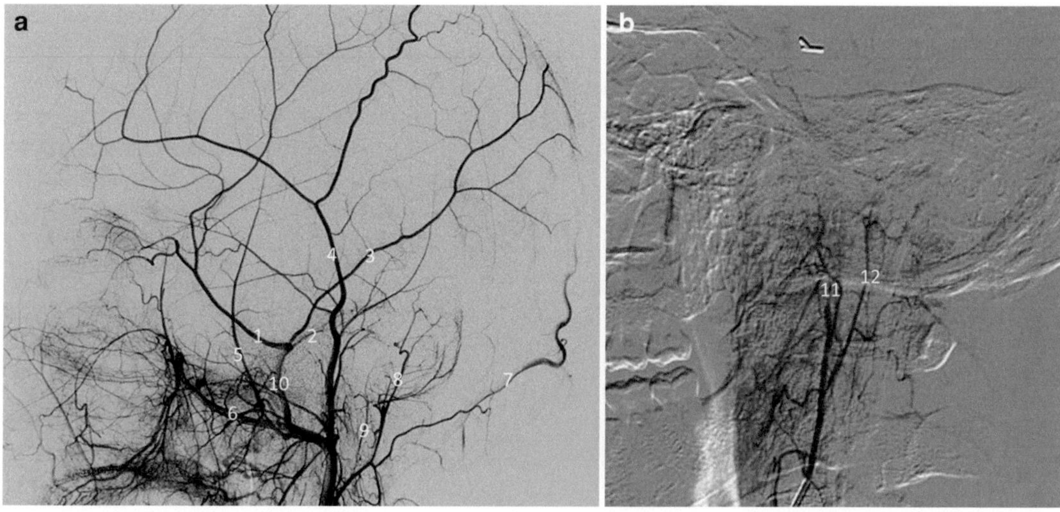

Fig. 19.4 lateral projection of external carotid artery (**a**) and ascending pharyngeal artery (**b**) injection shows their branches. 1—the anterior convexity branch of the middle meningeal artery, 2—petrosal branch of the middle meningeal artery, 3—the posterior convexity branch of the middle meningeal artery, 4—superficial temporal artery, 5—middle deep temporal artery, 6—internal maxillary artery, 7—occipital artery, 8—posterior auricular artery, 9—ascending pharyngeal artery, 10—middle meningeal artery, 11—the anterior branch of the ascending pharyngeal artery, 12—the posterior branch of the ascending pharyngeal artery (neuromeningeal trunk)

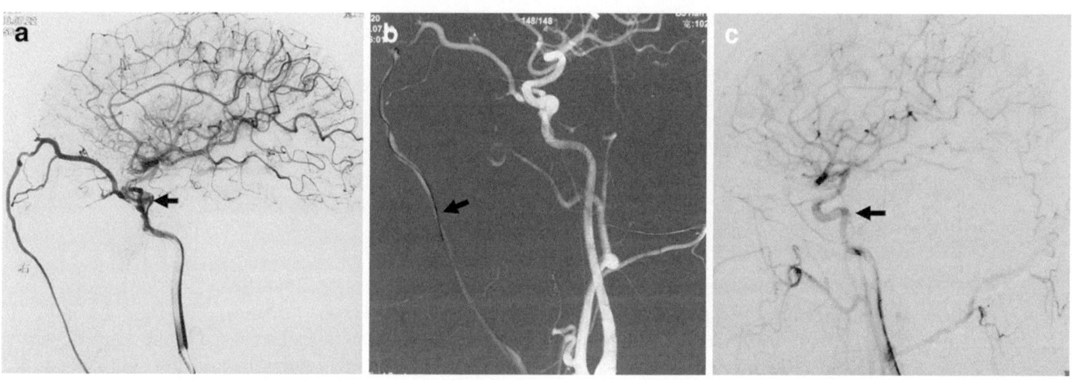

Fig. 19.5 A case of cavernous sinus DAVF treated with transvenous Onyx packing of the affected cavernous sinus. (**a**) Preoperative internal carotid angiogram (lateral view) shows the shunt in the cavernous sinus (arrow). (**b**) Internal carotid roadmap (lateral view) shows the facial vein was selected to access the affected cavernous sinus (arrow). (**c**) The postoperative common carotid angiogram (lateral view) shows complete occlusion of the fistula

feed the cranial nerves inside and outside the posterior fossa. The lower cranial nerves are supplied from the jugular branch of the ascending pharyngeal artery as it traverses the jugular foramen, and the hypoglossal branch supplies CN XII within the hypoglossal canal. Embolization of these branches can result in temporary or permanent cranial nerve palsies. The inferolateral and meningohypophyseal trunk of the internal carotid artery feed many cranial nerves and have a rich collateral anastomosis between external carotid artery. Transvenous Onyx packing of the cavernous sinus causes III, IV, V cranial nerve deficits, but they can recover after 3–4 months (Fig. 19.5) [11]. This mechanism may be the neurotoxicity of the DMSO (Dimethyl sulfoxide).

19.4 Cerebral Infarction

The dural branches of the external carotid artery have rich anastomosis with the dural and pial branches of the internal and vertebral arteries. Liquid embolic materials like NBCA (*n*-butyl cyanoacrylate) and Onyx, are easily migrating to the pial arteries via the network (Fig. 19.6) [12–14]. One must care about the most important and critical complications is cerebral ischemia resulting from the reflux of liquid embolic materials via the network between dural and pial arteries (Fig. 19.7). There are three regions that serve as the major extracranial–intracranial anastomotic pathways [15]:

1. The orbital region: via the ophthalmic artery is the interface between the internal maxillary and internal carotid arteries.
2. The petrous-cavernous region: via the inferolateral trunk (ILT), the petrous branches of the internal carotid artery (ICA), and the meningohypophyseal trunk to the carotid artery.
3. The upper cervical region: via the ascending pharyngeal, the occipital, and the ascending and deep cervical arteries to the vertebral artery (Fig. 19.8).

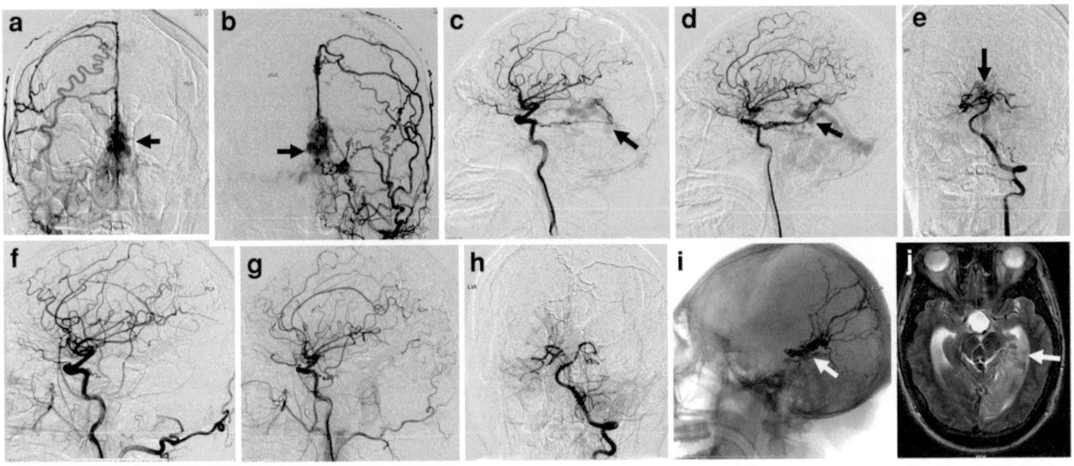

Fig. 19.6 A case of DAVF in the tentorium showing Onyx migration. (**a**) Anterior-posterior projection of the right external carotid artery injection. (**b**) Anterior-posterior projection of the left external carotid artery injection. (**c**) Lateral projection of the right internal carotid artery injection. (**d**) Lateral projection of the left internal carotid artery injection. (**e**) Anterior-posterior projection of the left vertebral artery injection. Shows dural fistula (arrow) fed by dural branches of the bilateral external carotid arteries, internal carotid arteries and bilateral arteries of Davidoff and Schechter with early filling of the vein of Galen (arrows). Post-embolization. (**f**) Lateral projection of the right common carotid artery injection. (**g**) Lateral projection of the left common carotid artery injection. (**h**) Anterior-posterior projection of the left vertebral artery injection. (**i**) Craniogram showing the Onyx cast (arrow). (**j**) Postoperative MRI indicates migration of the Onyx coming into the distal posterior cerebral artery via the artery of Davidoff and Schechter (arrow)

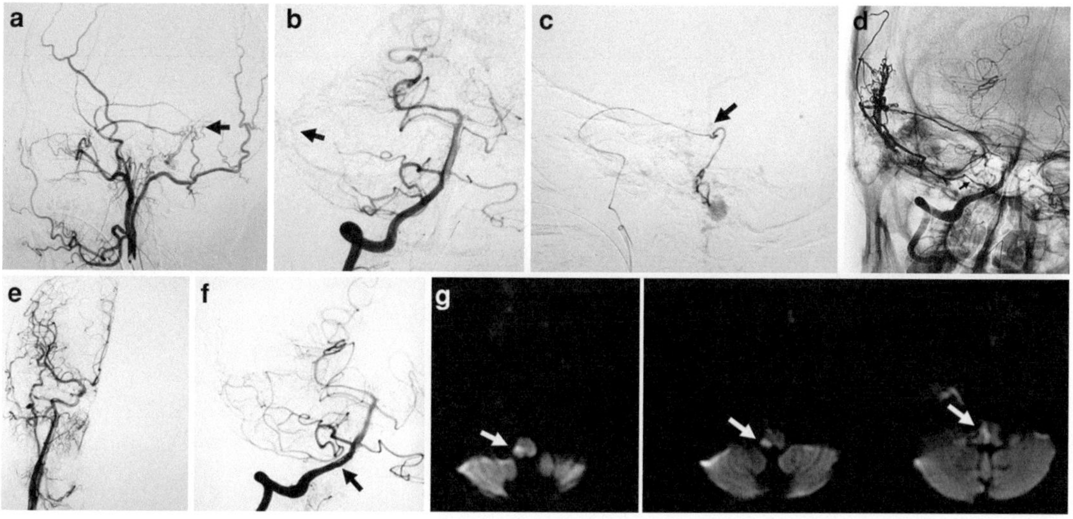

Fig. 19.7 A case with modified Borden II DAVF involving the sigmoid sinus. The shunt was obliterated with Onyx injection from the middle meningeal artery. (**a**) Preoperative lateral projection of the right external carotid artery angiogram. (**b**) Preoperative anterior-posterior projection of the right vertebral artery angiogram. Shows dural fistula (arrow) fed by dural branches of the right external carotid artery and the right posterior inferior cerebellar artery (arrows). (**c**) Lateral projection of a microcatheter injection within the posterior branch of the middle meningeal artery shows the early venous filling into the sigmoid sinus. (**d**) Postoperative craniogram shows the Onyx cast coming back to the posterior inferior cerebellar artery. (**e**) Postoperative common carotid angiogram. (**f**) Postoperative vertebral angiogram indicating complete obliteration of the shunt and disappearance of the posterior inferior cerebellar artery. (**g**) Postoperative MR imaging indicates dorsolateral medulla oblongata infarction

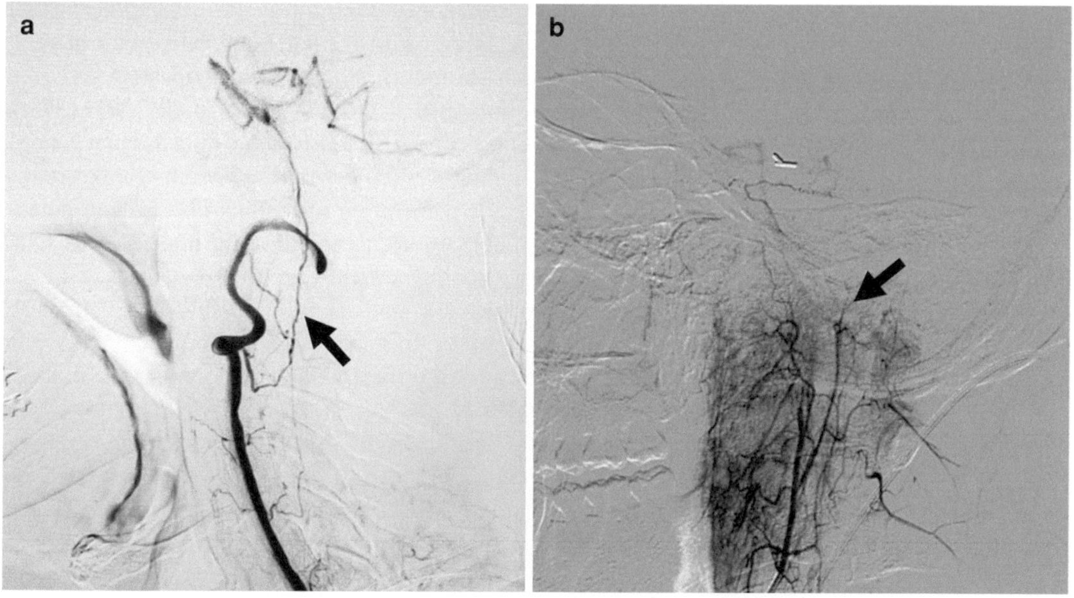

Fig. 19.8 Upper cervical regions (anastomoses to the vertebral artery). (**a**) Lateral projection of the vertebral artery injection shows the anastomoses between the vertebral artery and basilar artery in a case with vertebral artery occlusion is the posterior spinal artery (arrow). (**b**) Lateral projection of the ascending pharyngeal artery injection showing there is anastomoses between the ascending pharyngeal artery and the vertebral artery from the neuromeningeal trunk (arrow). (**c**, **d**) lateral projection of the vertebral artery injection showing the occipital artery is filled through the connection between the external carotid artery to the vertebral artery through the posterior anastomotic radicular branches at C2 levels (arrow)

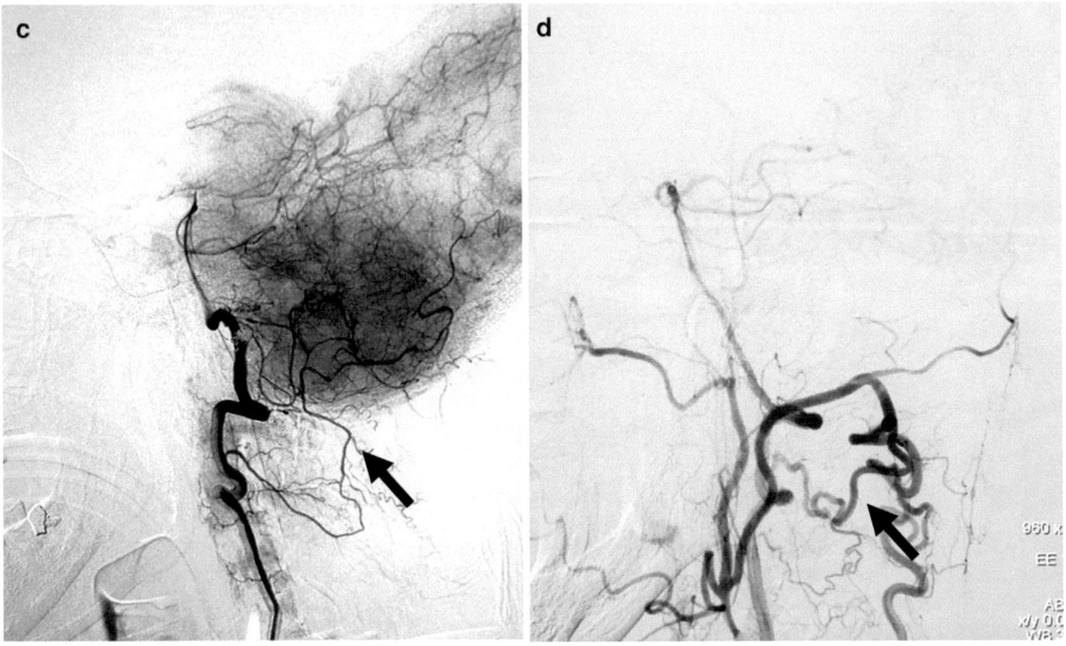

Fig. 19.8 (continued)

19.5 Venous Infarction and Venous Bleeding

Onyx can penetrate the dural arteriovenous fistula easily and go to the initial venous side. This penetration is the essential phenomenon for the curative treatment and is the most advantageous point of Onyx to the particulates. However, excessive penetration (migration) could occasionally result in the occlusion of the functioning cerebral veins, causing potential venous infarction [12–14, 16]. Premature venous occlusion or thrombosis developed from the partial DAVF embolization cause venous hypertension and venous rupture (Fig. 19.9) [12–14, 16]. If the fistula has pial arterial supply, in addition to dural arterial supply, a transvenous approach without retrograde penetration of pial feeders can result in hemorrhagic complication.

Venous infarction or rupture can be caused by blocking the normal venous drainage after transvenous sinus embolization. Transvenous sinus packing of these lesions have a potential complication of venous bleeding from excessive residual drainage to the cortical vein if the packing is incomplete. Therefore, the dangerous small draining veins like the uncal vein, petrosal vein, and bridging veins to the brain stem must be obliterated during transvenous approaches (Fig. 19.10). Similarly, if a fistula has pial venous drainage, a transvenous approach without retrograde penetration of feeding arteries can potentially convert the fistula to a higher grade with worsening cortical vein involvement. Visual loss, glaucoma and acute exophthalmos are also reported following transvenous approach via superior orbital vein for treatment of indirect CCF [13, 14].

Hemorrhagic complication after the endovascular treatment of the DAVFs has been reported up to 4.5%, which was not eligible in DAVF treatment [16]. Non-sinus location, the presence of pial arterial supplier, giant venous aneurysm and high Onyx volume in one session have been reported to be the risk factors hemorrhagic complication of DAVF embolization [16]. Knowledge of this potentially fatal complication is of importance during DAVF embolization.

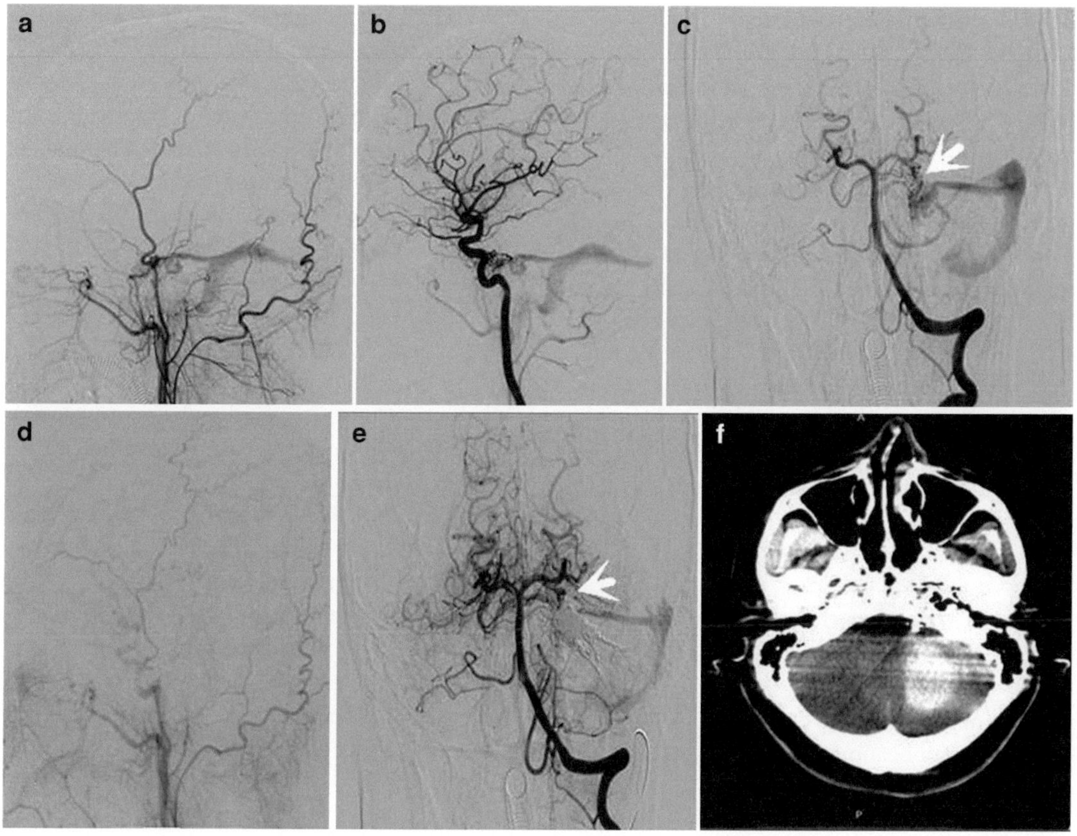

Fig. 19.9 A case with DAVF involving the superior petrosal sinus. (**a**) Lateral view of the right external carotid artery injection. (**b**) Lateral view of the internal carotid artery injection. (**c**) Anterior-posterior projection of the left vertebral artery injection. Shows a DAVF of the superior petrosal sinus fed by the left middle meningeal artery, posterior auricular artery, meningohypophyseal trunk of the internal carotid artery and the temporal branch of the left posterior cerebral artery, then drained into the superior petrosal sinus. Onyx embolization was performed via the middle meningeal artery. (**d**) The left common carotid artery angiogram. (**e**) Anterior-posterior projection of the left vertebral artery injection showed the small residual fistula fed by the temporal branch of the left posterior cerebral artery. After 6.5 h, the patient complained of numbness of the left limb and suffered a sudden onset of unconsciousness and acute CT scanning showed an intra-cerebellar hematoma (**f**)

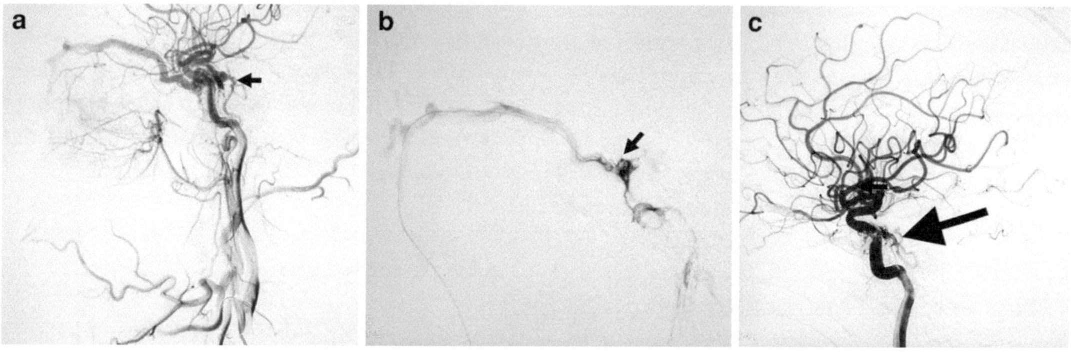

Fig. 19.10 An example of the dangerous draining veins. (**a**) Preoperative common carotid angiogram (lateral view) shows the shunt in the cavernous sinus (arrow). (**b**) Lateral projection of a microcatheter injection within the cavernous sinus shows the early venous filling into the superior ophthalmic vein and the inferior petrosal sinus. (**c**) The postoperative internal carotid angiogram (lateral view) shows small residual fistula drained into the transverse pontine vein and the patient died of brain stem infarction

19.6 Vessel Perforation

Arterial or venous perforation developed particularly during navigation of the wire or catheter [13, 14]. Advantages of transarterial embolization include decreased chance of flow redirection into an alternate venous pathway, ability to save functional venous system, avoidance of post-treatment de novo DAVF formation from venous hypertension and decreased complications specific to commonly used transvenous approaches (e.g., venous perforation from catheterisation and bleeding from premature venous occlusion). Vein perforation was reported during the transvenous approach by recanalization of the closed venous segment.

19.7 Cardiac and Pulmonary Embolism

Cardiac and pulmonary embolism are the other potential complications of DAVFs embolization during glue or Onyx injection in high-flow lesions [17–21]. Pulmonary embolization following embolization was also reported in spinal arteriovenous malformation [22]. Cardiac and pulmonary embolization is a potentially fatal complication of this therapy, and its risk should be known by all involved in the care of patients with DAVFs. Although asymptomatic pulmonary emboli are known to occur, these events are likely to result in clinical symptoms requiring treatment. Careful assessment of DAVF angioarchitecture for precise embolization is essential to determine endovascular strategies. The flow-arrest techniques should be considered when high-flow fistulas are known to be present. These precautions will help prevent migration of glue to the pulmonary circulation, as well as deposition in cerebral venous structures with associated complications.

19.8 Retained Microcatheter

Microcatheters may be trapped by both adhesive and nonadhesive liquid embolic material due to long time injection, long reflux or tortuous access route [13, 14]. Techniques for the retrieval of a trapped microcatheter include using a monorail snare technique to grasp the trapped catheter or advancing another catheter to apply countertraction. For firmly glued-in catheters, permanent implantation may be needed by cutting the catheter at the level of the femoral artery. The microcatheter will be pressed against the arterial wall by blood flow down the aorta, allowing it to become endothelialized over time. If a retained microcatheter is left in place, the patient should be kept on aspirin for 3 months. Pseudoaneurysm of the femoral artery or popliteal artery occlusion has been reported after cutting and leaving in place a glued-in catheter. If the microcatheter impairs cerebral blood flow, surgical extraction may be required. Microcatheter fractures above the level of the aorta may result in distal thrombosis and infarction. In these cases, a self-expanding stent can be used to trap the microcatheter against the parent artery wall or a microsnare can be used to grasp the fragment. If a stent is used, dual antiplatelet therapy is required.

19.9 Intracranial Abscess

Intracranial abscess has been reported after transvenous DAVF embolization using detachable coils [23]. A transverse sinus DAVF converted to retrograde filling of a cortical draining vein that was not seen on initial angiography after transvenous coil embolization. Two months after the embolization, the patient developed a cerebral abscess in the region of the previous cortical infarction. The abscess was successfully treated with antibiotic therapy and drainage. The authors speculated that the possible contribution of the cerebral abscess was the cortical draining vein.

19.10 Conclusion

Complications related to DAVF embolization include perforation or rupture of intracranial vessels, venous infarction, and worsening of venous hypertension. These post-embolization complications may lead to a decline in the quality of life and even endanger the patient's life. Therefore, for different location or types of DAVF, it is very important to choose an appropriate treatment method. Familiarity with these postoperative complications is of great significance to improve the prognosis of patients.

References

1. Ghobrial GM, Marchan E, Nair AK, Dumont AS, Tjoumakaris SI, Gonzalez LF, Rosenwasser RH, Jabbour P. Dural arteriovenous fistulas: a review of the literature and a presentation of a single institution's experience. World Neurosurg. 2013;80(1–2):94–102.
2. Lv X, Wang G, Wang J. Craniospinal vascular diseases and endovascular neurosurgery. New York: Nova Science; 2021.
3. Tsumoto T, Terada T, Tsuura M, Matsumoto H, Yamaga H, Masuo O, Itakura T. Analysis of complications related to endovascular therapy for dural arteriovenous fistulae. Interv Neuroradiol. 2004;10(Suppl 1):121–5.
4. Lv X, Li Y, Lv M, Liu A, Zhang J, Wu Z. Trigeminocardiac reflex in embolization of intracranial dural arteriovenous fistula. AJNR Am J Neuroradiol. 2007;28(9):1769–70.
5. Malik MH, Brinjikji W, Savastano LE. Asystole during Onyx embolization of 64-year-old patient with dural arteriovenous fistula. Neuroradiol J. 2021;19714009211047453 https://doi.org/10.1177/19714009211047453. Epub ahead of print.
6. Nicholson P, Hilditch C, Brinjikji W, Krings T. Asystole during onyx embolisation of a dural av fistula: the trigeminocardiac reflex. Interv Neuroradiol. 2019;25(2):132–4.
7. Lv X, Li Y, Jiang C, Wu Z. The incidence of trigeminocardiac reflex in endovascular treatment of dural arteriovenous fistula with onyx. Interv Neuroradiol. 2010;16(1):59–63.
8. Lv X, Jiang C, Zhang J, Li Y, Wu Z. Complications related to percutaneous transarterial embolization of intracranial dural arteriovenous fistulas in 40 patients. Am J Neuroradiol. 2009;30:462–8.
9. Lv X, Jiang C, Li Y, Wu Z. Results and complications of transarterial embolization of intracranial dural arteriovenous fistulas using Onyx-18. J Neurosurg. 2008;109:1083–90.
10. Tashiro N, Kawano H, Hiraoka F, Nakamura Y, Fukuda S, Yano S, Aikawa H, Go Y, Kazekawa K, Matsumoto Y. Iatrogenic middle meningeal arteriovenous fistula during embolization: two case reports and literature review. J Stroke Cerebrovasc Dis. 2021;30(8):105909.
11. Lv X, Jiang C, Li Y, Yang X, Wu Z. Recovery of opthalmoplegia associated with cavernous sinus dural arteriovenous fistulas after transvenous cavernous sinus packing. Eur J Radiol. 2010;75:139–42.
12. Lv X, Wu Z. The philosophy of 'unity of knowledge and action' in interventional neuroradiology teaching. Neuroradiol J. 2018;31(3):330–2.
13. Bentson J, Rand R, Calcaterra T, Lasjaunias P. Unexpected complications following therapeutic embolization. Neuroradiology. 1978;16:420–3.
14. Davis MC, Deveikis JP, Harrigan MR. Clinical presentation, imaging, and management of complications due to neurointerventional procedures. Semin Intervent Radiol. 2015;32(2):98–107.
15. Geibprasert S, Pongpech S, Armstrong D, Krings T. Dangerous extracranial-intracranial anastomoses and supply to the cranial nerves: vessels the neurointerventionalist needs to know. AJNR Am J Neuroradiol. 2009;30(8):1459–68.
16. Liu P, Chen X, You W, Li Y, Lv M, Lv X. Hemorrhagic risk factors of endovascular onyx embolization of intracranial dural arteriovenous fistulas. Interv Neuroradiol. 2020;26(5):643–50.
17. Pukenas BA, Satti SR, Bailey R, Weigele JB, Hurst RW, Stiefel MF. Onyx pulmonary artery embolization after treatment of a low-flow dural arteriovenous fistula: case report. Neurosurgery. 2011;68(5):E1497–500.
18. Herman TE, Siegel MJ, Vachharajani A, Masand P, Cross D. Cerebral arteriovenous fistula to pulmonary artery onyx embolization. J Perinatol. 2007;27(4):238–40.
19. Pelz DM, Lownie SP, Fox AJ, Hutton LC. Symptomatic pulmonary complications from liquid acrylate embolization of brain arteriovenous malformations. AJNR Am J Neuroradiol. 1995;16(1):19–26.
20. Kjellin IB, Boechat MI, Vinuela F, Westra SJ, Duckwiler GR. Pulmonary emboli following therapeutic embolization of cerebral arteriovenous malformations in children. Pediatr Radiol. 2000;30(4):279–83.
21. Kline JN, Ryals TJ, Galvin JR, Loftus CM, Hunter JH. Pulmonary embolization and infarction. An iatrogenic complication of transcatheter embolization of a cerebral arteriovenous malformation with polyvinyl alcohol sponge. Chest. 1993;103(4):1293–5.
22. Jablawi F, Nikoubashman O, Dafotakis M, Schubert GA, Hans FJ, Mull M. Treatment strategy and long-term outcome in patients with deep lumbosacral arteriovenous fistulas. A single center analysis in nineteen patients. Clin Neurol Neurosurg. 2020;188:105596. https://doi.org/10.1016/j.clineuro.2019.105596. Epub 2019 Nov 11.
23. Zurin AA, Ushikoshi S, Houkin K, Kikuchi Y, Abe H, Saitoh H. Cerebral abscess as an unusual complication of coil embolization in a dural arteriovenous fistula. Case report. J Neurosurg. 1997;87(1):109–12.

20 Hemorrhagic Complications After Endovascular Treatment for Intracranial Dural Arteriovenous Fistulas

Kun Hou and Jinlu Yu

Abstract

Dural arteriovenous fistulas (DAVFs) are arteriovenous shunts within the dural leaflet. Endovascular treatment (EVT) has become the first-line treatment for DAVFs. However, during or after EVT, disastrous hemorrhagic complications can occur. Little is known about the potential for severe hemorrhagic complications. Currently, EVT-associated hemorrhage may be considered associated with the rupture of a glomus-like structure around the draining vein, which is often supplied by a pial artery. In addition, excessive Onyx occluding the ostium of cortical veins may result in venous hypertension, which carries a risk of venous hemorrhage. Therefore, the major pial arterial supply should be occluded first, and patency of the involved sinus and its tributaries should be preserved. To decrease EVT-associated hemorrhagic complications, staged EVT may be helpful after occlusion of the risky draining vein. EVT-associated hemorrhagic complications are often disastrous due to the nature of venous hypertension. If the hemorrhage can be evacuated after urgent craniotomy, especially in cases of supratentorial or epidural hemorrhage, a good outcome can be achieved.

Keywords

Dural arteriovenous fistula · Endovascular treatment · Hemorrhagic complication

20.1 Introduction

Dural arteriovenous fistula (DAVFs) are arteriovenous shunts between dural arteries (or with pial arteries) and venous sinuses or/and cortical veins, and in most cases of DAVF, the shunt is located within the dural leaflet [1]. One or multiple DAVFs can occur anywhere in the intracranial dura [2]. Although the outcome of microsurgery for DAVFs is acceptable, it could be feasible as a second-line treatment option for DAVFs [3].

During the past two decades, beyond microsurgery, endovascular treatment (EVT), including transarterial and transvenous access to fistulous connections, has become the first-line treatment for DAVFs [4]. EVT is safe for most DAVFs, with a good prognosis, but rarely, disastrous hemorrhagic complications can occur [5, 6]. Hemorrhagic complications after EVT for DAVFs have been reported in recent literature, with an incidence rate of 0–3.8% [5]. Currently, little is known about the potential for severe hemorrhagic complications.

K. Hou · J. Yu (✉)
Department of Neurosurgery, First Hospital of Jilin University, Changchun, China
e-mail: jlyu@jlu.edu.cn

X. Lv (ed.), *Intracranial and Spinal Dural Arteriovenous Fistulas*,
https://doi.org/10.1007/978-981-19-5767-3_20

20.2 Classification of EVT-Associated Hemorrhage

EVT-associated hemorrhage can occur in various DAVFs, including those located in the tentorium, transverse-sigmoid sinus, cavernous sinus, superior sagittal sinus, petrosal region, etc. [7–10]. Hemorrhagic complications can often be associated with curative and complete EVT for DAVFs, and they can occur intraoperatively and early and late postoperatively [5, 11].

Immediate postoperative hemorrhages are usually due to rupture of the feeding artery, fistula point or draining vein due to the high-pressure casting of Onyx (Medtronic, Irvine, California, USA) [12]. In Jiang et al.'s report of EVT for tentorial DAVFs, one patient died as a result of venous rupture while undergoing Onyx injection [4]. Delayed postoperative hemorrhage often occurs during the first 24 h postoperatively due to unintended venous embolization followed by restricted venous outflow, which results in progressive venous hypertension [5, 13]. These delayed hemorrhagic complications may be similar to the mechanism of delayed hemorrhage after the procedure for cerebral arteriovenous malformations [14, 15].

In addition, according to the location of the hemorrhage, EVT-associated hemorrhages can include epidural, cerebral, cerebellar, and intraventricular hemorrhage [8, 9].

20.3 Angioarchitecture of EVT-Associated Hemorrhage

EVT-associated hemorrhage may originate from any structure with a DAVF, especially in cases of high Cognard and Borden grades [16–19]. However, the underlying causes are not thoroughly understood, and both a pial arterial supply and giant venous aneurysm may be risk factors [5].

20.3.1 Feeding Artery

Dural arteries are prominent feeders in DAVFs, while pial arterial involvement is less common. A pial arterial supply is defined as a supply from a pial artery to the DAVF [10, 11, 20]. The pial arterial supply may be the result of neovascularization in the setting of venous hypertension [20]. DAVFs associated with a pial arterial supply are more likely to be tentorial in location, especially galenic- and torcular-type DAVFs [20].

A pial arterial supply is present in 11.3–23.8% of all DAVFs [11]. The rate of a pial arterial supply has been reported in several large series. In a report by Osada et al., the rate on angiography was 10% [1]. In a report by Brinjikji et al., the rate on angiography was 13.4% [20]. In a report by Okamoto et al., the rate on microsurgery was 20% [11]. All intracranial arteries can send a pial arterial supply to a DAVF, the most common of which is the artery of Davidoff and Schechter, which is a dural branch arising from the posterior cerebral artery that supplies the region of the tentorial incisura (Fig. 20.1) [4, 20–23].

A pial arterial supply was divided into two types by Osada et al., including a dilated preexisting dural branch of the pial artery and a pure pial supply consisting of tortuous and fragile vessels [1, 20]. In EVT for DAVFs, a pial arterial supply increases the risk of hemorrhagic complications [11]. In a report by Wu et al. on EVT for tentorial DAVFs, the rate of hemorrhagic complications was 33%, and DAVF patients with post-EVT hemorrhage showed pial arterial supply involvement [8]. When the proximal draining vein of the DAVF is embolized, the restriction of venous outflow can lead to hemorrhage from residual pial arterial feeders [1]. In addition, flow-related aneurysm of the pial arterial supply can occur, which is dangerous (Fig. 20.1c).

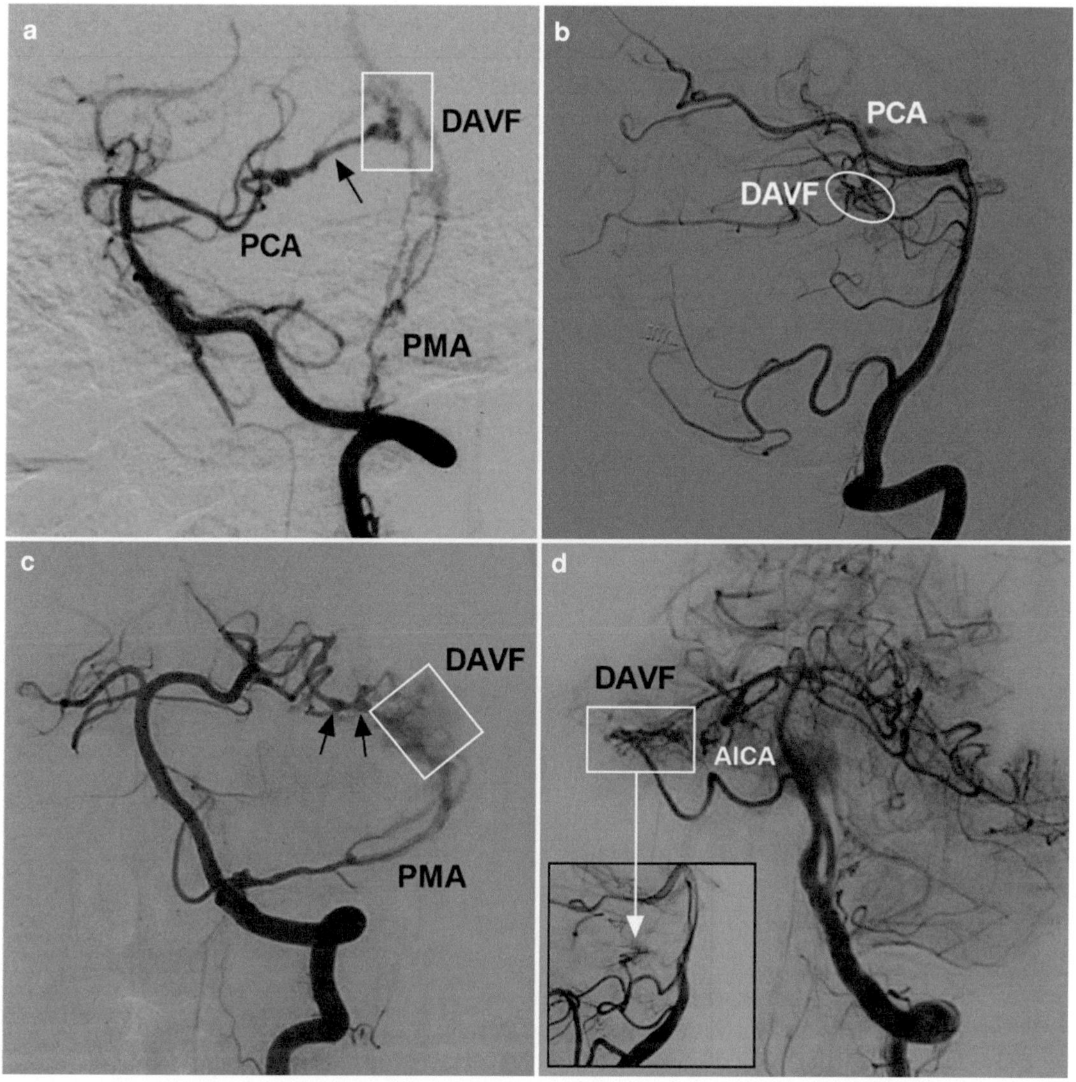

Fig. 20.1 Pial arterial supply in DAVF. (**a**) DSA of the VA showing that the DAVF (frame) was supplied by the meningeal branch of the PCA, which was dilated (arrow), as well as the PMA. (**b**) DSA of the VA showing that the PCA sent a pure pial supply to the DAVF (circle). (**c**) DSA of the VA showing that the PCA sent a dilated pial supply to the DAVF (frame), with flow-related aneurysms (arrows) in the pial supply; the PMA also supplied the DAVF. (**d**) DSA of the VA showing that the AICA sent a pure pial supply to the DAVF (frame). The inset shows the lateral view of the VA, and the arrow indicates the DAVF. *Abbreviations*: *AICA* anterior inferior cerebellar artery, *DAVF* dural arteriovenous fistula, *DSA* digital subtracted angiography, *PCA* posterior cerebral artery, *PMA* posterior meningeal artery, *VA* vertebral artery

20.3.2 Fistula Structure

Commonly, DAVFs are located in the dural leaflet, and they can be divided into sinus and nonsinus types according to the presence of communication with the sinus [1, 24]. DAVFs can result in venous hypertension; in turn, venous hypertension may promote DAVF growth [25]. Rarely, DAVFs may extend to the subdural space along the drainage route, presenting with a glomus-like structure around the drainage vein, which is often supplied by a pial artery [12]. The presence of a glomus-like structure increases the risk of EVT, so its identification is necessary. Due to the hypervascularized and complex angioarchitecture of DAVFs, such glomus-like structures may not be visible on angiography [12, 26]. In Okamoto et al.'s report on microsurgery for DAVFs, the detection rate of an angiographically occult pial arterial supply was estimated to be 6.7% [11]. In theory, the location and classification (sinus or nonsinus type) of DAVFs may be associated with the occurrence of hemorrhagic complications (Fig. 20.2). However, in report by Liu et al., no difference in EVT-associated hemorrhages was found between sinus and nonsinus DAVFs or by the location of DAVFs [5].

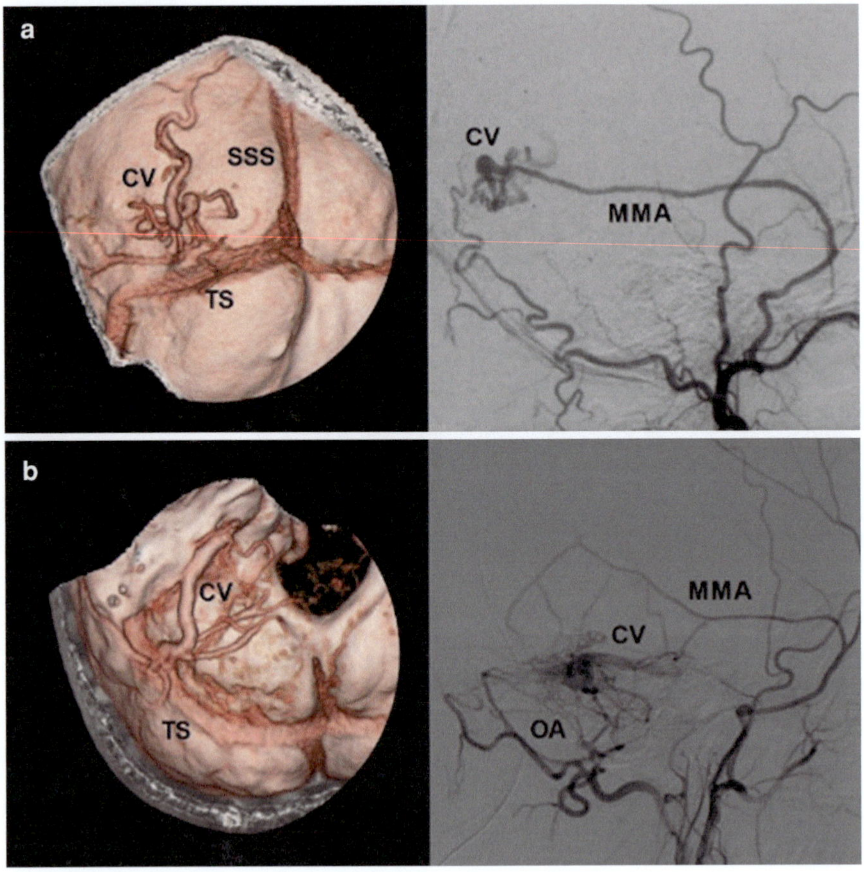

Fig. 20.2 Venous draining patterns in DAVFs. (**a**) Left, CTA showing a nonsinus-type DAVF located in the TS, with a tortuous draining vein; right, DSA showing the Cognard grade IV DAVF. In this DAVF, although the grade was high, the draining vein was not extensive, and EVT could be performed via the MMA safely, and complete EVT may not result in excessive venous occlusion. (**b**) Left, CTA showing a nonsinus-type DAVF located in the TS, with a dilated draining vein extended into the cerebellum; right, DSA showing the Cognard grade IV DAVF. In this DAVF, the draining vein was extensive, and EVT via the MMA would be dangerous, as it would result in excessive venous occlusion. (**c**) Left, CTA showing a sinus-type DAVF located in the TS, with a dilated draining vein; right, DSA showing the Cognard grade IIa + b DAVF and indicating that EVT may impact the TS. (**d**) Left, CTA showing a sinus-type DAVF located in the TS, with a dilated draining vein; right, DSA showing the Cognard grade IIb DAVF and indicating that EVT via the MMA may impact the TS. *Abbreviations*: *CTA* computed tomography angiography, *CV* cortical vein, *DAVF* dural arteriovenous malformation, *DSA* digital subtracted angiography, *EVT* endovascular treatment, *MMA* middle meningeal artery, *OA* occipital artery, *SSS* superior sagittal sinus, *TS* transverse sinus

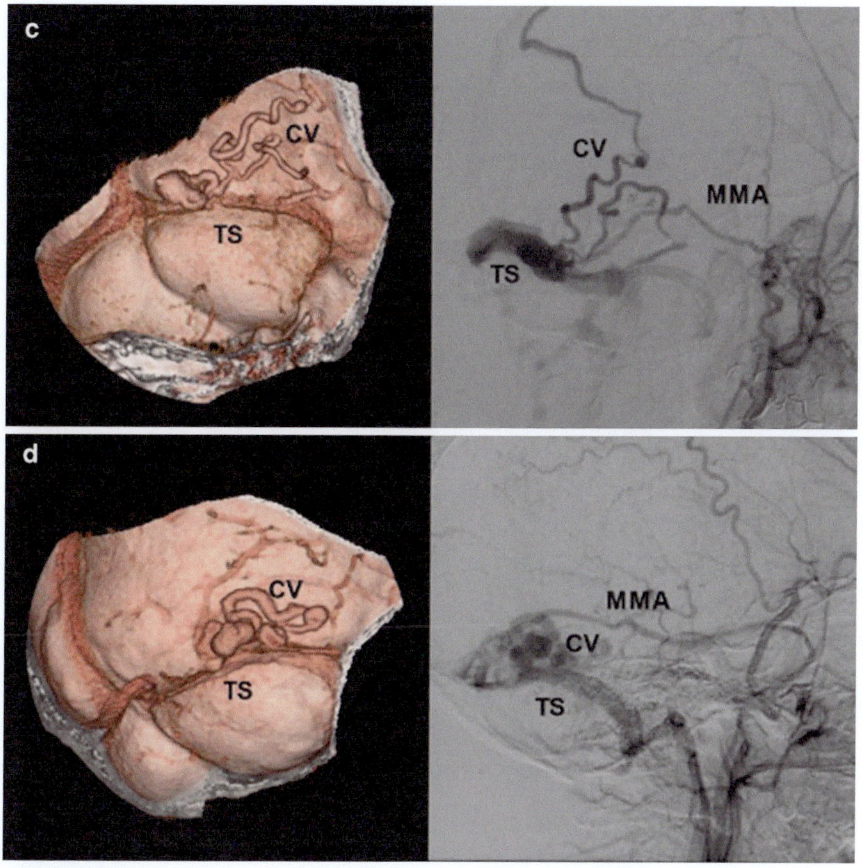

Fig. 20.2 (continued)

20.3.3 Draining Vein

In normal veins in the brain, many tributaries often share one trunk and flow into a sinus (Fig. 20.3) [27]. In cases of DAVF, venous hypertension results in draining vein arterialization, presenting with dilatation, varix formation, aneurysm formation and congestion [4, 20, 28]. Venous dilatation is defined as an increase in the normal vessel diameter, a varix is defined a vessel dilatation to more than twice that the diameter of veins proximal and distal to the varix, and venous congestion is defined as veins exhibiting a pseudophlebitic pattern (Fig. 20.4) [29]. DAVFs with a pial arterial supply are more likely to have these venous pathologies [20]. Venous hypertension in cases of DAVFs can result in dural sinus stenosis or occlusion and lead to an isolated venous sinus, which can be associated with EVT-associated hemorrhage [30].

During EVT, an excessive amount of Onyx may enter and penetrate these fragile venous structures. In addition, occlusion of the ostium of cortical veins may result in venous hypertension, and these veins tend to rupture [18, 31, 32]. After EVT, venous blood stagnation may occur, which is a very powerful trigger of the coagulation cascade and may also cause venous rupture [31]. Large or giant venous aneurysms may be more prone to lead to thrombosis after EVT, and they carry a risk for delayed rupture (Fig. 20.5) [5, 33, 34].

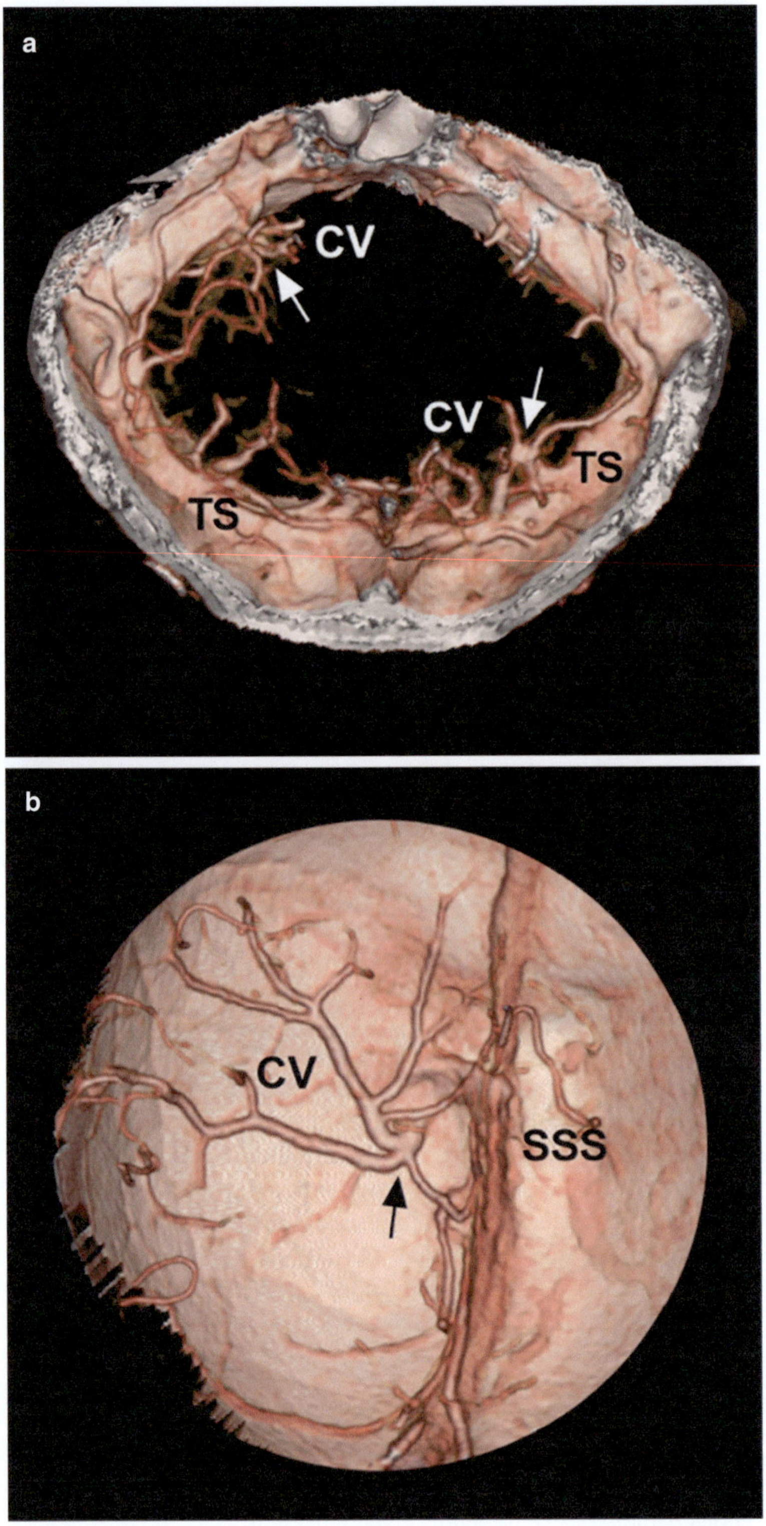

Fig. 20.3 Normal venous draining pattern in the brain. (**a**) CTA showing the venous draining pattern in the tentorium, with the veins flowing into one trunk (arrows). (**b**) CTA showing the venous draining pattern in the superior sagittal sinus, with the veins flowing into one trunk (arrow). *Abbreviations*: *CTA* computed tomography angiography, *CV* cortical vein, *SSS* superior sagittal sinus, *TS* transverse sinus

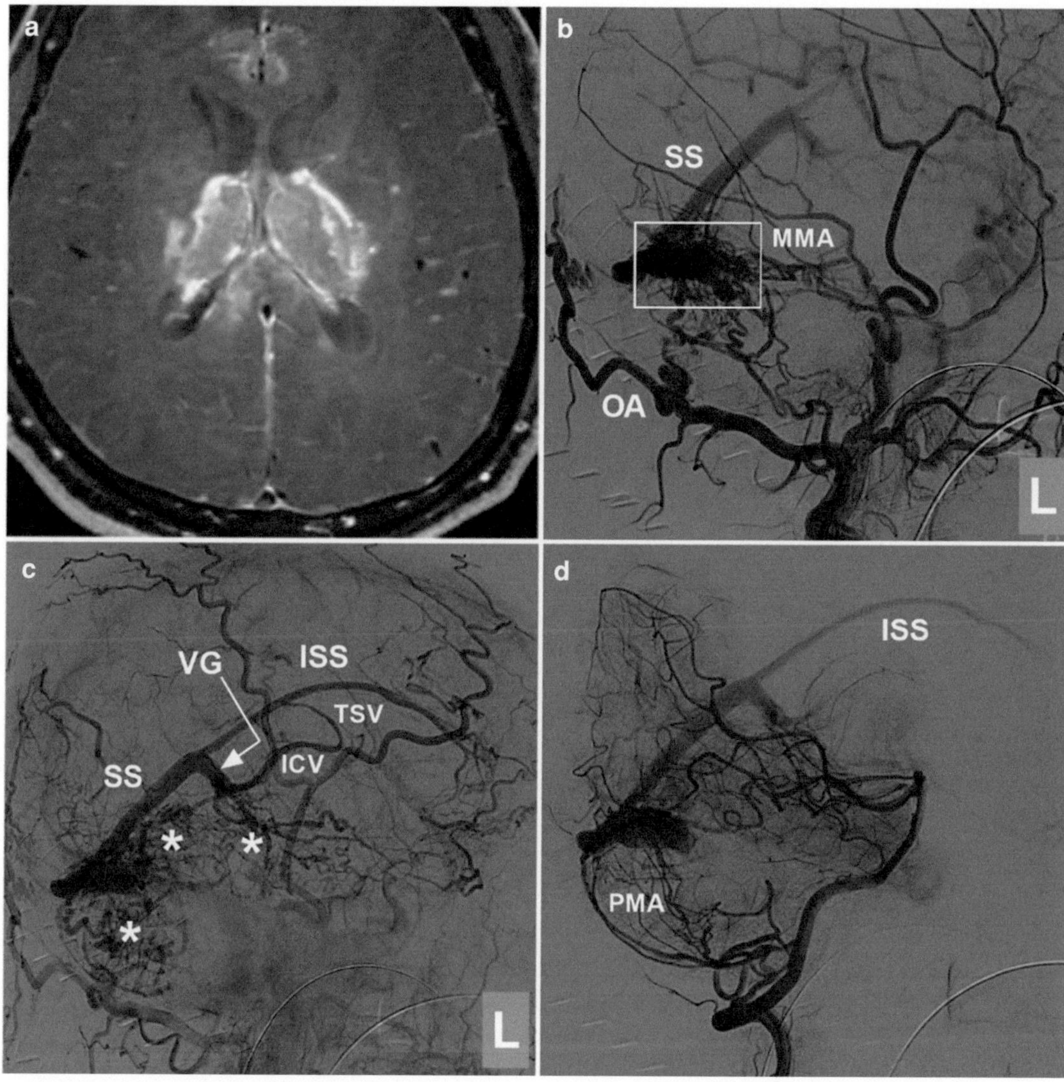

Fig. 20.4 Venous pseudophlebitic pattern in a case of DAVF. (**a**) MRI with a T1WI VISTA sequence showing the bilateral thalamus with a high signal indicating edema. (**b**, **c**) DSA of the left ECA showing the DAVF (frame in **b**) in the transverse sinus, with the MMA and OA as feeders and brain deep vein system congestion; the asterisks in (**c**) indicate the pseudophlebitic pattern. (**b**) Arterial phase. (**c**) Venous phrase. (**d**) DSA of the VA showing that the PMA was also feeding the DAVF. *Abbreviations*: *DAVF* dural arteriovenous fistula, *DSA* digital subtracted angiography, *ECA* external carotid artery, *ICV* internal cerebral vein, *ISS* inferior sagittal sinus, *L* left, *MMA* middle meningeal artery, *MRI* magnetic resonance imaging, *OA* occipital artery, *PMA* posterior meningeal artery, *SS* straight sinus, *TSV* thalamostriate vein, *VA* vertebral artery, *VG* vein of Galen

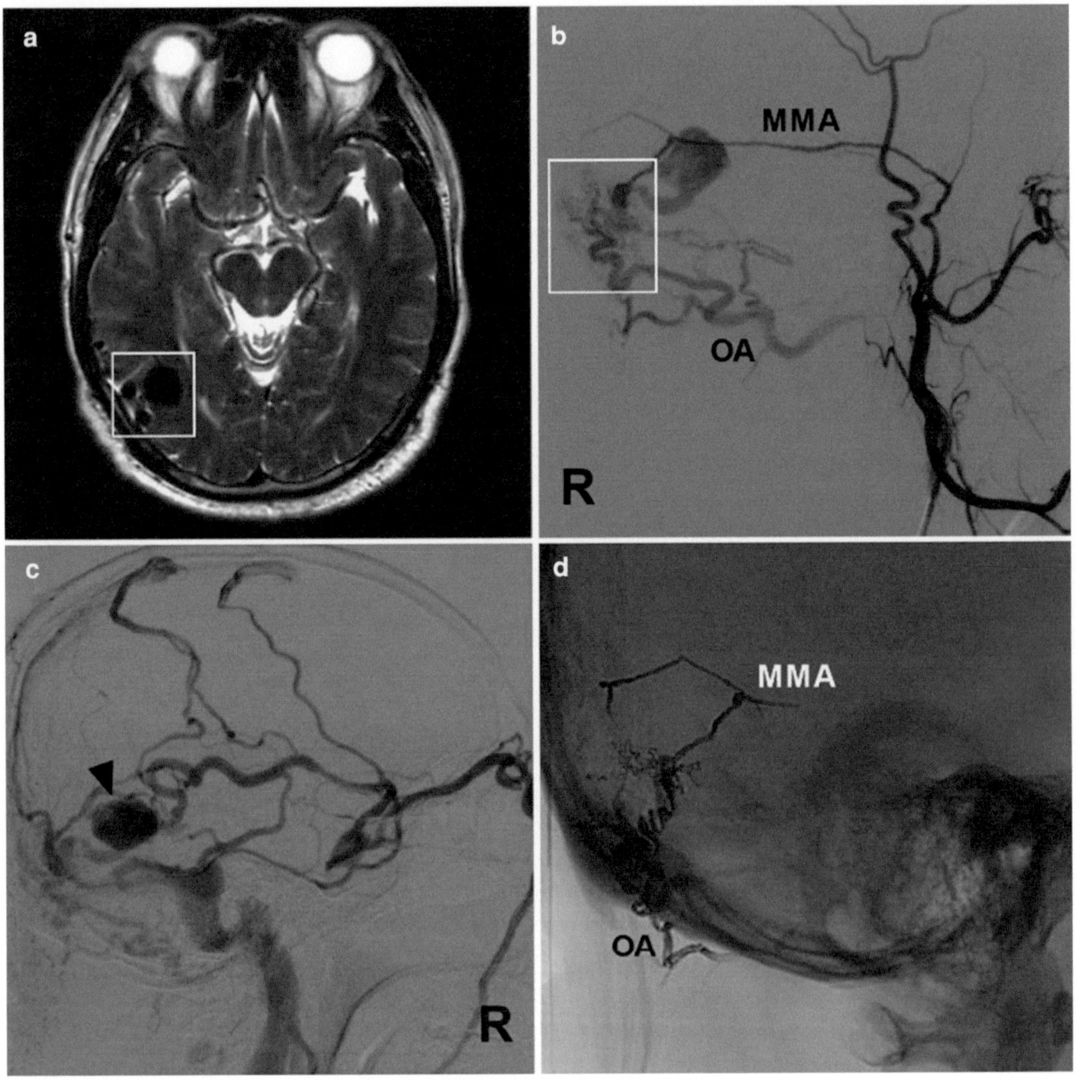

Fig. 20.5 Delayed hemorrhagic complication after TAE for a DAVF. (**a**) MRI with a T2WI sequence showing the venous lesion (frame) at right posterior temporal lobe. (**b**) Arterial-phase DSA of the right ECA showing the DAVF (frame) in the transverse sinus, with the MMA and OA as feeding arteries. (**c**) Venous-phase DSA of the right ECA showing that the draining veins were extensive and many superficial veins of the hemisphere were involved; the triangle indicates a venous aneurysm. (**d**) X-ray examination showing Onyx casted via the MMA and OA. (**e**) DSA of the right OA showing no visible DAVF with capillary-like termination of the OA (frame). (**f**) CT 2 h postoperatively showing hemorrhage in the posterior temporal lobe around the venous aneurysm (asterisk). *Abbreviations*: *CT* computed tomography, *DAVF* dural arteriovenous fistula, *DSA* digital subtracted angiography, *ECA* external carotid artery, *MRI* magnetic resonance imaging, *MMA* middle meningeal artery, *OA* occipital artery, *R* right, *TAE* trans-arterial embolization

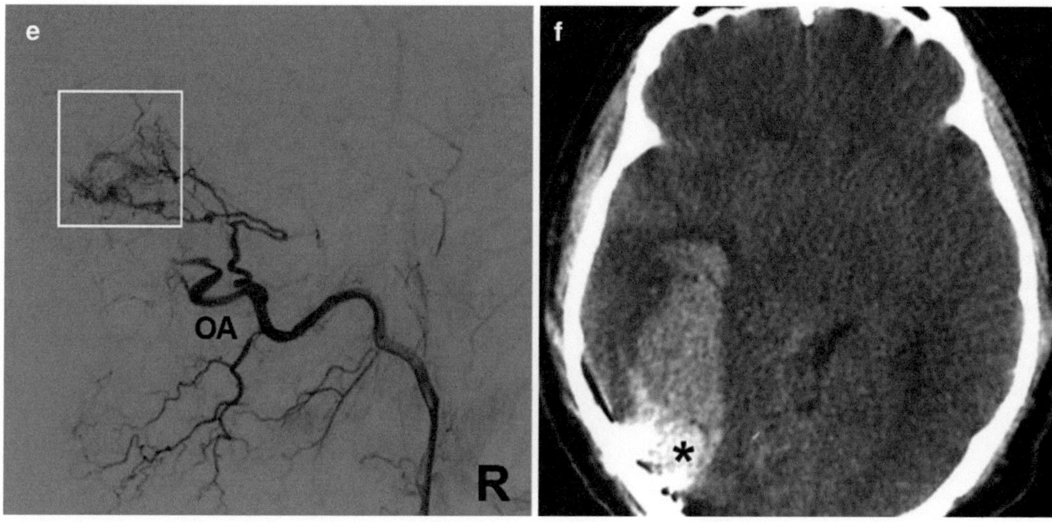

Fig. 20.5 (continued)

20.4 EVT Techniques, Risks, and Preventive Measures

Various EVT techniques can be used in the treatment of DAVFs, including transarterial embolization (TAE), transvenous embolization (TVE), or both in combination [35]. All of these methods are associated with hemorrhagic complications [7, 35, 36]. For instance, EVT-associated hemorrhages can occur in 7.7–33.3% of TAE procedures for DAVFs [11, 37].

20.4.1 General Considerations

EVT-associated hemorrhages are usually due to complete fistula occlusion [13]. If the Cognard grade is downgraded after EVT reduces the shunt volume or the size of the DAVF, staged EVT can become safer. Nontarget embolization has a high risk of post-EVT hemorrhage because it risks the occlusion of functional drainage veins, potentially leading to venous hemorrhage [38]. It is feasible to leave a small remaining fistula rather than risk severe secondary complications due to complete single-stage embolization [4].

In TVE, a sinus occlusion approach is crucial for obtaining an angiographic cure; however, normal drainage function can be affected, which is associated with post-EVT hemorrhage. Therefore, a sinus-preserving approach is attractive because it enables the physiological venous drainage of brain tissue. In addition, in DAVFs with sinus stenosis or occlusion, the restoration of sinus flow with cortical venous reflux was feasible [39].

EVT should not transfer blood flow into the veins of the cortex or brainstem or into the deep vein system, as this can result in post-EVT hemorrhagic complications. In a report by Mochizuki et al., after TVE for a cavernous sinus DAVF, delayed brainstem hemorrhage occurred because of partial obliteration of the drainage pathways exacerbated reflux of the prepontine bridging vein into the brainstem [7].

20.4.2 TAE, Risks and Preventive Measures

TAE can be considered in the treatment of all types of DAVFs; it requires distal catheterization of the feeding artery as much as possible, and then Onyx is used to penetrate the fistulous connection and proximal aspect of the venous receptacle [21]. During navigation, the feeding artery can rupture by microguidewire penetration [40]. Additionally, when the microcatheter tip is too far away from the fistula, complete EVT is difficult, and high-pressure Onyx casting could result in rupture of the path artery, resulting in epidural hemorrhage (Fig. 20.6). Therefore, the micro-

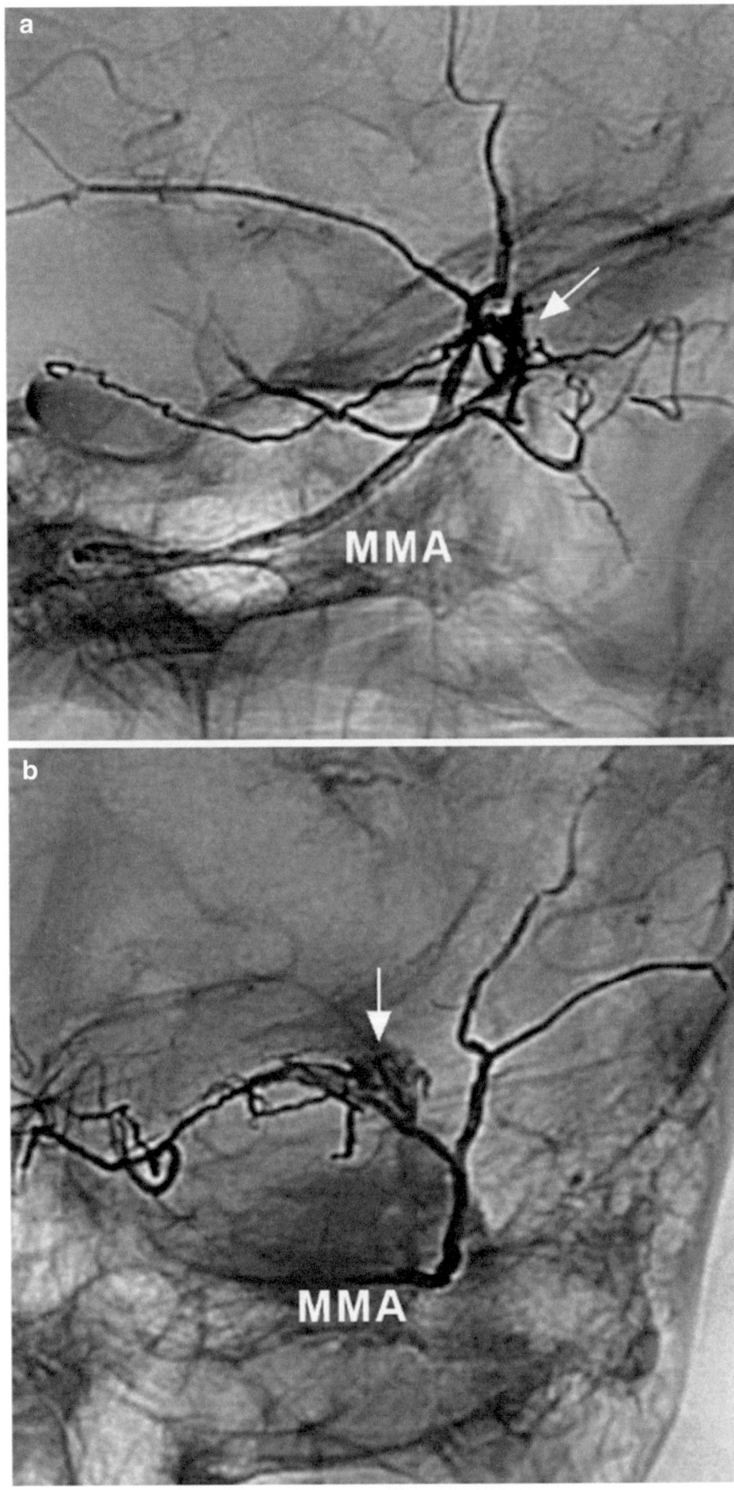

Fig. 20.6 MMA rupture during Onyx casting for DAVF. (**a**, **b**) X-ray examination showing Onyx casting in the MMA and its branches. During Onyx casting, the MMA ruptured; the arrows show the point of rupture. (**a**) Lateral view. (**b**) Anteroposterior view. *Abbreviations*: *DAVF* dural arteriovenous fistula, *MMA* middle meningeal artery

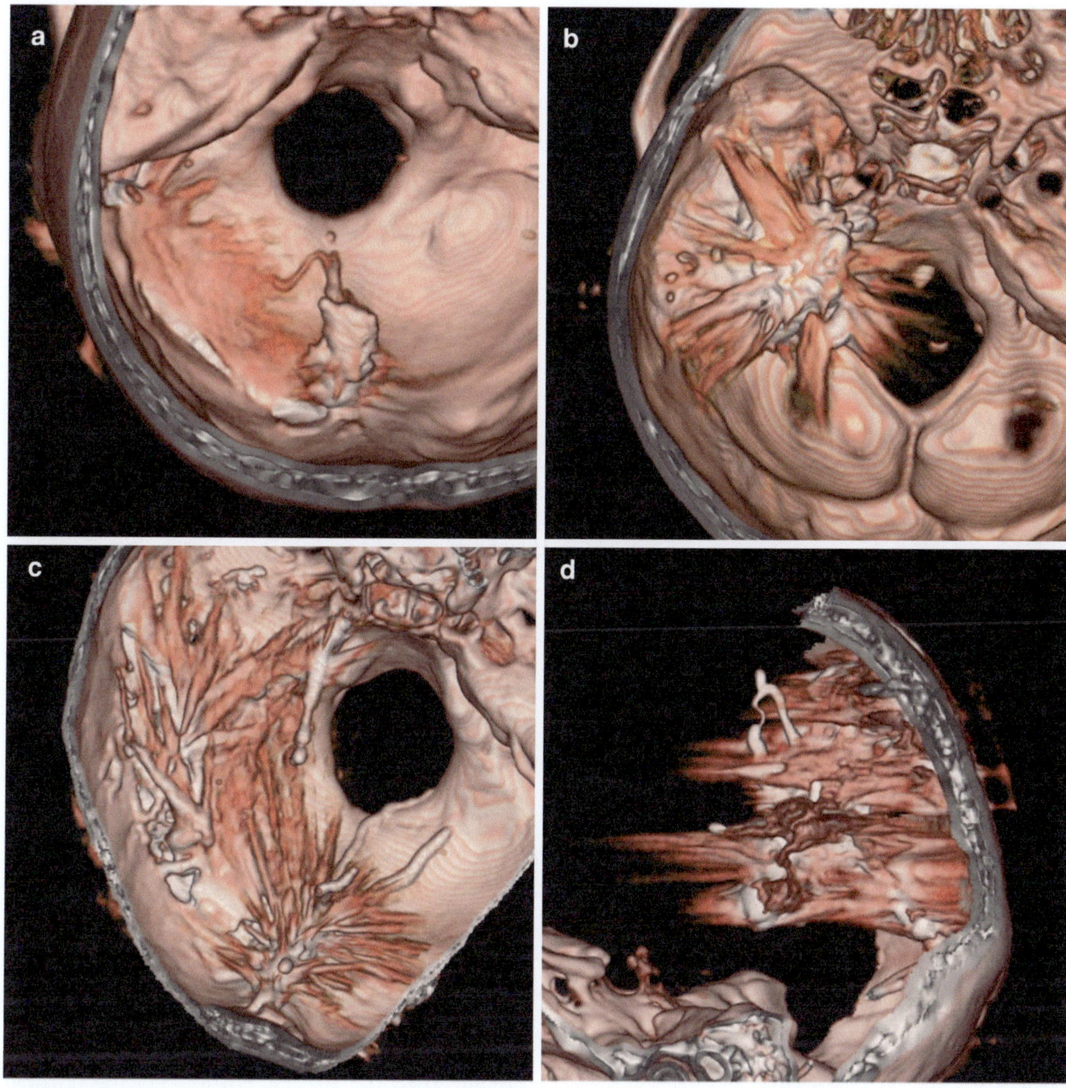

Fig. 20.7 Onyx casting for DAVFs on CTA. (**a–d**) CTA showing Onyx casting in DAVFs, with occlusion of the fistula and the origin of the draining vein. (**a**) A DAVF of a sinus confluence. (**b**) A DAVF in the tentorium. (**c**) Multiple DAVFs. (**d**) A DAVF in the cerebral falx. *Abbreviations*: *CTA* computed tomography angiography, *DAVF* dural arteriovenous fistula

catheter tip should be "wedged" into the feeding artery to access the DAVF.

When pursuing complete EVT via TAE, the ostium of cortical veins may be occluded by Onyx casting (Fig. 20.7). The angiographic view after Onyx casting should be superimposed at the end of the procedure on the initial angiographic view of the venous phase to verify that the Onyx did not contaminate the ostium of the veins. The patency of all involved sinuses and their tributaries should be preserved to avoid delayed hemorrhage. In addition, the volume of Onyx used in one session should be minimized. In a report by Liu et al. on EVT for DAVFs, an Onyx casting volume of more than 6 mL was a risk factor for EVT-associated hemorrhage [5].

A pial arterial supply is also a risk factor for hemorrhagic complications in EVT for DAVFs (Fig. 20.1). The stagnation of the pial feeding artery from EVT via other dural arteries may be insufficient to avoid EVT-associated hemorrhage. Therefore, at least major pial feeding arteries, and if possible, the entire pial network, should be obliterated before performing curative EVT. However, in general, gaining catheter access to the pial artery is difficult and sometimes dangerous due to its distal location and tortuous structure [11, 12].

Although the risk of a pial arterial supply is acceptable, whether it should be occluded remains controversial. In the Osada et al. study, postoperative bleeding did not occur even when the pial arterial supply was not obliterated, while the venous outflow was occluded [1]. In a report by Brinjikji et al., more than 10% of DAVFs had a pial supply, but this was not a contraindication to EVT; post-EVT hemorrhage related to pial arterial supply rupture was not found [20].

20.4.3 TVE, Its Risks, and Preventive Measures

TVE can be considered mainly in the treatment of sinus-type DAVFs, and either dural sinus occlusion or preservation can be used. However, whenever it is possible, sinus preservation should be preferred [39], especially when a specific sinus segment is essential for intracranial venous drainage [41].

20.4.3.1 Sinus Trapping

It is easy to perform dural sinus occlusion by trapping the sinus together with fistula points at the dural sinus wall. Coiling combined with Onyx casting is helpful, and after coiling to form the frame, the dural sinus can be completely occluded by casting Onyx. Trapping the dural sinus with TAE via arterial feeders is supposed to offer a higher rate of definite angiographic cure of DAVFs. However, occlusion of the dural sinus carries a risk of venous hemorrhage (Fig. 20.8). Iatrogenic sinus occlusion is never recommended because the complete obliteration of a dural sinus might impair normal venous drainage.

20.4.3.2 Sinus Preservation by Retrograde Catheterization

There are two approaches in TVE: one is catheterization to shunt the pouch through the dural sinus; the other is retrograde catheterization of the cortical vein.

A shunted pouch is a tubular or elliptic vascular structure that is separated from the main sinus lumen into which multiple feeding arteries converge and continue to the sinus. For DAVFs located within the dural sinus wall, TVE by coil deposition and/or Onyx casting has been reported to provide a higher likelihood of cure than TAE [42]. During TVE aimed at a shunted pouch, balloon-assisted sinus protection is helpful. By keeping a temporary balloon in the diseased sinus segment during EVT, the balloon can preserve the natural dural venous sinus drainage and allow better penetration of the fistula network by the Onyx [43].

Retrograde cortical vein catheterization is also an option for TVE. First, the DAVF can be embolized via TAE to reduce blood flow, and then the microguidewire can be carefully introduced and advanced to the fistular portion via the cortical draining vein, followed by the microcatheter [4]. However, navigation to reach the arteriovenous shunting point of a leptomeningeal vein is usually technically demanding and therefore riskier, and should be the last resort, as the draining vein may be perforated by the microguidewire [44].

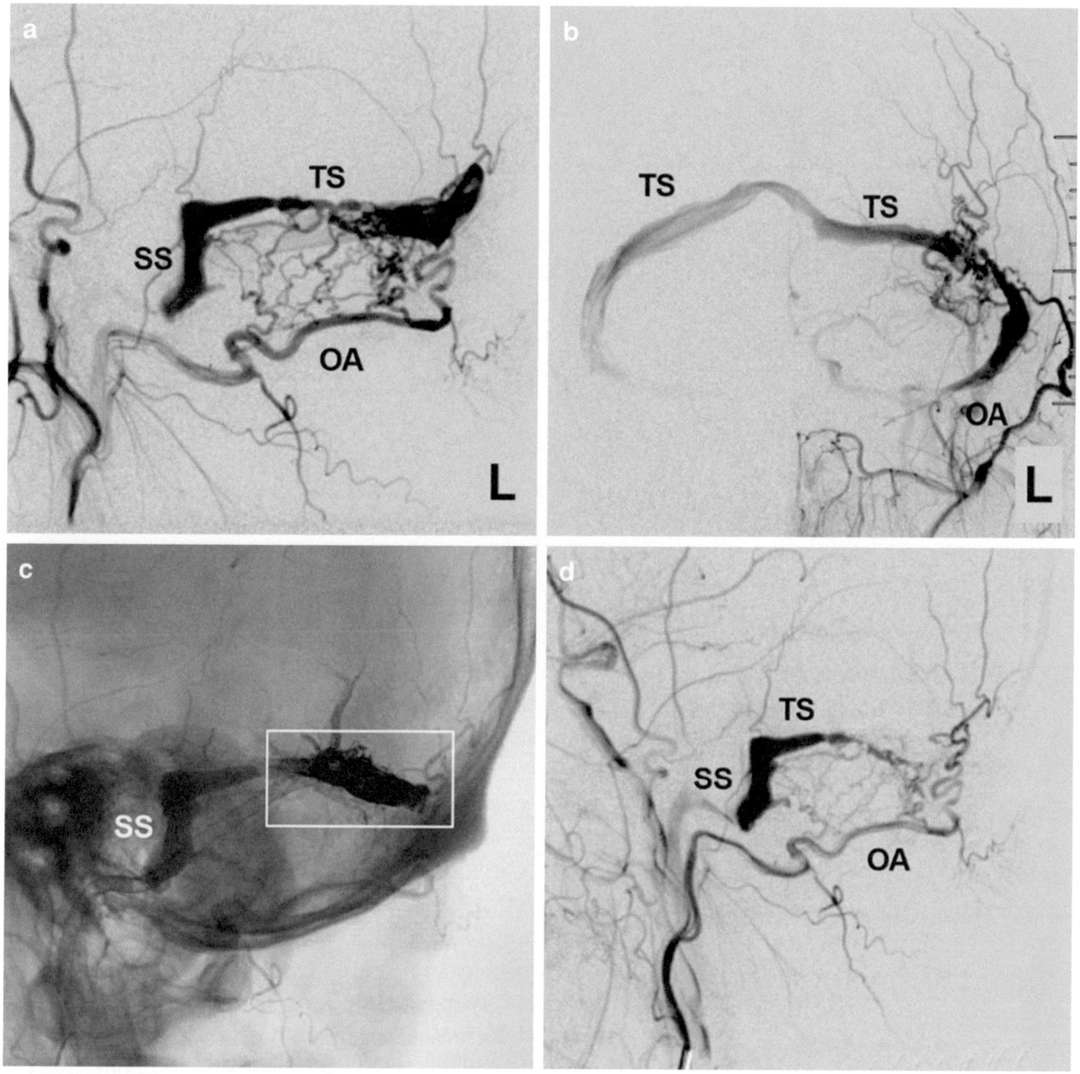

Fig. 20.8 Postoperative hemorrhage after TVE for a TS DAVF. (**a**, **b**) DSA of the left ECA showing the DAVF in the TS, occlusion of the SS, and draining toward the contralateral TS; the Cognard grade was IIa. (**a**) Lateral view. (**b**) Anteroposterior view. (**c**) X-ray examination showing occlusion of the DAVF via TVE with coiling and Onyx assistance (frame). (**d**) DSA of the ECA showing downgrading of the DAVF from grade IIa to grade I after TVE. (**e**) CT at 4 h postoperatively showing multiple cerebellar hemorrhages (asterisks). (**f**) CT reconstruction showing the casted Onyx in the cerebellar veins (frame). *Abbreviations*: *CT* computed tomography, *ECA* external carotid artery, *DAVF* dural arteriovenous fistula, *DSA* digital subtracted angiography, *L* left, *MMA* middle meningeal artery, *OA* occipital artery, *SS* sigmoid sinus, *TS* transverse sinus, *TVE* transvenous embolization

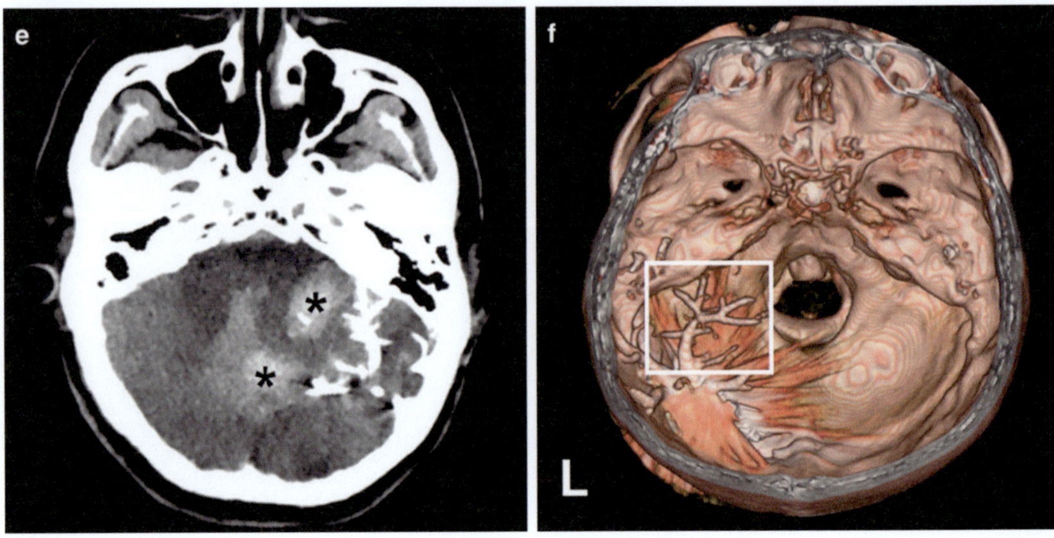

Fig. 20.8 (continued)

20.4.4 Combination of TAE and TVE with Balloon Protection

TAE under intrasinus balloon protection is an efficient treatment strategy for DAVFs, and the use of supercompliant balloons is important [45]. With this technique, Onyx casted via TAE can diffuse into arteriovenous shunts up to the area in communication with the normal sinus, and the balloon can preserve the natural dural venous sinus drainage and allow better penetration of the fistula network by the Onyx [43]. In addition, balloon-assisted sinus protection can prevent the unwanted embolization of nontarget veins.

However, balloon assistance has been a source of hemorrhagic complications due to the occlusion of normal veins by Onyx diffusing between the balloon and the sinus wall. In addition, even the stasis of a small vein can result in disastrous postoperative hemorrhage [46]. In a report by Guo et al. of EVT for 14 DAVFs, hemorrhagic complications, including epidural hematoma and cerebellar hematoma, occurred after the treatment of 14.3% of DAVFs due to temporary balloon obstruction [9].

Due to the drawbacks of balloon-assisted sinus protection, the balloon can be replaced with a stent. Guedon et al. reported that TAE for sinus-type DAVFs with Carotid WALLSTENT (Boston Scientific, Natick, MA, USA)-assisted sinus protection may be prioritized over that with balloon assistance. Before TAE, a Carotid WALLSTENT is semireleased in the sinus lumen to obstruct Onyx diffusion into the sinus; after EVT, the Carotid WALLSTENT is recaptured with some Onyx. Such stent-assisted sinus protection is effective in protecting the sinus without causing stasis or venous congestion that could lead to hemorrhagic complications [47].

The combination of TAE and TVE with balloon protection is controversial. In a report by Zamponi et al., TAE for DAVFs without transvenous balloon protection did not show an advantage over that with transvenous balloon protection, and TAE both with and without transvenous balloon protection was effective [48].

20.5 Treatment and Prognosis of Hemorrhagic Complications

Hemorrhagic complications are often disastrous due to the nature of venous hypertension. In the report by Liu et al. of post-EVT hemorrhagic complications in 12 patients, 2 patients died of severe intracranial hemorrhage, 2 patients suffered severe disability, and the other 8 patients recovered well

[5]. In Wu et al.'s report of EVT for tentorial DAVFs, intraoperative hemorrhage occurred in 2 of 6 patients with a pial arterial supply, and one patient died as a result of hemorrhage [8]. If the hemorrhage can be evacuated after urgent craniotomy, especially in cases of supratentorial or epidural hemorrhage, a good outcome can be achieved. In general, extensive cerebellar and brainstem hemorrhages may have poor outcomes.

20.6 Summary

Hemorrhagic complications of EVT for DAVFs are disastrous. These complications can be considered to be associated with the rupture of a glomus-like structure around the draining vein. Excessive Onyx occlusion of the ostium of cortical veins may also carry a risk of venous hemorrhage; thus, it is necessary to identify glomus-like structures before EVT. The major pial arterial supply should be occluded first, and patency of the involved sinus and its tributaries should be preserved. If hemorrhage can be evacuated after urgent craniotomy, especially in cases of supratentorial or epidural hemorrhage, a good outcome can be achieved.

Acknowledgments We thank our colleagues who provided the case images.

Funding None.

Conflicts of Interest The authors declare that they have no conflicts of interest.

Ethics Approval Ethics approval is not needed for review articles at our institution.

Informed Consent Informed consent was obtained from all individual participants included in the study or their legal guardians.

References

1. Osada T, Krings T. Intracranial dural arteriovenous fistulas with pial arterial supply. Neurosurgery. 2019;84:104–15.
2. Guo Y, Yu J, Zhao Y, Yu J. Progress in research on intracranial multiple dural arteriovenous fistulas. Biomed Rep. 2018;8:17–25.
3. Sugiyama T, Nakayama N, Ushikoshi S, Kazumata K, Okamoto M, Ito M, et al. Complication rate, cure rate, and long-term outcomes of microsurgery for intracranial dural arteriovenous fistulae: a multicenter series and systematic review. Neurosurg Rev. 2021;44:435–50.
4. Jiang C, Lv X, Li Y, Zhang J, Wu Z. Endovascular treatment of high-risk tentorial dural arteriovenous fistulas: clinical outcomes. Neuroradiology. 2009;51:103–11.
5. Liu P, Chen X, You W, Li Y, Lv M, Lv X. Hemorrhagic risk factors of endovascular onyx embolization of intracranial dural arteriovenous fistulas. Interv Neuroradiol. 2020;26:643–50.
6. Moenninghoff C, Pohl E, Deuschl C, Wrede K, Jabbarli R, Radbruch A, et al. Outcomes after Onyx embolization as primary treatment for cranial dural arteriovenous fistula in the past decade. Acad Radiol. 2020;27:e123–31.
7. Mochizuki Y, Iihoshi S, Tsukagoshi E, Kasakura S, Kohyama S, Kurita H. A rare brainstem hemorrhage due to incomplete transvenous embolization of the cavernous sinus dural arteriovenous fistula: a case report. Radiol Case Rep. 2021;16:2526–9.
8. Wu Q, Zhang XS, Wang HD, Zhang QR, Wen LL, Hang CH, et al. Onyx embolization for tentorial dural arteriovenous fistula with pial arterial supply: case series and analysis of complications. World Neurosurg. 2016;92:58–64.
9. Guo F, Zhang Y, Liang S, Liang F, Yan P, Jiang C. The procedure-related complications of transarterial onyx embolization of dural arteriovenous fistula using transvenous balloon protection. World Neurosurg. 2018;116:e203–10.
10. Volders D, Cora EA, Chaalala C, Cartier M, Tanaka M, Farzin B, et al. Fatal hemorrhagic complication after coil embolization of a petrosal arteriovenous shunt. Interv Neuroradiol. 2021; https://doi.org/10.1177/15910199211057705.
11. Okamoto M, Sugiyama T, Nakayama N, Ushikoshi S, Kazumata K, Osanai T, et al. Microsurgical findings of pial arterial feeders in intracranial dural arteriovenous fistulae: a case series. Oper Neurosurg (Hagerstown). 2020;19:691–700.
12. Sato K, Matsumoto Y, Endo H, Tominaga T. A hemorrhagic complication after Onyx embolization of a tentorial dural arteriovenous fistula: a caution about subdural extension with pial arterial supply. Interv Neuroradiol. 2017;23:307–12.
13. Ertl L, Bruckmann H, Kunz M, Crispin A, Fesl G. Endovascular therapy of low- and intermediate-grade intracranial lateral dural arteriovenous fistulas: a detailed analysis of primary success rates, complication rates, and long-term follow-up of different technical approaches. J Neurosurg. 2017;126:360–7.
14. Biondi A, Le Jean L, Capelle L, Duffau H, Marsault C. Fatal hemorrhagic complication following endovascular treatment of a cerebral arteriovenous malformation. Case report and review of the literature. J Neuroradiol. 2006;33:96–104.

15. Piao J, Luan T, Wang Y, Yu J. Imaging characteristics and endovascular treatment strategy for cerebellar arteriovenous malformations. Med Int. 2021;1:5.
16. Cognard C, Gobin YP, Pierot L, Bailly AL, Houdart E, Casasco A, et al. Cerebral dural arteriovenous fistulas: clinical and angiographic correlation with a revised classification of venous drainage. Radiology. 1995;194:671–80.
17. Borden JA, Wu JK, Shucart WA. A proposed classification for spinal and cranial dural arteriovenous fistulous malformations and implications for treatment. J Neurosurg. 1995;82:166–79.
18. Qureshi AM, Bhatia K, Kostynskyy A, Krings T. Clinical and angioarchitectural features of ruptured dural arteriovenous fistulas. World Neurosurg. 2021;147:e476–81.
19. Mendez-Ruiz A, Guerrero WR, Szeder V, Farooqui M, Zevallos CB, Quispe-Orozco D, et al. Endovascular embolization of high-grade cerebral dural arteriovenous fistulas—assessment of long-term recurrences. Interv Neuroradiol. 2022;28:411–8.
20. Brinjikji W, Cloft HJ, Lanzino G. Clinical, angiographic, and treatment characteristics of cranial dural arteriovenous fistulas with pial arterial supply. J Neurointerv Surg. 2021;13:331–5.
21. Su H, Xu K, Wang Y, Yu J. Is the middle meningeal artery the optimal path for dural arteriovenous fistula embolization? Front Neurol. 2021;12:675355.
22. Tong D, Chen X, Lv X, Li K, Xu K, Yu J. Current status of endovascular treatment for dural arteriovenous fistulae in the tentorial middle region: a literature review. Acta Neurol Belg. 2019;119:5–14.
23. Bhatia KD, Kortman H, Walchli T, Radovanovic I, Pereira VM, Krings T. Artery of Davidoff and Schechter supply in dural arteriovenous fistulas. AJNR Am J Neuroradiol. 2020;41:300–4.
24. Kuwayama N, Akioka N. Complications of endovascular treatment of intracranial dural arteriovenous fistulas. Acta Neurochir Suppl. 2021;132:123–7.
25. Buell TJ, Raper DM, Ding D, Chen CJ, Liu KC. Development of an intracranial dural arteriovenous fistula after venous sinus stenting for idiopathic intracranial hypertension. J Neurointerv Surg. 2018;10:e15.
26. Maki Y, Komuro T, Satow T, Ishibashi R, Miyamoto S. Mixed pial-dural arteriovenous malformation in the anterior cranial fossa mimicking dural arteriovenous fistula. Asian J Neurosurg. 2021;16:418–22.
27. Baltsavias G, Kumar R, Avinash KM, Valavanis A. Cranial dural arteriovenous shunts. Part 2. The shunts of the bridging veins and leptomeningeal venous drainage. Neurosurg Rev. 2015;38:265–71; discussion 72.
28. Baltsavias G, Spiessberger A, Hothorn T, Valavanis A. Cranial dural arteriovenous shunts. Part 4. Clinical presentation of the shunts with leptomeningeal venous drainage. Neurosurg Rev. 2015;38:283–91; discussion 91.
29. Willinsky R, Goyal M, terBrugge K, Montanera W. Tortuous, engorged pial veins in intracranial dural arteriovenous fistulas: correlations with presentation, location, and MR findings in 122 patients. AJNR Am J Neuroradiol. 1999;20:1031–6.
30. Shin NY, Kwon YS, Ha SY, Kim BM, Kim DI, Kim DJ. Venous angioarchitectural features of intracranial dural arteriovenous shunt and its relation to the clinical course. Neuroradiology. 2013;55:1119–27.
31. Hou K, Song Y, Guo Y, Yu J. Brain arteriovenous malformations and dural arteriovenous fistulas with extensive venous congestive encephalopathy. Acta Neurol Belg. 2022;122:1–9.
32. Hou K, Ji T, Luan T, Yu J. CT angiographic study of the cerebral deep veins around the vein of Galen. Int J Med Sci. 2021;18:1699–710.
33. Iki Y, Morofuji Y, Somagawa C, Yamaguchi S, Hamabe J, Horie N, et al. Surgical venous drainage disconnection from cavernous sinus dural arteriovenous fistula and ruptured varix. World Neurosurg. 2020;137:18–23.
34. Priola SM, Ku JC, Pasarikovski CR, Yang VXD, da Costa L. Angio-architecture of complex cranial dural arteriovenous fistulas: a single centre retrospective review of treatment modalities and outcomes. J Clin Neurosci. 2020;76:87–99.
35. Samaniego EA, Roa JA, Hayakawa M, Chen CJ, Sheehan JP, Kim LJ, et al. Dural arteriovenous fistulas without cortical venous drainage: presentation, treatment, and outcomes. J Neurosurg. 2021;136:942–50.
36. Hou K, Li G, Qu L, Liu H, Xu K, Yu J. Intracranial dural arteriovenous fistulas with brainstem engorgement: an under-recognized entity in diagnosis and treatment. Front Neurol. 2020;11:526550.
37. Li Y, Chen SH, Guniganti R, Kansagra AP, Piccirillo JF, Chen CJ, et al. Onyx embolization for dural arteriovenous fistulas: a multi-institutional study. J Neurointerv Surg. 2022; https://doi.org/10.1136/neurintsurg-2020-017109.
38. Sun L, Ren J, Wang L, Li J, He C, Ye M, et al. Preservation of coexisting normal superior petrosal vein in the microsurgical treatment of superior petrosal sinus dural arteriovenous fistulas assisted by indocyanine green video angiography. World Neurosurg. 2020;141:e836–43.
39. Lin YH, Lee CW, Liu HM. Clinical outcomes of adjunct sinus stenting in dural arteriovenous fistulas: role of flow restoration in steno-occlusion and cortical venous reflux. Clin Neuroradiol. 2022;32:455–64.
40. Hendriks EJ, Lynch J, Swaminathan SK, Nicholson P, Agid R, Radovanovic I, et al. Embolization strategies for intracranial dural arteriovenous fistulas with an isolated sinus: a single-center experience in 20 patients. J Neurointerv Surg. 2022;14:605–10.
41. Choi BJ, Lee TH, Kim CW, Choi CH. Reconstructive treatment using a stent graft for a dural arteriovenous fistula of the transverse sinus in the case of hypoplasia of the contralateral venous sinuses: technical case report. Neurosurgery. 2009;65:E994–6; discussion E6.
42. Xu K, Yang X, Li C, Yu J. Current status of endovascular treatment for dural arteriovenous fistula of the

transverse-sigmoid sinus: a literature review. Int J Med Sci. 2018;15:1600–10.
43. Kerolus MG, Chung J, Munich SA, Matsuda Y, Okada H, Lopes DK. An Onyx tunnel: reconstructive transvenous balloon-assisted Onyx embolization for dural arteriovenous fistula of the transverse-sigmoid sinus. J Neurosurg. 2018;129:922–7.
44. Roa JA, Dabus G, Dandapat S, Hasan D, Samaniego EA. Ethmoidal dural arteriovenous fistulas: endovascular transvenous embolization technique. J Neurointerv Surg. 2020;12:610.
45. Yabuzaki H, Terada T, Tsumoto T, Matsuda Y, Tanaka Y, Nakayama S, et al. Transarterial embolization in dural arteriovenous fistulas under sinus balloon protection using the SHOURYU supercompliant balloon. Interdiscip Neurosurg. 2022;27:101415.
46. Vollherbst DF, Ulfert C, Neuberger U, Herweh C, Laible M, Nagel S, et al. Endovascular treatment of dural arteriovenous fistulas using transarterial liquid embolization in combination with transvenous balloon-assisted protection of the venous sinus. AJNR Am J Neuroradiol. 2018;39:1296–302.
47. Guedon A, Elhorany M, Labeyrie MA, Civelli V, Saint-Maurice JP, Houdart E. Transarterial embolization of dural arteriovenous fistulas of the lateral sinuses with stent-assisted sinus protection. J Neurointerv Surg. 2021; https://doi.org/10.1136/neurintsurg-2021-018176.
48. Zamponi JO Jr, Trivelato FP, Rezende MTS, Freitas RK, de Castro-Afonso LH, Nakiri GS, et al. Transarterial treatment of cranial dural arteriovenous fistulas: the role of transarterial and transvenous balloon-assisted embolization. AJNR Am J Neuroradiol. 2020;41:2100–6.

MIX
Papier aus verantwortungsvollen Quellen
Paper from responsible sources
FSC® C105338

If you have any concerns about our products,
you can contact us on
ProductSafety@springernature.com

In case Publisher is established outside the EU,
the EU authorized representative is:
Springer Nature Customer Service Center GmbH
Europaplatz 3, 69115 Heidelberg, Germany

Printed by Libri Plureos GmbH
in Hamburg, Germany